Cardiac Bioelectric Therapy

Mechanisms and Practical Implications

Cardiac Bioelectric Therapy

Mechanisms and Practical Implications

Edited by

Igor R. Efimov, PhD
Washington University
St. Louis, MO

Mark W. Kroll, PhD
California Polytechnic University and
University of Minnesota
Minneapolis, MN

Patrick J. Tchou, MD
Cleveland Clinic Foundation
Cleveland, OH

Foreword by Raymond E. Ideker, MD, PhD

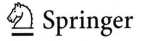 Springer

Igor R. Efimov, Ph.D.
Washington University
St. Louis, MO

Mark W. Kroll, Ph.D.
California Polytechnic University
and
University of Minnesota
Minneapolis, MN

Patrick J. Tchou, M.D.
Cleveland Clinic Foundation
Cleveland, OH

ISBN: 978-0-387-79402-0   e-ISBN: 978-0-387-79403-7

Library of Congress Control Number: 2008936096

Printed on acid-free paper

9 8 7 6 5 4 3 2 1

springer.com

Contents

Part I   History

Part II   Theory of Electric Stimulation and Defibrillation

Part III   Electrode Mapping of Defibrillation

Part IV   Optical Mapping of Stimulation and Defibrillation

Part V   Methodology

Part VI   Implications for Implantable Devices

Preface

Biomedical science has been driven in the eighteenth through the twentieth centuries by the promise to deliver lifesaving therapies against disease and to extend human life. Development of all branches of biomedical sciences, including cardiac electrophysiology, went through a periodic adherence to either reductionist or integration approaches. Cardiac electrophysiology strived to deliver therapy against arrhythmias, which are still responsible for one of four deaths in the industrialized world.

Reductionist Approach to Arrhythmia

A dramatic increase in understanding of the molecular mechanisms of normal and abnormal cellular electrophysiology led to development of new theories of arrhythmia. A number of these theories have been supported by a convincing empirical evidence "from cell to bedside."[1,2] And, as a result, the field has been propelled by promises to society of elegant, "silver bullet" pharmacological solutions against lethal cardiac arrhythmias. Nearly every generation of electrophysiologists has come up with a target of their own "silver bullet": sodium channel, calcium channel, potassium channel, gap junction, and so forth. Visions of several generations have crystallized into the recent development of theory of chanelopathies.[3]

According to one saying, every new thought is a long forgotten old one. The state of the arrhythmia research is reminiscent in some sense of an earlier history of the elementary particle physics. It appeared to many physicists at the time that the foundation of laws of matter can be eloquently explained by the interaction of very few elementary particles and very few fundamental laws governing these interactions. Yet, as more and more unexpected particles or peculiar properties of the existing particles were uncovered, the increasingly more sophisticated theories were produced, making irrelevant the elegance and eloquence of the earlier theories. And this process goes on.

Cardiac electrophysiology went along a very similar path in search of antiarrhythmia therapy. A giant of the field, Carl J. Wiggers, drafted a road map more than a half a century ago:

> As to the fundamental mechanisms of fibrillation we have plenty of theories, but none is universally accepted . . . they all center around two ideas, viz., (a) that the impulses arise from centers, or pacemakers, or (b) that the condition is caused by the re-entry of impulses and the formation of circles of excitation.[4]

The old ion channel–based theory seemed to have done a pretty good job explaining both focal and reentrant theories of arrhythmia. These early theories of arrhythmia, with their four classes of antiarrhythmic drugs, were almost Aristotelian. But they fell under the pressure of empirical evidence[5]: ever multiplying channel isoforms and subunits; alternative splicing variants of these proteins; mutations in genes encoding ion channels; numerous increasingly complex signaling pathways; unexpected proteins expressed and functioning in concert with channels. These important players had been unknown, overlooked, or neglected in the past and present new opportunities in the future.

Can a cardiac arrhythmia with broad clinical impact be explained within a framework based on a single channel biophysics or even a single cell physiology? And, most importantly, can a treatment be developed for it based on such a mechanism? Despite the explosion in the number of filed patents offering exactly such answers, it is becoming more and more apparent that these questions will not be so easy to answer. Integrative approaches are needed to synthesize the wealth of knowledge obtained by the reductionists.

Integrative Approach

Integrative physiologists looked at the arrhythmia from an opposite direction: How one can restore normal rhythm in hearts with failed sinoatrial or atrioventricular nodes using technological means available to us at the present time? How one can terminate lethal ventricular fibrillation using biomedical engineering approaches? Electrotherapy, including implantable devices and ablation, has emerged as the only effective therapeutic approach to treat arrhythmia, often without precise knowledge of the mechanisms of arrhythmia it treats. History of cardiac bioelectric therapy is long and fascinating, spanning several centuries, many countries, and several continents. Ideas to use electricity for treating cardiac disorders apparently have been born in the minds of the Italian, French, and British physicians and physiologists as evident from the numerous eighteenth-century publications in these languages, culminating in arguably the first report of a patient's treatment for cardiopulmonary arrest by electricity from Charles Kite. The nineteenth-century cardiac physiology has brought about both recognition of importance of arrhythmia as a direct cause of death and provided compelling evidence for the ability of electric stimulation to restore normal sinus rhythm in cases of both bradycardia and tachyarrhythmia. The twentieth century finally brought to fruition three centuries of research and developed an array of therapies that now save millions of patients worldwide with more than a million new implantations annually.

In this book major aspects of the development of this truly outstanding achievement are presented: bioelectric therapy of cardiac arrhythmia that allowed a significant extension of human life. Leading experts in the field contributed rigorous accounts of historical, theoretical, experimental, engineering, and clinical tracks of the development of implantable device therapy. A history of cardiac bioelectric therapy has not yet been written. However, let me conclude with a vision that was formulated by Hubert Humphrey in the U.S. Senate in October 13, 1962, after his meeting with Professors Vladimir Negovsky and Naum Gurvich that led to his recognition of importance of defibrillation and to subsequent increased federal and private financial support for this important field of physiology and medicine.[6]

I do, however, want to state that it is one of the most important of all phases of medical research. Why? Because it concerns the most universal interest of man; namely: the prolongation of human life, the postponement of death, and, yes, perhaps the greatest scientific frontier – the reversibility of death . . .

What do I urge, therefore? I urge establishing under NIH support of specialized centers or institutes on the physiology of death, on resuscitation and on related topics. I urge that the United States compete with the U.S.S.R. in bold research toward at least partial conquest of death. Already our scientists and Russian scientists are cooperating in categorical studies of heart ailments, cancer and other diseases. Now, let us recognize that a new category has emerged – the oldest category in the world – but one which commands our newest efforts – the category of death, itself . . .

COMMITTEE ON GOVERNMENT OPERATIONS
JOHN L. MC CLELLAN, ARK., CHAIRMAN

HENRY M. JACKSON, WASH. KARL E. MUNDT, S. DAK.
SAM J. ERVIN, JR., N.C. CARL T. CURTIS, NEBR.
HUBERT H. HUMPHREY, MINN. JACOB K. JAVITS, N.Y.
ERNEST GRUENING, ALASKA
EDMUND S MUSKIE, MAINE

WALTER L. REYNOLDS, CHIEF CLERK

H 10-15-62

SUBCOMMITTEE ON REORGANIZATION AND
INTERNATIONAL ORGANIZATIONS
HUBERT H. HUMPHREY, MINN., CHAIRMAN

JOHN L. MC CLELLAN, ARK. KARL E. MUNDT, S. DAK.
ERNEST GRUENING, ALASKA JACOB K. JAVITS, N.Y.
EDMUND S. MUSKIE, MAINE
  JULIUS N. CAHN.
DIRECTOR OF MEDICAL RESEARCH PROJECT

H 10-15-62

United States Senate

INTERNATIONAL HEALTH STUDY
(PURSUANT TO S. RES. 336, 87TH CONGRESS)

Room 162, Old Senate Office Bldg.
Washington 25, D. C.
Tel. CA 4-3121, Ext. 2308

Congressional Record

A7837

A7838

OCTOBER 25, 1962

An Important Phase of World Medical Research: Let's Compete With U.S.S.R. in Research on Reversibility of Death

EXTENSION OF REMARKS
OF
HON. HUBERT H. HUMPHREY
OF MINNESOTA

IN THE SENATE OF THE UNITED STATES
Saturday, October 13, 1962

Mr. HUMPHREY. Mr. President, the 87th Congress has enacted a number of landmark bills for the strengthening of American and international medical research.

However, at this time, I should like to comment upon one phase of medical research, which has not, unfortunately, received sufficient administrative attention by Federal agencies.

Because the hour is late in this session, I will not presume to take the time of the Senate to describe this subject in great detail.

LIFE AND DEATH—THE UNIVERSAL INTEREST

I do, however, want to state that it is one of the most important of all phases of medical research.

Why? Because it concerns the most universal interest of man; namely: the prolongation of human life, the postponement of death, and, yes, perhaps the greatest scientific frontier—the reversibility of death.

In my judgment, on this supreme

APPENDIX

NIH SUPPORT LACKS COORDINATION

Earlier I had communicated with the National Institutes of Health as regards present NIH support of the study of what might be called the physiology of death.

NIH does support numerous important investigations, both in basic and applied research on death processes.

There is, however, lacking a quality which I, for one, have, in all frankness,

repeatedly found wanting both here and in other areas of NIH support.

I refer to the missing ingredient of coordination, of integration, of evaluation, of systematic pooling of interdisciplinary knowledge under an emerging new category and by strong teams.

TRUE MEDICAL LEADERSHIP IS NOT PASSIVE

In all candor, I say that the National Institutes of Health have the idea that they discharge their obligations when they merely hand out money to a variety of good investigators.

If, for example, 20 investigators apply for money, if a study section and a grant council approve 10 or 15 of the studies, if the studies proceed, then NIH tends to rest content.

I, for one, do not feel satisfied with this limited, passive approach.

ITEMS TO BE REPRINTED IN THE RECORD

I have selected certain items which illustrate, I believe, the challenge confronting mankind.

One is an introduction to an article in the August 25, 1962 issue of Saturday Review, as written by John Lear, science editor.

The article itself comprised quotations from Professor Negovskii's latest book.

The second item is the preface to Professor Negovskii's book, as written by Professor Beck. Mr. Lear's brief introduction to Professor Beck's comments is also included.

The third item consists of a supplementary memorandum which I had invited from Professor Beck on this subject.

I ask unanimous consent that the items be printed at this point in the RECORD.

There being no objection, the items were ordered to be printed in the RECORD as follows:

THE REVERSAL OF DEATH

NEW FRONTIER IN SOVIET SCIENCE?

(EDITOR'S NOTE.—Almost unknown to the American people, there has been taking place in recent years, in various parts of the world, including this country, a revolutionary shift in the approach to the study of death. To the old and established ways of preventing death has been added the possibility of reversing death, and windows have been opened onto understanding of the infinite metabolisms involved in the process of dying. Although some of the very first steps in this

References

1. Zipes DP, Jalife J. *Cardiac Electrophysiology: From Cell to Bedside.* Philadelphia: W.B. Saunders Company; 1990
2. Zipes DP, Jalife J. *Cardiac Electrophysiology: From Cell to Bedside.* Philadelphia: W.B. Saunders Company; 2000
3. Marban E. Cardiac channelopathies. *Nature* 2002;415:213–218
4. Wiggers CJ. The mechanism and nature of ventricular fibrillation. *Am Heart J* 1940;20: 399–412
5. Are implantable cardioverter-defibrillators or drugs more effective in prolonging life? The Antiarrhythmics Versus Implantable Defibrillators (AVID) Trial Executive Committee. *Am J Cardiol* 1997;79:661–663
6. Hon. Hubert H. Humphrey. *An Important Phase of World Medical Research: Let's Compete With U.S.S.R. in Research on Reversibility of Death.* Congressional Records, Saturday, October 13, 1962:A7837–A7839

St. Louis, MO

Igor R. Efimov

List of Contributors

Hana Akselrod
Caritas St. Elizabeth's Medical Center of Boston, Tufts University School of Medicine,
Boston, MA, USA

Didier Allexandre
Department of Molecular Cardiology, Department of Biomedical Engineering, The Lerner
Research Institute, Cleveland Clinic, Cleveland, OH, USA

Edward J. Berbari
Biomedical Engineering Department, Indiana University – Purdue University Indianapolis,
Indianapolis, IN, USA

V. N. Biktashev
Department of Mathematics, University of Liverpool, UK

David J. Christini
Division of Cardiology, Weill Medical College of Cornell University, New York, NY, USA
Department of Physiology and Biophysics, Weill Graduate School of Medical Sciences of
Cornell University, New York, NY, USA

Derek J. Dosdall
Departments of Medicine, Biomedical Engineering, and Physiology, University of Alabama-
Birmingham, Birmingham, AL, USA

John H. Dumas
The University of North Carolina at Chapel Hill and North Carolina State University, NC,
USA

Igor R. Efimov
Department of Biomedical Engineering, Washington University, St. Louis, MO, USA

Vladimir G. Fast
University of Alabama at Birmingham, Birmingham, AL, USA

Jeff Gillberg
CRDM Research, Medtronic, Inc., Minneapolis, MN, USA

Robert F. Gilmour, Jr.
Department of Biomedical Sciences, College of Veterinary Medicine, Cornell University,
Ithaca, NY, USA

Craig S. Henriquez,
Department of Biomedical Engineering, Duke University, Durham NC, USA

Herman D. Himel
The University of North Carolina at Chapel Hill and North Carolina State University, NC, USA

Raymond E. Ideker
Departments of Medicine, Biomedical Engineering, and Physiology, University of Alabama-Birmingham, Birmingham, AL

Troy Jackson
CRDM Research, Medtronic, Inc., Minneapolis, MN, USA

José Jalife
Department of Internal Medicine, Center for Arrhythmia Research, University of Michigan, Ann Arbor, MI

Deborah L. Janks
Department of Physics, Oakland University, Rochester, MI, USA

Hrayr S. Karagueuzian
Cardiovascular Research Laboratories, David Geffen School of Medicine at UCLA, Los Angeles, CA, USA

Alain Karma
Department of Physics and Center for Interdisciplinary Research on Complex Systems, Northeastern University, Boston, MA, USA

Galina Kichigina
Institute of Medical Science, University of Toronto, Toronto, ON, Canada

Stephen B. Knisley
The University of North Carolina at Chapel Hill and North Carolina State University, NC, USA

Wanda Krassowska Neu
Department of Biomedical Engineering, Duke University, Durham, NC, USA

Mark W. Kroll
Department of Biomedical Engineering, University of Minnesota, Minneapolis, MN, USA

Mingyi Li
Department of Diagnostic Radiology, The Cleveland Clinic, Cleveland, OH, USA

Shien-Fong Lin
Krannert Institute of Cardiology, Indiana University School of Medicine, Indianapolis, IN, USA

Srijoy Mahapatra
Division of Cardiovascular Medicine, University of Virginia, Charlottesville, VA, USA

John C. Neu
Department of Mathematics, University of California at Berkeley, CA, USA

Vladimir P. Nikolski
CRDM Research, Medtronic, Inc., Minneapolis, MN, USA

Michael V. Orlov
Caritas St. Elizabeth's Medical Center of Boston, Tufts University School of Medicine, Boston, MA, USA

Niels F. Otani
Department of Biomedical Sciences, College of Veterinary Medicine, Cornell University, Ithaca, NY, USA

Gernot Plank
Department of Biomedical Engineering, Institute for Computational Medicine, Johns Hopkins University, MD, USA
Institute of Biophysics, Medical University Graz, Austria

Crystal M. Ripplinger
Department of Biomedical Engineering, Washington University in St. Louis, St. Louis, MO, USA

Bradley J. Roth
Department of Physics, Oakland University, Rochester, MI, USA

Vinod Sharma
New Therapies and Diagnostics, Medtronic Inc., Minneapolis, MN, USA

Haris Sih
Cardiac Surgery Division, Boston Scientific, St. Paul, MN, USA

Charles D. Swerdlow
Division of Cardiology, Department of Medicine, Cedars-Sinai Medical Center, Los Angeles, CA, USA

Liang Tang
Krannert Institute of Cardiology, Indiana University School of Medicine, Indianapolis, IN, USA

Natalia Trayanova
Department of Biomedical Engineering, Institute for Computational Medicine, Johns Hopkins University, MD, USA

Leslie Tung
Department of Biomedical Engineering, School of Medicine, The Johns Hopkins University, Baltimore, MD, USA

John P. Wikswo, Jr
Departments of Biomedical Engineering, Molecular Physiology and Biophysics, and Physics and Astronomy, The Vanderbilt Institute for Integrative Biosystems Research and Education, Vanderbilt University, Nashville, TN, USA

Wenjun Ying
Department of Biomedical Engineering, Duke University, Durham NC, USA

Paul Ziegler
CRDM Research, Medtronic, Inc., Minneapolis, MN, USA

Foreword

Since pacemakers and defibrillators were developed a little more than 50 years ago, their usage has grown rapidly, so that over 900,000 pacemakers and 200,000 defibrillators are implanted every year throughout the world. During this half century there have been astonishing advances in the efficacy and sophistication of these devices. Yet the devices still have major limitations. For example, with current pacemakers the heart contracts less efficiently with a paced beat than with a normal sinus beat so that pacing can hasten the development of heart failure. As another example, some evidence suggests that defibrillation shocks can damage the heart and contribute to mortality.

Many of the previous advances made in pacemakers and defibrillators have been accomplished through improvements in their hardware and software and by experimental trial and error. Further advances will probably require increased knowledge of the basic mechanisms by which electric fields interact with the myocardium. Although there are many books that deal with the practical aspects of pacing and defibrillation, there is a pressing need for a single source that presents current knowledge about the basic mechanisms of cardiac bioelectric theory. This book, edited by Efimov, Kroll, and Tchou, admirable fulfills this need. The chapters thoroughly and masterfully cover all aspects of this subject and are written by experts in the field. The book covers the history of the development of pacing and defibrillation, the theory of how electric fields affect the myocardium, the experimental techniques used to study this subject, and the implications of this subject for future implantable devices including speculative approaches such as those that involve nonlinear dynamics. I predict this book will be the standard source that will be consulted both by experienced workers in this area as well as by students and others who wish to learn more about this subject.

Birmingham, AL   Raymond E. Ideker

Part I

History

Chapter 1.1

History of Cardiac Pacing

Srijoy Mahapatra

Earl Bakken: One Version of the First Pacemaker Story

In 1954 Dr. C. Walton Lillehei, a cardiac surgeon at the University of Minnesota, made advances in the treatment of the blue baby syndrome. In blue baby syndrome there is an abnormal blood communication between the left and right chambers of the heart. As a part of the treatment, Lillehei typically closed holes in the septum between the left and right heart chambers. Because the normal conduction system is in this septum, one common complication of the surgery was complete heart blockage, which meant the patient had no pulse. This heart blockage often resolved over a period of weeks, but to keep the child alive until then, Lillehei used temporary epicardial pacing. These pacing pads were sewn onto the heart and power by a large cart-mounted electrical generator. The patients were effectively tethered to the wall plug. If nurses had to move them, the staff could walk only so far as the next electrical outlet, unplug the generator, and then replug it into the next outlet. This not only made it difficult for the patients to be active, it made it difficult to move them for tests. This system, while cumbersome, allowed Lillehei to keep many children alive, and by 1957 he was one of the busiest congenital cardiac surgeons in the nation.

On October 31, 1957, a 3-hour power outage in Minneapolis rendered these generators useless because the wards had no backup electrical generators. Although one version of the story is that a child died, in an interview with Earl Bakken, Lillehei reported no deaths. Nonetheless, Lillehei knew he needed something battery operated.[1] Soon after this, Lillehei contacted Bakken, an engineer who owned the Medtronic medical equipment service company. Bakken spent the next month working on a pacemaker generator that would be small enough to wear and be powered by batteries. As inspiration he used an electronic, transistor-based metronome that generated sound periodically.

As Bakken tells it on the Bakken Museum website "I dug out a back issue of *Popular Electronics* magazine in which I recalled seeing a circuit for an electronic, transistorized metronome. The circuit transmitted clicks through a loudspeaker; the rate of the clicks could be adjusted to fit the music. I simply modified that circuit and placed it, without the

Division of Cardiovascular Medicine, University of Virginia, Charlottesville, VA, USA, sm9cd@virginia.edu

I. R. Efimov et al. (eds.), *Cardiac Bioelectric Therapy: Mechanisms and Practical Implications.*
© Springer Science+Business Media, LLC 2009

loudspeaker, in a four-inch-square, inch-and-thick metal box with terminals and switches on the outside—and that, as they say, was that."

"That" was the first, wearable, transistorized pacemaker. Modern electrophysiologists would barely recognize it as a pacemaker. The generator was not implanted into the body, and the only programming options were the rate and output. The leads were epicardial, which required the chest to be opened to position them. However, its small size allowed patients for the first time to be free of the wall plug. Two years later, doctors in St. Paul, Minnesota, proposed using Bakken's pacemaker in Stokes-Adams seizures.

Bakken's Medtronic grew from there. In subsequent years, his ideas and former employees lead to the formation of Cardiac Pacemakers Inc. (now part of Boston Scientific) and Pacesetter (now part of St. Jude Medical, Inc, where Lillehei was a medical director). In the lore of the Twin Cities device companies, Earl Bakken and Walt Lillehei had spurred an entire industry.

In Minneapolis, along Lake Calhoun, stands the Bakken Museum dedicated to under-standing electricity. According to its website, Earl Bakken was honored by the National Academy of Engineers for "invention of the first human heart pacemaker."

However, although very important, Bakken's device was more evolutionary than revolu-tionary. To paraphrase Newton, Bakken had stood on the shoulder of giants who had been working on electrically stimulating the heart since 1774 and others later stood on Bakken's shoulders. In fact, no one person "invented" the pacemaker.

The Long List of Inventions and Observations that Led to the Pacemaker

Pulse Theory and Observations that Bradycardia Leads to Syncope

Today physicians and athletes routinely measure the pulse. Although it is fairly simple to measure, especially compared to our now sophisticated imaging tools like magnetic resonance imaging, the pulse is still considered one of the "vital" signs. The knowledge that the pulse was a critical sign of health goes back to the ancient Egyptians. In 1875 George Ebers purchased an Egyptian scroll written in 1553 BC that described the relationship between the pulse in various locations and the heart beat.[2]

By 317 AD, the Chinese went further and developed a system of pulse analysis that was in some ways more complex than our own. They observed pulse at 11 locations and measured pulse rate variability (or lack of it) differences in pulses in different limbs. Wang Su-He observed that if the pulse became perfectly regular "the patient will be dead in four days."[3,4] These were just two cultures that incorporated "pulse theory" as a key component of health care.

More recently, in 1580, Italian born Geronimo Mercuariale noted that a slow pulse was associated with syncope. In particular, he noted that patients that had either episodic or chronically low pulses while awake seemed more likely to have syncope. He did not, however, actually check the pulse during syncope, and thus could not show that the low pulse actually caused syncope.[5] That observation would have to wait two centuries until in 1761 Giovanni Morgagni, another Italian, noted a patient during syncope had a slow pulse.

Shortly thereafter, Irish physicians Robert Adams and William Stokes described in separate publications patients who had low pulses and syncope. They also noted that bradycardia leads to dizziness, short pauses to more dizziness, and longer pauses to visual aura, then to complete syncope, convulsions, and finally death. In other words, longer pauses led to more symptoms. Although, Morgagni and Mercuariale had already made less detailed observations, Stokes and Adams are generally credited with the observation that syncope could have bradycardic instead of neurologic origin.[6]

However, it was not clear how one could increase the pulse. It was also unclear that electricity could be used to change the pulse.

In 1783 Luigi Galvani was dissecting frog legs on the same table where he had previously done work on static electricity. When an errant spark from a scalpel hit the sciatic nerve, the frog leg moved. Later observations, both with frog legs and later hearts, showed that electricity could stimulate muscle. He published these observations in 1791 as "Commentary on the Effect of Electricity on Muscular Motion."[7] This may in part have served as an inspiration for Mary Shelley's novel *Frankenstein*.[8]

In 1800 Marie Bichat was able to stimulate the cardiac ventricles in patients soon after execution. Later in 1803 Pierre-Hubert Nysten observed that contractility of the left ventricle faded first and after death, while the right ventricle would contract with electrical stimulation 1 h after death. The atria would contract the longest. These observations were the first to show that direct electrical stimulation of the heart could lead to muscular contraction.

Early Cardiac Pacing

Given that bradycardia leads to syncope, and that electricity can be used to pace the heart, Giovani Aldini reasoned that electrical pacing of the heart could alleviate syncope. In 1804 he alleviated syncope by pacing the heart. He went on to recommend a combination of pacing and respiration to revive people.

In 1853 chloroform anesthesia was used during Queen Victoria's delivery of children, and the use of the anesthetic grew. Although, it was an advance, one major side effect of its use was cardiac arrest. A solution was needed to prevent this fatal side effect. Building on previous observations, F. Steiner in Germany was the first to perform needle electrode pacing in animals after chloroform induced cardiac arrest.[9] Direct current pulses were delivered via a 13-cm long, 1-mm thick needle with a metronome as a regulator. Steiner paced a woman who had suffered cardiac arrest by placing a needle electrode inserted to her ventricular apex.[10] This emergency temporary pacing may have saved her life. Later Greene in the United Kingdom paced the apex from a direct current battery and also paced the phrenic nerve to provide cardiac and respiratory support.[9]

In 1882 a Prussian woman named Catharina Serafin came to the attention of Hugo von Ziemssen. Serafin had a chest wall tumor that was removed, leaving her heart exposed under a thin layer of skin. This allowed for a series of important experiments (although likely unethical by today's standards). Using electrical stimulation on the ventricles, he was able to pace the ventricle and achieve a pulse between 120 and 180 beats per minute. He could also induce and then treat ventricular fibrillation. He noted that different pacing sites seems to create different kind of beating (probably pacing left versus right ventricle).[11]

Up until this point all cardiac pacing had been epicardial. However, in 1927 Marmostein paced the right atrium and ventricle using a transvenous approach.[12] Although this is the most common technique currently used, it was forgotten for years until rediscovered by S. Furman.[13]

Previous devices were basically leads hooked up to a power source where the current needed human control. To make the control automatic, in 1932 Albert Hyman built an external pacemaker generator and control box. His device generated electricity as determined by a clock. He hooked this generator up to an epicardial lead on the right ventricle first in animals, then in humans.[14]

Internal Pacemakers

Shortly after World War II, Drs. William Bigelow and John Callaghan in Toronto used cold temperatures to slow the heart down enough to perform open heart surgery. Although, this made surgery easier, they struggled with the problem of how to start the heart if it stopped and on how to restart the heart at the end. John Hopps, an electrical engineer, built an external device of vacuum tubes that was powered by 60 Hz wall current. The generator was hooked up to a lead attached to the right atrium in animals via the internal jugular vein.[15]

Paul Zoll was aware of the Toronto's group work when he developed his external ventricular pacemaker. Zoll was a cardiologist with the U.S. Army during World War II. At that time he observed that the heart was quite irritable to touch. When he returned to Boston he was struck by the death of a patient from Stokes-Adams seizures. In 1950 he used an esophageal probe to stimulate the ventricle of a dog. Two years later he used this external stimulation for 52 h in a patient with complete heart block. The device he created was called the PM-65. It was manufactured by Electrodyne and could both monitor and pace. The PM-65 was carried on a cart and had a top piece that was a monitor and a bottom piece that was meant to pace. It was large but was cart mounted so the patient could walk as long as the cart was tethered to a plug point. Unfortunately, this external pacing was quite painful. Thus, for the most part, pacing was done via epicardial wires placed during cardiac surgery.

It was the PM-65 that Dr. Lillehei used in Minnesota that failed when the power went out. In 1957 Bakken created his wearable battery powered pacemaker. The Medtronic device was wearable but not implantable.

William Greatbatch wanted to go one step further. Greatbatch had also served in World War II as a radio engineer. In 1952 he was worked on an animal physiology farm at Cornell when two Boston physicians came to a brown bag lunch with him. They told him about complete heart block, and Greatbatch instantly decided he could fix the problem. "When he described it, I knew I could fix it," hetold the MIT-Lemelson board years later. In 1956 he was working in Buffalo using transistors to record heart sounds. He apparently plugged the wrong transistor into his recording mechanism and created a generator that pulsed for 1.8 ms and then was silent for 1 s. This seemed ideal for heart stimulation.

On May 7, 1958, he and William Chardack, a surgeon at the Buffalo Veterans Hospital, implanted a variant of this pacemaker into a dog. The device was the first to use a lead (not patches) to pace the atrium and ventricle from the epicardium. It was controlled by an oscillating transistor and powered by mercury-zinc batteries.[9] Greatbatch's employer, however, was unwilling to pursue human trials. It was not until 2 year later that Chardack implanted a device into a 77-year-old patient. It was the first implantable pacemaker with a myocardial lead. Greatbatch left his company and a later device was licensed to Medtronic.

At almost the same time, in Stockholm Sweden, Rune Elmqvist developed an implantable pacemaker made with two newly developed silicone transistors and rechargeable nickel–cadmium batteries. Dr. Ake Senning of the Karolinska Heart Institute implanted this device in Arne Larrson, an engineer who developed complete heart block as a complication of hepatitis and myocarditis after eating raw oysters.[16]

Prior to pacer placement he was having multiple syncopal episodes per day and his wife urged him to go ahead with the experimental device. On September 8, 1958, the device was implanted (Senning Cardiac Pacing in Retrospect). The first device only lasted hours, but rapid improvements by Elmqvist extended the life of the next device to 6 weeks. He then went without a pacer for 2 years until 1960 when he received a longer lasting device. He lived a full life and became an ambassador for the pacemaker industry. The patient died in 2001 after 43 years and 26 battery change outs.

Interestingly, although Elmqvist was an engineer, he had considered going to medical school. His invention meant he had made contributions to both fields. The company that Elmqvist worked for, Elema, was later acquired by Siemens and then by St. Jude Medical, Inc. and Pacesetter. It is not surprising that while the Medtronic website emphasizes Bakken's first wearable pacemaker, St. Jude Medical, Inc. emphasizes Elmqvist's first implantable pacemaker.

Pacing for Nonsurgeons

Initially, pacing leads were epicardial and placed by surgeons. In 1958, Furman rediscovered the idea of transvenous pacing. He used it as a temporary pacemaker for weeks in patients with complete heart block. It was a radical innovation that made lead placement less traumatic.

However, it was not until 1965 that permanent transvenous pacing became popular. This was in part driven by a new flexible Medtronic lead. Gradually, more implanters adopted the transvenous access. The transvenous approach was not only less traumatic but encouraged the study of intracardiac electrograms, which helped bridge the gap with electrophysiology. Initially this transvenous approach used the internal jugular, but this was a nuisance since it required tunneling over the clavicle. Eventually, Furman advocated using the subclavian or axillary vein, which simplified the procedure.[17]

Nonetheless, this transvenous approach still required a cut down approach, usually to the cephalic vein. Thus, most pacemakers were still placed by surgeons. In 1979 P. Littleford reported using a peal away sheath to access the vein, place the lead, and then remove the sheath while leaving the lead intact. This allowed nonsurgeons to use the more familiar Seldinger technique to access the axillary or subclavian vein. The combination of the peel away sheath and more flexible leads is a major reason why most pacemakers are placed by cardiologists today.[18]

Power Innovations

Early in the 1960s it was noted that a major limitations of pacemakers was the short battery life. There were two solutions: a longer-lasting battery or a rechargeable battery.

The pacemaker Senning had received in 1958 had been intended to be rechargeable and used nickel–cadmium. However, it and other rechargeable batteries had a shorter life span, despite recharging, than the mercury batteries. Pacesetter Systems, a new company in California, introduced a longer lasting nickel–cadmium battery in 1973 that only needed to be recharged weekly at the patient's home.[19] The overall life of the battery was predicted to last 20 years. However, there were several concerns. One was liability if the patient should fail to properly charge the battery. Another was a fear that older patients could not be relied upon to charge the battery, or even if they could, might not want to be reminded of their dependence on a machine.

At around the same time, Greatbatch was also looking for a solution. In 1967 Catalyst Research invented the lithium–iodine battery that significantly increased the life span of batteries. They could not find a market for it until Greatbatch thought of using it in a pacemaker. In 1973 his own firm, Greatbatch Ltd., started making these batteries, which were first used by a new pacemaker company, CPI, in their first pacemaker. These lithium batteries not only lasted longer and were smaller, but also slowly reduced their output voltage as they approached their end of life, which gave physicians plenty of warning for the need to change batteries. Another advantage is they did not produce oxidizing gas that had plagued the older mercury-zinc batteries. This gas meant the box could not be sealed and body fluids could leak in and create short circuits.

Greatbatch Inc. is still one of the largest device battery companies. In 1996 Greatbatch won the MIT-Lemelson Lifetime Achievement award for his contribution to pacemaker engineering. He continued inventing for 30 years and in the 1990s, with John Sanford, was granted three patents related to acquired immunodeficiency syndrome (AIDS).

Programming

The original pacemakers had only two programmable options: rate and output voltage. Often the rate could only be set to one of two rates. Furthermore, changing these options sometimes required surgery to expose the pulse generator.

Cordis introduced noninvasive programming of pacemakers in 1972. The device, the Omnicor, had six rate choices and four output voltage choices. To program it, the physician would use a magnetic device to transmit a series of pulses to the device. The pulse would move a magnetic reed switch. Each time the switch moved it would increase a counter. Each value of the counter corresponded a particular output and rate (24 in all.)

Although Cordis's patents initially gave them a monopoly, eventually other manufacturers expand this idea and provided more programming options. The programming, however, simply told the device what to do. The device still did not communicate with the physician.

In 1978 Intermedics introduced two-way communication in its CyberLith. The device gave the operators multiple programming options, including sensitivity and pulse width, but the operators could also download information about battery voltage, lead impedance, and frequency of stimulation. This communication was facilitated by a new telemetry system that used a low-power, high-frequency signal. Changes in this frequency acted as a code to transmit information.[20] It too was activated by a magnetic reed switch.

Eventually, growth in the processing power allowed pacemakers to become minicomputers that not only had thousands of programming options but could also provide a wealth of information to the doctor, making the pacemaker a diagnostic tool. It could store information on tachycardia and bradycardia episodes. Nonetheless, even today approximately one third are not reprogrammed ever after implant. Many are implanted right out of the box.

Dual-Chamber Pacing

It was recognized in the 1950s that dual-chamber pacing was likely hemodynamically advantageous. This is especially helpful in patients with sick sinus syndrome who could get pacemaker syndrome from ventricular pacing. Although ventricular pacing alone kept these patients alive, they could experience headaches, fatigue, or dyspnea. Although atrial pacing alone could solve this problem, a small but definite percentage could develop heart block later.

In 1963 Cordis introduced an epicardial atrioventricular (AV) synchronous pacemaker. It sensed the right atrium (RA) and this triggered pacing of the right ventricle (RV) (ventricular activation time [VAT] mode). Even this relatively primitive version of dual-chamber pacing required complex circuitry. In particular, if there was an atrial tachycardia, it had to switch to 2:1 conduction. These decisions drained battery life. It had no way to pace the RA. It was most helpful in patients with AV block, but no sinus node dysfunction and no history of atrial arrhythmias.[21]

The first bifocal pacer was introduced by American Optical. It had two transvenous leads and worked by pacing the atrium then the ventricle after an AV delay if it did not sense a native RV depolarization (DVI mode.) Thus, it would not track an atrial tachycardia. However, it could not track an appropriate sinus tachycardia with exercise either. It was found to be useful in patients with both AV block and sinus node dysfunction or atrial arrhythmias.[22]

With further advances in battery life and circuit design, manufactures could squeeze the logic into the pacemaker brain to finally build a full dual-chamber pacemaker (DDD mode). In the United States, Cordis was the first to introduce a true DDD pacemaker in 1982. Soon other manufacturers, including Medtronic, followed. These devices could pace and sense both RV and RA but this meant having to take into account not only AV intervals, but also such intervals as postventricular atrial refractory times (PVARP) and upper rate limit behavior. They all had telemetry.[23]

Unfortunately, these new pacemakers also introduced the new concept of pacemaker-mediated tachycardia (PMT). In a common scenario, a premature beat in the ventricle (PVC) would conduct into the atria. This atrial beat would be sensed and trigger a ventricular paced beat. This beat would then be conducted to the atria and repeat the syndrome. Usually one could program around PMT, and modern pacemakers have ways to automatically avoid PMT. Dual-chamber pacers were also more complicated to program.

A major advance that made dual-chamber pacing more acceptable was the preformed J curve that made it easier to pace the atrium. In part because of this, by the mid-1980s DDD pacing was fairly standard, although most pacemakers were still single chamber.

Activity Rate Responders

Dual-chamber pacemakers allowed the ventricular rate to increase with exercise if the sinus node increased in rate. However, in patients with sinus node dysfunction, atrial fibrillation, or just poor atrial sensing, the ventricular rate was "stuck" at its base rate. The first rate-adaptive pacing was reported in 1976 and used changes in venous pH as a marker of exercise. Soon after this a system was introduced that allowed sensing of the QT interval. A shorter QT suggested activity and thus the system paced further. One problem with these systems is that they did not have a quick onset and were slow to raise the rate. The QT sensors were influenced by drugs.

In 1983 Medtronic introduced a DDDR (rate-responsive) pacer that used a piezoelectric crystal. This crystal used no power, but when the patient moved it generated a signal that told the pacemaker to pace faster. The higher the frequency of the patient's movements, the faster the pacemaker paced. It was the first method of rate-adaptive pacing to be widely adopted.

However, the piezoelectric crystal sensor responded more to certain types of exercise than others (running than rowing). Later devices used more advanced accelerometers and minute ventilation, other surrogates for lung tidal volume, and evoked potentials to determine the pacing rates. These advances have allowed many patients to resume their normal lifestyles.

Implantable Cardiac Defibrillators

Today we tend to think of implantable cardiac defibrillators (ICDs) as an extension of a pacemaker, one with a capacitor that allows the delivery of a defibrillator charge. It seems only natural that once a pacemaker was built, an ICD would also be built. However, the development path for early ICDs was mostly separate from pacemakers and was, unlike pacemakers, developed by a single group. In fact, even as pacemaker use was growing, the very idea that and ICD could work was greeted with skepticism by many experts.

Michel Mirowski

Michel Mirowski was born in Poland in 1924. During World War II he was forced to flee the Nazis. The Holocaust took the lives of all other members of his family. After the war, he did his medical and cardiology training in Lyon, Israel, Baltimore, and Mexico City. He then returned to Israel where in 1967 a colleague died of recurrent ventricular tachycardia (VT).[24] Mirowski became convinced that an implantable defibrillator, by shocking the patient out of VT quickly, would have saved his friend. Since the device should be able to both defibrillate ventricular fibrillation (VF) and cardiovert VT he called it an implantable cardioverter-defibrillator. Later, since few noncardiologist knew the difference between cardioversion and defibrillation, manufacturers would rename it an implantable cardiac defibrillator.

In 1968 he returned to Baltimore and started working on the ICD with Morton Mower. Although ICDs are now known to have saved thousands of lives, at the time the idea of internal defibrillation was met with skepticism. The concerns included the difficulty of detecting VT and VF, the difficulty of terminating VF with a battery-powered system, as well as the need to test the device by inducing VF, a concern that continues today. In 1972 Bernard Lown (who at the time was a powerful figure in cardiology) denounced the idea as "impossible" and "unethical."

The U.S. National Institutes of Health rejected his grant application and an initial study on a dog with defibrillation of just 20 J was rejected from the *New England Journal of Medicine*. Mirowski ended up funding his own project.[25]

The opposition was so strong that although Earl Bakken of Medtronic was initially excited about the dog studies showing that ICDs could work, Medtronic decided not to pursue the idea because of this opposition in the medical community. In essence, they thought it would take 20 years to convince the medical community to use ICDs, and this was beyond their time horizon. It would take Mirowski 13 years. He seemed to find the opposition inspiring and told his biographer John Kastor he pushed ahead since "it couldn't be done."

In 1975 they completed 25 chronic canine implants and made dramatic films showing that the device could induce VF and the dog would collapse. Then the device would detect VF and shock the dog to sinus rhythm. Within a few minutes the dog was awake and wagging its tail. When Earl Bakken asked what would happen if the ICD was disconnected, Mirowski disconnected it and the dog died.[26] Despite these dramatic results, much of the cardiology community discounted the devices as dangerous and unworkable. Some even thought the dogs were trained actors.

However, after much work, on February 4, 1980, a 57-year-old woman with multiple episodes of recurrent VF with syncope who had failed multiple drugs underwent an ICD implantation. The surgeon was Levi Watkins and the device was attached to the epicardium with patches.

In 1985 the device won U.S. Food and Drug Administration approval. The initial ICDs required large patches to be placed on the epicardium via a thoracotomy. This carried a high morbidity risk, and generally ICDs were only placed when patients needed to have a thoracotomy anyhow. This high morbidity may be one reason that the CABG-PATCH trail was negative. Eventually, however, just as with pacing, the combination of a peel-away sheath and a flexible defibrillation lead allowed nonsurgeons to place the ICD.

Originally ICDs were just rate detectors. If the rate is greater than a determined rate, it would shock. However, recently multiple algorithms were used to minimize inappropriate shocks. However, these algorithms must be designed to avoid missing VF since the most inappropriate shock is the one not given for VT. Other innovations include quicker charge times, antitachycardia pacing to minimize shocks, and the addition of multiple pacemaker options. These innovations have made the ICD both more effective and somewhat more likely to deliver inappropriate shocks.

Conclusion

The invention of the pacemaker occurred more in a series of steps rather than in a eureka moment. It began with the worldwide observation that the pulse (or lack thereof) seemed to related to syncope and fatigue. Next multiple scientists were able to stimulate muscle with electrical impulses. From, there investigators stimulated live hearts, both in open chests and later in transvenous models. These leads were then hooked up to metronome like pacemakers.

In the recent years there have been many modifications made to the basic structure of pacemakers, the most important of which was the introduction of peel-away sheaths, flexible leads, and more flexible programming. Also, biventricular pacing with ICDs has improved or saved countless lives.

Future improvements will likely include reintroduction of epicardial pacing especially for LV pacing from a less invasive route, leadless pacemakers, and the reintroduction of rechargeable batteries.

References

1. Jefferey K. *Machines in Our Hearts.* Baltimore: JHU; 2001:68
2. Luderitz B. *History of the Disorders of Cardiac Rhythm.* Armonk: Futura Publishing; 2002:4
3. Cheng TO. Decreased heart rate variability as a predictor for sudden death was known in China in the third century AD. *Eur Heart J* 2000;21:2081–2082
4. Cowan MJ. Measurement of heart rate variability. *Western Journal of Nursing Research* 1995;17:32–48
5. Luderitz B. *History of the Disorders of Cardiac Rhythm.* Armonk: Futura Publishing; 2002:27
6. Adams R. (1791–1875) Morgagni–Adams–Stokes syndrome. *JAMA* 1968;206:639–640
7. Galvani L. *Commentary on the Effects of Electricity on Muscular Motion.* Trans. by Foley MG. Norwalk: Burdy Libarary; 1953
8. Wikipedia Search Lugi Galvani on Aug 11, 2007
9. Gedes LA, Bakken E. *IEEE Engineering in Medicine and Biology* 2007;26:77–79
10. Luderitz B. *History of the Disorders of Cardiac Rhythm.* Armonk: Futura Publishing; 2002:68
11. Luderitz B. *History of the Disorders of Cardiac Rhythm.* Armonk: Futura Publishing; 2002:120

12. Marmorstein M. Contribution of l'etude des excitation electriques localisees sur le Coeur en rapport avec la topographie de l'innervation de coeur chez le chien. *J Physiol (Paris)* 1927;25:617
13. Luderitz B. *History of the Disorders of Cardiac Rhythm.* Armonk: Futura Publishing; 2002:125
14. Hyman AS. Resuscitation of the stopped heart by intracardial therapy, II: experimental use of an artificial pacemaker. *Arch Int Med* 1932;50:283–305
15. Callaghan JC, Bigelow W. An electrical artificial pacemaker for standstill of the heart. *Ann Surg* 1951;134:8–17
16. Jefferey K. *Machines in Our Hearts.* Baltimore: JHU; 2001:90
17. Jefferey K. *Machines in Our Hearts.* Baltimore: JHU; 2001:123
18. Parsonnet V, Littleford P. *PACE* 1981;1:109–112
19. Silver AW. *Annals Thoraic Surgery* 1:380–388
20. Jeffery K. *Machines in Our Hearts.* Baltimore: JHU; 2001:138
21. Furman S. Therapeutic uses of atrial pacing. *Am Heart J* 1973;73:835–840
22. Castillo C. Bifocal demand pacing. *Chest* 1971;59:360–364
23. Belott PH. A variation on the introducer technique for unlimited access to the subclavian vein. *PACE* 1981;4:43–48
24. Kastor JA. Michel Mirowski and the automatic implantable defibrillator. *Am J Cardiol* 1989;63:977–982 and 1121–1126
25. Jefferey K. *Machines in Our Hearts.* Baltimore: JHU; 2001:239

Chapter 1.2

History of Defibrillation

Hana Akselrod, Mark W. Kroll, and Michael V. Orlov

Introduction: Defibrillation and Its Creators

Sudden cardiac death is believed to be involved in nearly a quarter of all human deaths, with ventricular fibrillation being its most common mechanism.[1] One of the first descriptions of ventricular fibrillation and its link to sudden cardiac death belongs to the British physiologist John A. McWilliam, a former student of the famous Carl Ludwig, who was working at the University of Aberdeen. He wrote in the late 1880s[2] that ventricular fibrillation wreaks chaos across the fibers of the heart, trapping the organ in a helpless quiver and depriving the body of oxygen, bringing about death within a matter of minutes. The story of how modern medicine and technology came together first to understand, and then to defeat fibrillation, is enlightening on many levels. It begins with astounding cures that seem to predate the discovery of the phenomenon itself; dives into the gothic with grisly experiments on executed criminals; rises into the light as the understanding of both electricity and cardiac pathophysiology increases; and flows vigorously into the modern blossoming of cardiopulmonary medicine and intensive care. It involves lessons transmitted across academic generations and geopolitical divisions, and discoveries made possible by cooperation of fields as dissimilar as surgery and electrical engineering. However, it also abounds with examples of great gaps of understanding, lengthy detours, and misdirected research; many key discoveries were preceded by periods of stagnation, while others were in fact set aside and had to be rediscovered altogether many decades later. However, as this chapter shows, the delays were seldom arbitrary and the detours seldom fruitless. It was the result of efforts by many devoted experts, many of them working in parallel or in competition, that led to the creation of defibrillation as we know it today. The case of the divergent investigations of alternating- versus direct-current electric shock therapy is particularly illustrative.

All along its length, the development of defibrillation was tightly coupled to developments in other fields of science and medicine and to changes in public understanding and demand

Michael V. Orlov

Caritas St. Elizabeth's Medical Center of Boston, Tufts University School of Medicine, Boston, MA, USA, mvorlov@pol.net

I. R. Efimov et al. (eds.), *Cardiac Bioelectric Therapy: Mechanisms and Practical Implications.*
© Springer Science+Business Media, LLC 2009

for certain types of procedures, often pushing to the limit assumptions—medical and popular alike—about the line separating life and death themselves. Many of these aspects are beyond the scope of the present publication; nevertheless, a detailed examination of the emergence of defibrillation is an intriguing insight into over three centuries of changes in medicine and society. According to many views, the window for defibrillation was opened as the more conservative medical predilections for pharmaceutical treatments began to shift in response to the growth in variety and success of surgical interventions.[3] Key factors in the boom in pacing and defibrillation research in the mid-twentieth century included an improved understanding of arrhythmias, experience with open-chest defibrillation, rising expertise in cardiac surgery, and a post–World War II cultural change that redefined the hospital as a technological center equipped and intended for the delivery of intensive care to critically ill patients.[4] Finally, biomaterials and microcircuit electronics were vital in opening new possibilities for medical research and vice versa: refinement of life-saving devices provided a demand for the development and production of advanced power sources, insulation materials, circuit components, and technical support. Defibrillation not only fed off the boom of cardiology as a complex specialty after the 1970s, but itself contributed to the building of optimism and confidence about medical technology as the means to conquer heart disease.[4]

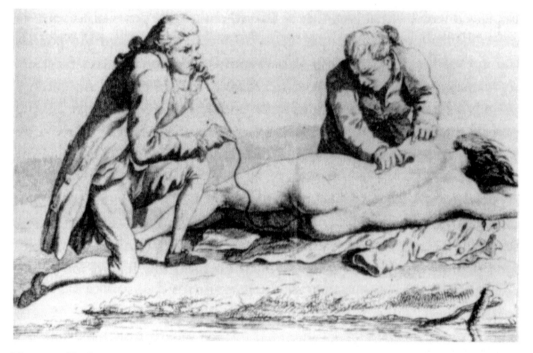

Figure 1: Early resuscitation recommendation. An eighteenth-century approach to resuscitating a human patient by blowing smoke into the anus and applying electrodes to the chest cavity. Other methods employed electrodes moistened with conductive fluids and inserted into the patient's orifices

In order to appreciate the historical setting we point out Fig. 1 which shows that nicotine smoke stimulation was part of the standard of care for resuscitation in the 1700s.

Mysteries of Early Research: Abdilgaard's Chickens and Kite's Successes

The history of electric defibrillation starts at the beginning of human manipulation of electricity. The first "electricity machine" was invented in 1660, and the first capacitor capable of collecting the charge from an electricity machine, storing it in a glass container, and delivering it as a static shock in 1745. This type of capacitor, used extensively in experiments during this period, was most often known as a Leyden jar. Almost as soon as it was invented, the Leyden jar saw use for the electrocution of small animals, first performed by van Pieter Musschenbroek. The nascent field was quick to intrigue many of the foremost scientific minds across Europe, and one, in the famously curious person of Benjamin Franklin, across the Atlantic.[5] Franklin made several important contributions to the understanding and design of capacitors, and himself experimented with delivering electric shocks to turkey tissues in 1750. In 1752, following his fabled kite experiment, he published the account of his near-electrocution.[6] Recent historical research now suggests that Franklin was too smart to engage in such a dangerous experiment and only suggested it to get revenge on a British scientist who was stealing his ideas. Sadly, Professor Georg Richmann in St. Petersburg was killed in front of his family when he tried to "duplicate" the experiment.

Shortly after, in 1755, Giovanni Bianchi applied various electrical shocks to dogs, managing to alternately induce seizures, stop respiration, and revive the animals.[7]

One of the long-standing mysteries in the history of defibrillation concerns the experiments of Danish veterinarian P. C. Abdilgaard. In his report, published in the 1775 *Proceedings of the Medical Society of Copenhagen*, Abdilgaard describes killing chickens by means of an electric shock to the head, and then reviving them with a subsequent shock to the chest:

> With a shock to head, the animal was rendered lifeless and arose with a second shock to the chest; however, after the experiment was repeated rather often, the hen was completely stunned, and walked with some difficulty, and did not eat for a day and night; then later is very well and even laid an egg.[8]

Abdilgaard observed that the chickens killed in such a way exhibited little damage to internal organs, and that no spontaneous remission occurred. Both of these observations suggest induced fibrillation as the cause of the chickens' deaths, and therefore defibrillation as the mechanism of the cure. A Leyden jar has a capacitance on the order of 100 pF. With a 50 kV charge, 125 J could be stored, which could be enough to defibrillate. However, the stored charge is only 5 mC, which is probably insufficient to defibrillate externally even a small animal. Of greater concern is the fact that even with a 1 kΩ resistance, the time constant of the shock would only be 100 μs, which is about 2 orders of magnitude too small for effective charging of the cardiac myocyte membrane needed for defibrillation. With lower resistances to increase the current, the shock time is even smaller. Unpublished animal data demonstrate that such very short shocks result in either asystole or have no effect.

Thus, although it is tempting to fix the origins of defibrillation at this early date, there are several arguments that point to the contrary: first, the spherical electrodes used at the time had prohibitively high impedances; second, the Leyden jar device itself is unlikely to have possessed an adequate charge storage for defibrillation; third, shocks to the head would not necessarily have caused fibrillation of the heart; and fourth, the chicken heart might have undergone spontaneous conversion, especially if prompted by chest contraction and motor neuron stimulation from the shocks. Indeed, as the classical review by Comroe and Dripps suggests, Abdilgaard's experiments could have well been an instance of neurogenic shock and spontaneous conversion, rather than fibrillation and defibrillation.[5] Hearts as small as the chickens do not maintain fibrillation well. In conclusion, there is much doubt that this episode was truly the first recorded electrical defibrillation.

Abdilgaard was but one of several scientists working in parallel at the time who were looking into the effects of electricity on animals; some reported similar results to his, while others could not reproduce them. Another Dutch-born scientist, Daniel Bernouilli, successfully used electrostatic sparks to revive drowned birds. The Italian scientist Felice Fontana, on the other hand, noted that the discharges from a Leyden jar killed young lambs and chickens outright or caused them to enter a state of irreversible petrifaction. In 1796 the Prussian naturalist Alexander von Humboldt revived an unconscious bird by passing a current between electrodes inserted in its beak and anus. The method was subsequently attempted on human patients, along with other "highly imaginative" modes of application: binding patients in metal chains, and immersing them in metallic bathtubs filled with brine.[3]

The possibility of human triumph over death became an interest of the Medical Societies, the scientific organizations of the time. The most famous of these was the Royal Humane Society of London, which in 1774 published the first documented case of a successful resuscitation by electricity, often debated as the first possible documented case of defibrillation. The case of 3-year-old Sophia Greenhill, who was pronounced dead of a fall, but saved through the intervention of an ingenious neighbor, is reported as follows:

> A child three years old, fell from a one-pair-of-stairs window, upon the pavement, and was taken up without any signs of life. An apothecary being sent for, he declared that nothing could be done, and that the child was irrecoverably dead; but a gentleman who lived opposite to the place, proposing a trial with Electricity, the parents consented. At least twenty minutes elapsed before he could apply the shock, which he gave to various parts of the body without any appearance of success. At length, on sending a few shocks through the chest, a small pulsation became perceptible; soon after the child began to sigh, and to breathe, though with great difficulty: in about ten minutes, she vomited. A kind of stupor remained for some days; but she was restored to perfect health and spirits in about a week.[9]

In 1787 the Royal Humane Society reported a highly similar case of a young boy who fell from a second-story window onto the ground, was pronounced dead, then on being carried home was given electric shocks by an experimenter, and revived. Such reports portrayed the use of electricity as an experimental means to be tried when contemporary medicine had given up, or in an emergency when ordinary medical attention could not be procured.[3] In a 1792 review of resuscitation cases, the British scientist James Curry describes the following procedure, uncannily prefiguring modern defibrillation protocols:

When the several measures recommended above have been steadily pursued for an hour or more, without any appearance of returning life, Electricity should be tried... Moderate shocks are found to answer best, and these should, at intervals, be passed through the chest in different directions, in order, if possible, to rouse the heart to act.[9]

Curry recommends that the patient's body be isolated by placing it on a slab of nonconductive material (e.g., on a door supported by a number of empty, dry bottles); that the lungs of the patient be artificially filled with and emptied of air between shocks; and that shocks to the brain be avoided altogether. For the positioning of the electrodes, he recommends the following: the spherical tip of one discharging rod placed above the right collar bone, and the tip of the second rod above the floating ribs on the left side of the patient, "in order more certainly to pass the shock through the heart," rather near the position of the paddles of a modern emergency external defibrillator, and suggests varying the positions of the rods if no results are obtained.[9]

The apparatus Curry investigated was a Leyden jar–based device, described earlier by the inventor Charles Kite in his *Essay on the Recovery of the Apparently Dead*, written for the Royal Humane Society in 1788.[10] It is believed that the resuscitation cases described by the Royal Humane Society employed devices (Fig. 2) highly similar to Kite's.[9,10] Kite's Leyden jar could produce up to 50,000 V, with a capacitance of 6.29×10^{-10} F and discharge in a spark of about 3 cm.[11] However, the same concerns about the applicability of the Kite device for defibrillation plague these cases as they do Abdilgaard's. Furthermore, there is a considerable debate over whether a fall from a first-story window could cause cardiac

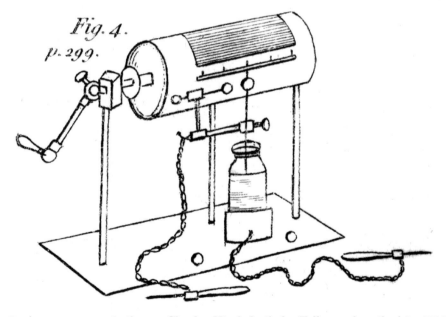

Figure 2: An apparatus similar to Charles Kite's built by Fell was described in 1792 issue of the *Gentleman's Magazine*. Courtesy to Mark Gulezian, Takoma Park

fibrillation in a child and the timelines suggest that any fibrillation would have degraded to asystole or pulseless electrical activity.

In 1802 the Royal Humane Society published a lengthy report praising the potential of electric resuscitation and suggested that the application of electric shock be used as the definitive test for distinguishing real from apparent death. Also working in London in the early 1800s, John Aldini, nephew of the renowned Italian physician Luigi Galvani, who published his watershed papers on "animal electricity" and contraction of muscle in the 1790s, took up his uncle's research. Aldini experimented on bodies of hanged criminals, causing the bodies to convulse "as if the wretched man was on the eve of being restored to life. This however was impossible."[3] Aldini believed that electric resuscitation should be combined with the technique of artificial breathing and argued against the prevalent view, which held that electricity should only be administered after rescue breathing has been provided continuously and unsuccessfully for two entire hours. In 1807 a report by William Babington published in the prestigious *Medico-Chirurgical Transactions* provided the first conclusive evidence for the increased effectiveness of electric resuscitation with concurrent administration of artificial respiration.[3] Still, in the following years the importance of this research would be ignored, until voiced again by Carl Wiggers in 1936.[5] This is a perfect example of an empirical breakthrough that, due to the absence of corresponding theoretical understanding at the time, would not be utilized for further development of resuscitation techniques for many years to come.

Aldini's experiments proved unpopular in the public opinion and were criticized in the press as morbid and satanic in nature.[3] Mary Shelley's novel *Frankenstein*, published in 1818, with its fearsome vision of the reanimated dead as an allegory for irresponsible invention and out-of-control evil, still provides some of the most recognizable imagery of fears about the modern world. The macabre aura of electric experiments was reinforced by the role of electrocution as capital punishment. Later, however, with the growth of the electric power grid, electrocution also became an increasingly common cause of accidental deaths. Its mechanism was eventually understood to be fibrillation. The injuries and fatalities suffered by electrical workers in particular would later motivate electric companies to invest money toward heart conduction and defibrillation research.[12]

With the invention of the voltaic battery, amateur and scientific "galvanism" grew in popularity during the nineteenth century (Fig. 3). According to some sources, it was considered fashionable for physicians who followed current research to carry canes with battery components hidden in special hollow compartments to allow quick assembly of a galvanic mechanism in case of an emergency. Along with these early precursors of portable defibrillators, the same time period saw the first precursors of "do not resuscitate" (DNR) orders: people wary of being experimented upon by vigilante galvanists were known to sew labels into their clothing, bearing requests to be left unelectrified if fallen unconscious. Ever on the borderline between desire and discomfort, electric resuscitation continuously struggled for legitimacy in the public comprehension, against allegations of sorcery on one side and quackery on the other. Later in the nineteenth century, with several key authorities on toxicology voicing their approval, electric resuscitation machines became a fixture in European surgery rooms, where they were used as backup measures for reviving patients suffering from poisoning by anesthetics.[12] Still, the field suffered from a grave setback: the

PLATE I.

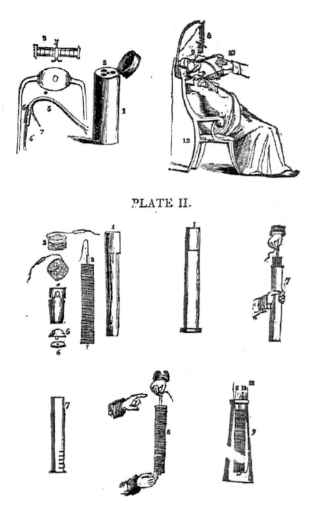

PLATE II.

•₊• This Apparatus is sold at the Medical Hall, 171. Piccadilly.

Fig. 2A. In the 1820 and 1824[20] editions of his book, Richard Reece depicted the paraphernalia and position most apt for restoring persons from suspended animation. Plate I shows a partitioned satchel with individual compartments for a bellows, constituents of a galvanic pile, laryngeal cannula, gastric tube, forceps for pinching the nose, and bottles of nitric acid, ether, and brandy. Also indicated is how these implements were to be applied to best advantage. Plate II shows the kit and assembly of the battery.

Figure 3: Portable galvanic resuscitation mechanism, nineteenth century

general lack of explanation for what the current was doing to the heart and how. Further advances would have to wait until the elucidation of the physiological mechanism. With greater understanding would come greater efficiency, and also greater acceptance by medical practitioners and patients alike.

Elucidating the Mechanism, Imagining the Cure

The mechanism of electric conduction in the heart through specialized fibers in the ventricles was first described by Jan Purkinje in 1839. It continued to be investigated throughout the nineteenth and early twentieth centuries, through the efforts of Stannius, Koliker and Muller, Engelmann, McWilliam, His, and others. The electrocardiogram (ECG) was developed in the late decades of the nineteenth century (using amplifiers designed to detect the weak transatlantic telegraph signals); by 1920 it had been refined for diagnosis of different arrhythmias in humans.[5] Meanwhile, the most threatening of these arrhythmias had already become the focus of much attention. In 1849 the German scientist Carl Friedrich Wilhelm Ludwig and his student Moritz Hoffa became the first to document the onset of ventricular fibrillation, by inducing it in a dog's heart with electric current applied directly to the ventricles.[13,14] For many years, fibrillation was considered a phenomenon that had little relevance to human clinical situations, although it was a topic of some debate whether the heart could recover from fibrillation.[12] Most physiologists believed that the uncontrollable contractions were caused by abnormal impulse generation and conduction within the network of nerve fibers. The Swiss physiologist Edmé Vulpian was the first to suggest the myogenic model of arrhythmia, thus pointing subsequent research in the right direction.[15] He was also responsible for the minting of the term *fibrillation*, in reference to the disorderly movements of the heart fibers, and described the event as a progression of distinct stages (Fig. 4).

The British physiologist John McWilliam confirmed Vulpian's conclusions independently and suggested the great importance of ventricular fibrillation in human deaths. Between 1887 and 1889, McWilliam published a series of articles in the *British Medical Journal*, in which he distinguished between different types of sudden cardiac failure, and wrote the first classic, detailed description of fibrillation in the English language:

> The normal beat is at once abolished, and the ventricles are thrown into a tumultuous state of quick, irregular, twitching action; at the same time there is a great fall of blood pressure. Ventricles become distended with blood, as the rapid quivering movement of their walls is wholly insufficient to expel their contents. . . . Instead of a coordinated contraction leading to a definite narrowing of the ventricular cavity, there occurs an irregular and complicated arrhythmic oscillation of the ventricular walls. . . . This condition is very persistent.[16]

The next breakthrough was made by a team of two physiologists, Jean Louis Prevost and Frederic Battelli, at the University of Geneva. In the 1899 issue of the *Journal de Physiologie et de Pathologie Generale*, Prevost and Battelli reported that it was possible to arrest heart contractions altogether by delivering a strong electric shock (2,400–4,800 V) to the body of an animal.[17] Furthermore, they found that they could stop not only regular heart rhythm in this way, but also fibrillation induced by application of a weaker current a short time

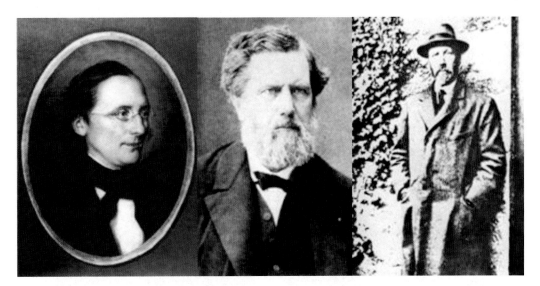

Figure 4: Ludwig, Vulpian, McWilliam

(15 s) earlier. The electrodes were placed in the mouth and the small intestine of the animal, and the shock delivered for up to 1 s in duration. Thus, Prevost and Battelli performed the first true, internal defibrillation. They did not manage to provide a mechanistic explanation for the phenomenon of defibrillation following the shock, although they did note that a refractory period in the activity of the myocardium followed the electric discharge. Working with capacitor discharges, Prevost and Battelli encountered difficulties in inducing the desired effect on the heart; this was one of the reasons the method was shelved until some decades later, when alternating teams of Russian and American scientists would apply new lessons about heart conduction to solving this problem (Fig. 5).

Although Prevost and Battelli were experimenting with dogs and internal electrodes, another scientist, Louise Robinovitch, very nearly invented both the external pacemaker and the transthoracic defibrillator. Working on cases of respiratory and cardiac arrest due to chloroform poisoning between 1906 and 1909, Robinovitch found that existing methods of resuscitation took too long to set up while the patient was deprived of oxygen.[18] She suggested using electrical current to induce both respiration and heartbeat without opening the chest cavity, and in fact designed a device that could be carried by an ambulance and plugged into the household electricity grid. However, as in the case of her predecessors, the work was crippled by the lack of scientific understanding of the mechanism of fibrillation. After Prevost and Battelli, and Louise Rabinovitch, the trail of discoveries in fibrillation research cooled off for a number of years. According to Eisenberg's *Life in the Balance* the significance of the work and its relevance to humans went underappreciated at the time; electric defibrillation was pronounced impracticable, and chemical defibrillation research was given greater priority. The Electric Light Association funded some research on electricity

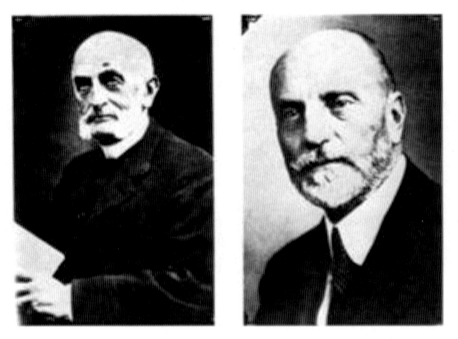

Figure 5: Prevost and Batelli

and fibrillation in 1913, but few important discoveries in the field can be traced to the years of World War I.[12]

In the 1920s scientists picked up on the possibility of electric defibrillation again. The Rockefeller Institute funded more research on the cause of electrocutions, distributing money to several academic centers and laboratories, including Johns Hopkins University, where physicians Orthello Langworthy and Donald Hooker were working with engineering professor William Kouwenhoven and accidentally rediscovered defibrillation as well as what would eventually become cardiopulmonary resuscitation (CPR).[19,20] By the 1930s results were being published again, more promising than before. Hooker, Kouwenhoven, and Langworthy were initially unaware of Prevost and Battelli's experiments. They began by placing the electrodes directly in the chest cavity of the dogs, against the myocardium of the ventricles. In 1933 they succeeded in arresting the fibrillation when they accidentally gave a second current application, hence the term *countershock*. Later they found the Prevost and Battelli papers and acknowledged them. When they pushed paddles hard against the chest to lower the impedance, they noticed an arterial pressure increase and thus also discovered chest compressions. In 1936 another team of cardiologists and electric engineers—Ferris, King, Spence, and Williams—defibrillated sheep by applying a current of 3,000 V across the animals' closed chests.[21]

Meanwhile, former students of the earlier pioneers were continuing their work far from its places of origin. In the United States, Carl Wiggers at Western Reserve University was pursuing the line of investigation he began in his student days under his mentor, W.P.

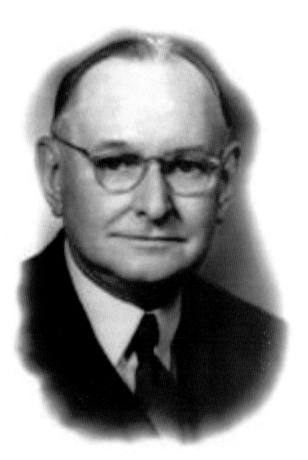

Figure 6: Carl J. Wiggers

Lombard, who himself had been a student of Carl Ludwig. He set out to untangle the basic causes and mechanisms of fibrillation; the research paid off. In 1940 Wiggers published a landmark paper, giving for the first time a mechanistic explanation for the induction of ventricular fibrillation, through the concept of the vulnerable period.[22] According to the Wiggers-Wégria model, fibrillation can occur if a second heartbeat is initiated before the natural end of the preceding contraction is reached. This period coincides with the appearance of the T wave on the ECG. A distinctive property of the vulnerable period is such that it responds in the same fashion to stimulation of different sorts: fibrillation may result from artificial stimulation by electricity, or from more "natural" physiological triggers (Fig. 6).

Wiggers is often credited with resurrecting the line of inquiry into electrical defibrillation, not only because of his scientific breakthrough, but also because of his assiduous efforts to fight institutional reluctance to investigate human defibrillation further. However, Wiggers was quite skeptical on the subject of transthoracic defibrillation, believing that the risks of the method of applying 3,000 V at 25–30 A to a patient's body can cause severe burns, disrupt the function of the central nervous system, and induce dangerous spasms in the respiratory system were too high. Also, he believed that the limited time (2–3 min after the beginning of fibrillation) during which defibrillation was useful posed a problem, as it was difficult to produce a confident diagnosis in so short a time, and delivering a shock in the absence of a definitive diagnosis was unacceptably dangerous. Therefore, Wiggers's recommendation was to restrict the use of electric defibrillation to the operating room, for cases when the chest cavity was already opened and the electrodes could be placed directly on the heart. In such cases, current from the wall outlets would be sufficient to defibrillate, and direct heart massage could be used to reduce hypoxia and aid the resumption of heart contractions.[23] Transthoracic defibrillation, it was clear, would wait for the coming of yet newer advances: the development of cardiopulmonary resuscitation, and the invention of a safer way to defibrillate.

Defibrillation: From Russia and the Soviet Block

While Hooker and Kouwenhoven were racing their competitors to the development of alternating current (AC) defibrillation, Dr. Lina Solomonovna Schtern, a former student of Prevost and Battelli, was heading research into the effects of electric shocks on the induction of arrhythmias and defibrillation in Moscow. She assigned this task to her graduate student Naum L. Gurvich. In his work toward a Ph.D. he investigated the efficacy of AC shocks in defibrillation, and discovered that direct current (DC) shocks were significantly more efficacious and less damaging. In 1938–1939, Gurvich and his colleague Yuniev from Schtern's laboratory developed a method for transthoracic defibrillation using condenser (capacitor) discharge.[24] Experimenting on over 650 dogs, sheep, and goats, they placed metal electrodes, covered by gauze moistened with saline solution, on both sides of the thorax, in line with the position of the heart, and passed alternating current through them to induce fibrillation. They then used the same electrodes to deliver a shock of 2,000–6,000 V (depending on the size of the animal) from a capacitor to the chest. Cardiac function was restored if defibrillation was performed within 1–1.5 min of fibrillation onset; if the defibrillation was prefaced by close-chest cardiac massage, this time window could be extended by several minutes. Gurvich proceeded to determine the thresholds for capacitance and voltage that were needed for the procedure to be effective in each type of animal. He also discovered that when an inductor was included in the circuit of the condenser apparatus, the thresholds of voltage were lowered. Their results were first published in English by the Moscow Institute of Physiology, USSR Academy of Sciences in 1945.[25,26]

There were several advantages to the use of direct rather than alternating current. In order to produce the AC current of 2,000–3,000 V and 25–30 A needed to cause defibrillation across the chest of an animal with a chest the size of a large dog or a human, it is necessary to have a very powerful, very bulky current generator or transformer on hand. The strong chest contractions often broke ribs. Such high-tension AC is dangerous to the technicians and sometimes to the patient, for a number of reasons: electrocution, a technical glitch can causing the current to be lowered at the surface of the patient's body, causing it to produce further fibrillation in the heart instead of stopping it, etc. The DC discharge,

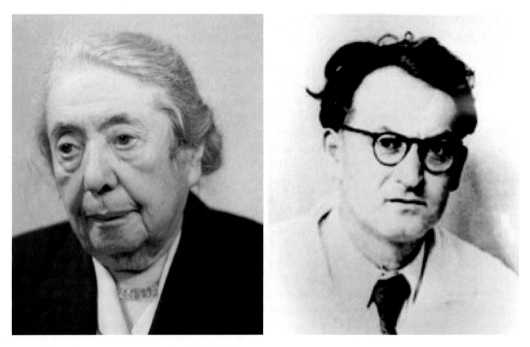

Figure 7: Lina S. Shtern and Naum L. Gurvich

on the other hand, is much less likely to cause fibrillation, even after repeated trials, a significant advantage, given that a single shock is often insufficient to defibrillate.[25] In a later publication, Gurvich noted that the prolonged exposure of the heart to AC reduced its functionality, following the defibrillation procedure, often making it necessary to restart heart contractions by artificial means. In contrast, heartbeat was shown to be more likely to restart spontaneously after defibrillation with a DC shock (Fig. 7).[23]

Naum Gurvich went on to become the key twentieth-century figure in the field of electrophysiology in Russia and the Soviet Union, remaining mostly unknown in the West. A member of the USSR Academy of Medical Sciences in Moscow, he focused his research career on the mechanisms of initiation and maintenance of fibrillation and defibrillation. In the 1940s he combined his observations about the capacitor-inductor circuit experiments with the newly published Wiggers-Wégria model of the vulnerable period, and proposed a radically new physical element of defibrillation: the biphasic waveform discharge. He also introduced the hypothesis of defibrillation as the stimulation of the myocardium by shock (in contrast to the prevalent theories that defibrillation incapacitated the myocardium), and introduced the concept of leading reentry circuits in the heart as the sustaining elements of fibrillation.[23] However, it was his concept of the biphasic waveform that had the most direct impact on the design of transthoracic, and, later, implantable, defibrillators. His condenser defibrillator model was first tried for clinical use in cardiac surgery units in 1952. Following the work of Alexander Vishnevsky in the late 1950s, the model was successfully tested in large-scale clinical studies.[27]

However, it is important to remember that developments in science followed an unpredictable course during the era of Stalin. Lina Schtern was tried by an infamous anti-Semitic Soviet trial during the last years of Stalin's rule. She was sentenced to death among several prominent Jewish celebrities. However, she was the only survivor among them, due to a personal pardon from Stalin, who according to legends believed that she could bring people back from the dead. Gurvich also was not exempt from the dangers of the time. He miraculously escaped persecution during this time, being protected by his new employer, director of the Institute of Reanimatology Vladimir Negovsky. But his work remained underappreciated by the Soviet state for many years. Nonetheless, in 1970 Gurvich was awarded the National Award of the USSR for his compendium of work. By his death in 1981, the biphasic defibrillator he had created was ubiquitous in emergency and cardiac care units in hospitals, across the USSR and in Europe.

The inclusion of an inductor into the DC defibrillator circuit, as introduced by Gurvich, had the effect of prolonging the time of discharge of the capacitor while moderating its peak voltage, thus stretching the pulse duration to more optimal values. It also reduced the damage to heart tissues from the procedure, thus increasing overall survival rates. The electric impulse delivered by such circuits takes the form of a biphasic wave, in which a first crest is followed by a second one of variable magnitude. Although not understood then, the second phase heals several proarrhythmic side effects of the first phase by discharging virtual electrodes, discharging partially charged membranes, and probably reducing electroporation stunning.[28] Defibrillation could now be accomplished using only 60% of the energy required by the monophasic wave. Furthermore, the part of the wave that was known to be the most dangerous to the patient, the high peek current of the electric discharge at the beginning of the shock, was altogether removed in the biphasic form. The overall procedure was much safer for the patient and was soon accepted as standard practice in emergency rooms. Remarkably, Gurvich first reported using the rounded biphasic waveform for defibrillation as early as 1939 (Fig. 8).[5]

The next major defibrillation advances in Europe were made by the Czech scientist Bohumil Peleška of the Institute for Clinical and Experimental Surgery in Prague, who visited Gurvich in Moscow and was familiar with his research. In a 1957 paper in the *Rozhledy v chirurglii* (Surgical Research) journal, he reported on his work in the development and optimization of DC defibrillation, in both the transthoracic and the direct approaches.[29] Histological studies showed that repeated discharges with increased voltage produce greater morphological damage to the myocardium; Peleška was responsible for optimization of the procedure using lower voltages. He also introduced the use of electrodes with larger surface area, proving that these produced a more even distribution of current and a more regular defibrillation of the entire organ. After confirming the reliability and safety of the transthoracic method in animals, Peleška then performed it on humans.[29] In subsequent work, Peleška untangled some of the complications that DC defibrillation could cause. It had been observed that DC shocks could in some instances cause arrhythmias, which would gradually transition into another cycle of ventricular fibrillation. Peleška's findings showed that fibrillation was most likely to follow a DC shock if the shock is delivered during the relative refractory period of the cardiac cycle, the T wave.[30] However, he showed the case to be different for condenser defibrillators with induction coils included in the circuit: the

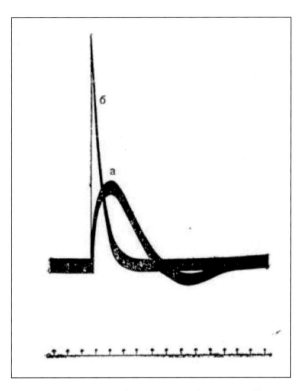

Figure 8: Early experiments on the biphasic waveform by Gurvich. Graph shows the comparative amplitude and length of the electric discharge in defibrillation of the heart of a dog (**a**) using a capacitor-inductor circuit and (**b**) using a capacitor only. (Gurvich and Yuniev 1947)[26]

electrical resistance of the coil lowered the peek current and increased the duration of the pulse to something closer to the defibrillation chronaxie, and fewer arrhythmias occurred.[31] Thus, the biphasic DC waveform was found to have additional advantages over both AC and the simple condenser discharge.

Across the Atlantic, the original Gurvich and Yuniev paper was reprinted in the *American Review of Soviet Medicine* in 1946 and 1947, and soon became part of an international dialogue on electrophysiology research, a dialogue characterized at once by shared scientific respect and by Cold War competition. In 1958 the U.S. senator and future vice president of the United States Hubert H. Humphrey went on to visit the USSR and was amazed by how advanced the research on resuscitation was in that country. He received a detailed demonstration of Gurvich's experiments at the Institute lead by Negovsky, which triggered subsequent congressional hearings: "Let's compete with U.S.S.R. in research on reversibility of death."[32] These hearings spurred U.S. research efforts in this area and also resulted in collaboration between both countries. One of the most well-known collaborative programs was the U.S.-Soviet cooperative research project that remained active for many years.

In 1953 the American research team of R. Stuart MacKay and Sanford Leeds reported in the *Journal of Applied Physiology* on their success using an experimental DC defibrillation protocol in dogs, similar to Gurvich and Yuniev's experiments.[33] Unlike AC, they write, DC, by virtue of its constant amplitude, can be expected to remain safely outside the range in which further fibrillation can be induced:

> The previous work [with DC by Prevost and Battelli, Gurvich and Yuniev, and Hooker and Kouwenhoven] has indicated that there is a critical current below which fibrillation is produced and above which defibrillation is produced, but never fibrillation. . . . The probable reason is that if a shock is strong enough to produce a uniform, all-over contraction rather than a localized or incomplete stimulation, there will resume a normal co-ordinated beat.[33]

MacKay and Leeds pointed out similar arguments as the Russians about the advantages of DC shocks from condenser discharges over AC for defibrillation, and reported on the relative safety of the DC method, including its relative safety for the central nervous and the respiratory systems. The authors proceeded to apply parameters and observations from experiments by Kouwenhoven et al. and Zoll et al. to make suggestions about possible use of DC defibrillation on humans.[33]

Defibrillation: AC to DC, in America and Beyond

Meanwhile, in the United States, defibrillation research had been following a different path altogether, the path of AC and surgical applications. One of the colleagues who paid attention to Wiggers's research at Western Reserve University was Dr. Claude S. Beck, professor of cardiovascular surgery. Beck developed an interest in fibrillation after losing a young patient to ventricular fibrillation in the late 1920s, and closely followed Hooker's and Kouwenhoven's experiments on open-chest defibrillation on animals throughout the 1930s. He performed experiments himself as well and developed a procedure that worked in dogs and monkeys. In 1947 Beck successfully performed the first documented defibrillation on a human patient. Richard Heyard, aged 14, was undergoing surgery to correct a "hollow chest" breastbone malformation. Near the end of the procedure, his heart suddenly entered ventricular fibrillation. The surgeon immediately started direct heart massage, keeping Heyard's blood in circulation, but the fibrillation showed no indication of stopping spontaneously. Beck requested permission to perform his experimental procedure, connecting two electrodes directly to Heyard's exposed heart. After four shocks of 110 V, the fibrillation ceased, and this time mere seconds of heart massage sufficed to restore heartbeat. Richard made a complete recovery, and the case became a deservedly publicized news item, under a variety of titles such as "How Science Brings Americans Back from the Dead."[34,35] The case was also published in *JAMA* by Beck, Pritchard, and Feil.[36] Beck continued his research on mechanical means of resuscitation, pioneered the use of a combined defibrillator and heart massage device, and designed the first program to teach laypeople CPR (Fig. 9).

Although Beck was successful with AC defibrillation applied directly to the heart, research on transthoracic defibrillation was beset by more difficulties. After his initial success with open-chested defibrillation of dogs, William Kouwenhoven, dean of the School

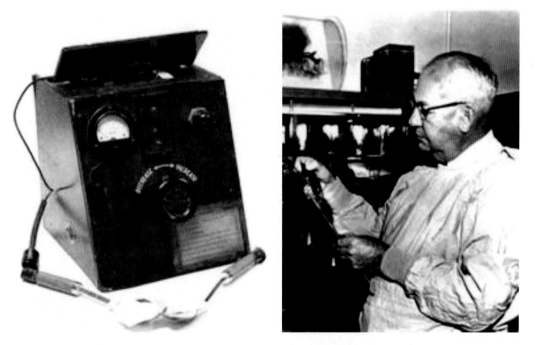

Figure 9: Beck's first defibrillator, Claude Beck

of Engineering at Johns Hopkins University and bearer of an honorary medical degree from its medical school, directed his research toward developing a portable external defibrillator. After initial attempts with DC designs in the early 1950s, he had to abandon the idea; batteries powerful enough to create the necessary charge simply did not exist at the time. Switching to AC-powered models instead, Kouwenhoven found success in 1951, with a device funded by the Edison Electric Institute. In 1957 he developed a closed-chest defibrillator that used AC to deliver repeated shocks of 480 V to the adult heart without damaging the myocardium. The device weighed 120 kg and was used on two patients.[37] Ironically, while Kouwenhoven spent decades studying defibrillation, he was beaten to the publication date by a Boston cardiologist, Paul Zoll.[38] Kouwenhoven's enduring fame would come from his achievements in the development of another nonsurgical method of heart activation: external cardiac compression, the basis of CPR, which would play a great role in the spread of defibrillation procedure in subsequent years. For his work, Kouwenhoven would be awarded the American Medical Association Scientific Achievement Award in 1972 (Fig. 10).[12,40]

Zoll, the Harvard researcher who independently scooped Kouwenhoven on transthoracic AC defibrillation, came to defibrillation research from a different beginning: after working in cardiac surgery in the U.S. army during World War II, he came back to civilian practice and soon became fascinated by the case of a patient with recurrent Stokes-Adams attacks. Zoll started to perform experiments on external cardiac pacing and defibrillation in animals, and first used an external pacer in a patient in 1952. Although the prevailing medical opinion at

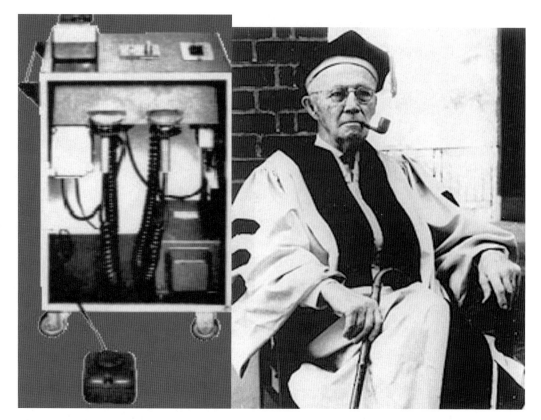

Figure 10: Kouwenhoven defibrillator, 120 kg, William Kouwenhoven

the time held that external defibrillation would never work because the necessary electric current was believed to be so high that significant damage to the patient would be caused before it reached the heart, Zoll based his experiments on the same research from the 1930s as Kouwenhoven did, and also believed the prevailing opinion to be wrong. He had a model for human external defibrillation built by Electrodyne, successfully used it in 1955, and published the results in *NEJM* in 1956.[38] Prohibitively large and heavy, the Electrodyne defibrillator, like its cousin made by Edison Electric, was only portable to the extent to which it could be wheeled into the emergency room, its most bulky component being a transformer that could convert the wall outlet supply to 1,000 V.[12]

These advances were being made at a time when a great surge was beginning in the development of lifesaving emergency methods and procedures. Claude Beck had declared that battling sudden cardiac death should be a national priority, and the idea proved popular; his associate Dr. David Leighninger famously stated that "many hearts die that are too good to die."[39] Autopsy studies performed at the time showed that nearly 70% of sudden cardiac death cases showed no new pathology in the heart tissue, but had stopped due to electrical problems that could be fixed by electric pacing or defibrillation. At the same time, the development of quality prehospital care and intensive emergency procedures inspired greater interest of both the medical authorities and the general public; interest fueled funding and development; and these in turn generated results, which attracted further interest. Intensive care in nonmilitary hospitals developed toward the middle of the twentieth century, following along with advances in medical technology and surgery. It started with setting aside a specially monitored room for patients recovering from high-risk surgical operations. During the poliomyelitis epidemic in the 1950s, for instance, many hospitals designated new intensive care units for patients needing artificial or assisted respiration. The young specialty of cardiac surgery especially required nonstop monitoring of their patients by trained personnel and sensitive equipment. Therefore, as the new inventions of pacemakers, defibrillators, and cardioverters appeared, they could be immediately provided to cardiac patients undergoing intensive care at the hospital.[5,12]

Although civilian ambulance services began in some American cities in the 1900s as a transport service, most communities did not develop them until the 1940s. The modern emergency medical services system was established with the passage of the National Highway Safety Act in 1966, and professional standards for emergency medical technicians were first standardized in 1970.[41] In the 1960s Kouwenhoven's closed-chest heart massage (now CPR) became standard practice for emergency rescue services, and in the 1970s the American Heart Association approved training laypersons in the technique.[12] Thus, during the 1960s and 1970s, it became possible to imagine the fulfillment of the predictions of James Curry and Carl Wiggers: a patient would be kept alive by competent provision of oxygen to the tissues and defibrillated promptly by a portable defibrillator. Only one link in the chain was incomplete: a defibrillator that was truly portable and safe.

In the United States, that final link was created by Dr. Bernard Lown of Brigham and Women's Hospital in Boston. Lown used Zoll's apparatus to correct persistent ventricular tachycardia in a patient; the technique was successful initially, but the AC procedure later induced ventricular fibrillation. Finding alternating current to be thus unsuitable for cardioversion, Lown began investigating the possibility of using condenser discharges instead. In a 1962 *JAMA* paper, Lown, Amarasingham, and Neuman reported their success with the transthoracic treatment of nine ventricular tachycardia patients by monophasic DC shocks, where all patients reverted successfully with a single discharge. Commenting on their results, they cited previous work with DC defibrillation of human patients by both Gurvich and Peleška. They explained the difficulties encountered by other teams of scientists, Kouwenhoven and Milnor, Guyton and Satterfield, in trying to reproduce the results by lack of consistency in circuit design and current shape, noting that more research would be necessary.[42] Already the team was investigating the possibilities, placing electrodes inside the chests of dogs and defibrillating them using different capacitor-inductor currents, in a resounding echo of earlier experiments. Seemingly unaware that the optimal DC waveform had already been discovered on the other side of the Iron Curtain, they wrote that "at the present time, there is no physiological basis for predicting the wave form which is optimal for defibrillation."[43] Lown would pursue this line of research for many years, finally succeeding with the biphasic waveform model several years later.

The external DC defibrillator used by the Lown research team was first constructed in 1961 by the Hungarian engineer Barouh Berkovits and patented in the name of the American

Optical Company.[44] Berkovits came to the United States after World War II and could have been familiar with research by Gurvich and Peleška on the other side of the Atlantic. Moreover, future model of Lown's "Cardioverter" was based on Gurvich's schematic.[45,46] Berkovits then went on to solve the problem of pacemaker-induced ventricular fibrillation and to create the demand pacemaker in the 1960s–1970s.[4]

It was at that time that the subfield of defibrillation came to join paths with another emergent branch of cardiology research: cardioversion and cardiac pacing, the history of which is described elsewhere in this book. Defibrillators and pacemakers became sufficiently sophisticated to work together, sustaining heart rhythm inside the human body. The development of the implantable cardioverter-defibrillator (ICD) began with its inventor, Michel Mirowski, who came up with the idea of the device in the late 1960s after his mentor died of a heart arrhythmia, and he succeeded with the first human implantation in 1980.[47,48] John Schuder published the idea of ICD at the same time, but he did not pursue its validation and development.[49] Thus, Mirowski deserves most of the credit for ICD. A Polish Jew who left home at age 14 to escape the Nazis, Mirowski attended medical school in France, completed residency in Israel, and finished his cardiology fellowship in the United States. After living in Israel for several years, Mirowski returned to the United States in 1968 to become the coronary care director at Sinai Hospital in Baltimore and to conduct his research on the ICD as an alternative to surgery and drugs.[50] This bold idea faced considerable opposition from the medical community of the early 1970s: prominent authorities in the field, including B. Lown, were concerned about the technical difficulties, less than clear indications, high costs, and possible dangers of the new technology, and skeptical that its use would be anything but very narrow.[51]

Nevertheless, Mirowski and his teem succeeded: the first human implant, employing a defibrillator device the size of a deck of cards and weighing 250 grams, was performed in 1980. Subsequent research would reduce the size and cost of the device, and the end of the twentieth century would witness the astounding boom of the technology, with hundreds of thousands of patients having implantable defibrillators worldwide.[50] In 1982 the cardioversion function was fused with the internal defibrillator, and in 1985 the ICD received U.S. Food and Drug Administration approval. As it happened, this part of the chronology is where the waveform conundrum was finally solved in the West. The efficacy of an ICD is limited by the maximum energy supplied by the accompanying power source; in their quest for the minimal size of the device, the inventors of the ICD eventually chose the more effective biphasic waveform over the higher monophasic current used in transthoracic devices at the time.

It was thus that the biphasic waveform, as first described by Gurvich and used in external defibrillators in Russia,[52] finally was incorporated into Western external defibrillators in the late 1990s. In fact, it was first proven to be more effective in implantable defibrillators, and only then made its remarkable comeback to external ones. This is another example of an eminent idea being circumvented for decades but finally winning the day due to superiority of design. With the final development of single-button automatic external defibrillators (AED),[53] defibrillation became not only ubiquitous but even safe and available for use by laypersons. Popularized along with advanced CPR and first aid training, it has brought about far better odds of survival for victims of out-of-hospital cardiac arrest.

Conclusion

Comroe and Dripps, in their classic review of developments in cardiopulmonary medicine, note that cardiac defibrillation had a relatively long time lag between initial discovery of the phenomenon and its successful clinical application.[5] As we have seen, a remarkably clear prototype of resuscitation from sudden death, through delivery of electric shock and artificial respiration, emerged as early as the threshold of the nineteenth century, with the reports of Curry and Babington. Even if we disregard the early experiments as haphazard and fortuitous, another half a century elapsed between the first modern success, by Prevost and Battelli, and its human application by Beck, longer still if we decide to wait for the first widely used application, with the invention of first stationary and then portable transthoracic defibrillators. The history of cardiac defibrillation is punctuated with gaps, where discoveries were set aside due to lack of scientific understanding, resource availability, or general interest, only to be repeated years or decades later, after some new leap in understanding. Additional lags were incurred across the divide of the Iron Curtain, delaying the development of safe and portable defibrillation by a number of years. We can understand this pattern of lags and leaps by classifying the discoveries described in this chapter into the following rough framework:

1. *The early experiments: the late 1700s and early 1800s.* This was the period of the initial, tantalizing reports published by Abdilgaard, Kite, Aldini, and others. Characterized by a nebulous understanding of the physiology involved, it nevertheless yielded results that pointed clearly toward the possibilities of the new science and showed the direction for future research.

2. *The rising popularity of electricity: the 1800s.* The century that started with Franken-stein's monster would see public opinion grow increasingly comfortable with the idea that electricity might participate in normal human health. It imparted a colorful tableau of quackery, fashionable "galvanism," and legitimate scientific achievements in the understanding of electricity.

3. *Understanding the heart's wiring: the 1800s.* Even as electricity was becoming promi-nent in everyday life and health, discoveries by Purkinje, Ludwig, Vulpian, McWilliam, and others were elucidating the processes by which it made the heart contract, or cease to contract. By 1899 Prevost and Battelli could put together the new advances in electricity and cardiology and perform the first proven cardiac defibrillation. During this period, research grew more standardized, according to the scientific method, and results became accordingly clearer.

4. *The great delay: the 1900s–1920s.* This was the period in which fibrillation was set aside, due to reasons of both economics and science. No advances were made in fibrillation research beyond Prevost and Battelli's. However, other scientists at the time were making advances in surgery, reanimation, and cardiology, including important refinement of arrhythmia diagnostics by ECG, which set the stage for the next cluster of breakthroughs.

5. *New possibilities through surgery and cardiology: the 1930s–1950s.* As is often the case, that period of stagnation was followed by a time of vibrant discovery on the defibrillation front. Great leaps in understanding of the mechanism of fibrillation were made, first by Wiggers in the United States, and then by Gurvich in Russia. Meanwhile, progress in surgery made more successful open-chest work possible, both on test animals and on human patients. These advances helped the teams of Wiggers, Kouwenhoven, and Gurvich, and culminated in the performance of the first successful human open chest defibrillation by Beck.

6. *Improving design and leaving the chest cavity: the 1950s–1960s.* With the foundation of human cardiac defibrillation firmly established, the discipline reached a stage when designs were revised and redesigned, different forms of current chosen between, and protocols optimized. The work of Gurvich, Kouwenhoven, Zoll, Peleška, and finally Lown culminated in the creation of first the transthoracic defibrillator, then the safe transthoracic defibrillator, and finally the portable safe transthoracic defibrillator familiar to us today.

7. *Implantable defibrillators: the 1960s–1980s.* Despite considerable opposition from various parties, including the medical society of the day, the teams of Mirowski and Schuder invented and implanted the first internal defibrillator in 1980, later fusing it with the implantable cardioverter. Further refinements created the small, sophisticated ICD of today, one of the most effective lifesaving therapies in cardiology.

8. *Infrastructure and popularity: the midcentury to present time.* The last pieces of the story have to do with the creation of the infrastructure that permitted defibrillation to become the ubiquitous presence it is today. With the development of modern cardiopulmonary resuscitation methods by Kouwenhoven and others, and the creation of the modern emergency response system by federal and state governments, defibrillation by AED devices gained a truly unprecedented reach, and it is now responsible for saving numerable lives every year.

In closing, the common pattern that explains the punctuations and delays in the development of defibrillation stems from the dyssynchronies in the respective development of scientific knowledge, changes in the perception of clinical need for that knowledge, and interest in applying the clinical discoveries widely. These obstacles were overcome by a continuity of research throughout generations of academicians, continuing from Ludwig to Lombard and then Wiggers, and crossing the Atlantic in the process to spread across the world. In addition to vertical continuity, a great horizontal variety of approaches were pursued in competition as well as cooperation: Kouwenhoven, Beck, Zoll, and other teams were motivated and helped by the others' discoveries. Post–World War II mobility greatly increased the international spread of the research being done; Berkovits and Mirowski continued their work far from their lands of origin. Despite the Cold War, key developments did become available to leading medical researchers across the Iron Curtain: Gurvich built upon Wiggers's discoveries, and his work in turn fed into the research of scientists in America. Although significant delays in the field occurred in the early 1900s when the electrical industry considered safe transthoracic defibrillation to be unattainable, later it

History of Defibrillation – Major Contributions

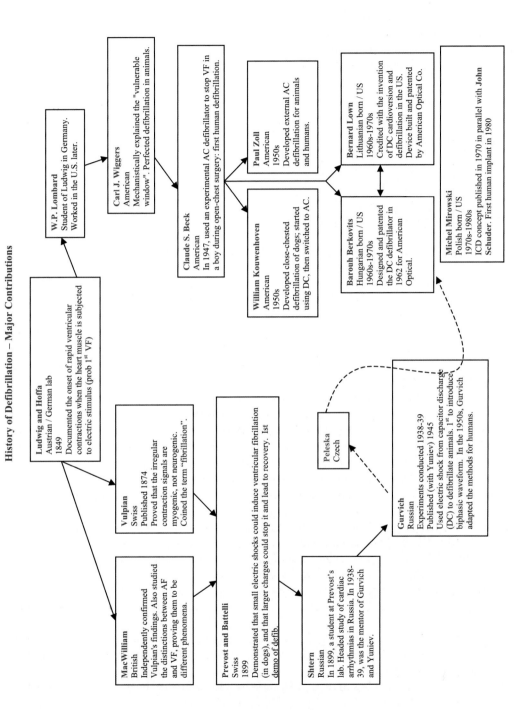

would be funding, resources, and technical expertise of companies like Edison Electric, Electrodyne, and American Optical that would make the creation of defibrillators possible. In the end, it was a great example of cooperation between scientists, surgeons, and engineers that made most, if not all, of the story possible.

References

1. Turakhia M, Tseng ZH. Sudden cardiac death: epidemiology, mechanisms, and therapy. *Curr Probl Cardiol* 2007;32:501–546
2. McWilliam JA. Fibrillar contraction of the heart. *J Physiol* 1887;8:296–310
3. Schechter DC. Early experience with resuscitation by means of electricity. *Surgery* 1971;69:360–372
4. Jeffrey K. Pacing the heart: growth and redefinition of a medical technology, 1952–1975. *Technol Cult* 1995;36:583–624
5. Comroe JH, Dripps RD. *The Top Ten Clinical Advances in Cardiovascular-Pulmonary Medicine and Surgery Between 1945 and 1975: How They Came About.* Bethesda, MD: National Heart and Lung Institute; 1977:10
6. Stillings D. Benjamin Franklin's celebrated kite experiment. *Med Instrum* 1973;7:234
7. Bianchi G. Réponse á la lettre du Docteur Bassani. *J Méd* 1756;4:46
8. Abilgaard N. *Communication*, vol. 2. Amsterdam: Societies Medicae Havniensis Collectanea; 1775:157–161
9. Stillings D. The first defibrillator? *Med Prog Technol* 1974;2:205–206
10. Kite C. *An Essay on the Recovery of the Apparently Dead.* London: C. Dilly, 1788:166
11. Kuhfeld E. Curator of Instruments, The Bakken. In personal communication with Mark Kroll, Ph.D., Feb. 01, 2002. Used with permission of Dr. Kroll
12. Eisenberg MS. *Life in the Balance: Emergency Medicine and the Quest to Reverse Sudden Cardiac Death.* New York: Oxford University Press; 1997
13. Hoffa M, Ludwig C. Einige neue Versuche über Herzbewegung. *Z Rationelle Med* 1850;9:107–144
14. Schröer H. Carl Ludwig. *Begründer der messenden Experimental-Physiologie 1816–1895.* Stuttgart: Wissenschaftliche Verlagsgesellschaft; 1967:67–71
15. Vulpian FA. Notes sur les éffets de la faradisation directe des ventricules du coeur chez le chien. *Arch Physiol Norm Path* 1874;6:975–982
16. McWilliam JA. Cardiac failure and sudden death. *Br Med J* 1889:6–8
17. Prevost JK, Battelli F. La mort par les déscharges électriques. *J Physiol* 1899;1:1085–1100
18. Robinovitch LG. Induction coil specifically constructed according to our indication for purposes of resuscitation of subjects in a condition of apparent death caused by chloroform, morphine, electrocution, etc. *J Mental Pathol* 1909;8:129–145
19. Hooker DR, Kouwenhoven WB, Langworthy OR. The effects of alternating electrical currents on the heart. *Am J Physiol* 1933;103:444–454

20. Kouwenhoven W, Hooker DR. Resuscitation by countershock. *Electrical Eng* 1933;52:475–477
21. Ferris LP, King BC, Spence PW, Williams HP. Effect of electric shock on the heart. *Electrical Eng* 1936;55:498–515
22. Wiggers CJ, Wegria R. Ventricular fibrillation due to single, localized induction and condenser shocks applied during the vulnerable phase of ventricular systole. *Am J Physiol* 1940;128:500–505
23. Gurvich NL. In Savchuk BD, ed. *Osnovniyi Printzipy Defibrillatziyi Serdtza.* Moscow: Medicine; 1975
24. Gurvich NL, Yuniev GS. O vosstanovlenii normalnoi deyatelnosti fibrilliruyuschego serdza teplokrovnih posredstvom kondensatornogo razryada. *Bull Exp Biol I Med* 1939;8:55–59
25. Gurvich NL, Yuniev GS. Restoration of regular rhythm in mammalian fibrillating heart. *Am Rev Soviet Med* 1946;3:236–239
26. Gurvich NL, Yuniev GS. Restoration of heart rhythm during fibrillation by a condenser discharge. *Am Rev Soviet Med* 1947;4:252–256
27. Vishnevsky AA, Zuckerman BM, Smelovsky SI. Ustranenie merzatelnoi aritmii metodom elektricheskoi defibrillyazii predserdii. *Klinicheskaya Medizina* 1959;37:26
28. Kroll MW. A minimal model of the single capacitor biphasic defibrillation waveform. *Pacing Clin Electrophysiol* 1994;17:1782–1792
29. Peleška B. Transthoracic and direct defibrillation. *Rozhl Chir* 1957;36:731–755
30. Peleška B. Cardiac arrhythmias following condenser discharges and their dependence upon strength of current and phase of cardiac cycle. *Circ Res* 1963;13:21–32
31. Peleška B. Cardiac arrhythmias following condenser discharges led through an inductance: comparison with effects of pure condenser discharges. *Circ Res* 1965;16:11–17
32. U.S. Senate. International health study. *Congr Rec* 1962;A7837–A7839
33. Mackay RS, Leeds SE. Physiological effects of condenser discharges with application to tissue stimulation and ventricular defibrillation. *J Appl Physiol* 1953;6:67–75
34. Associated Press. Revive "Dead" Boy, 14. *New York Daily News,* Dec 12, 1947
35. Associated Press. Dying Boy Revived by Voltage. *Denver Post,* Dec 12, 1947
36. Beck CS, Pritchard WH, Feil HS. Ventricular fibrillation of long duration abolished by electric shock. *JAMA* 1947;135:985–986
37. Kouwenhoven WB, Milnor WR, Knickerbocker GG, Chesnut WR. Closed chest defibrillation of the heart. *Surgery* 1957;42:550–561
38. Zoll PM, Linenthal AJ, Gibson W, Paul MH, Norman LR. Termination of ventricular fibrillation in man by externally applied electric countershock. *NEJM* 1956;254: 727–732
39. Beck CS, Leighninger DS. Death after a clean bill of health. So-called "fatal" heart attacks and treatment with resuscitation techniques. *JAMA* 1960;174:133–5
40. Lasker Foundation: http://www.laskerfoundation.org/awards/obits/kouwenhovenobit. shtml Originally in print in *The New York Times.* Obituary, William Kouwenhoven. November 12, 1975
41. Limmer D, O'Keefe MF, Dickinson ET. *Emergency Care,* 10th edn. Upper Saddle River, NJ: Pearson Prentice Hall; 2005

42. Lown B, Amarasingham R, Neuman J. New method for terminating cardiac arrhythmias. Use of synchronized capacitor discharge. *JAMA* 1962;182:48–55

43. Lown B, Neuman J, Amarasingham R, Berkovits BV. Comparison of alternating current with direct current electroshock across the closed chest. *Am J Cardiol* 1962;10:223–233

44. Berkovits BV. Defibrillator. 1966. U.S. Patent No. 3,236,239. Washington, DC, United States Patent and Trademarks Office

45. Negovskii VA, Gurvich NL. On possibility of resuscitation after electric injury. *Feldsher I Akusherka* 1952;6:6–13

46. Negovskii VA, Gurvich NL, Semenov VN, Tabak VY, Makarycheva VA. *Theoretical Aspects of Electro Impulse Therapy of Several Forms of Cardiac Arrhythmias.* Moscow: Novoe v kardiohirurgii; 1966:105–108

47. Mirowski M, Mower MM, Staewen WS, Tabatznik B, Mendeloff AL. Standby automatic defibrillator: an approach to prevention of sudden coronary death. *Arch Intern Med* 1970;126:158–161

48. Mirowski M, Reid PR, Mower MM, Watkins L, Gott VL, Schauble JF, Langer A, Heilman MS, Kolenik SA, Fischell RE, Weisfeldt ML. Termination of malignant ventricular arrhythmias with an implanted automatic defibrillator in human beings. *N Engl J Med* 1980;303:322–324

49. Schuder JC, Stoeckle H, Gold JH, West JA, Keskar PY. Experimental ventricular defibrillation with an automatic and completely implanted system. *Trans Am Soc Artif Intern Organs* 1970;16:207–212

50. National Inventors Hall of Fame. Inventor Profile: Michel Mirowski. United States Patent and Trademark Office. http://www.invent.org/Hall_Of_Fame/175.html. 2007

51. Lown B, Axelrod P. Implanted standby defibrillators. *Circulation* 1972;46:637–639

52. Venin IV, Gurvich NL, Tabak VY, Sherman AM. Scheme for forming bipolar defibrillation impulse. *Nov Med Priborostr* 1973;84–90

53. Olson KF, Gilman BL, Anderson KH, Kroll KJ. Automated external defibrillator operator interface. 1998. U.S. Patent No. 5,792,190. Washington, DC, United States Patent and Trademarks Office

Chapter 1.3

Ventricular Fibrillation: A Historical Perspective

Galina Kichigina and José Jalife

He who calls departed ages back again into being enjoys a bliss like that of creation.

Carl Wiggers[1]

Introduction

This chapter explores some scientific and technological aspects of the emergence of modern cardiology in the late nineteenth century that were important to the formation of cardiac electrophysiology, which rose into prominence in the 1940s–1950s. The chapter features the historical growth of ideas, concepts and understanding of ventricular fibrillation (VF) as a distinct clinical condition among the disturbances of the heart's rhythm.

To describe the ideas, concepts, and technical methods that led to modern understanding of VF, we shall touch on some of the important developments in cardiovascular physiology and instrumentation, which were to reshape the clinical conception of cardiac arrhythmias. Much of this work took place in continental Europe, most notably in the laboratories of Carl Ludwig in Leipzig and of Étienne Jules Marey in Paris. At the end of the nineteenth century much of the physiological research that became essential to modern conceptions of arrhythmias concentrated on the problem of the heart's rhythmic activity. There also appeared a number of anatomical and histological studies crucial for the deeper understanding of the specialized cardiac conduction system. The fundamental physiological

Galina Kichigina, Ph.D.

Institute for the History and Philosophy of Science and Technology, University of Toronto, 91 Charles St W Toronto, Ont, Canada M5S 1K7, gkichigi@chass.utoronto.ca

José Jalife, M.D.

Center for Arrhythmia Research, University of Michigan, 5025 Venture Drive, Ann Arbor, MI 41808, USA, jjalife@umich.edu

I. R. Efimov et al. (eds.), *Cardiac Bioelectric Therapy: Mechanisms and Practical Implications.*

concepts of the heart action were also paralleled by transformations in clinical medicine. Clinicians began to focus their attention specifically on heart rhythm disorders, drawing extensively on physiological work on rhythmicity and using instruments adapted or devised for this particular purpose. A watershed event occurred in the early twentieth century, when a new and promising approach for recording the heart's action through its electrical activity was set forth by Willem Einthoven in Leiden and Thomas Lewis in London. It was during these years that most of the cardiac arrhythmias were described, the electrocardiographic basis of atrial fibrillation (AF) was established, and AF and VF were clearly distinguished.

Extensive studies to explain the mechanism of fibrillation centered around two competing theories: *circus movement reentry* and so-called *tachysystole* from a single focus. Electrophysiological investigations with the use of increasingly sophisticated technologies done in the late 1940s dismissed the circular movement hypothesis, which had been dominant for nearly 30 years, later used as an explanatory model in more elaborated and sophisticated form. Yet, the intellectual vitality of the basic concepts of the nineteenth- and early twentieth-century cardiovascular physiology for understanding ventricular fibrillation would always ensure interest and fascination of modern researchers.

Concepts, Instruments, and Institutions: Nineteenth-Century Legacy

The heartbeat and its relation to the pulse have interested physicians for some 3,000 years or more. The intellectual history of heart rhythm disorders customarily begins with the mention of the pulse by the Edwin Smith papyrus of 3500 B.C. and by the Ebers papyrus of 1500 B.C.:

> When the heart is diseased, its work is imperfectly performed: the vessels proceeding from the heart become inactive, so that you cannot feel them. . . . If the heart trembles, has little power and sinks, the disease is advancing and death is near.[2]

To begin the history with the Egyptian papyri, mythical in large part, or with William Harvey's *De Motu Cordis*, is to construct a respectable, positive lineage for a modern complex of medical ideas, practices, and institutions, and to assert the continuity of modern studies with those of the predecessors.[3] A system of medical ideas that dominated Western medicine up to 1800 in large part went back to the writings of Hippocrates (circa 400 B.C.) and Galen (circa 130–201 A.D.) and played a major role in the understanding and treatment of health and disease.[4]

By the nineteenth century, however, this tradition no longer carried the same force or occupied so central a position within medicine. The difference between the medical world of twenty-first century and that of the turn of the eighteenth century, to go no further back, is so dramatically different that one can think of discontinuity between the modern medical science and the past. Yet, paradoxically, few writers of medical papers can resist the temptation to look at the previous developments in their field in retrospect that set their current studies in its historical context. Although there is little or nothing in the ancient medical writings that points to any knowledge of heart disease as we understand it today, this must not be taken to imply that the ancient physicians did not observe accurately enough symptoms and syndromes that would suggest heart rhythm disorders to the modern physician. For instance, the description of a *pulse caprizans* by Herophilus (circa 300 B.C.), the leading anatomist of Alexandrian school, is suggestive that he observed extrasystole.[5] Galen's description of the irregularity of the pulse and his diagnosis of blockage as the result of a narrowing of the passage of a large artery in the lung point unequivocally to the atrial fibrillation associated with mitral valve stenosis.[6] The *De morbis acutis* of the Roman physician Caelius Aurelianus (fifth century A.D.) contains an exact description of the vascular collapse from ventricular fibrillation.[7] However, we shall use the second half of the nineteenth century as a working landmark for the beginning of new science, when the emerging field of experimental physiology began to reshape and restructure the perception of cardiac diseases, arrhythmias, in particular.

By the mid-nineteenth century there had been a rich investigative and explanatory structure for the study of heart diseases composed largely of physical diagnosis and pathological anatomy. Bedside techniques for localizing cardiac pathology, which form the basis for many modern concepts of heart diseases, had been developed mainly in France by the Paris school. Although symptoms associated with an irregular pulse could not be correlated with postmortem findings, irregular pulse was a subject of attention for the eighteenth-century French clinician, Jean Baptiste de Sénac, physician to King Louis XV, and for the early nineteenth-century doctors Jean Nicolas Corvisart and Jean Baptiste Bouillaud. Sénac's *rebellious palpitation* (later known as *delirium cordis* and *pulsus irregularis perpetuus*) was often associated with mitral valve disease and heart failure and observed to respond to digitalis.[8] The introduction of the stethoscope in the 1820s by René Laennec allowed synchronization of the audible cardiac rhythm with palpation of the pulse, and Bouillaud applied the new instrument to the heart. Both Corvisart, who reintroduced Leopold Auenbrugger's method of percussion and applied it to the heart, and Bouillaud published influential treatises on cardiac pathologies.[9] These texts, however, did not include descriptions of heart rhythm disorders, which were recognized clinically but could not be defined anatomically. The same tendency persisted into the end of the nineteenth century. William Osler's *The Principles and Practice of Medicine* of 1892 included such conditions as palpitation and arrhythmias, but it largely treated heart diseases as structural rather than functional entities.[10] Palpation, percussion and auscultation of the chest, and the volume and strength of the pulse, rather than its rhythm, were still the cornerstone of cardiac practice. Until the turn of the twentieth century, clinical practice was still essentially perceived as an art, to which the basic science and instruments and methods associated with them had little to offer.[11]

Paris teachings of the 1820s–1840s turned the hospital morgue into a site for cutting-edge pathological anatomy, for which the Paris school became so famous. By the 1850s, the laboratory had begun to challenge the hospital as the major site of medical discovery. The new laboratory disciplines, experimental physiology, and cellular pathology offered perspectives on bodily functions and malfunctions that previously seemed impossible. Nineteenth-century laboratory leaders created a distinct scientific medicine based on microscopy, vivisection, and chemical investigations in uniquely controlled experimental environments. They used sophisticated instruments, devices, and methods translated from mechanics, optics, physics, and organic chemistry that began to reshape medical education and clinical medicine. The changes in nineteenth-century medicine that made it emblematic of modern development have often been explained through medicine's close relationship with the basic sciences. One reason for this trend was that, by 1840, the two physical sciences in which quantitative methods became most pervasive—physics and chemistry—offered methods and technologies more effectively applicable to physiological phenomena than had ever before been available.[12]

There were also related institutional developments. Technological improvements mean little without matching career opportunities, and German universities provided such openings. Specialized scientific institutes within the university system developed into prestigious research centers, excellently staffed, equipped, and lavishly funded by the government on a level that was unthinkable for the institutions in France and Britain. From 1847 onward German physiology was dominated by Hermann Helmholtz in Heidelberg, Emil du Bois-Reymond in Berlin, and Ernst Brücke in Vienna, all three students of the brilliant and versatile Johannes Müller and Carl Ludwig in Leipzig. All of them in turn taught large numbers of students who propagated their methods wherever physiology was practiced. This group of physiologist-physicists took a reductionist approach based primarily on qualitative, analytic, and physicochemical methods and techniques that was the centerpiece of their experimental practice. Among German physiologists, it was Carl Ludwig who became the supreme teacher at the Physiological Institute in Leipzig, an institution on a grand scale that housed departments of histology, anatomy, physical physiology, and physiological chemistry. In France, Claude Bernard, the premier physiologist and teacher, despite severe budgetary and institutional limitations, ran the laboratory at the Paris Collège de France, which, like the best German laboratories, attracted many young investigators. Bernard powerfully influenced physiological research and practice on a very broad range of problems and developed an explicit methodological and epistemological discussion of experimental medicine in his famous *Introduction à l'étude de la medecine expérimentale* of 1865.[13]

Nineteenth-century physiology had multiple relationships with clinical medicine. With its experimental approach, instruments, and measuring devices, which reflected the ideals of quantification, precision, and objectivity, physiology became a model for clinical medicine, although it was never fully accepted or applied in all its aspects. Entire generations of doctors acquired an idea of scientific medicine through laboratory work, and in this respect the laboratory served as a site of medical innovation and acquired an increasing significance in medical practice. Clinicians who had worked in the laboratories of Claude Bernard in Paris, Carl Ludwig in Leipzig, or Michael Foster in Cambridge oriented their clinical practices toward the laboratory, formulating new scientific questions and promoting new research projects relevant to the clinic.

The Clinic and the Laboratory

By the end of the nineteenth century clinicians with a special interest in heart rhythm disorders and a new approach to bedside practice began to make their mark in continental and British medicine. What distinguished their work was an appreciation of the results obtained by cardiovascular physiologists, along with the use of pulse recording devices such as sphygmograph and polygraph, and subsequently the newest technology such as the electrocardiograph, in their clinical practice. These were the very laboratory instruments through which new experimental knowledge was gained and which, applied in the clinic, proved seminal in reconceptualizing heart rhythm disorders.

Among the instruments that were developed during the second half of the nineteenth century, the sphygmograph, literally a pulse writer, was the first one aimed to make the salient features of the action and pathology of the human heart accessible to both the physiologist and the physician. The forerunner of the sphygmograph was the kymograph, devised in 1846 by Carl Ludwig to measure and record variations in fluid pressure. The kymograph, however, could not estimate accurately characteristics of the pulse, such as its frequency, and could not produce a tracing of the human pulse without having to open a blood vessel. To obviate these difficulties, Karl Vierord, professor of physiology at Tübingen, redesigned kymograph in 1853–1855. His sphygmograph was useful for collecting data on the pulses from the well and the sick, but it failed to display any features of the pulse except frequency. However, the sphygmograph, as Vierord pointed out, was an example of the characteristic direction of modern medicine, with its search of the objective signs of the disease by the use of chemical, physical, and physiological techniques.[14] In France, it was the Parisian physiologist Étienne-Jules Marey who, after visiting Ludwig in Vienna, became an enthusiast for *la méthode graphique*. In 1859 Marey designed a new version of the sphygmograph, which could write a short but clear record showing some interesting features of the normal pulse. Although Marey presented tracings of "senile pulse" (later defined as atrial fibrillation) from the patients with aortic and mitral insufficiency in his *Physiologie médical* of 1863, he was not essentially interested in clinical correlations, using his instrument mainly in experiments on animals.[15]

About that time, in the early 1850s, few German physiologists attempted to reproduce du Bois-Reymond's experiments demonstrating electrical phenomena in the living tissue. Du Bois-Reymond's basic concepts and the instruments, multiplier, induction apparatus, and nonpolarizable electrodes opened new possibilities for the study of bioelectricity, and electrophysiological research swept over German physiological laboratories. In 1855, at Würzburg University, Rudolf A. Kölliker and Heinrich Müller, both fundamentally histologists, demonstrated that each beat of the frog's heart produced a definite electric current.[16] Although Kölliker established for the first time the occurrence of action currents resulting from cardiac activity, his experiments did not attract attention at the time, until 1874, when Theodor Wilhelm Engelmann, a Ludwig student, and by then a professor of physiology at Utrecht, performed a series of experiments using the latest in electrical recording instruments, the differential rheotome. This instrument was designed by Julius Bernstein, a student of du Bois-Reymond and Helmholtz, to eliminate the sluggishness of du Bois-Reymond's sensitive galvanometer.[17] Although the curves obtained by Engelmann from the rheotome applied to a stimulated frog's heart were still rather confusing, the researchers began to get some idea of the propagation of the electrical activity in the heart.[18]

The first 30 years of the physiologists' recording the electrical activity of the heart, from 1855 to the mid-1870s, were the investigation of phenomena that had as yet no defined physiological or clinical significance. In 1875 Marey, by then professor at the Collège de France, came across an instrument that, as he believed, had great promise in studying the heart. This was the capillary electrometer, which used a new physical principle to

measure electrical potential and its changes. The concept behind the instrument had been
worked out by the French physicist Gabriel Lippmann in the famous physical laboratory
of Gustav Kirchoff at Heidelberg. The new instrument was both sensitive and quick,
which made it vastly superior to the standard galvanometer. In 1876 Marey conducted
numerous experiments with excised frog hearts using Lippmann's capillary electrometer
and adequate optical and photographic systems, which detected electrical variation with
precision impossible with any other previous instruments. These experiments, which began
to define the electrical activity of the heart, earned Marey a reputation as a technical
genius.[19]

In London, at his laboratory at St. Mary Hospital, the clinician Desiré Waller, an
enthusiastic student of Ludwig, took the lead in using a capillary electrometer in experiments
on the excised mammalian heart. In the late 1880s Waller recorded the first human
electrocardiogram using the capillary electrometer. His was a fundamentally physiological
approach: his classical diagram of tilted electrical axes of the human heart, his published
electrocardiogram, and his interpretation of "the electromotive properties of the heart" were
highly acclaimed. He was awarded the most prestigious European *Prix Montyon* in physiology by the French Académie des Sciences and demonstrated the human electrocardiogram
at the First International Congress of Physiologists in Basel in 1889.[20]

Waller realized, however, that his instrument was too clumsy to allow its use in a
clinical setting. Clinician-scientists interested in heart rhythm disorders preferred to use
the sphygmograph to record the patients' pulses and to correlate the graphic patterns with
those obtained from experimental animals. By 1906 Thomas Lewis at University College
London had published a number of articles reporting new results in the fundamentals of
sphygmography.[21] Arthur Cushny, a professor of pharmacology at the University College,
who had studied experimental technique under Hugo Kronecker, reported in 1906 that auricular fibrillation known to develop acutely in dogs under certain (open chest) experimental
conditions, might be a distinct and clinically important arrhythmia. This observation was
suggested to him by the correlation of the experimental results with the clinical findings
based on arterial pulse tracings from the sphygmograph in a patient with the so-called
delirium cordis.[22] In 1908 Lewis began using a new instrument, the polygraph, developed
by the provincial doctor James MacKenzie, who had moved to London to work with Lewis.
The polygraph could simultaneously record not only arterial but also venous pulse, which
allowed analyzing different kinds of relationship between auricular and ventricular action.

By that time a superior instrument, the string galvanometer, had been invented by
the Leiden physiologist Willem Einthoven, who had a talent for both developing theory
and the construction of instruments. The optical and photographic systems of the new
instrument were identical to those used in the capillary electrometer, but as a scientific
instrument it used so many recently invented components and processes that it would have
been impossible 20 years before. It was exceedingly sensitive and accurate, and the records
it produced were of an elegance and precision more often found in the physical sciences than
in physiology and medicine.[23] In 1903 Einthoven began publishing the first physiological
studies using his string galvanometer. The fascinating instrument attracted attention of
physiologists and clinicians engaged in studies of arrhythmias with the polygraph. Heinrich Hering, professor of physiological pathology in Prague,[24] and Carl Rothberger and

Heinrich Winterberg,[25] clinicians in Vienna made important contributions in the 1910s to the electrocardiographic investigation of atrial fibrillation using the string galvanometer. In 1908 Lewis together with Waller applied the new string galvanometer to the patient and correlated the obtained results with those recorded by Mackenzie's polygraph. The electrocardiogram confirmed precisely with greater clarity the results of the polygraph. At this point Lewis began to realize the admirable potentialities of the string galvanometer not only in defining physiological and clinical pictures of arrhythmias but also in physiological understanding of cardiac conduction.

Lewis was well aware of a series of important studies during the late 1890s and early 1900s that had led to more precise knowledge of the specialized conduction system in the heart. In 1907 Arthur Keith, an anatomist at the London Hospital School of Medicine, and a medical student Martin Flack described the sinoauricular node. Their finding correlated with the auricular-ventricular node described a year earlier by Sunao Tawara during his stay at Marburg University, and the auricular-ventricular bundle discovered by Wilhelm His, Jr., in Leipzig, in 1893, and the long-known Purkinje system. Although the original definition of these structures was anatomical and histological, physiologist clinicians, such as Lewis, using the string galvanometer and a series of experimental techniques, began to acquire a more precise understanding of the functional role of the conduction system and of the relationship between cardiac conduction and arrhythmias.[26] Still, however, electrical activity and conduction within the heart was such a new and poorly understood concept that no one had conceived of it as the basis of any disease state.

Ventricular Fibrillation: Experimental Evidence and Basic Concepts, 1880s–1920s

It is generally accepted that the first experimentally induced fibrillation of the heart was the work of Carl Ludwig, then at the physiological laboratory of Zurich University, in 1850. During these years in Zurich Ludwig wrote the first volume of his famous *Lerhbuch der Physiologie des Menschen*, which treated diffusion and osmosis, acoustics and optics, hemodynamics and animal electricity, all topics of medical physics, which came to the fore through Ludwig's research. Apparently Ludwig became interested in application of du Bois-Reymond's newly devised electrophysiological methods to the animal heart. He and his collaborator Moritz Hoffa Ludwig demonstrated that a strong constant (faradic) current applied directly to the rabbit ventricle produced irregular and weak contractions, which they called *Flimmern*. Ludwig, however, did not continue his experiments on the electrical activity in the heart because the "fundamental action," he believed, could not be apprehended with the methods and instruments available.[27]

Although physiologists took the lead in studying electrical phenomena in living tissue, clinicians, interested in experimental research, too were keen in applying electricity as a therapeutic modality. The prestigious *Prix Montyon* of the French Académie des Sciences had a special category for the works in electrotherapy. Felix Édme Alfred Vulpian, professor of pathological anatomy at Paris University and staff physician at the Charité hospital, took a special interest in the action of the faradic current on the heart. A fine experimentalist, Vulpian showed that direct faradization applied directly to the ventricle of the dog heart caused irregular tremulous chaotic muscular movements of the ventricle, which he called *mouvement fibrillaire*, while the auricle continued to beat normally. Similarly, direct current applied to the auricle also led to fibrillary contractions, *fremissement fibrillaire*. Since Vulpian's experiment of 1874 the term fibrillation came into use to describe the phenomenon.[28] Another eminent clinician at the Paris Faculté de Médecine, Germain Sée reported in 1879 that he induced ventricular fibrillation in the dog by occluding its coronary arteries.[29]

During that time, in the 1870s and 1880s, the controversy was ranging over the nature of cardiac automatism, whether the heartbeat was myogenic, that is, due to inherent excitation by the heart muscle itself, or neurogenic, that is, due to either neural or local ganglionic control. Since the discovery of the sympathetic and parasympathetic nerves and ganglia inside and outside the heart, and following the lead of Alfred Volkmann at Halle University, who suggested that the cardiac ganglia were the centers of automaticity, the neurogenic theory became ultimately dominant both in Germany and France. Studies on the effect of electrical stimulation of the nerves on the heart also provided convincing proofs of neurogenicity. Claude Bernard contributed, although indirectly, to the neurogenic theory through his demonstration of a reflex nervous mechanism in the endocardium and his "ganglionic" theory of vasomotor action. Alfred Vulpian, in his acceptance of neurogenic theory, depended heavily on the presumed analogy between cardiac inhibition and vasodilation.[30] The leading center of the neurogenic view was Germany, since German physiological institutes led the field in general. Ludwig's institute, where important research on the innervation of the heart was pursued, became the major stronghold of neurogenicity. In Britain, Michael Foster was the major proponent of the myogenic theory. In fact, it was at his laboratory at Cambridge that Walter Gaskel performed experiments that appeared to definitively prove the myogenic theory. Before his work in Foster's laboratory, Gaskel had studied the innervation and vagal stimulation of the heart and the vasomotor control of blood flow in skeletal muscle arteries at Ludwig's laboratory. In Cambridge, Gaskel, working with an isolated strip of tortoise ventricular muscle devoid of ganglion and nervous connections, showed that the strip continued to pulsate at a rate similar to the intact heart. These experiments suggested to him that the rhythm of the heart beat depended on the persistence of a primitive condition of heart muscle but not on the presence of ganglion cells.[31]

Myogenic theory had its opponents, however, and they too had worked with Ludwig. Hugo Kronecker, Ludwig's collaborator for many years, and Ilia Cyon, with whom Ludwig discovered the depressor nerve, the vasodilator branch of the vagus nerve, back in 1866, were the most influential opponents among cardiovascular physiologists. Oskar Langendorff at the University of Königsberg also preferred the neuroganglionar explanation over the myogenic hypothesis. Only a few German physiologists believed in myogenicity: Theodor Engelmann at Utrecht University studying cardiac automatism and conduction established it in the isolated ventricular beat. Wilhelm His, Jr., in Leipzig contributed fundamentally to extending Gaskel's results from the lower vertebrate to the mammalian heart. The most impressive claim of the myogenecists was the appearance of rhythmicity in the absence of differentiated nervous elements. But the neurogenesists had an equally strong argument, the obvious influence of nervous action on the intact heart beat.[32]

Most of experimentalists working with the mammalian heart were well familiar with ventricular fibrillation. It was generally treated as an experimental curiosity and definitive proof that atrial fibrillation, separate from ventricular fibrillation, was still lacking. Fibrillar contractions were referred to as *delirium cordis*. In 1899 Arthur Cushny clarified the terminology: in physiology *delirium cordis* referred to fibrillar contractions that arrest the circulation and prove rapidly fatal, whereas clinically, the term referred to extreme irregularity of the pulse.[33]

The first important research that treated VF with deeper insight into its pathophysiology was the work by John A. MacWilliam, a physiologist at Aberdeen University, who had, like every other physiologist, studied at Ludwig's laboratory. He was there at the same time as Walter Gaskel and Henry Bowditch of Harvard. In 1887–1889 MacWilliam published results of his experiments on ventricular fibrillation. He was convinced that the arrhythmia occurred independently of "any mechanical relation of the ventricles to the rest of the heart, and of any nervous relation of the ventricles to the rest of the heart or to the extra-cardiac nerves." He demonstrated that fibrillary movements of the heart were the result of the lack of harmony in the contraction and relaxation of the minute muscular fibers that compose the myocardium, thus supporting the myogenic character of VF.[34] The general appearance of VF was well known, but MacWilliam's accurate and colorful description claimed both a new clinical significance for VF as a cause of sudden death, and its dependence on the changes within the "ventricular substance": "The cardiac pump is thrown out of gear, and the last of its vital energy is dissipated in the violent and prolonged turmoil of fruitless activity in the ventricular walls."[35] In his review on electrical stimulation of the heart, MacWilliam differentiated cardiac arrest caused by asystole from that caused by VF. He suggested that fibrillation results from a rapid succession of uncoordinated peristaltic contractions, described the relationship of the refractory period to these changes, and presented evidence of the effect of certain poisons, which when injected into the blood stream, caused fibrillation of the ventricles.[36]

MacWilliam pointed out that although VF was known to be fatal in experimental animals, he sometimes managed to restore normal rhythm "by applying rhythmical compression of the ventricles with hand and administering pilocarpine intravenously."[37] He referred to the previous investigation by the Berlin physician Hugo von Ziemssen on alterations in heart rhythm and rate induced by the application of electrical shock either directly to the heart open for surgery or through the thorax. MacWilliam's experiments also showed that electric shocks applied through a large pair of electrodes, one located on the ventricular apex and the other over the sixth or seventh dorsal vertebra, could be used to terminate VF in man. However, as MacWilliam pointed out, von Ziemssen's work of 1882 remained largely unnoticed, because the suggested technique was virtually impossible to use in the clinical setting.[38] MacWilliam's ideas on cardiac resuscitation would only be appreciated and fully developed many years later by Carl Wiggers at the Western Reserve University.

Although MacWilliam's conception of the pathophysiology and clinical significance of VF was quite advanced, his work did not receive very much recognition during its publication.

Much later, in 1915 Lewis acknowledged that MacWilliam was the first to draw attention to the important fact that sudden death was often caused by VF.[39]

Several researchers around this time were attempting to study ventricular fibrillation in man using the new technique of electrocardiography. In 1911 Lewis and Levy used the electrocardiograph to demonstrate that when ventricular fibrillation occurred during chloroform anesthesia, it was often preceded by the appearance of multiform ventricular extrasystole or ventricular tachycardia.[40] In 1912 Augustus Hoffmann published the electrocardiographic record of a patient with ventricular fibrillation, which occurred at the end of a period of paroxysmal ventricular tachycardia.[41] The same year Canby Robinson of Washington University at St. Louis published electrocardiograms recorded from seven patients at the time of death, including two tracings, which were consistent with ventricular fibrillation.[42] Explaining difficulties in documenting VF in humans Lewis wrote in 1915: "Remarkably, practically every form of irregularity, which has been produced experimentally in the mammalian heart, has now been recorded in clinical cases. But there is one notable exception.... Why is fibrillation of the ventricles so uncommon an experience? For a good reason: fibrillation of the ventricles is incompatible with existence.... If it occurs in man it is responsible for unexpected and sudden death."[43]

With the understanding of AF as a uniquely atrial rhythm responsible for what was called *arrhythmia perpetua*, and the demonstration in the 1910s that it was distinct from VF, the question of the mechanism underlying fibrillation came into focus. Intensive studies on the experimentally induced fibrillation brought out several hypotheses. Hugo Kronecker argued that fibrillation resulted from the disturbance of a hypothetical cardiac "coordination center" regulated by nervous impulse; his experiments showed that a needle inserted into the upper third of the ventricular septum destroyed this center and induced VF.[44] Surprisingly, Kronecker's hypothesis was not widely accepted, even though he was a greatly respected figure in the field of cardiac research, and many foreign physiologists studied at his institute in Bern. Kronecker and his students worked on problems concerned with virtually every area of cardiac physiology such as vascular innervation, cardiac poisons, irritability, and functional capacity of the heart. In 1895 Theodor Engelmann suggested that each heart fiber independently becomes rhythmical, and each is a focus of its own impulse formation due to increased excitability.[45] Heinrich Winterberg further developed Engelmann's theory of multiple heterotopic centers in 1906.[46] Lewis too supported the idea that activity from one or more heterogeneous centers may account for a single premature beat and for incoordinated activity during fibrillation.[47] In 1915 the Viennese clinician Carl Rothberger and Winterberg proposed a contrasting theory of "tachysystole," which attributed fibrillation to extremely rapid discharge of a single focus, possibly due to vagal influence.[48] In the 1920s these theories were replaced by the so-called circus movement theory, developed by the Cambridge physiologist George Ralph Mines[49] and subsequently adopted by Lewis, who published a series of papers demonstrating the mechanism of circus movement in cases of AF and atrial flutter and their differentiation.[50] Lewis based his idea of circus movement on the original studies on the umbrella of the jellyfish by the American zoologist Alfred Mayer. In 1906 Mayer demonstrated that a chemical or mechanical stimulus of the quiescent ring resulted in a band of contraction that went about the circuit in one direction for hours.[51]

There were two important contributors to the circus movement theory, George Mines and the American physiologist Walter Garrey. Assistant demonstrator at the Cambridge physiological laboratory, Mines was a fine and clever experimentalist. After visiting Marey's Institute in Paris in the early 1900s, where he saw Marey's invention, the first moving image camera, Mines used the novel method in his studies of cardiac contractions. While working at the Roscoff biological station in France, Mines became interested in developing Mayer's idea to explain the mechanism of fibrillatory contraction of the myocardial tissue. In 1913 Mines proved that "If a closed circuit of muscle is provided, of considerably greater length than the wave of excitation, it is possible to start a wave in this circuit that will continue to propagate itself round and round the circuit for an infinite number of times."[49] Mines applied the idea of reentry to myocardial tissue and demonstrated it in his classical diagram showing normal tissue with rapid conduction and no reentry, and abnormal tissue with delayed conduction permitting reentry to occur. He formally pointed to the conditions necessary for reentry to occur: unidirectional block; recirculation of the impulse to its point of origin; and elimination of the rhythm by cutting the pathway.[52] Interested in studying the onset of VF, Mines modified the technique by applying single shocks to the rabbit heart instead of the repeated electrical shocks as was usually done. By timing single shocks precisely at various periods during the cardiac cycle, he identified a narrow zone fixed within electrical diastole during which the heart was extremely vulnerable to fibrillation. Mines believed that stimuli, either external or from within the heart, could trigger fatal arrhythmia if the stimuli fell within this zone, and could cause death by disruption of what he called "dynamic equilibrium of the heart."[53]

Walter Garrey at Tulane University independently developed the circus movement theory and reentry mechanism as possible substrates for the generation of arrhythmias. He showed that when a fibrillating chamber was cut into four pieces, each fragment continued to fibrillate. He reasoned that the fragments were not dependent on a single tachysystolic center, the hypothesis proposed by Carl Rothberger. On the other hand, Garrey found that although portions of the isolated heart muscle were able to fibrillate, a critical amount of muscle mass was needed. He showed that a piece cut from any part of ventricular tissue obtained from mammals or turtles would cease fibrillating if its surface area was less than four square centimeters. These observations ultimately undermined the individual or multiple heterotopous centers theory. Moreover, if the ring was made thin enough, the uncoordinated fibrillatory contractions organized themselves into rotating waves that followed each other successively and repeatedly around the ring, in a manner similar to that described by Mines for circus movement reentry. Garrey provided the first mechanistic description of the arrhythmia as "intramuscular ringlike circuits," with resulting "circus contractions," which are fundamentally essential to the fibrillary process.[54] He also pointed to the possibility of setting up vortex-like reentrant circuits around a stimulated region without any anatomical obstacle, an idea that was later dismissed by some theorists,[55] but more recently confirmed by experimentalists.[56]

Although some continental physiologists, Carl Rothberger for example,[57] were critical of the circus movement theory of fibrillation, this theory remained dominant for nearly 30 years, particularly in Britain. It had some very heavyweight supporters, such as Lewis. The theory was further developed to explain the complexity of experimental findings, including such concepts as a single "mother ring," which propagated the arrhythmia and generated "daughter rings," and multiple independent rings. Garrey, one of the early supporters of circular movement, argued in 1924 that the circuit, although present, could no longer be presented as a simple circuit due to blocks to its conduction: "[T]he impulse is diverted into different paths, weaving and inter-weaving through the tissue mass, crossing and recrossing old paths again to course over them or to stop short as it impinges on some barrier of refractory tissue."[58]

From Wiggers to Moe: The Multiple Wavelet Hypothesis

In 1930 Wiggers[59] conducted high-speed cinematographic studies on the evolution of VF produced by an electric shock in the dog heart and demonstrated that the uninter-rupted arrhythmia goes through four stages: (1) undulatory, lasting for a second or two; (2) convulsive incoordination, which lasts from 15 to 40 s; (3) tremulous incoordination, lasting 2–3 min; (4) atonic fibrillation, which usually develops 2–5 min after the onset of VF. During the undulatory and convulsive incoordination stages, the ventricular activation frequency is very high (about 10 Hz), whereas in the tremulous incoordination and atonic fibrillation stages, the activation rate gradually slows as a result of ischemia.[59] Based on these and other observations, Wiggers[60] concluded that both formation of limited circuits and reentry occur throughout the evolution of fibrillation. Most important, he was first to bring attention to the fact that "inasmuch as sequential reentrant excitations travel over a bulky mass of ventricular muscle, one must not think in terms of two-dimensional rings or circuits, but rather of massive wave fronts spreading in three dimensions."[61]

By the 1950s there seemed to be general agreement that atrial or ventricular tachycardias could certainly be produced either by repetitive discharges from an ectopic focus[62] or by the circulation of a wave front around an obstacle.[55] In either case, it was proposed that under certain conditions, the impulse initiated at the reentrant circuit or at the pacemaker source could occur so rapidly that neighboring tissues would be unable to respond regularly, thus giving rise to the apparently chaotic electrocardiogram pattern of fibrillation.

In 1956, however, Moe[63] proposed that the mechanism of fibrillation was fundamentally different from that of tachycardia. His observations led him to contend that during fibril-lation there was total disorganization of activity. He envisioned the arrhythmia as being the result of randomly wandering wave fronts, ever changing in number and direction. Subsequently, in 1959 Moe and Abildskov[64] demonstrated that atrial fibrillation could exist as a stable state, self-sustained and independent of its initiating agency, but also that such an independent survival of the arrhythmia was possible only in the presence of inhomogeneous repolarization. In 1962 Moe[65] postulated the "multiple wavelet" hypothesis of atrial fibrillation, in which randomness in the temporal and spatial distribution of membrane properties plays a dominant role. In 1964 Han and Moe[66] carried out a series of important experiments testing the effects of various agencies on the refractory period of the ventricular muscle and established the importance of heterogeneity in the relatively refractory period in the induction of cardiac fibrillation. The same year, the multiple wavelet hypothesis was crystallized by the development of the first computer model of cardiac fibrillation in two-dimensional myocardium.[67] It demonstrated that without heterogeneous distribution of refractory periods reentrant activity remained periodic and the arrhythmia did not degenerate into fibrillation. Yet, experimental support for the multiple wavelet hypothesis had to wait about 20 years, until the development of high-resolution electrode mapping technology.

In the 1970s invasive electrophysiological techniques emerged, sophisticated computer modeling and multiple electrode mapping technologies were introduced, and new hypotheses were proposed to explain fibrillation. All these developments and changes are rooted in the classical research of the nineteenth and early twentieth centuries. In 1985 Allessie et al.[68] mapped the spread of excitation in the atria of a dog heart during acetylcholine-induced atrial fibrillation and provided the first in vivo demonstration of multiple propagating wavelets giving rise to turbulent atrial activity.

Although Moe's computer model was intended to simulate atrial fibrillation, a large body of experimental literature has subsequently appeared in which it is assumed that the multiple wavelet hypothesis also applies to the mechanism of ventricular fibrillation.[69–72] Thus, the traditional consensus is that although focal activation may play a role in the initiation of the arrhythmia, maintenance of fibrillation in the three-dimensional ventricles involves multiple wandering wavelets of activation whose pathways usually change randomly from one cycle the next.[67]

Modern Concepts of Ventricular Fibrillation

In recent years, the use of computer modeling, together with newer and more advanced high-resolution mapping technology, has led to the reemergence of an old controversy: Are the complex dynamics of VF the result of the random occurrence and propagation of multiple independent wavelets?[65,67] Or are multiple wavelets a consequence of the sustained activity of a single or a small number of dominant reentrant sources activating the ventricles at exceedingly high frequencies?[73–75]

The experimental work of Allessie et al.[76–78] in the 1970s gave birth to the so-called *leading circle* concept and was an essential initial step toward our current understanding of the phenomenon of functional reentry in cardiac tissue; that is, reentry without the involvement of an anatomical obstacle. At about the same time, work conducted by Soviet scientists using the Belousov-Zhabotinsky reaction[79,80] and its numerical counterparts led to the idea that two-dimensional spiral autowaves could be a possible mechanism of cardiac arrhythmias.[81,82] Subsequently, the notion of spiral autowaves was brilliantly expanded into the third dimension by the Arthur T. Winfree,[83–85] who in fact coined the term "rotor" to signify the actual vortex that generates the spiral (scroll) wave activity, which led to the virtual abandonment of the use of the term leading circle. Thereafter, much work focused on rotors as the underlying mechanism of ventricular tachycardia and VF.

The advancements of experimental and computational techniques validated the view of Moe regarding the mechanism of VF, but they also revived the hypothesis that VF may be attributable to impulse reentry around a functional or anatomical obstacle. To date, the debate is by no means settled. It remains controversial whether a large number of multiple wavelets propagating about the heart in a random fashion maintain VF or if the mechanism is one of few sustained reentrant circuits that result in fibrillatory conduction.

Concluding Remarks

This chapter does not attempt to cover every study and every factor that contributed to the formation of modern concepts on ventricular fibrillation. Nor does it encounter some important institutional and social factors that catalyzed the growth of the field of cardiac electrophysiology, its concepts, and techniques. Rather, the intention was to indicate the breadth of view necessary to write the history of ventricular fibrillation within the context of general development of cardiac physiology. This chapter touched on its major concepts, methods, and instruments, as well as its institutions and contending schools of thought.

References and Notes

1. Wiggers C. Some significant advances in cardiac physiology during the nineteenth century, *Bul Hist Med* 1960;34:1–15
2. Breasted JH. *The Edwin Smith Surgical Papyrus*, 2 vols, v.1. Chicago: University of Chicago Press; 1930:105
3. Lawrence C. Moderns and ancients: the "new cardiology" in Britain 1880–1930. In Bynum W, Lawrence C, Nutton V, eds. *The Emergence of Modern Cardiology*. London: Wellcome Institute for the History of Medicine; 1985:1–33
4. Conrad L, Neve M, Nutton V, eds. *The Western Medical Tradition 800 BC to AD 1800.* Cambridge, UK: Cambridge University Press; 1995:3–7
5. Vierordt H. Geschichte der Herzkrankheiten. In Puschmann T. *Handbuch der Geschichte der Medizin*, 2 vols, v.2. Jena: Gustav Fisher; 1903:631–647. Horine EF. An epitome of ancient pulse lore, *Bull Hist Med* 1941;10:209–249
6. Galen C. On the Affected Parts. In Harris CR. *The Heart and the Vascular System in Ancient Greek Medicine*. Oxford, UK: Clarendon; 1973:448
7. Aurelianus C. De morbis acutis, In Harris CR, *The Heart and the Vascular System in Ancient Greek Medicine*. Oxford, UK: Clarendon Press; 1973:437
8. In his famous treatise on the structure, function and diseases of the heart Jean-Baptiste de Sénac (1693–1770) gave accurate description of the 'rebellious palpitation', which he correlated with post mortem findings of mitral valve disease and dilatation of the left ventricle. Sénac JB. *Traité de la structure du coeur, de son action et ses maladies*, 2 vols, v. 1. Paris: J. Vincent; 1749:524
9. Corvisart JN. *Essai sur les maladies et les lesions organiques du coeur et des gros vaisseux*. Paris, 1818; idem., *Nouveau method pour reconnâitre les maladies internes de la poitrine*, Paris, 1808; Bouillaud JB. *Traité clinique des maladies du couer*, 2 vols, Paris: JB Bailliére; 1835

10. Osler W. *The Principles and Practice of Medicine.* New York: D. Appleton; 1892:592–662

11. Lawrence, op. cit. (note 3), p. 6

12. Hager M. Scientific Medicine. In Cahan D, ed. *From Natural Philosophy to the Sciences: Writing the History of Nineteenth-Century Science.* Chicago: Chicago University Press; 2003:49–87

13. Colemann W. The cognitive basis of the discipline Claude Bernard on Physiology. *Isis* 1985;76:49–70

14. Vierord K. *Die Lehre vom Arterienpuls in gesunden und kranken Zustnden. Gegründed auf eine neue Methode der bildlichen Darstellung des menschlichen Pulses* Braunschweig: Vieweg and Sohn; 1855:4–12

15. Marey JE. *Physiologie médicale de la circulation du sang.* Paris: Delahaye; 1863. Marey is credited with the discovery of the refractory period of the heart muscle in 1875. On Marey and his studies on the heart with capillary electrometer, see R. Frank. The telltale heart: physiological instruments, graphic methods, and clinical hopes, 1854–1914. In Coleman W, Holmes F. *The Investigative Enterprise Experimental Physiology in Nineteenth-Century Medicine.* Berkeley: University of California Press; 1988:211–290

16. Kölliker A, Müller H, Nachweis der negative Schwankung des Muskelstroms am natürlich sich kontrahierenden Muskel. *Verhandl Phys Med Gesellsch* 1856;6:528–533

17. Lenoir T, Models and instruments in the development of electrophysiology, 1845–1912. In *Historical Studies in the Physical and Biological Sciences.* Los Angeles: University of California Press; 1986:1–54

18. Engelmann Th.W. Über das elektrische Verhalten des thätigen Herzens. *Pflügers Archiv für gesamte Physiologie des Menschen und der Tiere* 1878;17:68–99. Rothschuh KE. Theodor Wilhelm Engelmann. *Dictionary of Scientific Biography*, vol. 4, 1970:371–373. Meijler FL, ed. *Th. W. Engelmann, Professor of Physiology, Utrecht (1889–1897).* Amsterdam: Rodopi; 1984

19. Hopley IB, Lippmann GJ. In *Dictionary of Scientific Biography*, vol. 8, 387–388. Frank, op. cit. (note 15)

20. Waller A. A demonstration on man of electromotive changes accompanying the heart's beat. *J Physiol* 1887;8:229–234

21. Lewis T. The interpretation of the primary and first secondary wave in sphygmograph tracings. *J Anat Lond* 1907;1:137–140

22. Cushny AR, Edmunds CW. Paroxysmal irregularity of the heart and auricular fibrillation. In Bulloch W, ed. *Studies in Pathology.* Scotland: Aberdeen; 1906:95–110

23. Burnett J. The origins of the electrocardiograph as a clinical instrument. In Bynum WF, Lawrence C, Nutton V, eds. *The Emergence of Modern Cardiology.* London: Wellcome Institute for the History of Medicine; 1985:53–76

24. Hering HE. Das Electrokardiogram des Pulsus irregularis perpetuus. *Dtsch Arch klin Med* 1908;94:205–208

25. Rothberger CJ, Winterberg H. Vorhofflimmern und Arhythmia perpetua. *Wien klin Wchnschr* 1909;22:839–844

26. Lewis T. Observations upon disorders of the heart's action. *Heart* 1912;3:279–300. Some aspects on Lewis's studies of arrhythmia are mentioned in Krickler D. The development

of the understanding of arrhythmias during the last 100 years. In Bynum et al., eds. *Emergence of Modern Cardiology*, op. cit. (note 23), pp. 77–81

27. Hoffa M, Ludwig C. Einige neue Versuche über Herzbewegung. *Z rationewlle Med* 1850;9:107–144. Schröer H, *Carl Ludwig. Begründer der messenden Experimental-physiologie 1816–1895*. Stuttgart: Wissenschaftliche Verlagsgesellschaft; 1967:67–71

28. Vulpian EFA. Notes sur les éffets de la faradisation directe des ventricules du coeur chez le chien. *Arch Physiol Norm Path* 1874;6:975–982. Vulpian was basically a neurophysi-ologist and together with his collaborator Jean-Martin Charcot exerted great influences on nineteenth-century French medicine. Together with Charcot, Vulpian founded the journal *Archives de physiologie normale et pathologique* in 1868

29. Sée G. *Du diagnostic et du traitement des maladies du coeur et en particulier de leurs formes anomales*. Paris: JB Bailliére; 1879

30. On Bernard's endocardial reflex in support of neurogenicity, see W. Rutherford, Lectures on Experimental Physiology. *Lancet* 1871;2:841. On Vulpian's acceptance of neurogenic theory, see Vulpian FA. *Leçons sur l'appareil vasomoteur (physiologie et pathologie)*, Carville HC, ed., 2 vols, Paris: JB Bailliére; 1875:v. 1, 321–322. On myogenic-neurogenic debate, see Geison G. *Michael Foster and the Cambridge School of Physiology*. Prince-ton, NJ: Princeton University Press; 1978:342–347

31. On Gaskel and his research, see Geison, op. cit. (note 30), pp. 247–252; 280–289

32. On the acceptance of the myogenic theory by German physiologists, see His W Jr. A story of the atrioventricular bundle with remarks concerning embryonic heart activity. *J Hist Med* 1949; 4:319–333

33. Cushny AR. On the interpretation of pulse-tracing. *J Exp Med* 1899; 4:327–347

34. MacWilliam JA. Fibrillar contraction of the heart. *J Exp Physiol* 1887; 8:296–310

35. MacWilliam JA. Cardiac failure and sudden death. *Br Med J* 1889; 1:6

36. MacWilliam JA. Fibrillar contraction of the heart. *J Physiol* 1887; 8:296–310

37. MacWilliam JA. On the rhythm of the mammalian heart. *Proc R Soc Lond* 1888; 44:206

38. Ziemssen H. Studien über die Bewegungsvorgänge am menschlichen Herzen, sowie über die mechanische und elektrische Erregbarkeit des Herzens und des Nervus Phrenicus, angestelt an dem freiligenden Herzen der Catharina Serafin. *Dtsch Arch clin Med* 1882; 30:270; MacWilliam JA, Electrical stimulation of the heart in man. *Br Med J* 1889; 1:348

39. Lewis T. *Lectures on the Heart*. New York: Paul B. Hoeber; 1915

40. Levy AG, Lewis T. Heart irregularities, resulting from the inhalation of low percentages of chloroform vapour, and their relationship to ventricular fibrillation. *Heart* 1911; 33:99–112

41. Hoffmann A, Fibrillation of the ventricles at the end of an attack of paroxysmal tachycardia in man. *Heart* 1912; 3:213–218

42. Robinson GC. A study with electrocardiograph of the mode of death of the human heart. *J Exp Med* 1912; 16:291–302. Robinson GC, Bredeck JF, Ventricular fibrillation in man with cardiac recovery. *Arch Int Med* 1917; 20:725–738

43. Lewis T. *Lectures on the Heart*. New York: Paul B. Hoeber; 1915

44. Kronecker H, Schmey F, Das Coordinationscentrum der Herzkammerbewegung, *Berliner Klinische Wochenschrift* 1884; 21:738–739. Kronecker improved the proofs for

the all-or none law applied for the heart in 1873, worked out the method of the isolated heart, and almost simultaneously with Marey described the refractory period of the heart in 1874. A device for measuring the pressure of the isolated heart is named after him. Rothschuh K in Gillispie Ch, ed. *Dictionary of Scientific Biography.* New York: Scribner; 1970–1980:504–505

45. Engelmann TW, Über den Einfluss der Systole auf der motorische Leitung in der Herzkammer, mit Bemerkungen zur Theorie allorhythmischer Herzstorungen. *Arch ges Physiol* 1896;62:543–566

46. Winterberg H. Ueber Herzflimmern und seine Beeinflussung durch Kampher, *Zeitschrift f experimentalle Pathologie und Therapie* 1906;3:182–208

47. Lewis T, Schleiter HG. The relation of regular tachycardias of auricular origin to auricular fibrillation. *Heart* 1912;3:173–193

48. Rothberger CJ, Winterberg H. Der Vorhofflimmern und Vorhofflattern. *Pflügers Archiv für die gesamte Physiologie des Menschen und der Tiere* 1915;160: 42–90

49. Mines GR. On dynamic equilibrium in the heart. *J Phyiol* 1913;46:349–383. DeSilva RA, Mines GR. Ventricular fibrillation and the discovery of the vulnerable period. *J Am Coll Cardiol* 1997; 29:1397–1402

50. Lewis T, Schleiter HG. The relation of regular tachycardias of auricular origin to auricular fibrillation. *Heart* 1912; 3:173–193

51. Mayer AG. *Rhythmical Pulsation in Scyphomedusae*, vol. 47. Washington DC: Carnegie Institute of Washington; 1906:1–62

52. Mines GR. On circulating excitation in heart muscle and their possible relations to tachycardia and fibrillation. *Proc Trans R Soc Canada* 1914; 8:43–52

53. Mines. 1913, op. cit. (note 49)

54. Garrey WE. The nature of fibrillatory contractions of the heart: its relation to tissue mass and form. *Am J Physiol* 1914;33:397–414

55. Weiner N, Rosenblueth A. The mathematical formulation of the problem of conduction of impulses in a network of connected excitable elements, specifically in cardiac muscle. *Arch Inst Cardiol Mex* 1946;16:205–265

56. Davidenko J, Pertsov A, Salomonsz R, Baxter W, Jalife J. Stationary and drifting spiral waves of excitation in isolated cardiac muscle. *Nature* 1991;355:349–351

57. Rothberger CJ. Neue Theorien über Flimmern und Flattern. *Wien Klinische Wochenschrift* 1922;1:82–87; idem., Bemerkungen zur Theorie der Kreisbewegung beim Flimmern', *Wien Klinische Wochenschrift* 1923; 2:1407–1409

58. Garrey WE. Auricular fibrillation. *Physiol Rev* 1924;4:215–250

59. Wiggers CJ. Studies on ventricular fibrillation produced by electric shock. II. Cinematographic and Electrocardiographic observations of the natural process in the dog's heart. *Am Heart J* 1930;5:351–365

60. Wiggers CJ. The mechanism and nature of ventricular fibrillation. *Am Heart J* 1940;20:399–412

61. Wiggers CJ. Fibrillation. *Am Heart J* 1940;20:399–422

62. Scherf D, Schott A. *Extrasystoles and Allied Arrhythmias.* New York: Grune and Stratton; 1953

63. Moe GK. Introductory remarks to part III of experimental methods for the evaluation of drugs in various disease states. *Ann NY Acad Sci* 1956;64:540–542

64. Moe GK, Abildskov JA. Atrial fibrillation as a self-sustaining arrhythmia independent of focal discharge. *Am Heart J* 1959;58:59–70

65. Moe GK. On the multiple wavelet hypothesis of atrial fibrillation. *Arch Int Pharmacodyn* 1962;CXL:183–188

66. Han J, Moe GK. Nonuniform recovery of excitability in ventricular muscle. *Circ Res* 1964;14:44–60

67. Moe GK, Rheinbolt WC, Abildskov JA. A computer model of atrial fibrillation. *Am Heart J* 1964;67:200–220

68. Allessie MA, Lammers WEJEP, Bonke FIM, Hollen J. Experimental evaluation of Moe's multiple wavelet hypothesis of atrial fibrillation. In Zipes DP, Jalife J, eds. *Cardiac Electrophysiology and Arrhythmias*. Orlando, FL: Grune and Stratton; 1985:265–275

69. Downar E, Harris L, Mickelbrough LL, Shaigh N, Parson I. Endocardial mapping of ventricular tachycardia in the intact human ventricle: evidence for reentrant mechanisms. *J Am Col Cardiol* 1988;11:703–714

70. Janse MJ, Wilms-Schopman FJG, Coronel R. Ventricular fibrillation is not always due to multiple wavelet reentry. *J Cardiovasc Electrophysiol* 1995;6:512–521

71. Witkowski FX, Leon LJ, Penkoske PA, Giles WR, Spano ML, et al. Spatiotemporal evolution of ventricular fibrillation. *Nature* 1998;392:78–82

72. Epstein AE, Ideker RE. Ventricular fibrillation. In Zipes DP, Jalife J, eds. *Cardiac Electrophysiology: From Cell to Bedside*, 2nd edn. Philadelphia: Saunders; 1995:927–933

73. Gray RA, Jalife J, Panfilov AV, Baxter WT, Cabo C, et al. Mechanisms of cardiac fibrillation. *Science* 1995;270:1222–1225

74. Jalife J, Gray RA. Drifting vortices of electrical waves underlie ventricular fibrillation in the rabbit heart. *Acta Physiol Scand* 1996;157:123–131

75. Jalife J, Gray RA, Morley GE, Davidenko JM. Self-organization and the dynamical nature of ventricular fibrillation. *Chaos* 1998;8:79–93

76. Allessie MA, Bonke FIM, Schopman FJC. Circus movement in rabbit atrial muscle as a mechanism of tachycardia. *Circ Res* 1973;33:54–62

77. Allessie MA, Bonke FIM, Schopman FJC. Circus movement in rabbit atrial muscle as a mechanism of tachycardia. II. The role of nonuniform recovery of excitability in the occurrence of unidirectional block as studied with multiple microelectrodes. *Circ Res* 1976;39:168–177

78. Allessie MA, Bonke FIM, Schopman FJC. Circus movement in rabbit atrial muscle as a mechanism of tachycardia. III. The "leading circle" concept: a new model of circus movement in cardiac tissue without the involvement of an anatomical obstacle. *Circ Res* 1977;41:9–18

79. Belousov BP. A periodic reaction and its mechanism. *Compilation Abstr Radiat Med* 1959;147:145

80. Zhabotinsky AM. Periodic processes of malonic acid oxidation in a liquid phase. Biofizika 1964;9:306–311

81. Gul'ko FB, Petrov AA. Mechanism of the formation of closed pathways of conduction in excitable media. *Biophysics* 1972;17:271–281
82. Krinsky VI. Mathematical models of cardiac arrhythmias (spiral waves). *Pharmacol Ther B* 1978;3:539–355
83. Winfree AT. *When Time Breaks Down.* Princeton, NJ: Princeton University Press, 1987
84. Winfree AT, Strogatz SH. Organizing centres for three-dimensional chemical waves. *Nature* 1984;311:611–615
85. Winfree AT. Electrical turbulence in three-dimensional heart muscle. *Science* 1994;266:1003–1006

Part II

Theory of Electric Stimulation and Defibrillation

Chapter 2.1

The Bidomain Theory of Pacing

Deborah L. Janks and Bradley J. Roth

Introduction

The implantable cardiac pacemaker is one of the most important medical innovations of the twentieth century.[1] Yet until recently researchers have not understood the basic mechanisms governing how a pacemaker excites the heart. The development of a mathematical model describing the electrical properties of cardiac tissue – the bidomain model – helped unravel these mechanisms. This chapter outlines several important predictions of the bidomain model related to pacing. Several other chapters in this book examine related topics.

The bidomain model[2,3] represents cardiac tissue as a multidimensional cable that can be represented by a network of resistors and capacitors. Figure 1 shows a network equivalent to the two-dimensional bidomain model. The lower grid of resistors represents the intracellular space, and the upper grid represents the extracellular space. The two spaces are coupled by resistors and capacitors representing the membrane. The electrical properties of cardiac muscle are markedly anisotropic; in Fig. 1 the resistors in the x direction may be different from the resistors in the y direction. Moreover, the degree of anisotropy differs within the intracellular and extracellular spaces. The ratio of conductivities in the x and y directions in the extracellular space is on the order of two, but in the intracellular space it is about ten, indicating the intracellular space is more anisotropic than the extracellular space.[4] This condition of "unequal anisotropy ratios" leads to many of the interesting phenomena predicted by the bidomain model.[5]

Unipolar Stimulation

Sepulveda et al.[6] calculated the transmembrane potential in a passive two-dimensional sheet of cardiac tissue having unequal anisotropy ratios when a constant current is delivered

Bradley J. Roth
Department of Physics, Oakland University, Rochester, MI, USA, roth@oakland.edu

I. R. Efimov et al. (eds.), *Cardiac Bioelectric Therapy: Mechanisms and Practical Implications.*
© Springer Science+Business Media, LLC 2009

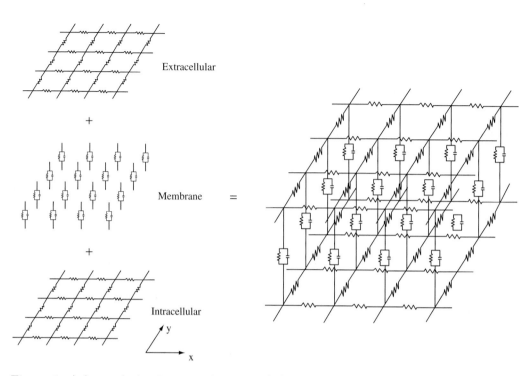

Figure 1: A lumped circuit approximation of the two-dimensional bidomain model. The lower and upper networks represent the electrical properties of the intracellular and extracellular spaces. The vertical resistors and capacitors represent the electrical properties of the membrane. The tissue is anisotropic, so the resistors parallel to the x axis are different than the resistors parallel to the y axis. (Roth 1992)[3]

through a unipolar cathode (Fig. 2). The calculation predicted a "dog bone" shaped region of depolarization around the cathode with adjacent weaker regions of hyperpolarization (called virtual anodes) along the fiber direction. This prediction has been verified experimentally[7-9] and has important implications during electrical stimulation of the heart.[10-12]

Make and Break Excitation

What is the mechanism by which an electrical current through a unipolar electrode excites cardiac tissue? Why can excitation occur near an anode as well as a cathode? Why can excitation be initiated by turning a stimulus off (break) as well as by turning it on (make)? The key to answering these questions is to realize that there are four distinct mechanisms responsible for the excitation of cardiac tissue: cathode make, anode make, cathode break, and anode break. These types of excitation have been known for decades,[13-15] but the mechanism responsible for this behavior was not understood until the incorporation of an active membrane into the bidomain model.[10]

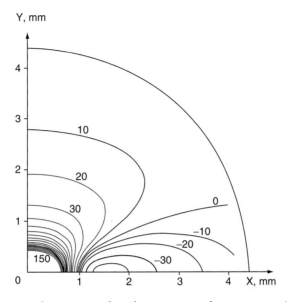

Figure 2: The isopotential contours for the transmembrane potential, calculated using unequal anisotropy ratios. The fibers are along the x axis. The current is applied cathodally with an extracellular electrode at the origin, with strength $4\,\mathrm{mA/mm}$. The isopotential contours near the source become very close together and are not drawn. Only one quadrant of the x–y plane is shown. The membrane is passive and the transmembrane potential represents deviations from the resting potential. (Sepulveda et al. 1989)[6]

Figure 3 shows the transmembrane potential distribution after the start of a cathodal stimulus (cathode make excitation). Each panel is a contour plot of the transmembrane potential as a function of the position z (along the fibers) and ρ (perpendicular to the fibers) at one instant (3, 6, 9, and 12 ms). Excitation begins at the electrode (black rectangle) and propagates outward as an elliptical wave front. A virtual anode exists, but the hyperpolarization (approximately 1 mV) is so small that it plays little or no role in the wave front dynamics (it is too weak to appear in Fig. 3).

During anode make excitation (Fig. 4), the tissue near the anode is strongly hyperpolarized following the start of a stimulus. An area of depolarization (a virtual cathode) develops about 1 to 2 mm from the anode in the direction parallel to the fibers. Excitation arises at the virtual cathode and propagates outward.

To understand cathode break excitation (Fig. 5), consider the transmembrane potential distribution following a long cathodal stimulus. Just before the end of the stimulus pulse the tissue is in steady state (top left panel, 0 ms), and is strongly depolarized under the cathode. About 2 mm from the electrode in the direction parallel to the fibers, the tissue at the virtual anode is hyperpolarized by more than 10 mV. Cardiac tissue is not excitable unless the sodium channel inactivation gate is open. The steady state inactivation curve implies that this gate is open where the transmembrane potential is more negative than

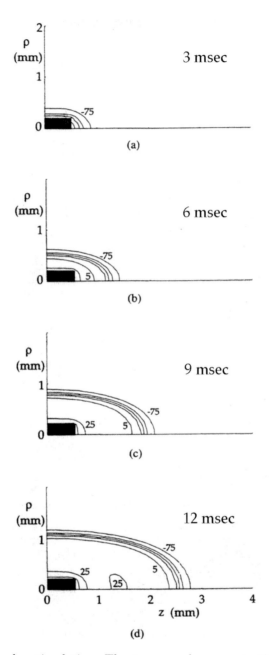

Figure 3: Cathode make stimulation. The transmembrane potential as a function of z (parallel to the fibers) and ρ (perpendicular to the fibers), 3, 6, 9, and 12 ms after the start of a long cathodal stimulus (0.06 mA). Only one quadrant of the $\rho - z$ plane is shown. The electrode size and position are indicated by the *black box*. Contour lines are drawn in increments of 20 mV. (Roth 1995)[10]

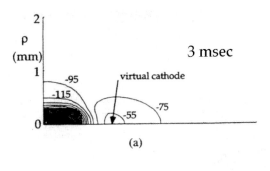

(a)

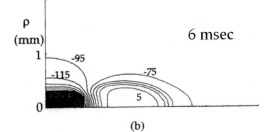

(b)

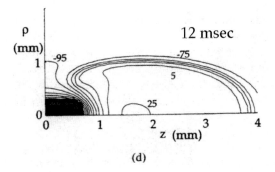

(c)

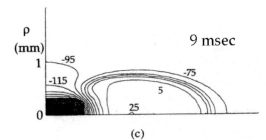

(d)

Figure 4: Anode make stimulation. The transmembrane potential as a function of z (parallel to the fibers) and ρ (perpendicular to the fibers), 3, 6, 9, and 12 ms after the start of a long anodal stimulus (0.6 mA). Only one quadrant of the $\rho - z$ plane is shown. The electrode size and position are indicated by the *black box*. Shading indicates hyperpolarization more negative than -215 mV. Contour lines are drawn in increments of 20 mV. (Roth 1995)[10]

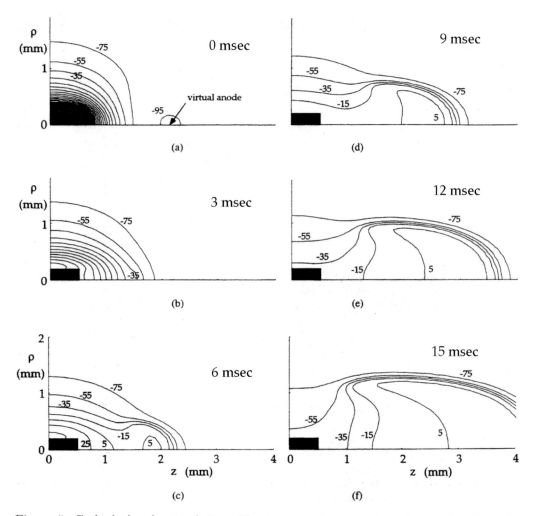

Figure 5: Cathode break stimulation. The transmembrane potential as a function of z (parallel to the fibers) and ρ (perpendicular to the fibers), 0, 3, 6, 9, 12, and 15 ms after the end of a long cathodal stimulus (0.7 mA). Only one quadrant of the $\rho - z$ plane is shown. The electrode size and position are indicated by the *black box*. Shading indicates depolarization more positive than 205 mV. Contour lines are drawn in increments of 20 mV. (Roth 1995)[10]

about -70 mV. Therefore, the depolarized tissue under the cathode is not excitable, although the tissue around the virtual anode is. After the stimulus ends, the transmembrane potential distribution decays and diffuses. The diffusion process is particularly important because it causes the strong depolarization under the cathode to diffuse outward into the virtual anode (3 ms). The excitable tissue at the virtual anode is depolarized to threshold by

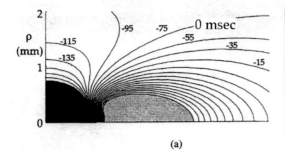
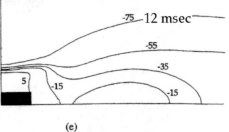
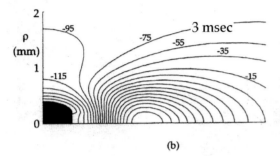
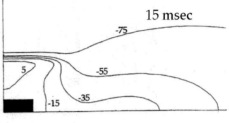

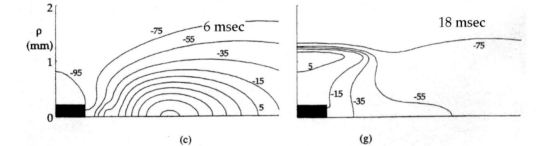
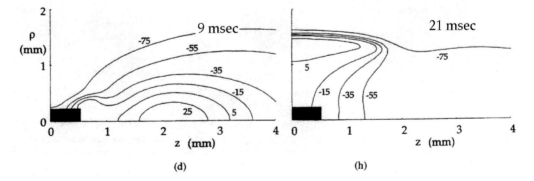

Figure 6: Anode break stimulation. The transmembrane potential as a function of z (parallel to the fibers) and ρ (perpendicular to the fibers), 0, 3, 6, 9, 12, 15, 18, and 21 ms after the end of a long anodal stimulus (7 mA). Only one quadrant of the $\rho - z$ plane is shown. The electrode is indicated by the *black box*. *Light shading* indicates depolarization more positive than 205 mV, and *dark shading* indicates hyperpolarization more negative than −215 mV. Contour lines are drawn in increments of 20 mV. (Roth 1995)[10]

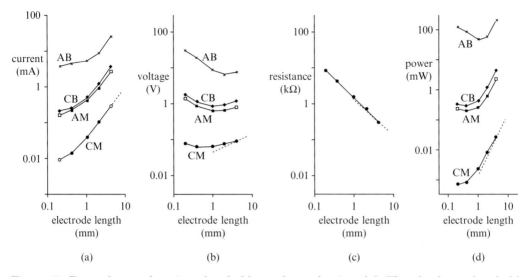

Figure 7: Dependence of pacing threshold on electrode size. (a) The rheobase threshold current for cathode make (CM), anode make (AM), cathode break (CB), and anode break (AB) stimulation as a function of electrode length. The corresponding (b) steady-state electrode voltage, (c) pacing resistance, and (d) power dissipation. The *dotted lines* have slopes of (a) 1.5, (b) 0.5, (c) −2, and (d) 2. (Roth 1995)[10]

6 ms. The resulting wave front propagates in the positive z direction, but cannot propagate back toward the electrode because the tissue in that direction is unexcitable.

Figure 6 shows the transmembrane potential distribution following a long anodal stimulus, resulting in anode break excitation. In steady state, the tissue under the anode is extremely hyperpolarized, and the tissue at the virtual cathode is depolarized (top left panel, 0 ms). When the stimulus ends, the transmembrane potential decays and diffuses. The depolarization at the virtual cathode decays more slowly than the hyperpolarization under the anode. By 6 ms, the now dominant depolarization diffuses inward toward the anode and excites the originally hyperpolarized (and therefore excitable) tissue. The resulting wave front propagates in the ρ direction but cannot propagate in the z direction because the tissue there is unexcitable.

Cathode make has the lowest threshold for excitation (Fig. 7). The threshold depends on electrode size, but for a small electrode the threshold can be as low as 0.01 mA, consistent with measurements by Lindemans and Denier van der Gon.[16] Anode make and cathode break have intermediate thresholds, about an order of magnitude higher than the cathode make threshold. The anode break threshold is higher yet, over 1 mA. This order of excitation threshold is consistent with experiments.[14,16] For a more complete comparison of theory and experiment, see Roth.[17]

Strength-Interval Curves

A strength-interval curve describes the refractoriness of cardiac tissue. The curve is generated by applying two sequential stimuli, S_1 and S_2. S_1 is only strong enough to induce propagation of an action potential within resting tissue. The strength-interval curve is constructed by varying the interval between S_1 and S_2 and noting the threshold S_2 strength. At longer intervals, threshold is lower because the tissue has nearly recovered from the S_1 action potential. At shorter intervals, S_2 is applied earlier in the repolarization phase of the S_1 action potential, and threshold increases because the tissue is refractory.

Dekker[14] stimulated a dog heart and measured strength-interval curves associated with each mechanism: cathode make, anode make, cathode break, and anode break. His make curves decrease monotonically with the interval, while his break curves contain a dip: a section in which the threshold increases paradoxically as the interval increases. The dip is particularly prominent in the anodal strength-interval curve.[18,19] What is the mechanism for this dip, and why is it often present during anodal stimulation but rarely observed during cathodal stimulation? Simulations based on the bidomain model provide answers to these questions.[11]

Figure 8 shows the calculated cathodal and anodal strength-interval curves for different S_2 pulse durations. In Fig. 8a, the 20 ms cathodal curve falls abruptly at 318 ms, with the threshold stimulus strength decreasing by a factor of six over a 4 ms window. Figure 9 provides an explanation for why this discontinuity occurs. Both columns of Fig. 9 contain contour plots of the transmembrane potential at five different times after the start of the S_2 pulse (the 20 ms stimulus pulse ends between the second and third panels in each column). In the left column, the S_2 stimulus has an interval of 316 ms and strength of 0.45 mA. During the S_2 pulse a make wave front is almost but not quite initiated; the tissue is still too refractory to support propagation. After the end of the pulse, however, the depolarization under the cathode diffuses into the virtual anode, triggering a break wave front (the hyperpolarization at the virtual anode is too weak to appear in the contour plots, but it is there). In the right column, the S_2 stimulus has an interval of 320 ms (4 ms later than the left column) and a strength of 0.065 mA. In this case, the S_2 pulse excites a make wave front, which initially propagates perpendicular to the fibers, but quickly becomes a closed wave front propagating outward with a nearly elliptical shape. The threshold strength, the site and time of initial excitation, and the initial direction of propagation are dramatically different between the two simulations, even though they correspond to a mere 4 ms difference in interval. This behavior arises from a change in the mechanism of stimulation from make to break.

The threshold for make stimulation is lower than for break stimulation as long as the interval is large enough that the tissue is excitable at the onset of the 20 ms stimulus pulse (> 318 ms). The change in threshold near 318 ms reflects the increase in refractoriness of the tissue near the end of the action potential. For intervals < 318 ms, the tissue near the cathode is refractory when the stimulus turns on; therefore, make excitation does not occur. However, the hyperpolarized tissue at the virtual anode may recover from refractoriness during the pulse. As a result, at the end of the pulse the tissue at the virtual anode is

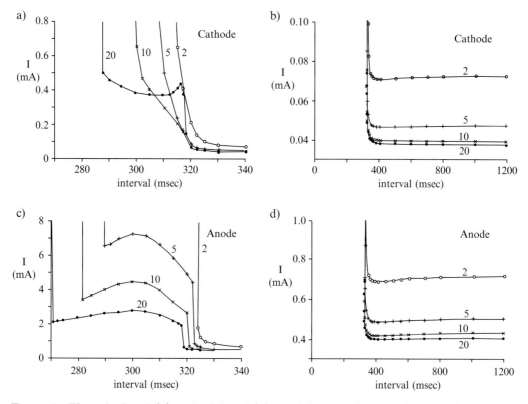

Figure 8: The calculated (**a**) cathodal and (**c**) anodal strength-interval curves for S_2 pulse durations of 2, 5, 10, and 20 ms. The same data for (**b**) cathodal and (**d**) anodal stimulation are plotted on different scales to highlight the behavior of the strength-interval curve at long intervals. (Roth 1996)[11]

excitable and can support action potential propagation if excited by the break mechanism. For intervals from 285 to 318 ms, break excitation is the low threshold mechanism, resulting in a wave front propagating through the excitable tissue at the virtual anode. However, for very short intervals (< 285 ms), once this wave front leaves the region of the virtual anode, the surrounding tissue is still refractory and propagation fails.

The anodal strength-interval curves are more complex than the cathodal curves. The 5, 10, and 20 ms anodal curves in Fig. 8c each contain an abrupt fall (almost a discontinuity) near 320 ms. This behavior can be explained by examining the wave front dynamics during and following a threshold-strength S_2 stimulus (Fig. 10). The left column corresponds to a threshold stimulation using a 20 ms duration, anodal S_2 stimulus with an interval of 318 ms. Depolarization at the virtual cathode initiates a weak wave front (note the closely spaced contour lines for -55, -35, and -15 mV at 323 ms), but the tissue is too refractory for the wave front to propagate (by 343 ms, no sign of the wave front is apparent). However, following the end of the pulse the depolarization at the virtual cathode diffuses toward

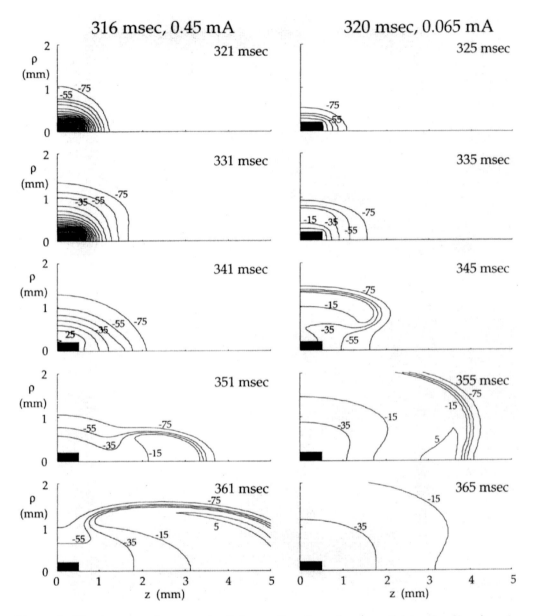

Figure 9: The transmembrane potential as a function of z (parallel to the fibers) and ρ (perpendicular to the fibers) during and following a 20 ms duration, cathodal S_2 stimulus. In the left column, S_2 has a strength of 0.45 mA and is applied at 316 ms. In the right column, S_2 has a strength of 0.065 mA and is applied at 320 ms. Only one quadrant of the z–ρ plane is shown. The *black box* indicates the electrode. *Shading* indicates depolarization more positive than 205 mV. Contour lines are drawn in increments of 20 mV. (Roth 1996)[11]

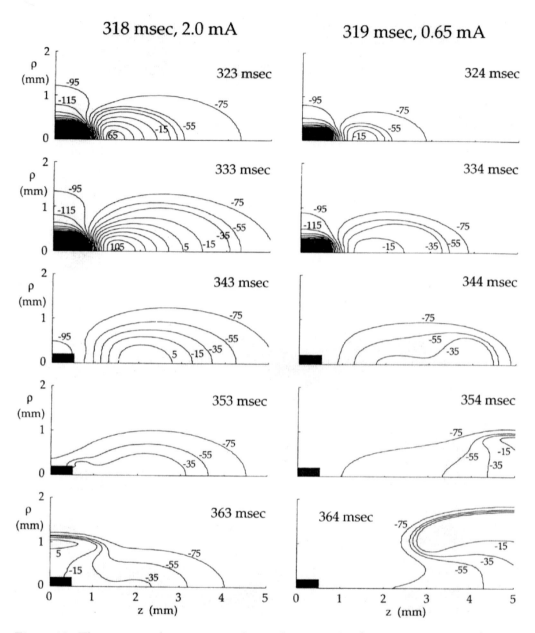

Figure 10: The transmembrane potential as a function of z (parallel to the fibers) and ρ (perpendicular to the fibers) during and following a 20 ms duration anodal S_2 stimulus. In the left column, S_2 has a strength of 2.0 mA and is applied at 318 ms. In the right column, S_2 has a strength of 0.65 mA and is applied at 319 ms. Only one quadrant of the z–ρ plane is shown. The *black box* indicates the electrode. *Shading* indicates hyperpolarization more negative than −215 mV. Contour lines are drawn in increments of 20 mV. (Roth 1996)[11]

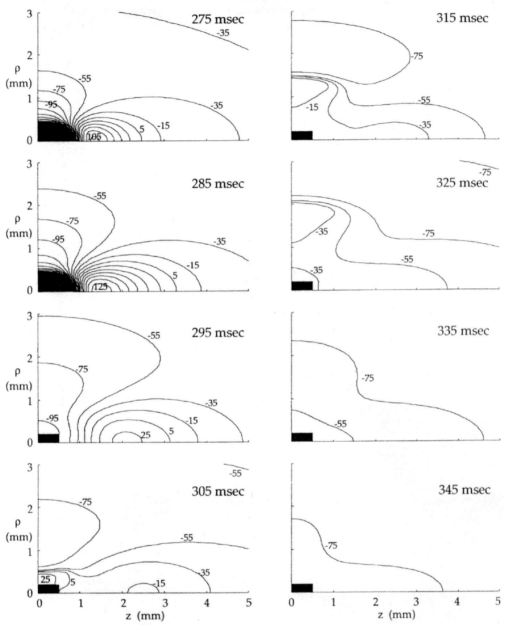

Figure 11: The transmembrane potential as a function of z (parallel to the fibers) and ρ (perpendicular to the fibers) during and following a 20 ms duration anodal S_2 stimulus. The stimulus has a strength of 2.5 mA and is applied at 270 ms. Only one quadrant of the $z - \rho$ plane is shown. The *black box* indicates the electrode. Shading indicates hyperpolarization more negative than -215 mV. Contour lines are drawn in increments of 20 mV. (Roth 1996)[11]

the anode and triggers a wave front by the break mechanism. The right column of Fig. 10 shows the wave front dynamics if a stimulus is applied only 1 ms later (319 ms). A wave front initiated at the virtual cathode propagates outward in the z direction. Propagation is slow because the tissue is relatively refractory but is ultimately successful. By 354 ms, the wave front propagates out of the region shown in the plot.

The abrupt fall in the 20 ms anodal strength-interval curve at 319 ms reflects the transition from make to break excitation. The division of the strength-interval curve into make and break sections is more distinct for anodal stimulation than it is for cathodal stimulation because of the different directions of propagation following anode make and anode break excitation. For make excitation, initial propagation occurs parallel to the fibers; conversely for break excitation initial propagation occurs perpendicular to the fibers. During cathodal stimulation, the difference in the direction of propagation is not as dramatic.

Between 300 and 320 ms, the anode-break threshold decreases with increasing interval (Fig. 8c). One cause of this "dip" in the strength-interval curve is that depolarization near the anode just before the S_2 pulse is greater for shorter intervals (the S_1 action potential is repolarizing). The tissue at the virtual cathode, therefore, is depolarized partially when the S_2 stimulus begins. The limiting factor in anode break excitation is not having sufficient hyperpolarization under the anode (the strong hyperpolarization there is more than sufficient to render the tissue excitable), but instead is having sufficient depolarization at the virtual cathode. Decreasing the interval tends to increase the depolarization at the virtual cathode, thereby decreasing the threshold and causing the "dip."

A minimum interval exists below which the anode break mechanism does not excite the tissue. This minimum interval depends on the duration of the S_2 pulse in such a way that the end of the S_2 pulse (interval plus pulse duration) occurs at about 290 ms (Fig. 8c). For shorter intervals, the break mechanism initially causes a wave front to propagate away from the anode. Once this wave front propagates several millimeters, however, it reaches tissue that was affected negligibly by the stimulus. This tissue is still refractory, and the wave front cannot propagate further (Fig. 11).

Sidorov et al.[20] verified experimentally the predicted shapes of the anodal and cathodal strength-interval curves, and confirmed that an abrupt fall in a curve corresponds to the transition from make to break excitation.

No-Response Phenomenon

The *no-response phenomenon* in cardiac tissue occurs when an increase in stimulus strength abolishes excitation. This phenomenon has been observed experimentally during anodal stimulation[19] and is explained by the bidomain model.[12,21] Figure 12 shows the response to an anodal S_2 stimulus, with an interval of 273 ms, for three different stimulus currents. A current of 2 mA is too weak to cause break excitation, and no wave front develops (left column). For 3 mA, break excitation triggers a wave front (center column). For 4 mA, a break wave front is launched (right column, 310 ms), but it then

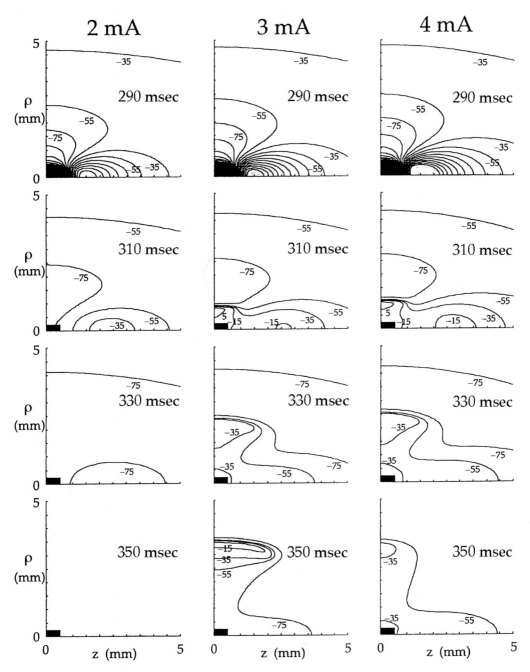

Figure 12: The transmembrane potential as a function of z (parallel to the fibers) and ρ (perpendicular to the fibers) during and following a 20 ms duration anodal S_2 stimulus. The stimulus has a strength of 2, 3, or 4 mA and begins at 273 ms. Only one quadrant of the z–ρ plane is shown. The *black box* indicates the electrode. *Light shading* indicates hyperpolarization more negative than -215 mV and *dark shading* indicates depolarization more positive than 145 mV. Contour lines are drawn in increments of 20 mV. (Roth 1997)[12]

decays (right column, 350 ms). A wave front can propagate as long as it is in recovered tissue. The tissue hyperpolarized by the stimulus at the virtual anode is excitable and can support propagation. Once the wave front reaches the edge of the virtual anode, however, it enters tissue that may or may not be excitable. A stronger stimulus may make the tissue within the virtual anode recover more completely, resulting in faster propagation. Because the wave front traverses the virtual anode in less time, it reaches the edge of the virtual anode more quickly. Tissue outside the virtual anode has insufficient time to recover from refractoriness and cannot be excited. Once the wave front reaches the edge of the virtual anode, it decays. The no-response phenomenon is important because for defibrillation-strength shocks, a similar mechanism is responsible for the "upper limit of vulnerability."[22,23]

Effect of Potassium on Pacing

High extracellular potassium favors break over make excitation. Figure 13 shows the anodal strength-interval curves for four extracellular potassium concentrations.[24] The make section of the curve has a threshold strength of about 0.25 mA for each concentration, but the break

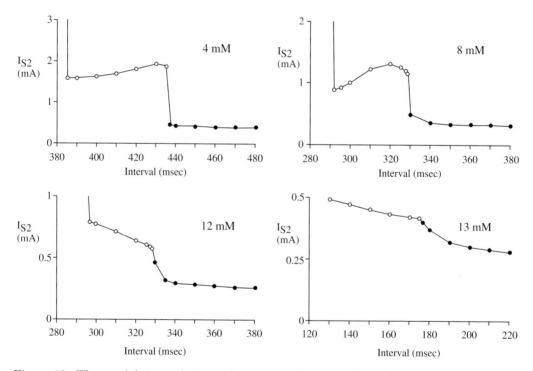

Figure 13: The anodal strength-interval curve calculated for S_2 pulse duration of 20 ms and extracellular potassium ion concentrations of 4, 8, 12, and 13 mM. *Open circles* indicate break excitation, and *filled circles* indicate make excitation. (Roth and Patel 2003)[24]

threshold drops from 2 to 0.5 mA as the concentration increases from 4 to 13 mM. For a concentration of 13.3 mM (not shown), the break threshold is so low that break, rather than make, is the mechanism for exciting resting tissue. High potassium raises the resting potential, depolarizing the tissue. The limiting factor in break excitation is depolarization at the virtual cathode. The depolarized resting potential supplies additional depolarization, making break excitation easier. Sidorov et al.[25] observed similar effects experimentally.

The "dip" in the anodal strength-interval curve disappears at high concentrations (Fig. 13). High potassium causes "postrepolarization refractoriness": the tissue remains refractory for a time, even though the transmembrane potential has returned to its resting value.[26] The mechanism of the dip discussed previously was that depolarization at the virtual cathode caused by an S_2 stimulus is augmented by the repolarization of the S_1 action potential, lowering the threshold for break excitation. If postrepolarization refractoriness is present, then shortening the interval does not result in additional depolarization because the transmembrane potential is already at its resting value, thereby eliminating the "dip." A "dip" in the anodal strength-interval curve exists only if the break section of the curve occurs during the repolarization phase of the S_1 action potential.

Time Dependence of the Anodal and Cathodal Refractory Periods

Mehra et al.[27] observed that immediately following implantation of a pacemaker the anodal refractory period was shorter than the cathodal refractory period, but after several weeks the cathodal refractory period became shorter than the anodal refractory period. Figure 14 suggests one hypothesis to explain this observation.[28] After a pacemaker electrode is implanted, tissue adjacent to the electrode is healthy and excitable. However, within a few weeks a region of inexcitable scar tissue surrounds the electrode, making its effective size larger. Larger electrodes require a stronger current to trigger an action potential. Suppose a stimulator has a maximum current it can provide, as did the stimulator used by Mehra et al.[27] As scar tissue increases the effective size of the electrode, the threshold can increase so much that the entire break section of the strength-interval curve requires a stronger stimulus than the stimulator can produce. In that case, the strength-interval curve rises abruptly when the mechanism of excitation changes from make to break, and the experimentalist will naturally define the time of this rise as the end of the "refractory period." If the stimulator were more powerful, it would become apparent that this rise is associated with the make/break transition, and the true end of the "refractory period" is much earlier. In other words, the apparent "anodal refractory period" changes from the point where the break section becomes vertical (about 255 ms in Fig. 14b) to the point where the make section rises abruptly (315 ms). Thus, the anodal refractory period does not really change with time, but it appears to change because the stimulator is not powerful enough to trace out the break section of the strength interval curve. The observation is an artifact of the particular stimulator used, and does not represent a fundamental change in the behavior of the tissue.

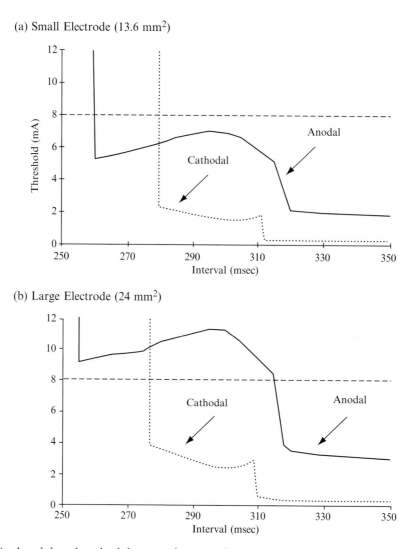

(a) Small Electrode (13.6 mm^2)

(b) Large Electrode (24 mm^2)

Figure 14: Anodal and cathodal strength-interval curves calculated using a 20 ms S_2 duration. (a) Small electrode with surface area of 13.6 mm^2. Note that both the anodal and cathodal curves lie below 8 mA shown by the *dashed line*. (b) Large electrode with surface area of 24 mm^2. The entire cathodal curve lies below 8 mA, but the break section of the anodal curve lies above 8 mA. If the stimulator had a maximum output of 8 mA, the break section of the anodal curve would be observed in (a) but not in (b). (Bennett and Roth 1999)[28]

Conclusion

Simulations based on the bidomain model have provided key insights into how an electrical stimulus excites cardiac tissue. They have helped resolved decades-old questions about the mechanisms of make and break excitation and the shape of the strength-interval curve. Bidomain simulations are also important in understanding in the induction of reentry. Reentry can be induced in cardiac tissue using trains of weak pulses: each pulse having a strength similar to a pacemaker stimulus.[29] The bidomain properties of cardiac tissue are also crucial in predicting the response of cardiac tissue to strong shocks and can cause "quatrefoil reentry"[12,30,31] (see the Wikswo and Roth chapter). They influence how the heart responds to defibrillation.[32] Trayanova and Plank discuss these effects in the next chapter.

Acknowledgments

This research was supported by the National Institutes of Health and the American Heart Association. We thank Laura Janks for her assistance in preparing this chapter.

References

1. Jeffrey K. *Machines in Our Hearts: The Cardiac Pacemaker, the Implantable Defibrillator, and American Health Care*. Baltimore: Johns Hopkins University Press; 2001
2. Henriquez CS. Simulating the electrical behavior of cardiac tissue using the bidomain model. *Crit Rev Biomed Eng* 1993;21:1–77
3. Roth BJ. How the anisotropy of the intracellular and extracellular conductivities influences stimulation of cardiac muscle. *J Math Biol* 1992;30:633–646
4. Roth BJ. Electrical conductivity values used with the bidomain model of cardiac tissue. *IEEE Trans Biomed Eng* 1997;44:326–328
5. Roth BJ. How to explain why "unequal anisotropy ratios" is important using pictures but no mathematics. *28th Annual International Conference of the IEEE Engineering in Medicine and Biology Society*, Aug. 30–Sept. 3, 2006, New York
6. Sepulveda NG, Roth BJ, Wikswo JP Jr. Current injection into a two-dimensional anisotropic bidomain. *Biophys J* 1989;55:987–999
7. Neunlist M, Tung L. Spatial distribution of cardiac transmembrane potentials around an extracellular electrode: dependence on fiber orientation. *Biophys J* 1995;68:2310–2322
8. Knisley SB. Transmembrane voltage changes during unipolar stimulation of rabbit ventricle. *Circ Res* 1995;77:1229–1239
9. Wikswo JP Jr, Lin S-F, Abbas RA. Virtual electrodes in cardiac tissue: A common mechanism for anodal and cathodal stimulation. *Biophys J* 1995;69:2195–2210
10. Roth BJ. A mathematical model of make and break electrical stimulation of cardiac tissue by a unipolar anode or cathode. *IEEE Trans Biomed Eng* 1995;42:1174–1184

11. Roth BJ. Strength-interval curves for cardiac tissue predicted using the bidomain model. *J Cardiovasc Electrophysiol* 1996;7:722–737

12. Roth BJ. Nonsustained reentry following successive stimulation of cardiac tissue through a unipolar electrode. *J Cardiovasc Electrophysiol* 1997;8:768–778

13. Goto M, Brooks C McC. Membrane excitability of the frog ventricle examined by long pulses. *Am J Physiol* 1969;217:1236–1245

14. Dekker E. Direct current make and break thresholds for pacemaker electrodes on the canine ventricle. *Circ Res* 1970;27:811–823

15. Lindemans FW, Heethaar RM, Denier van der Gon JJ, Zimmerman ANE. Site of initial excitation and current threshold as a function of electrode radius in heart muscle. *Cardiovasc Res* 1975;9:95–104

16. Lindemans FW, Denier van der Gon JJ. Current thresholds and liminal size in excitation of heart muscle. *Cardiovasc Res* 1978;12:477–485

17. Roth BJ. Artifacts, assumptions, and ambiguity: Pitfalls in comparing experimental results to numerical simulations when studying electrical stimulation of the heart. *Chaos* 2002;12:973–981

18. van Dam RTh, Durrer D, Strackee J, van der Tweel LH. The excitability cycle of the dog's left ventricle determined by anodal, cathodal, and bipolar stimulation. *Circ Res* 1956;4:196–203

19. Cranefield PF, Hoffman BF, Siebens AA. Anodal excitation of cardiac muscle. *Am J Physiol* 1957;190:383–390

20. Sidorov VY, Woods MC, Baudenbacher P, Baudenbacher F. Examination of stimulation mechanism and strength-interval curve in cardiac tissue. *Am J Physiol* 2005;289:H2602–H2615

21. Roth BJ. A mechanism for the "no-response" phenomenon during anodal stimulation of cardiac tissue. *19th Annual International Conference of the IEEE Engineering in Medicine and Biology Society*, Chicago, Oct. 30–Nov. 2, 1997

22. Cheng Y, Mowrey KA, van Wagoner DR, Tchou PJ, Efimov IR. Virtual electrode-induced reexcitation: a mechanism of defibrillation. *Circ Res* 1999;85:1056–1066

23. Rodriguez B, Trayanova N. Upper limit of vulnerability in a defibrillation model of the rabbit ventricles. *J Electrocardiol* 2003;36(Suppl):51–56

24. Roth BJ, Patel SG. Effects of elevated extracellular potassium ion concentration on anodal excitation of cardiac tissue. *J Cardiovasc Electrophysiol* 2003;14:1351–1355

25. Sidorov VY, Woods MC, Wikswo JP. Effects of elevated extracellular potassium on the stimulation mechanism of diastolic cardiac tissue. *Biophys J* 2003;84:3470–3479

26. Rodriguez B, Tice BM, Eason JC, Aguel F, Trayanova N. Cardiac vulnerability to electric shocks during phase 1A of acute global ischemia. *Heart Rhythm* 2004;1:695–703

27. Mehra R, McMullen M, Furman S. Time dependence of unipolar cathodal and anodal strength-interval curves. *PACE* 1980;3:526–530

28. Bennett JA, Roth BJ. Time dependence of anodal and cathodal refractory periods in cardiac tissue. *PACE* 1999;22:1031–1038

29. Janks DL, Roth BJ. Quatrefoil reentry caused by burst pacing. *J Cardiovasc Electrophysiol* 2006;17:1362–1368

30. Saypol JM, Roth BJ. A mechanism for anisotropic reentry in electrically active tissue. *J Cardiovasc Electrophysiol* 1992;3:558–566
31. Lin S-F, Roth BJ, Wikswo JP Jr. Quatrefoil reentry in myocardium: an optical imaging study of the induction mechanism. *J Cardiovasc Electrophysiol* 1999;10:574–586
32. Efimov IR, Gray RA, Roth BJ. Virtual electrodes and de-excitation: new insights into fibrillation induction and defibrillation. *J Cardiovasc Electrophysiol* 2000;11:339–353

Chapter 2.2

Bidomain Model of Defibrillation

Natalia Trayanova and Gernot Plank

Introduction

Defibrillation of the heart by high-intensity electric shocks is currently the only reliable procedure for termination of ventricular fibrillation. Despite the critical role that defibrillation therapy plays in saving human life, elucidating the mechanisms by which electric shocks halt life-threatening arrhythmias has been a long and arduous process. Uncovering how electric current delivered to the heart to terminate lethal arrhythmias traverses myocardial structures and interacts with the wavefronts of fibrillation has been enormously challenging. Of particular importance has been obtaining insight into the mechanisms by which the shock fails since reinitiation of fibrillation is related not only to the effect of the shock on the electrical state of the myocardium, but also to the intrinsic properties of the tissue that lead to destabilization of postshock activations and their degradation into electric turbulence. The complexity of the relationships and dependencies to be teased out and dissected in this quest has been staggering.

Although over the years defibrillation devices have become smaller and their batteries longer lasting, defibrillation remains a traumatic experience, often resulting in myocardial dysfunction and damage. Furthermore, recent meta-analysis of industrial reports concluded that thousands of patients have been affected by high-voltage component implantable cardioverter-defibrillator (ICD) malfunctions, causing severe psychological trauma.[1] A significant reduction in shock energy can only be achieved by full appreciation of the mechanisms by which a shock interacts with the heart and then exploiting them to devise novel therapeutic approaches. Thus, comprehensive mechanistic insight into defibrillation remains a major scientific frontier. This chapter examines an important tool in the quest to understand the defibrillation mechanisms, the three-dimensional (3D) bidomain model of defibrillation.

Natalia Trayanova

Department of Biomedical Engineering and Institute for Computational Medicine, Johns Hopkins University, Baltimore, MD 21218, USA, ntrayan1@jhu.edu

I. R. Efimov et al. (eds.), *Cardiac Bioelectric Therapy: Mechanisms and Practical Implications.*
© Springer Science+Business Media, LLC 2009

Advancements Leading to the Development of the Bidomain Model of Defibrillation

Historically, overwhelming electrical artifacts had prevented researchers from recording during as well as shortly after the shock. A breakthrough in mapping cardiac activity associated with defibrillation occurred during the last decade of the twentieth century with the introduction of potentiometric dyes, which allowed continuous recording of activity before, during, and after the shock. At the same time, the theoretical electrophysiology community adopted a novel modeling methodology, the *bidomain model*; its theoretical underpinnings and applications are comprehensively explored in this book. The bidomain model (see the chapter by Henriquez and Ying for more details) is a continuum representation of the myocardium that takes into consideration current distribution resulting from a particular characteristic of cardiac tissue—the fact that the two spaces comprising the myocardium, the intra- and extracellular, are both anisotropic but to a different degree. The myocardium is thus characterized with "unequal anisotropy ratios." Since the bidomain model accounts for the current flow in the interstitium, it became instantly a powerful modeling tool in the study of stimulation of cardiac tissue (see the chapter by Janks and Roth), where current delivered in the extracellular space finds its way across the membranes of cardiac cells.

The first significant achievement of this new approach was the study of the passive (i.e., the ionic currents are not accounted for) shock-induced change in transmembrane potential following a strong unipolar stimulus (near-field effects). Bidomain simulations by Sepulveda et al.[2] demonstrated that the tissue response in the vicinity of a strong unipolar stimulus involved simultaneous occurrence of positive (depolarizing) and negative (hyperpolarizing) effects in close proximity. This finding of virtual electrodes was in stark contrast with the established view that tissue responses should only be depolarizing (hyperpolarizing) if the stimulus was cathodal (anodal).[3] Optical mapping studies that followed convincingly confirmed these theoretical predictions.[4] Since then, virtual electrode polarization (VEP) has been documented in experiments involving various stimulus configurations.[5–9]

The next big contribution of passive bidomain modeling was the detailed analysis of VEP etiology and its dependence on cardiac tissue structure and the configuration of the applied field; both were shown to be major determinants of the shape, location, polarity, and intensity of the shock-induced polarization.[7,10–14] In particular, theoretical considerations led to the recognition of two types of VEP: (1) *surface* VEP, which penetrates the ventricular wall over a few cell layers, due to current redistribution near the boundaries separating myocardium from blood cavity or surrounding bath, and (2) *bulk* VEP throughout the ventricular wall.[11,15] Analysis of the bidomain equations revealed that a necessary condition for the existence of the bulk VEP is the unequal anisotropy in the myocardium. Sufficient conditions include either spatial nonuniformity in applied electric field or nonuniformity in tissue architecture, such as fiber curvature, fiber rotation, fiber branching and anastomosis, and local changes in tissue conductivity due to resistive heterogeneities. Additional detail regarding the formation of VEP and the structural mechanisms that drive it can be found in the chapter by Tung.

How do cells respond to externally imposed changes in their transmembrane potential, such as those predicted by the passive bidomain model? The cellular response to shock-induced VEP depends on its magnitude and polarity, as well as on the electrophysiological state of the cell at the time of shock delivery. Action potential duration can be either extended (by positive VEP) or shortened (by negative VEP) to a degree that depends on VEP magnitude and shock timing, with strong negative VEP completely abolishing (deexciting) the action potential, thus creating postshock excitable areas in the virtual anode regions. Two-dimensional (myocardial sheet) simulations with the bidomain model that incorporated for the first time ionic fluxes through cell membranes (active bidomain modeling) resulted in the recognition of the importance of the distribution of transmembrane potential established by the shock to the origin of the postshock activations. Analyzing results of two-dimensional (2D) bidomain simulations of near-field behavior (behavior in the vicinity of a stimulus), Roth[16] demonstrated that the close proximity of a deexcited region and a virtual cathode could result in an excitation at shock end, called *break excitation* (i.e., at the break of the shock); the virtual cathode serves as an electrical stimulus, eliciting a regenerative depolarization and a propagating wave in the newly created excitable area. Break excitations arise at the borders between oppositely polarized regions provided that the transmembrane potential gradient across the border spans the threshold for regenerative depolarization.[17] The finding of break excitations, combined with the fact that positive VEP can result in regenerative depolarization in regions where tissue is at or near diastole (make excitation; takes place at the onset of the shock), resulted in a novel understanding of how a strong stimulus can result in the development of new activations.

These findings provided the background for the development of a comprehensive set of mechanisms aiming to explain the success or failure of a defibrillation shock based on the application of the bidomain model. This set of mechanisms includes the generating of VEP in the 3D ventricles by the defibrillation electrodes (far-field effects) and the initiation of postshock activations, the origin of which, if any, depends on shock strength and waveform. Developing this understanding required large-scale simulations of defibrillation in the whole heart, where geometry and fiber orientation play a major role in activity during and after the shock. This necessitated technological advancement in the application of the bidomain model and the numerical approaches employed in simulating defibrillation. The sections below present the algorithms used to solve the bidomain equations in 3D as well as examples of mechanistic insight obtained from the analysis of the simulations.

Bidomain Equations and Numerical Approaches for Large-Scale Simulations in Shock-Induced Arrhythmogenesis and Defibrillation

The quest to unravel how shocks could succeed in terminating fibrillation or how they could reinstate arrhythmia has driven the technological aspects of computer simulations of 3D bidomain activity. In order to be able to simulate postshock arrhythmogenesis in the ventricles, computational research has managed to overcome tremendous difficulties associated with obtaining solutions of very large systems of unknowns, involving stiff equations and computational meshes of irregular geometry. A brief overview of the computational approaches involved in conducting simulations of postshock arrhythmogenesis and defibrillation is presented below.

Governing Equations

The bidomain equations describe the electrical behavior of cardiac tissue as a syncytium, where all tissue parameters are accounted for in an averaged sense.[18] The domains of interest, intracellular and extracellular, and the cellular membranes, which physically separate the two domains, are distributed over the entire tissue volume. The bidomain equations state that currents that enter the intracellular or extracellular spaces by crossing the cell membrane represent the sources for the intracellular potential, ϕ_i, and the extracellular potential, ϕ_e:

$$\nabla \cdot \bar{\sigma}_i \nabla \phi_i = \beta I_m, \tag{1}$$

$$\nabla \cdot \bar{\sigma}_e \nabla \phi_e = -\beta I_m - I_e, \tag{2}$$

$$I_m = C_m \frac{\partial V_m}{\partial t} + I_{ion}(V_m, \vec{\eta}) - I_{stim}, \tag{3}$$

$$V_m = \phi_i - \phi_e, \tag{4}$$

where $\bar{\sigma}_i$ and $\bar{\sigma}_e$ are the intracellular and extracellular conductivity tensors, respectively, β is the membrane surface to volume ratio, I_m is the transmembrane current density, I_{stim} is the current density of the transmembrane stimulus used to initiate an action potential, I_e is the current density of the extracellular stimulus, C_m is the membrane capacitance per unit area, V_m is the transmembrane potential, and I_{ion} is the density of the total current flowing through the membrane ionic channels, pumps, and exchangers, which depends on the transmembrane potential and on a set of state variables $\vec{\eta}$. If at the tissue boundaries electrical isolation is assumed, it is accounted for by imposing no-flux boundary conditions on ϕ_e and ϕ_i.

If, however, cardiac tissue is surrounded by a conductive medium, such as blood in the ventricular cavities or a perfusing bath (Tyrode solution) in which the heart is submerged, then Laplace equation has to be additionally solved:

$$\nabla \cdot \sigma_b \nabla \phi_e = 0, \tag{5}$$

where σ_b is the isotropic conductivity of the conductive medium. In this case no-flux boundary conditions are assumed at the boundaries of the conductive medium, whereas continuity of the normal component of the extracellular current and continuity of ϕ_e are enforced at the tissue-bath interface. The no-flux boundary conditions for ϕ_i remain in place.

For most applications the bidomain equations are recast into other forms by substituting (4) into (1) and (2) and executing algebraic transformations. Several ways to recast the bidomain equations have been proposed; a systematic overview of the different linear transformations is found in Hooke et al.[19] A widely used transformation is to add (1) and (2) and replace ϕ_i by $V_m + \phi_e$:[20]

$$\nabla \cdot (\bar{\sigma}_i + \bar{\sigma}_e)\nabla \phi_e = -\nabla \cdot \bar{\sigma}_i \nabla V_m - I_e, \tag{6}$$

$$\nabla \cdot \bar{\sigma}_i \nabla V_m = -\nabla \cdot \bar{\sigma}_i \nabla \phi_e + \beta I_m, \tag{7}$$

which retains V_m and ϕ_e as the independent variables. For comparison of tissue and organ level simulations with experimental data, this is advantageous since ϕ_e can be measured via electrical and V_m via optical mapping techniques.

Computational Considerations

Large-scale computational studies employing the bidomain model in general, and defibrillation studies in particular, have remained a challenge, although computer speed and memory have dramatically increased. Several factors render any numerical solution of the bidomain equations computationally challenging:

- The fast rate of rise of action potential upstroke translates into a steep propagating wavefront in space where the wave of depolarization extends only a few hundred micrometers. Hence, both spatially fine-grained computational grids and a high temporal resolution are mandatory to faithfully capture wavefront propagation.

- To study cardiac arrhythmias, a discretized domain of interest has to be chosen that is large enough to support reentrant wave propagation. With constraints on spatial discretization, as mentioned above, the result is a large system, on the order of 10^5 to 10^7 degrees of freedom.

- The maximum size of the time step is either limited by the time constants of the ordinary differential equations (ODE) in the ionic models or by the mesh ratio (which becomes the limiting factor when fine spatial discretization, well below $100\,\mu\text{m}$, is used). Since most physiological processes of interest take place over seconds or minutes, temporal step size limits necessitate a large number of time steps, typically in the range from tens to hundreds of thousands.

Additional challenges specific to defibrillation simulations include:

- For defibrillation studies, the use of unstructured grids for anatomically realistic models of the heart is mandatory as to allow smooth representation of the organ's surfaces. Jagged boundaries, which inevitably form along the organ surfaces when regular structured or block structured grids are employed, cause spurious polarizations upon delivery of a defibrillation-strength shock.

- Fine spatial discretization becomes even more important for defibrillation since large transmembrane potential gradients are induced by the shock; for instance, in a passive

2D bidomain study,[21] a voltage drop of 1 V over a distance as short as $100\,\mu\mathrm{m}$ has been reported.

- State-of-the-art ionic models incorporate over 20 state variables of ever increasing stiffness. These models are developed for the normal physiological range of action potential variables. For defibrillation, however, even when ionic models are equipped with additional currents that limit the rise of V_{m},[22,23] transmembrane voltages can increase significantly beyond the physiological range of the parameters and undesirable behavior of the model equations could ensue. Typically, modifications are required to render an ionic model suitable for defibrillation studies.[24,25]

- Fast transients in state variables during shock onset enforce even smaller time steps, which make computations during the shock more burdensome.

- Due to the nature of defibrillation, where shock success depends on a multitude of parameters, most importantly shock strength and timing, but also pulse shape, polarity, electrode geometry, and location, a large number of simulations are required to sweep the parameter space. In the simplest case where only N timings and M shock strengths are tested to construct a vulnerability grid, a total of $N \times M$ simulations need to be performed.

Numerical Schemes

Among the possible castings of the bidomain equations, the one presented as (6) and (7) is the most popular. In the most general case, where a conducting medium is in contact with the myocardium, the bidomain equations are written as

$$\begin{bmatrix} -\nabla \cdot (\bar{\sigma}_{\mathrm{i}} + \bar{\sigma}_{\mathrm{e}})\nabla\phi_{\mathrm{e}} \\ -\nabla \cdot \sigma_{\mathrm{b}}\nabla\phi_{\mathrm{e}} \end{bmatrix} = \begin{bmatrix} \nabla \cdot \bar{\sigma}_{\mathrm{i}}\nabla V_{\mathrm{m}} \\ I_{\mathrm{e}} \end{bmatrix}, \tag{8}$$

$$\frac{\partial V_{\mathrm{m}}}{\partial t} = \frac{1}{\beta C_{\mathrm{m}}}(\nabla \cdot \bar{\sigma}_{\mathrm{i}}\nabla V_{\mathrm{m}} + \nabla \cdot \bar{\sigma}_{\mathrm{i}}\nabla\phi_{\mathrm{e}}) - \frac{1}{C_{\mathrm{m}}}I_{\mathrm{ion}}(V_{\mathrm{m}}, \vec{\eta}), \tag{9}$$

$$\frac{\mathrm{d}\vec{\eta}}{\mathrm{d}t} = g(V_m, \vec{\eta}). \tag{10}$$

Numerically, the bidomain equations can be solved as a coupled system[26] or alternatively, operator splitting techniques are applied[27] to decouple the computing scheme into three components: an elliptic partial differential equation (PDE), a parabolic PDE, and a set of nonlinear ODEs. It has been shown that the decoupled scheme converges quickly against the coupled scheme by employing a Block Gauss-Seidel iteration.[28] However, in most studies the components are essentially treated as independent. Solutions are then found by leap-frogging between the decoupled components, where either V_{m} in (8) or Φ_{e} in (9) are considered as constant. In Vigmond et al.[26] it has been found that with small error tolerances, the differences between coupled and decoupled approaches are negligible.

Discretizing the decoupled bidomain equations leads to a three-step scheme, which involves a solution of the parabolic PDE, the elliptic PDE, and the nonlinear system of ODEs at each time step. In the simplest case, both parabolic PDE and the nonlinear ODE systems can be solved with an explicit forward Euler scheme:[26]

$$V^{k*} = (1 - \Delta t A_{\mathrm{i}})V^k - \Delta t A_{\mathrm{e}}\phi_{\mathrm{e}}^k, \qquad (11)$$

$$V^{k+1} = V^{k*} + \frac{\Delta t}{C_{\mathrm{m}}} I_{\mathrm{ion}}\left(V^{k*}, \vec{\eta}^k\right), \qquad (12)$$

$$\vec{\eta}^{k+1} = \vec{\eta}^k + \Delta t g\left(V^{k+1}, \vec{\eta}^k\right), \qquad (13)$$

$$(A_{\mathrm{i}} + A_{\mathrm{e}})\Phi_{\mathrm{e}}^{k+1} = A_{\mathrm{i}}V^{k+1} + I_{\mathrm{e}}, \qquad (14)$$

where A_ξ is the discretized $-\nabla \cdot (\bar{\sigma}_\xi \nabla)/(\beta C_{\mathrm{m}})$ operator with ξ being either i or e; Δt is the time step; V^k, ϕ_{e}^k, and $\vec{\eta}^k$ are the temporal discretizations of V_{m}, ϕ_{e}, and $\vec{\eta}$, respectively, at the time instant of $k\Delta t$. In the case of a fine mesh, when the integration time step has to be reduced below the time step limit imposed by the ODE solver, it is advantageous to employ the more expensive semi-implicit Crank-Nicholson scheme instead of the forward Euler to solve the parabolic PDE:

$$\left[1 + \frac{1}{2}\Delta t A_{\mathrm{i}}\right] V^{k+1} = \left[1 - \frac{1}{2}\Delta t A_{\mathrm{i}}\right] V^k - \Delta t A_{\mathrm{e}}\phi_{\mathrm{e}}^k + I_{\mathrm{ion}}\left(V_{\mathrm{m}}^k, \vec{\eta}^k\right), \qquad (15)$$

thus replacing (11) and (12).

Typically, additional Dirichlet boundary conditions have to be enforced for the elliptic PDE, which is a singular system otherwise. This is usually achieved by adding a grounding electrode (i.e., choosing nodes in the mesh where ϕ_{e} is set to zero). With some iterative solver techniques, for instance, Krylov subspace methods such as conjugated gradients (CG), this is not necessarily required.[29]

Linear Solvers

Although the PDEs are solved most efficiently with direct methods, this is possible for small grids only;[26,30] otherwise memory demands increase quickly, which, in turn, significantly increases the required number of operations per solver step. Although direct methods have been implemented to run in parallel environments,[31,32] typically they are harder to parallelize due to the fine-grained parallelism, which is communication intense. For large systems, iterative methods are required.

When executing bidomain simulations on sequential computers, the main computational burden can be attributed to the solution of the elliptic problem and the set of ODEs. Typically, with simple ionic models, the elliptic problem contributes more than 90% to the overall workload, whereas with recent ionic models involving very stiff ODEs,[33,34] the ODE solution may even begin to dominate the computations. The parabolic problem is typically less of a concern. On coarser meshes, where time steps are limited by the ODEs, simple forward Euler steps can be employed to update V_{m}. In this case, the contributions of the diffusional component (PDE) and the local membrane component to changes in V_m can be updated separately, which renders the PDE linear. On finer grids, semi-implicit Crank-Nicholson schemes perform well. Even when relatively cheap iterative solvers are employed, the parabolic portion can be updated efficiently due to the diagonal dominance of the linear system.

For large systems, on the order of several hundreds of thousands of unknowns, parallel computing approaches are necessary to reduce execution times. The parallel computing context alleviates the problem of solving the set of ODEs. State variables in an ionic model do not diffuse, which qualifies the ODEs as an embarrassingly parallel problem. No communication between processors is required to update the state variables, and thus the parallel scaling of the ODE portion is linear. The parabolic problem is efficiently solved in parallel as well. Either only a forward Euler step is required (essentially a matrix-vector product for which good scalability is expected), or the well-posed diagonally dominant linear system is solved efficiently with relatively cheap iterative methods, such as the preconditioned CG. Typically, with an incomplete LU (ILU) preconditioner for the iterative CG solver, the parabolic problem can be solved in less than ten iterations.

The elliptic PDE is the most challenging problem. Standard iterative solvers such as ILU-CG typically require several hundreds of iterations to converge (Fig. 1a), which makes this solution significantly more expensive than that of the parabolic system, although both systems share the same sparsity pattern. The parallel scaling of standard iterative solvers is fairly good.[30] For instance, a parallel ILU-CG solver, where the system is decomposed by a Block Jacobi preconditioner with ILU(0) (i.e., an incomplete LU factorization with zero fill-in levels that preserves the sparsity pattern of the original matrix), used as a subblock preconditioner, exhibits good parallel scaling (Fig. 1b).[30] With fewer number of processors, ILU(N) with N levels of fill-in tends to be more efficient; however, with an increasing number of processors, the efficiency of the preconditioning deteriorates since the preconditioner is applied to the main diagonal block only (Fig. 1d). Employing overlapping block preconditioners such as additive Schwarz methods can circumvent this; however, they increase the communication burden, which, depending on the particular hardware, may be undesirable.

It has been demonstrated in several recent studies that multilevel preconditioners for CG methods both significantly improve the overall performance (Fig. 1c) and show reasonable parallel efficiency (better than 80%) for up to 128 processors.[30,35,36] A generally applicable algebraic multigrid preconditioner (AMG) in conjunction with an iterative Krylov solver reduces the number of iterations per solver step by almost two orders of magnitude compared to ILU-CG (Fig. 1a). Although a single iteration with AMG is significantly more expensive than with ILU, the reduction in number of iterations clearly favors a multilevel approach. In Plank et al.,[30] a speedup of six was reported (Fig. 1c). Using AMG-CG is, to date, the most efficient method for solving the elliptic portion of the bidomain equations. The method is particularly well suited for defibrillation studies since it is computationally efficient and handles unstructured grids straightforwardly.

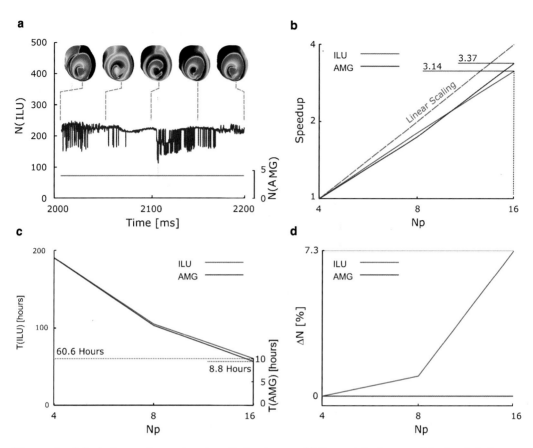

Figure 1: (**a**) A figure-8 reentrant activity in a rabbit ventricular model simulated over 200 ms employing either incomplete LU (ILU) or algebraic multigrid (AMG) preconditioner with an iterative conjugated gradient (CG) solver to compute the solution of the elliptic portion of the bidomain equations. The number of iterations per solver step needed to achieve convergence, N, was measured at each time step. A large variation in N as a function of $-\nabla \cdot \bar{\sigma}_i \nabla V_m$ was observed with the ILU preconditioner (with min/mean/max N of 137/201/377), whereas with the AMG preconditioner, N remained constant and equal to 4 for all time steps. (**b**) Scaling with the two preconditioners. The execution times were reduced by factors of 3.37 and 3.14 for AMG and ILU, respectively, when the number of processors, N_p, was increased from 4 to 16. (**c**) Decrease in execution time with increasing N_p for both methods. Although the trend is similar for both preconditioners, AMG outperformed the ILU preconditioner at least by a factor of 6 (note the differences in time scales at the left and right vertical axes). With 16 processors execution time was 60.6 h with ILU versus 8.8 with AMG. (**d**) Increasing N_p increased the number of iterations N by about 7.3% when using ILU preconditioning, whereas the efficiency of the AMG preconditioner was unaffected by parallelization. (Images are based on figures published in Plank et al.)[30]

Models of the Heart in Vulnerability and Defibrillation Studies

This section provides an overview of the remainder of the modeling tools used in bidomain studies of defibrillation.

Description of Myocardial Geometry and Fiber Architecture

The 3D organ-level simulations of defibrillation have used Vetter and McCulloch's[37] 3D model of anatomically based rabbit ventricular geometry and fiber orientation. The original geometry was defined in prolate spheroidal coordinates, which were then translated into Cartesian. MSC Patran (MSC-Software Corporation) was used to generate the computational grids. The surfaces and the "solids" of the mesh were created with Patran functions. Additional "solids" were generated to represent the ventricular cavities and the perfusing bath; the conductivity of these regions was assigned the value of blood. Using Patran, surfaces and solids were meshed to create unstructured triangular and tetrahedral meshes, respectively, with an average element edge length of 300–500 µm in the tissue and 1 mm in cavities and perfusing bath. Once the entire mesh was complete, files containing node coordinates, elemental connectivity, and the original finite element to which each tetrahedral element in the new mesh belongs, were generated. This information was then used to determine, with the combination of two multidimensional root-finding algorithms, fiber orientation at the centroid of each tetrahedron. Local material properties were assigned to each element using the fiber orientations. Fig. 2 illustrates the 3D geometry and fiber orientation in the rabbit ventricles as determined by this algorithm.

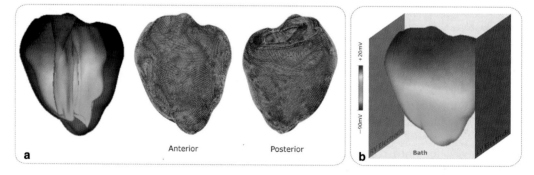

Figure 2: (a) Geometry (semitransparent rendering) and posterior and anterior views of epicardial fiber orientation (*short white lines*) in the rabbit ventricular model. (b) Configuration of the perfusing chamber (3.92 cm wide) and shock electrodes. The ventricles are paced at the apex, and the colors represent the distribution of transmembrane voltage during a paced beat

Representation of Ionic Currents and Membrane Electroporation

As already discussed above, for defibrillation studies, all membrane models need to be modified to ensure stability during the shock, when a dramatic change in transmembrane potential takes place.[24] It is important to understand, however, that defibrillation shocks induce complex changes in transmembrane potential, some of which have been consistently observed in experiments, but never reproduced by membrane models. Some of these observed phenomena are listed below. First, strong shocks applied during action potential plateau in isolated guinea pig papillary muscle,[38] cultured neonatal rat myocyte strands,[39] and isolated guinea pig myocytes[23] induce asymmetrical changes in transmembrane potential, V_m, with the negative transmembrane potential change, ΔV_m, being larger than the positive (i.e., $\Delta V_m^- > \Delta V_m^+$). Second, with increase in shock strength, ΔV_m magnitude does not increase proportionally but instead saturates.[38,39] Third, for large shock strengths ΔV_m^- exhibits non-monotonic behavior with initial rapid increase and then a decrease.[23,39] None of the available membrane models reproduce these responses to strong shocks, necessitating modifications in the available membrane models.

Using a recent version of the Luo-Rudy dynamic (LRd) model, Faber and Rudy[40] found that the negative bias in ΔV_m asymmetry could not be reproduced by the natural addition of electroporation (model LRd + EP), the latter documented to always take place following strong shocks.[41] Only when the outward current activated upon strong shock-induced depolarization was incorporated, I_a, first suggested by Cheng et al.,[23] that a match between simulation and experiment was achieved (Fig. 3), provided it was assumed that I_a was part of the K$^+$ flow through the L-type Ca$^+$-channel augmented LRd, or (aLRd model). With the use of the new aLRd model it was possible to reproduce the experimentally observed rectangularly-shaped positive ΔV_m transient, negative-to-positive ΔV_m ratio near 2,[39,42] stronger electroporation at the anode,[43] and dependence of the ΔV_m magnitude on field strength (compare Fig. 3 to Fast et al.[39] and Cheek et al.)[42] To conduct simulations with the rabbit ventricular model, similar changes were incorporated in the Puglisi-Bers ventricular myocyte ionic membrane model.[44] Being equipped with a membrane model that can accurately reproduce the membrane responses to shocks is essential to simulate tissue and organ behavior observed experimentally, and thus, to provide insight about behavior in the depth of the tissue that cannot be assessed by the current experimental techniques.

Shock Electrodes and Waveforms

In the rabbit model, shock electrodes are represented as 3D iso-current density or iso-voltage surfaces within the 3D computational grid (ventricles plus perfusing bath and blood in cavities); these are chosen to mimic geometry and location of electrodes in optical mapping experiments (far-field). The examples included in this chapter use external plate (at the boundaries of the perfusing chamber) electrodes; a right ventricle (RV) catheter and a return electrode in the posterior bath as well as cuff electrodes have also been implemented.[45,46] The shock waveforms include square waves as well as truncated-exponential (62% tilt) mono- and biphasic shocks of different polarities and durations.[47–52] All shocks were given

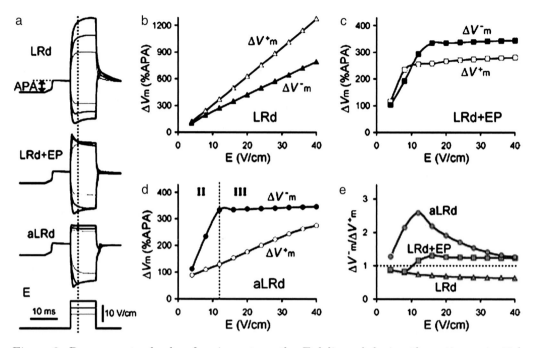

Figure 3: Responses to shocks of various strengths E delivered during the action potential plateau (coupling interval of 10 ms) in an 800 μm-long fiber. (a) Superposition of shock-induced virtual electrode polarization (VEP) at the fiber ends. Membrane kinetics is represented by the LRd, LRd with electroporation (LRd + EP), and augmented LRd (aLRd) models. Shock duration is 10 ms and strengths are 8, 12, and 16 V/cm^{-1} (*thin, thicker,* and *thickest solid lines*, respectively). APA, action potential amplitude. *Vertical dotted line* indicates time of ΔV_m (change in transmembrane potential V_m) measurement, 3 ms after shock onset. (b–d) Shock-induced positive and negative ΔV_m and ΔV_m as a function of shock strength for the three models. Characters II and III denote types of nonlinear responses, as per Fast et al.[39] (e) $\Delta V_m^-/\Delta V_m^+$ ratio as function of shock strength in the three models. (Figure modified from Ashihara and Trayanova)[25]

to ventricles paced eight to ten times at the apex of a basic cycle length of 300 ms. The shocks were administered at various coupling intervals with respect to the last paced beat.

Arrhythmia Induction with an Electric Shock and Defibrillation

The mechanisms of cardiac defibrillation have been strongly linked to cardiac vulnerability to electric shocks. A large body of research has demonstrated that an electric shock can induce ventricular arrhythmias if it is given during the "vulnerable window" within the normal cardiac cycle.[53–55] Furthermore, shocks that result in induction of arrhythmia are bound by a minimum and a maximum strength, termed the lower and upper limits of vulnerability (LLV and ULV).[56] Fabiato et al.[56] were the first to suggest that the mechanisms of ventricular fibrillation (VF) induction and termination may be similar. This suggestion is now supported by the correlation between ULV and defibrillation threshold (DFT).[57] For a defibrillation shock to succeed, it must extinguish existing VF activations throughout the myocardium (or in a critical mass of it), as well as not initiate new fibrillatory wavefronts. Extinguishing existing VF activations is not sufficient; the shock may still reinitiate VF by the mechanism it induces VF if applied during the vulnerable window. Therefore, understanding cardiac vulnerability to electric shocks is a route to understanding defibrillation and arrhythmogenesis by failed shocks. In this light, the present chapter provides a review of the application of the 3D bidomain model to the study of vulnerability to electric shocks, as published in several articles.[11,21,49,50,52,58,59] Finally, this chapter follows the direction of numerous electrical and optical mapping studies of VF induction and defibrillation: it focuses on the mechanisms that govern the responses to the shock in the normal isolated heart preparations as a necessary step in solving the riddles of clinical defibrillation.

Postshock Activity in the Ventricles

VEP Induced by the Shock in the 3D Volume of the Ventricles

Figure 4a presents VEP at the end of 4 ms-long square-wave shocks of different strengths, applied at a coupling interval of 105 ms. In each case the distributions of transmembrane voltage on the anterior epicardium and endocardium and in a transmural view of the midmyocardium are shown. VEP on the surfaces exhibits two main areas of opposite polarization: the RV epicardium, which is near the cathode, is depolarized, while the left ventricle (LV) epicardium is deexcited (postshock excitable area). A zone of intermediate voltage levels (green and yellow colored areas) is created between oppositely polarized areas; increasing shock strength reduces the width of this zone, resulting in larger spatial gradients between areas of opposite membrane polarity. These gradients act to provide the stimulus for the break excitations at shock end. In contrast to the surface VEP, transmural views present a more complex distribution of transmembrane voltage throughout the midmyocardium. In all cases, the LV free wall exhibits a wide excitable area that extends toward the base with an increase in shock strength. In contrast, the RV free wall and the septum are mostly depolarized at shock end. As determined by our simulation studies,[11,15] differences in VEP between ventricular surfaces and midmyocardium emanate from the different mechanisms that govern surface polarization and polarization in the tissue bulk and result in different postshock electrophysiological behavior on the surfaces and in depth, as demonstrated below. For weak shocks such as $1.0 \, \mathrm{V/cm^{-1}}$, the electric field is unable to reset the preshock state of the tissue, and dispersion of refractoriness in the apex-base direction, resulting from the preshock beat, can still be observed. However, with increasing shock strength, the remnants of the paced beat in the end-shock transmembrane voltage distribution disappear.

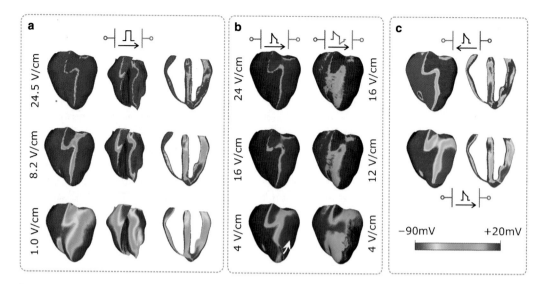

Figure 4: Transmembrane potential distribution at shock end for various shock waveforms, strengths, and polarities. Waveforms and polarities are indicated at the top of each panel. The color scale is saturated (i.e, the transmembrane potentials above 20 mV and below 90 mV appear as 20 mV and 90 mV, respectively). (a) Shocks are monophasic, 4-ms long, and of strengths shown in the figure; they are applied at a coupling interval of 105 ms. For each case, the anterior epicardium and endocardium and a transmural view of the ventricles are shown. (Images are based on figures published in Rodriguez and Trayanova)[62] (b) Truncated-exponential (62% tilt) monophasic and biphasic shocks are of 10 ms duration and of strengths shown in the figure. Biphasic shock polarity reverses at 6 ms. *White arrow* at the bottom image indicates the location and direction of initial postshock propagation. (c) Truncated-exponential monophasic shocks of reversed polarity and strength 5 V/cm^{-1}. Anterior epicardium and transmural views of the ventricles are shown. (Images are based on figures published in Rodriguez et al.)[52] The color scale is saturated (i.e, the transmembrane potential above 20 mV and below 90 mV appear as 20 mV and 90 mV, respectively)

Figure 4b compares the response of the ventricles to mono- and biphasic truncated-exponential shocks (same as those used in clinical practice) of different strengths and 10 ms duration. For the biphasic shock, VEP induced by the 6-ms-long first pulse reversed sign following the 4-ms-long second pulse. In this case transmembrane potential gradient between virtual anodes and cathodes at shock end was markedly lower than that at the end of the monophasic shock, indicating decreased likelihood that new activations will originate at the end of the shock.

The effect of polarity reversal on VEP is illustrated in Fig. 4c. For left-to-right direction of the applied field, regardless of shock strength and coupling interval of shock application, the main postshock excitable area is always within the LV wall (5 V/cm^{-1} shock episode illustrated in Fig. 4c). At shock end, the septum is either mildly or strongly positively (depending on shock strength) polarized and is not an avenue for postshock propagation. The shock-end negative polarization in the RV is a thin stripe in a thin wall; thus, the RV is not a major structure for postshock propagation (as discussed below).

Postshock Activations in the 3D Volume of the Ventricles

The inquiry into the 3D mechanisms governing shock-induced arrhythmogenesis (and thus, the failure of defibrillation) has been hampered by the inability of current experimental techniques to resolve, with sufficient accuracy, electrical behavior confined to the depth of the ventricles during and after the shock. Mapping the entire epicardial surface of the ventricles, the current state-of-the-art in optical imaging, does not reveal the global 3D activity that follows the shock since activations could propagate intramurally, without a signature on the epicardial surface. Most importantly, as discussed above, there is a dramatic difference between the magnitude and pattern of shock-induced VEP in the surface layers and in the depth of the myocardium. Such differences in VEP could result in different electrophysiological behavior on the surfaces and in depth, with midmyocardial postshock activity remaining confined to the depth of the ventricular wall and detached from surface postshock behavior for stretches of time. A major breakthrough in understanding of these mechanisms resulted from 3D bidomain simulations.

Figure 5 presents an episode of arrhythmia induction following a truncated-exponential monophasic shock of $3.2\,\mathrm{V/cm^{-1}}$ applied at a coupling interval of 96 ms. Following the shock, a transmural wave emanating from a break excitation at shock end in the region of the LV apex (where the largest gradient between shock-induced positive and negative polarization is formed) propagates toward the base through the remaining excitable area (24 and 42 ms panels). The wave returns toward the apex through the RV wall and the septum, and once tissue there has recovered (79 ms panel), it reenters, establishing a stable reentrant circuit (112 ms), with one spiral wave on the anterior (*white arrow*), and another on the posterior (not shown).

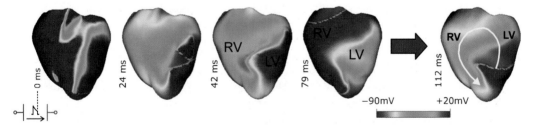

Figure 5: Evolution of shock activity from shock end until the end of the first cycle of a figure-8 reentry with the isthmus located at the apex. The shock is $3.2\,\mathrm{V/cm^{-1}}$ truncated exponential of 8-ms duration and is applied at a coupling interval of 96 ms. Transmembrane voltage distribution on the anterior epicardium is shown. The *arrow* indicates direction of propagation of the stable reentrant circuit. (Images are based on figures published in Rodriguez et al.)[58]

ULV and LLV

To determine the ULV for a given shock electrode configuration and polarity, vulnerability areas (i.e., areas on a 2D grid that encompass episodes of reentry induction for various shock strengths and coupling intervals) must be constructed. ULV is estimated from the vulnerability area as the highest shock strength that induces sustained arrhythmia. The 3D bidomain simulations have been crucial in understanding what causes the existence of ULV. As Fig. 6 illustrates, a shock succeeds in not initiating (new) reentry if elicited break excitations manage to traverse the shock-induced excitable areas in the LV before the remaining ventricles recover from shock-induced depolarization (presence of unidirectional block).[6,52,60] The episode presented in Fig. 6b top is the same as in Fig. 5, where postshock propagation takes place through the large postshock excitable area in the LV, initiating arrhythmia; this shock is thus below the ULV. The latency in the onset of a postshock activation, its propagation velocity through the excitable area, and shock-induced extension of refractoriness in the depolarized areas (which serve to block propagation) determine how quickly postshock activity subsides following successful shocks.[17,60,61] In Fig. 6a top the shock is stronger ($9.6\,\mathrm{V/cm^{-1}}$) and therefore the activation is initiated earlier than in Fig. 6b due to stronger gradients at the apex between positive and negative polarization (see 20 ms panels), and the postshock excitable area is quickly traversed; the wavefront dies out upon encountering refractory tissue in the shock-induced depolarized areas. This episode is above the ULV.

Figure 6 bottom presents episodes similar to those in Fig. 6 top; however, the shock polarity is reversed. Although the mechanisms responsible for the ULV are the same (compare panels in Fig. 6a to panels in Fig. 6b), these simulation results underscore the importance of accounting for the geometry of the ventricular chambers in the quest to understand generation of postshock arrhythmias. The difference in the thickness of the ventricular walls is ultimately manifested as a preferential location of the postshock excitable area; the postshock excitable areas are shown by these simulations[52] to be always located in the thick LV and septum, but never in the thin RV. One can speculate that identifying the location of the main postshock excitable area could be very important for improving clinical defibrillation efficacy since its eradication can be specifically targeted by auxiliary small-magnitude shocks, resulting in a dramatic decrease in defibrillation threshold. In addition, the location of the postshock excitable area determines the types of postshock reentrant circuits (compare panels in Fig. 6b). For the polarity shown in the top panel of Fig. 6, two rotors are induced, one counterclockwise and one clockwise, on the anterior and posterior sides of the ventricles, respectively, with a common pathway in the apex. In contrast, in the bottom panel, the reentrant circuit is a figure-8 on the anterior and another on the posterior with a common pathway in the LV. The pattern of the reentry is determined by the initial postshock propagation, here through the septum, resulting in subsequent activation through both free walls.

Vulnerability grids are also characterized with an LLV, the lowest shock strength below which arrhythmia is not induced. The failure to induce reentry in the paced ventricles with shocks of strength below the LLV is due to the absence of unidirectional block, which occurs in the RV (LV) free wall for the shock polarity used in Fig. 6, top (bottom) episodes. In this case (for instance $1\,\mathrm{V/cm^{-1}}$ shock; episode not shown, see Rodriguez and Trayanova),[62]

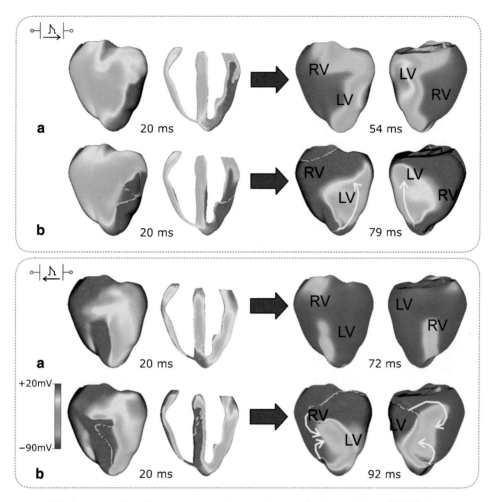

Figure 6: Mechanisms for the existence of upper limit of vulnerability (ULV) demonstrated through the evolution of postshock activity for shocks of reversed polarity (*top* and *bottom panels*). In both panels, episodes shown as (**a**) refer to responses to a shock above the ULV, while the ones shown in (**b**) refer to responses to a shock below the ULV. Anterior epicardial and transmural views of transmembrane potential distribution are shown on the *left*, whereas anterior and posterior views are rendered on the *right*. For the *top panel* polarity, the ULV is $9.6\,\text{V/cm}^{-1}$, while for the bottom panel polarity, it is $12.7\,\text{V/cm}^{-1}$. *White arrows* represent direction of propagation. (Images are based on figures published in Rodriguez et al.)[52]

shock-induced depolarization is weak, and the myocardium there is refractory only for the first few milliseconds following the shock. As a consequence of this, the wavefront initiated at the apex propagates simultaneously through both ventricular walls and the septum, depolarizing the entire heart and ultimately dying out at the base.

Shock-Induced Phase Singularities and Filaments

Initiation of shock arrhythmias is often examined in terms of the dynamics of the phase singularities, the organizing centers of reentry. The onset of a break excitation is associated with the formation of a (VEP-induced) phase singularity;[63] it forms at a point along the boundary between shock-induced depolarization and deexcitation[63,64] and is independent of the preshock state of the myocardium. If these phase singularities survive, allowing a spiraling wavefront to develop, the shock results in the (re)initiation of reentrant arrhythmia.

A phase singularity is typically observed on the ventricular surface (epicardium), since reentrant activity (spiral waves) is typically imaged there. However, in the context of the 3D geometry of the ventricles, a phase singularity represents the intersection of a scroll-wave filament, the 3D organizing center of reentry, with the ventricular surface. Clearly, 3D bidomain simulations of postshock behavior are important in elucidating the dynamics of the postshock filaments. Figure 7 presents two postshock episodes, one above the ULV (top) and one below it (bottom). In both cases, the shock induces a large number of filaments of complex geometry. At 15 ms postshock, there are fewer and smaller filaments following the stronger shock. In both cases, the number of the filaments decreases with time postshock (middle panels). In the stronger shock episode, at 95 ms, there is only one remaining filament; it is O-shaped (*black arrow*). O-filaments are unstable and collapse on themselves, such as in the case shown in the figure, leading to termination of the reentrant activity. In contrast, in the weaker shock episode, a single filament persists, causing the establishment of a sustained ventricular tachycardia. This is a U-shaped filament (a U-shaped filament is a filament, both ends of which are in contact with the same, endo- or epicardial surface), with both ends attached to the epicardium that underlies the same reentrant circuit, as shown in Fig. 5. Results from bidomain simulations have also provided important insights into how the 3D postshock reentrant circuits established soon after a failed shock can further degrade into ventricular fibrillation.[65]

Induction of Arrhythmia with Biphasic Shocks

The issue of induction of arrhythmia in a paced heart with a biphasic shock (and for that matter, failure of defibrillation with a biphasic shock) is particularly intriguing. Reversal of shock polarity during the shock has been found to improve defibrillation efficacy in both humans[66,67] and animal models,[68–71] and it is the current standard in clinical defibrillation. The mechanisms underlying the superiority of biphasic shock waveforms in achieving defibrillation success has been the subject of much debate.[70,72–74] Advancement of VEP theory for arrhythmia induction and termination offered new insights into the improved efficacy of biphasic waveforms. Studies of isolated rabbit hearts by Efimov et al.[6,64] demonstrated that the second phase of the biphasic shock reversed positive and negative polarization asymmetrically, as shown in Fig. 4b. The latter is owed to the rectification properties of the voltage-dependent ionic channels; an appropriate ("optimal") countershock[6,64,70] reverses the negative VEP while partially preserving the positive, and an overall weaker depolarization is achieved through most of the ventricles. Consequently, any phase singularities that

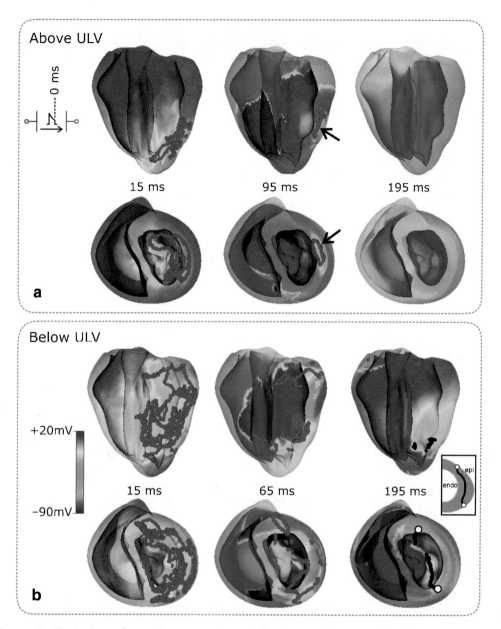

Figure 7: Evolution of postshock activity and filament dynamics for shocks above the upper limit of vulnerability (ULV) (a) and below the ULV (b). Transmembrane potential distributions are shown in anterior epicardial (*top rows* in each panel) and apex-to-base (*bottom rows* in each panel) views with the ventricles rendered semitransparent. Scroll-wave filaments are shown in *pink*, with the filament corresponding to the sustained reentrant circuit depicted in *black*. Inset in (b) shows that the filament is attached with both ends (small *white circles*) to the epicardial surface (U-shaped filament). *Black arrows* in (a) point toward the O-shaped filament. (Images are based on figures published in Arevalo et al.)[59]

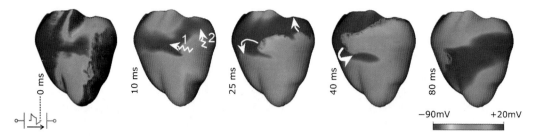

Figure 8: Induction of a postshock arrhythmia with a biphasic shock of strength $4\,\mathrm{V/cm}^{-1}$ and duration $10\,\mathrm{ms}$ ($6/4\,\mathrm{ms}$). Anterior epicardial views of transmembrane potential distribution are shown. *Zigzag arrows* 1 and 2 denote propagated graded responses. *White arrows* represent direction of propagation. (Images are based on figures published in Ashihara et al.)[77]

might be generated by the first shock phase are erased by the second. Biphasic shocks thus do not result in the formation of phase singularities at the end of the shock, which could underlie their increased efficacy.

How do biphasic shocks fail? Insight into this issue was also obtained from 3D bidomain simulations and is based on the recognition that some postshock activations could originate much later than the end of the shock. These activations were termed VEP-induced propagated graded responses[75,76] and were shown to occur in regions of intermediate VEP magnitude (green areas in the biphasic shock response shown in Fig. 4b). An example of arrhythmia induction with a $4\,\mathrm{V/cm}^{-1}$ biphasic shock (the shock strength is below the biphasic ULV) via the VEP-induced propagated graded response mechanism is shown in Fig. 8. Although the spatial gradient in transmembrane potential at the borders between oppositely polarized regions (0 ms panel) is again the stimulus that elicits the postshock activation, this activation occurs at an instant much later than shock end, when the mildly negatively polarized region repolarizes enough to "pick up" the stimulus. Thereafter, activations of low amplitude slowly propagate (*zigzag arrows*, 10-ms panel), emerging later as full-blown wavefronts (25 ms panel). The activations resulted in a transmural spiral wave, degenerating later into fibrillation.

Conclusion

The information and examples presented in this chapter regarding the development, achievements, and mechanistic insight provided by the 3D models of shock-induced arrhythmogenesis and defibrillation underscore the power of realistic modeling and simulations. Simulations are particularly useful in revealing electrical behavior hidden within the cardiac wall. Insights into vulnerability and defibrillation, such as these presented here, cannot be achieved with experimental methodology alone. When supported by experimental observations of behavior during and after the shock over the cardiac surfaces, realistic whole-organ simulations become invaluable in providing mechanistic insight. In general, such models can be successfully employed to study any aspect of arrhythmogenesis and serve as a test bed for new potential antiarrhythmia therapies.

Acknowledgments

This work was supported by NIH awards HL063195 and HL082729 (N.A.T.), by a Marie Curie Fellowship MC-OIF 040190 from the European Commission, and the SFB grant F3210-N18 from the Austrian Science Fund FWF (G.P.).

References

1. Maisel W. Pacemaker and ICD generator reliability: meta-analysis of device registries. *JAMA* 2006;295:1929–1934
2. Sepulveda NG, Roth BJ, Wikswo JP Jr. Current injection into a two-dimensional anistropic bidomain. *Biophys J* 1989;55:987–999
3. Hodgkin AL, Rushton WAH. The electrical constants of the crustacean nerve fiber. *Proc Roy Soc Lond* 1946;133:444–479
4. Wikswo JP Jr, Lin SF, Abbas RA. Virtual electrodes in cardiac tissue: a common mechanism for anodal and cathodal stimulation. *Biophys J* 1995;69:2195–2210
5. Efimov IR, Cheng Y, Biermann M, Van Wagoner DR, Mazgalev TN, Tchou PJ. Transmembrane voltage changes produced by real and virtual electrodes during monophasic defibrillation shock delivered by an implantable electrode. *J Cardiovasc Electrophys* 1997;8:1031–1045
6. Efimov IR, Gray RA, Roth BJ. Virtual electrodes and deexcitation: new insights into fibrillation induction and defibrillation. *J Cardiovasc Electrophys* 2000;11:339–353
7. Knisley SB, Trayanova NA, Aguel F. Roles of electric field and fiber structure in cardiac electric stimulation. *Biophys J* 1999;77:1404–1417
8. Evans FG, Ideker RE, Gray RA. Effect of shock-induced changes in transmembrane potential on reentrant waves and outcome during cardioversion of isolated rabbit hearts. *J Cardiovasc Electrophysiol* 2002;13:1118–1127
9. Efimov IR, Aguel F, Cheng Y, Wollenzier B, Trayanova NA. Virtual electrode polarization in the far field: implications for external defibrillation. *Am J Physiol* 2000;279:H1055–H1070
10. Sobie EA, Susil RC, Tung L. A generalized activating function for predicting virtual electrodes in cardiac tissue. *Biophys J* 1997;73:1410–1423
11. Trayanova NA, Skouibine K, Aguel F. The role of cardiac tissue structure in defibrillation. *Chaos* 1998;8:221–233
12. Trayanova NA. Far-field stimulation of cardiac tissue. *Herzschrittmacher Ther Electrophys* 1999;10:137–148
13. Fast VG, Sharifov OF, Cheek ER, Newton JC, Ideker RE. Intramural virtual electrodes during defibrillation shocks in left ventricular wall assessed by optical mapping of membrane potential. *Circulation* 2002;106:1007–1014

14. Trayanova NA. Concepts of defibrillation. *Phil Trans Roy Soc Lond A* 2001;359:1327–1337

15. Entcheva E, Trayanova NA, Claydon F. Patterns of and mechanisms for shock-induced polarization in the heart: a bidomain analysis. *IEEE Trans Biomed Eng* 1999;46:260–270

16. Roth BJ. A mathematical model of make and break electrical stimulation of cardiac tissue by a unipolar anode or cathode. *IEEE Trans Biomed Eng* 1995;42:1174–1184

17. Cheng Y, Mowrey KA, Van Wagoner DR, Tchou PJ, Efimov IR. Virtual electrode induced re-excitation: a mechanism of defibrillation. *Circ Res* 1999;85:1056–1066

18. Plonsey R. Bioelectric sources arising in excitable fibers (ALZA lecture). *Ann Biomed Eng* 1988;16:519–546

19. Hooke N, Henriquez CS, Lanzkron P, Rose D. Linear algebraic transformations of the bidomain equations: implications for numerical methods. *Math Biosci* 1994;120:127–145

20. Pollard AE, Hooke N, Henriquez CS. Cardiac propagation simulation. *Crit Rev Biomed Eng* 1992;20:171–210

21. Aguel F, DeBruin KA, Krassowska W, Trayanova NA. Effects of electroporation on the transmembrane potential distribution in a two-dimensional bidomain model of cardiac tissue. *J Cardiovasc Electrophys* 1999;10:701–714

22. DeBruin KA, Krassowska W. Electroporation and shock-induced transmembrane potential in a cardiac fiber during defibrillation strength shocks. *Ann Biomed Eng* 1998;26:584–596

23. Cheng DKL, Tung L, Sobie EA. Nonuniform responses of transmembrane potential during electric field stimulation of single cardiac cells. *Am J Physiol* 1999;277:H351–H362

24. Skouibine K, Trayanova NA, Moore PK. A numerically efficient model for simulation of defibrillation in an active bidomain sheet of myocardium. *Math Biosci* 2000;166:85–100

25. Ashihara T, Trayanova N. Asymmetry in membrane responses to electrical shocks: insight from bidomain simulations. *Biophys J* 2004;87:2271–2282

26. Vigmond EJ, Aguel F, Trayanova NA. Computationally efficient methods for solving the bidomain equations in 3D. In: *Engineering in Medicine and Biology Society, Proceedings of the 23rd Annual Conference of the IEEE/EMBS*; Vol 1. 2001:348–351

27. Keener JP, Bogar K. A numerical method for the solution of the bidomain equations in cardiac tissue. *Chaos* 1998;8:234–241

28. Pennacchio M, Simoncini V. Efficient algebraic solution of reaction-diffusion systems for the cardiac excitation process. *J Comp Appl Math* 2002;145:49–70

29. Potse M, Dube B, Richer J, Vinet A, Gulrajani RM. A comparison of monodomain and bidomain reaction-diffusion models for action potential propagation in the human heart. *IEEE Trans Biomed Eng* 2006;53:2425–2435

30. Plank G, Liebmann M, Weber dos Santos R, Vigmond EJ, Haase G. Algebraic Multigrid Preconditioner for the Cardiac Bidomain Model. *IEEE Trans Biomed Eng* 2007;54:585–596

31. Li X, Demmel J. SuperLU DIST: a scalable distributed-memory sparse direct solver for unsymmetric linear systems. *ACM Trans Math Softw TOMS* 2003;29:110–140

32. Amestoy P, Duff IS, L'Excellent JY, Koster J. Mumps: a general purpose distributed memory sparse solver. In: *PARA '00: Proceedings of the 5th International Workshop on Applied Parallel Computing, New Paradigms for HPC in Industry and Academia.* London: Springer; 2001:121–130

33. Iyer V, Mazhari R, Winslow RL. A computational model of the human left-ventricular epicardial myocyte. *Biophys J* 2004;87:1507–1525

34. Cortassa S, Aon MA, O'Rourke B, Jacques R, Tseng HJ, Marban E, Winslow RL. A computational model integrating electrophysiology, contraction, and mitochondrial bioenergetics in the ventricular myocyte. *Biophys J* 2006;91:1564–1589

35. Weber dos Santos R, Plank G, Bauer S, Vigmond E. Parallel multigrid preconditioner for the cardiac bidomain model. *IEEE Trans Biomed Eng* 2004;51:1960–1968

36. Austin TM, Trew ML, Pullan AJ. Solving the cardiac bidomain equations for discontinuous conductivities. *IEEE Trans Biomed Eng* 2006;53:1265–1272

37. Vetter FJ, McCulloch AD. Three-dimensional analysis of regional cardiac function: a model of rabbit ventricular anatomy. *Prog Biophys Mol Biol* 1998;69:157–183

38. Zhou X, Rollins DL, Smith WM, Ideker RE. Responses of the transmembrane potential of myocardial cells during a shock. *J Cardiovasc Electrophysiol* 1995;6:252–263

39. Fast VG, Rohr S, Ideker RE. Nonlinear changes of transmembrane potential caused by defibrillation shocks in strands of cultured myocytes. *Am J Physiol* 2000;278:H688–H697

40. Faber GM, Rudy Y. Action potential and contractility changes in $[Na^+]_i$ over-loaded cardiac myocytes: a simulation study. *Biophys J* 2000;78:2392–2404

41. Al-Khadra AS, Nikoloski V, Efimov IR. The role of electroporation in defibrillation. *Circ Res* 2000;87:797–804

42. Cheek ER, Ideker RE, Fast VG. Nonlinear changes of transmembrane potential during defibrillation shocks: role of Ca2+ current. *Circ Res* 2000;87:453–459

43. Cheek ER, Fast VG. Nonlinear changes of transmembrane potential during electrical shocks: role of membrane electroporation. *Circ Res* 2004;94:208–214

44. Puglisi JL, Bers DM. LabHEART: an interactive computer model of rabbit ventricular myocyte ion channels and Ca transport. *Am J Physiol* 2001;281:C2049–C2060

45. Trayanova NA, Eason JC, Aguel F. Computer simulations of cardiac defibrillation: a look inside the heart. *Comput Vis Sci* 2002;4:259–270

46. Constantino J, Blake R, Marshall M, Trayanova N. Decreasing LV postshock excitable gap lowers the upper limit of vulnerability. *Heart Rhythm* 2006;3:S225–S226

47. Trayanova NA, Bray MA. Membrane refractoriness and excitation induced in cardiac fibers by monophasic and biphasic shocks. *J Cardiovasc Electrophysiol* 1997;8:745–757

48. Anderson C, Trayanova NA, Skouibine K. Termination of spiral waves with biphasic shocks: the role of virtual electrode polarization. *J Cardiovasc Electrophysiol* 2000;11:1386–1396

49. Anderson C, Trayanova NA. Success and failure of biphasic shocks: results of bidomain simulations. *Math Biosci* 2001;174:91–109

50. Rodriguez B, Tice BM, Eason JC, Aguel F, Ferrero JM Jr, Trayanova N. Effect of acute global ischemia on the upper limit of vulnerability: a simulation study. *Am J Physiol* 2004;286:H2078–H2088

51. Rodriguez B, Tice B, Eason J, Aguel F, Trayanova N. Cardiac vulnerability to electric shocks during phase 1 a of acute global ischemia. *Heart Rhythm* 2004;6:695–703

52. Rodriguez B, Li L, Eason JC, Efimov IR, Trayanova N. Differences between left and right ventricular chamber geometry affect cardiac vulnerability to electric shocks. *Circ Res* 2005;97:168–175

53. Wiggers CJ. Studies of ventricular fibrillation caused by electric shock: cinematographic and electrocardiographic observations of the natural process in the dog's heart: its inhibition by potassium and the revival of coordinated beats by calcium. *Am J Physiol* 1930;5:351–365

54. King BG. The effect of electric shock on heart action with special reference to varying susceptibility in different parts of the cardiac cycle. Ph.D. thesis, Columbia University; 1934

55. Moe GK, Harris AS, Wiggers CJ. Analysis of the initiation of fibrillation by electrographic studies. *Am J Physiol* 1941;134:473–492

56. Fabiato A, Coumel P, Gourgon R, Saumont R. Le seuil de rponse synchrone des fibres myocardiques. Application la comparaison exprimentale de l'efficacit des diffrentes formes de chocs lectriques de dfibrillation. *Arch Mal Cur* 1967;60:527–544

57. Chen PS, Shibata N, Dixon EG, Martin RO, Ideker RE. Comparison of the defibrillation threshold and the upper limit of ventricular vulnerability. *Circulation* 1986;73:1022–1028

58. Rodriguez B, Eason JC, Trayanova N. Differences between left and right ventricular anatomy determine the types of reentrant circuits induced by an external electric shock. A rabbit heart simulation study. *Prog Biophys Mol Biol* 2006;90:399–413

59. Arevalo H, Rodriguez B, Trayanova N. Arrhythmogenesis in the heart: multiscale modeling of the effects of defibrillation shocks and the role of electrophysiological heterogeneity. *Chaos* 2007;17:015103

60. Skouibine K, Trayanova NA, Moore P. Success and failure of the defibrillation shock: insights from a simulation study. *J Cardiovasc Electrophysiol* 2000;11:785–796

61. Trayanova NA, Eason JC, Anderson C, Aguel F. Computer modeling of defibrillation II: why does the shock fail? In: Cabo C, Rosenbaum D, eds. *Quantitative Cardiac Electrophysiology.* New York: Marcel Dekker; 2002:235

62. Rodriguez B, Trayanova N. Upper limit of vulnerability in a defibrillation model of the rabbit ventricles. *J Electrocardiol* 2003;36[Suppl]:51–56

63. Efimov IR, Cheng Y, Van Wagoner DR, Mazgalev TN, Tchou PJ. Virtual electrode-induced phase singularity: a basic mechanism of defibrillation failure. *Circ Res* 1998;82:918–925

64. Efimov IR, Cheng Y, Yamanouchi Y, Tchou PJ. Direct evidence of the role of virtual electrode-induced phase singularity in success and failure of defibrillation. *J Cardiovasc Electrophysiol* 2000;11:861–868

65. Trayanova N, Aguel F, Larson C, Haro C. Modeling cardiac defibrillation: an inquiry into post-shock dynamics. In: Zipes D, Jalife J, eds. *Cardiac Electrophysiology: From Cell to Bedside*, 4th ed. Philadelphia: WB Saunders; 2004:282–291

66. Bardy GH, Ivey TD, Allen MD, Johnson G, Mehra R, Greene HL. A prospective randomized evaluation of biphasic versus monophasic waveform pulses on defibrillation efficacy in humans. *J Am Coll Cardiol* 1989;14:728–733

67. Saksena S, An H, Mehra R, DeGroot P, Krol RB, Burkhardt E, Mehta D, John T. Prospective comparison of biphasic and monophasic shocks for implantable cardioverter-defibrillators using endocardial leads. *Am J Cardiol* 1992;70:304–310

68. Chapman PD, Wetherbee JN, Vetter JW, Troup P, Souza J. Strength-duration curves of fixed pulse width variable tilt truncated exponential waveforms for nonthoracotomy internal defibrillation in dogs. *Pacing Clin Electrophysiol* 1988;11:1045–1050

69. Dixon EG, Tang ASL, Wolf PD, Meador JT, Fine MJ, Calfee RV, Ideker RE. Improved defibrillation thresholds with large contoured epicardial electrodes and biphasic waveforms. *Circulation* 1987;76:1176–1184

70. Feeser SA, Tang ASL, Kavanagh KM, Rollins DL, Smith WM, Wolf PD, Ideker RE. Strength-duration and probability of success curves for defibrillation with biphasic waveforms. *Circulation* 1990;82:2128–2141

71. Kavanagh KM, Tang ASL, Rollins DL, Smith WM, Ideker RE. Comparison of the internal defibrillation thresholds for monophasic and double and single capacitor biphasic waveforms. *J Am Coll Cardiol* 1989;14:1343–1349

72. Schuder JC, Gold JH, Stoeckle H, McDaniel WC, Cheung KN. Transthoracic ventricular defibrillation in the 100 kg calf with symmetrical one-cycle bidirectional rectangular wave stimuli. *IEEE Trans Biomed Eng* 1983;30:415–422

73. Tang ASL, Yabe S, Wharton JM, Dolker M, Smith WM, Ideker RE. Ventricular defibrillation using biphasic waveforms: the importance of phasic duration. *J Am Coll Cardiol* 1989;13:201–214

74. Kroll MW. A minimal model of the single capacitor biphasic defibrillation waveform. *Pacing Clin Electrophysiol* 1994;17:1782–1792

75. Bourn DW, Trayanova NA, Gray RA. Shock-induced arrhythmogenesis and iso-electric window. *Pacing Clin Electrophysiol* 2002;25(Pt II):604

76. Bourn DW, Gray RA, Trayanova NA. Characterization of the relationship between preshock state and virtual electrode polarization-induced propagated graded responses resulting in arrhythmia induction. *Heart Rhythm* 2006;3:583–595

77. Ashihara T, Constantino J, Trayanova NA. Tunnel propagation of postshock activations as a hypothesis for fibrillation induction and isoelectric window. *Circ Res* 2008;102:737–745, 2008

Chapter 2.3

The Generalized Activating Function

Leslie Tung

Introduction

Insight into the biophysical processes associated with electrical stimulation of the heart is important for the understanding of electrical pacing and defibrillation. When electrodes are physically placed on the myocardium, not only do they induce polarization changes in the cell membrane in regions in proximity to the electrodes, but they also induce polarization changes remote to the electrodes. How applied electrical currents are transduced into changes in cellular transmembrane potentials has been called the "missing link,"[1] and many mechanisms have been proposed, including the so-called sawtooth pattern arising from discontinuities in fiber conductivity,[2] "dog-bone" pattern arising from the anisotropic bidomain properties of cardiac tissue,[3] surface polarization,[4] fiber curvature,[4] fiber rotation,[5] and heterogeneities in intracellular volume fraction[6] (also see reviews[7–9] that describe the similarities among nerve, brain, and cardiac stimulation). More recently, studies of cardiac cell cultures grown in user-designed patterns[10] have permitted detailed investigations of electric field-induced responses of linear strands,[11] intercellular cleft spaces,[12] fiber branches, expansions and bends,[13] and curved fibers.[14]

The concept of the activating function was proposed by Rattay[15] for electrical excitation of unmyelinated nerve axons (based on earlier ground-breaking work by McNeal[16] on myelinated axons), where a nerve fiber is stimulated by an externally applied electric field. The electric field generates a gradient of electrical potential in space, which is impressed upon the outer surface of the axon. Depending on the distribution of potential, an electromotive force can arise across the surface membrane that causes the flow of membrane current, which in turn perturbs the transmembrane potential. The details of this process are most easily understood for the case of a one-dimensional fiber lying in a three-dimensional volume conductor, as described in the next section. The definition of the activating function will then be generalized for cardiac tissue, followed by examination of the generalized activating function for a number of examples.

Department of Biomedical Engineering, School of Medicine, The Johns Hopkins University, Baltimore, MD 21205, USA, ltung@jhu.edu

I. R. Efimov et al. (eds.), *Cardiac Bioelectric Therapy: Mechanisms and Practical Implications.*
© Springer Science+Business Media, LLC 2009

The Activating Function

In a seminal analysis of external stimulation of unmyelinated nerve axons, Rattay[15] advanced the idea of an activating function that determines the excitation of the axon. In a slight modification of his original work, the nerve fiber can be represented as a cylindrical, one-dimensional cable located a distance z_0 beneath the surface of a semi-infinite three-dimensional slab of tissue (Fig. 1a). An electrode (cathode) is placed on the surface, and its location is defined as the origin of the coordinate system.

The electrical representation for the fiber is shown in Fig. 1b. Unlike the conventional form of the core-conductor model used to describe a one-dimensional fiber lying in one-dimensional space,[17] the extracellular potential Φ_e for the one-dimensional fiber lying in three-dimensional space is considered to be *imposed* and is an *input* forcing function that produces a change in transmembrane potential, v_m. Thus, as derived in the Appendix,

$$I_{ion} + C_m \frac{\partial v_m}{\partial t} - \frac{1}{r_i} \frac{\partial^2 v_m}{\partial x^2} = \frac{1}{r_i} f, \tag{1}$$

where f is the activating function,[15] defined to be

$$f(x,t) = \frac{\partial^2 \Phi_e}{\partial x^2} = -\frac{\partial}{\partial x} E_x, \tag{2}$$

and the electric field E_x is the negative gradient of Φ_e. Thus, gradients in extracellular electric field (second derivatives of extracellular potential) directed along the axis of the fiber act as virtual sources that drive the electrical cable. Apart from its mathematical definition as a source, the activating function also gives insight into the initial polarization pattern of the fiber.[18] This is because prior to the onset of the stimulus, v_m, its spatial derivatives, and I_{ion} are zero. Thus, (1) reduces to

$$C_m \frac{\partial v_m}{\partial t} = \frac{1}{r_i} f. \tag{3}$$

Hence, the polarity of the initial response of the fiber follows that of f.

For the fiber located a distance z_0 from the point electrode as shown in Fig. 1a, it is readily seen that the equipotential lines are not uniformly parallel to the fiber axis. This implies that there exists a gradient in electric field along the fiber axis, and a nonzero activating function will develop. Φ_e and f are plotted in Fig. 1c for the case where $z_0 = \lambda$ (the fiber space constant), and their mathematical expressions are given in the Appendix. Directly under the cathode in the region $|x| < \sqrt{2}\lambda/2$, the activating function is greater than 0 (and can be called a virtual cathode), which from (3) leads to membrane depolarization and activation, whereas outside this region the activating function is less than 0 (a virtual anode), leading to membrane hyperpolarization. Figure 1d shows the response h of the fiber to an intracellular point source of current applied at $x = 0$, and thus the v_m response of the fiber (Fig. 1e) to f is the convolution of f and h (see the Appendix). As with f, v_m is positive and decays with distance along x in the region directly under the electrode (neighborhood of $x = 0$), similar to the response of a one-dimensional core-conductor model to an extracellular cathode or intracellular anode (Fig. 1d).[17] However, in contrast to the one-dimensional

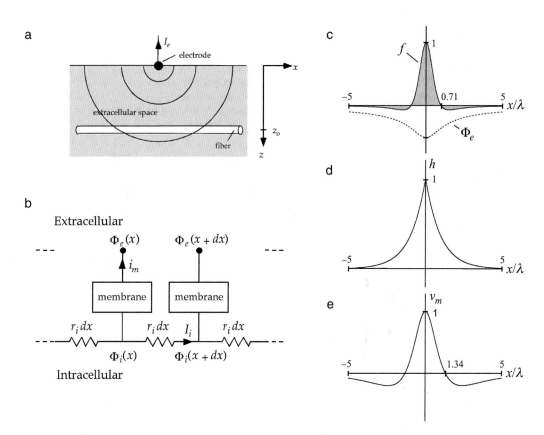

Figure 1: Point stimulation of a one-dimensional fiber lying in a semi-infinite, three-dimensional volume conductor. (**a**) Schematic of electrode location with respect to fiber. Equipotential surfaces are indicated by the *circular lines*. (**b**) Equivalent circuit for fiber membrane. The extracellular potential Φ_e is imposed on the fiber by the potential gradient in the volume conductor. This acts to drive current i_m across the cell membrane and I_i along the intracellular pathway, resulting in a gradient in Φ_i, which if not matched to the gradient in Φ_e produces a gradient in transmembrane potential $v_m (= \Phi_i - \Phi_e)$. Intracellular resistance r_i is assumed to be constant in this situation. (**c**) Plot of Φ_e (*dashed line*) on the fiber surface and of the activating function f (*solid line*), equal to the second spatial derivative of Φ_e. The function f has been normalized to its maximum value. When the point electrode is a cathode (as is the case here), the activating function has a positive value (virtual cathode) in the center flanked by negative values (virtual anodes) on either side. (**d**) Plot of h, the steady-state v_m response to an intracellular point source of current at $x = 0$, normalized to its maximum value. (**e**) Convolution of f and h, giving the steady-state v_m response to the stimulus current of (**a**). The v_m response has been normalized to its maximum value

core-conductor model, there exist side lobes of opposite polarity (membrane hyperpolarization) that are generated by the virtual anodes shown in Fig. 1c. These lobes may be significant during stimulation with a physical cathode because they can cause conduction block of the electrical impulse. Conversely, during stimulation with an extracellular anode, the side lobes become positive in sign and at sufficiently large intensities can lead to fiber excitation. In the cardiac literature, the regions of opposite polarity were initially described by Hoshi and Matsuda[19] and Bonke.[20]

The Generalized Activating Function

One of the fundamental differences between cardiac muscle and nerve fibers is that heart cells are electrically interconnected by low resistance gap junctions, which result in a tissue that behaves as an integrated syncytium. Thus, electrical propagation can occur parallel and also perpendicular to the cardiac fiber direction. Tissue responses to electrical stimuli are no longer adequately described by one-dimensional fiber responses, but rather, by the bidomain model, which describes current flow in the intracellular space, extracellular space, and the cell membrane, together with three potentials defined at every point in space: Φ_i, Φ_e, and v_m.[21] Generalization of (1) to three dimensions using the bidomain model (see Appendix) results in

$$\beta \left(I_{ion} + C_m \frac{\partial v_m}{\partial t} \right) - \nabla \cdot (\mathbf{G}_i \nabla v_m) = S, \tag{4}$$

where β is the membrane surface-to-volume ratio, $\mathbf{G}_i$ is the intracellular conductivity tensor relating currents in the x-, y-, and z-directions to the potential gradients along those directions, and S is the generalized activating function[*]

$$S = \nabla \cdot (\mathbf{G}_i \nabla \Phi_e). \tag{5}$$

Note that unlike the original formulation of the activating function f, tissue properties (i.e., $\mathbf{G}_i$) are incorporated into S, because these are just as important in generating virtual electrode effects as are gradients in electric field.

Equation (5) can be interpreted as follows. First, $\mathbf{G}_i$ consists of the intracellular conductivities along the three orthogonal axes of a tissue having orthotropic anisotropy, adjusted for fiber angle in the tissue (see the Appendix). Second, S can be rewritten as the sum of two components (see the Appendix) that take the general form,

$$S = \sum_k (\text{gradients of intracellular conductance})(\text{gradients of } \Phi_e)$$

$$+ \sum_k (\text{intracellular conductances})(\text{second derivatives of } \Phi_e) \tag{6}$$

---

[*] The term generalized activating function has also been used by Rattay[22] to describe an activating function for neurons that incorporate fiber diameter, intracellular resistance, and membrane capacitance together with the second derivative of extracellular surface potential along the fiber axis.

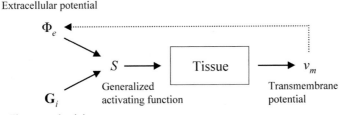

Figure 2: Schematic showing the relationships among Φ_e, $\mathbf{G}_i$, S, and v_m. See text for description

or alternatively,

$$S = \sum_k (\text{gradients of intracellular conductance})(\text{components of applied field})$$

$$+ \sum_k (\text{intracellular conductances})(\text{gradients of applied field}), \tag{7}$$

where the gradient of Φ_e is taken to be the applied field, and the index k in the sums is varied over the three orthogonal directions. Equation (7) tells us that sources can result either from the extracellular field weighted by spatial gradients of intracellular conductivity (the first term), or by spatial gradients of the extracellular field weighted by the intracellular conductivities (the second term). Thus, in the absence of spatial variations in intracellular conductivity, a uniform field cannot excite the tissue.

The relationships among Φ_e, $\mathbf{G}_i$, S, and v_m are summarized in Fig. 2. S, the generalized activating function, is the stimulus source that acts on the tissue to produce changes in transmembrane potential v_m. S is determined by the spatial distributions of extracellular potential, Φ_e, and intracellular conductivities, $\mathbf{G}_i$. According to (5), the generalized activating function depends on the actual spatial profile of the extracellular potential, which may differ somewhat from that associated with the applied field. For example, the presence of the cardiac fibers will perturb the applied electric field, but because their diameters are small compared with the typical distance to the electrode, this effect is relatively minor.[23] More significantly, the extracellular potential distribution will be perturbed by the transmembrane currents that flow in response to the developing v_m (dashed pathway in Fig. 2). Thus, the actual profile of Φ_e (and thus, S and v_m) should take into account the influence of v_m on Φ_e, whereas with the concept of the generalized activating function, Φ_e is assumed to be known, and an approximate solution for v_m is obtained by disregarding the dashed path of Fig. 2. Because the accuracy of the approximate solution is a critical issue in the use of the generalized activation function, the spatial profiles of v_m for both the exact and approximate solutions will be compared in some of the examples that follow.

Examples

For simplicity, the examples that will be discussed are two dimensional, which retains the salient features of the generalized activating function. The first example (Fig. 3) is the well-documented "dog-bone" shape of polarization that is produced by a point electrode applied to the surface of cardiac tissue.[3] The intracellular domain has been assumed to have a conductivity ten times greater in the longitudinal direction (x axis) than in the transverse direction (y axis), whereas the extracellular domain has been assumed to have equal longitudinal and transverse conductivities.[†] This situation of differing anisotropy in the intracellular and extracellular domains is referred to as unequal anisotropy. Because of symmetry about the origin, only one quadrant of the tissue is shown. Isovalue contours of S (Fig. 3a) show positive values (which have been called the virtual cathode)[‡] in a dog-bone shape along the y axis, flanked by negative values (the virtual anode) on the x axis. Figure 3b shows the response of the tissue to a unitary current injected at the origin (the impulse response of the system, h), which decays with distance from the origin and thus, resembles a low-pass spatial filter as was the case in Fig. 1d for the one-dimensional fiber. Because in this example the tissue is homogeneous (spatially invariant in its properties), h is shift-invariant, and therefore v_m at any location is given by the convolution of the generalized activating function with the impulse response.[24] Figure 3c shows that v_m is qualitatively similar to S, but with isopotential contours that are less tightly clustered about the origin, as expected if v_m is a spatially low-pass version of S. The contour lines in the transverse (y-) direction exhibit the characteristic dog-bone shape.

The concepts embodied in the unequally anisotropic case of Fig. 3 can be extended to the case of isotropic tissue (Fig. 4) and lends a novel perspective into the v_m response. The conditions are the same as in Fig. 3, except that the intracellular conductances now have the same value in the longitudinal and transverse directions. The generalized activating function is shown in Fig. 4a and b, broken down into its x and y components. Each component contains oppositely polarized regions, but when added together to give the complete activating function, a monotonic function is obtained (Fig. 4c). This in turn produces a monotonic v_m response that decays with distance from the origin (Fig. 4d), which is the well-known response of an isotropic tissue to extracellular point stimulation. However, under conditions of unequal anisotropy, the x and y components of S will no longer contribute equally to the overall function, and sources of opposite polarity may now emerge that coexist side by side. In the extreme case of complete transverse uncoupling (i.e., setting g_y to zero), the dog-bone pattern is most pronounced,[25] and the activating function consists of only its x component.

Another well-known example from the cardiac literature is that of a finite length, quasi-one-dimensional muscle strip (e.g., trabecular muscle) stimulated by electrodes at both

---

[†] Roth[25] has shown that in the general case of anisotropy, a spatial scaling process can be used to equalize the conductivities in one of the domains, as was assumed here for the extracellular domain.

[‡] Note that the usage in this section of the terms virtual cathode and anode follows that commonly used in the literature, where they are linked to the sign of membrane polarization, as opposed to the sign of the generalized activating function, as mentioned earlier.

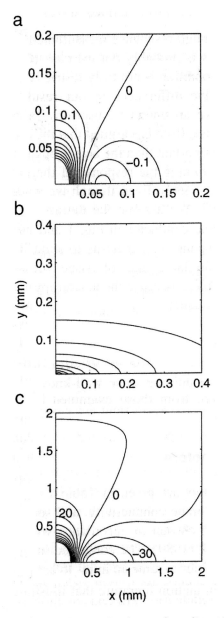

Figure 3: Point stimulation of an anisotropic sheet of cardiac tissue. Stimulating cathode is located $50\,\mu m$ above the surface of a semi-infinite, isotropic volume conductor, and intracellular conductance is ten times higher in the x direction than in the y direction. (a) Contours of the generalized activating function S, normalized to its peak value, in increments of 0.1. (b) Response h of the tissue to a unitary current injected at the origin, normalized to its peak value. (c) Contours of induced transmembrane potentials v_m, in $10\,mV$ increments (Adapted with permission from Sobie et al.)[24]

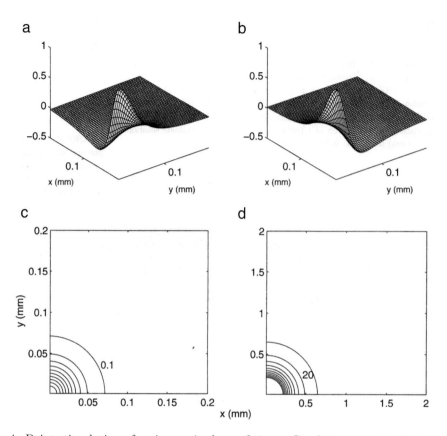

Figure 4: Point stimulation of an isotropic sheet of tissue. Conditions are identical to Fig. 3, except that intracellular x and y conductances are equal. (a) Surface plot of the normalized x component of the generalized activating function, $g_x \partial^2 \Phi_e / \partial x^2$. (b) Surface plot of the normalized y component of the generalized activating function, $g_y \partial^2 \Phi_e / \partial y^2$. (c) Contours of the complete generalized activating function, normalized to its peak value, in increments of 0.1. (d) Contours of induced transmembrane potentials, in 10 mV increments (Adapted with permission from Sobie et al.)[24]

sealed ends (Fig. 5).[26] The field strength and intracellular conductance are assumed to be uniform along the x axis, so no sources develop in the bulk of the tissue. Sources arise only at the ends of the strip, where longitudinal intracellular conductance undergoes a step change to zero.[27] Consequently, a virtual, intracellular current sink exists at the left edge, and an equal amplitude, virtual intracellular current source exists at the right edge. The resulting v_m is shown in Fig. 5c and is an example of surface polarization. The approximate and exact steady-state solutions for v_m overlap completely.

Yet another example that has been extensively studied in the literature is the "sawtooth" pattern, proposed to be a mechanism underlying field stimulation in the bulk myocardium

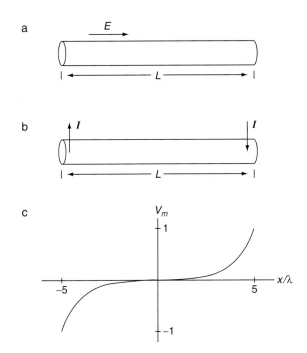

Figure 5: One-dimensional muscle strip subjected to an extracellular electric field. (**a**) Geometry. The tissue is of finite length, L, with electrodes at both ends. (**b**) Generalized activating function. Equivalently, field stimulation can be represented as intracellular current injection at the ends. Current injection magnitude and locations are defined by the generalized activating function, so $I = E\left(\partial g_i/\partial x\right)$. Both formulations produce the same results in terms of passive and active tissue responses to field stimulation. (**c**) Tissue response. Plotted is v_m (normalized to its maximum value), which decays exponentially from its values at the ends. L has been assumed to be 10 times the space constant λ. The approximate solution (*solid line*) fully masks the exact bidomain solution (*dashed line*)

in regions remote from the electrodes.[2,28] It arises from spatially periodic discontinuities in intracellular conductivity, as might be associated with gap junctions interconnecting the cardiac cells, bundles of myocardial fibers, or sheets of cardiac cells that form the laminar structure of the heart. In the example shown in Fig. 6, a uniform electric field is imposed on a sheet of tissue with uniform fiber direction and a periodic drop in intracellular conductance (Fig. 6a). According to the generalized activating function, virtual sources take the form of dipoles that are located at every location with depressed conductivity (Fig. 6b). The v_m response of the tissue takes on a periodic, sawtooth pattern (Fig. 6c). As with the previous example, the approximate and exact steady-state solutions completely overlap. It is also clear that the distribution of virtual sources based on the polarity of S (Fig. 6b) differs significantly from that based on the polarity of v_m (Fig. 6c).

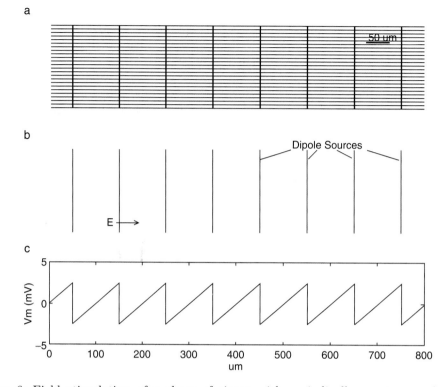

Figure 6: Field stimulation of a sheet of tissue with periodically varying conductivity. (a) Geometry. Intracellular conductivity is reduced by a factor of 1,000 every 100 μm, as indicated by the *thick vertical lines*. A uniform 1 V/cm field is applied to the tissue as shown. (b) Generalized activating function. Each gap junction, or periodic reduction in conductivity, causes a dipole source. (c) Tissue response. The approximate solution (*solid line*) masks the bidomain solution (*dashed line*) (Sobie et al.)[24]

Other situations exist in which discontinuities in intracellular conductivity give rise to virtual sources. Consider the case of a tissue containing a region of depressed conductivity (Fig. 7a), as might arise during ischemia. For a uniform electric field, the generalized activating function defines a positive virtual source at the left edge and negative virtual source at the right edge of the depressed region (Fig. 7b). The tissue response resembles that of a dipole potential at distances far from the region (Fig. 7c). If conductivity in the region is reduced to zero, the gradient in conductivity at the edges of the region increases, and the magnitude and extent of the v_m response increases (Fig. 7d). In both cases, the approximate and exact solutions are very similar, although not identical, to each other. The results in Fig. 7c compare favorably with experimental measurements conducted in cultured cell monolayers containing intercellular cleft spaces.[12]

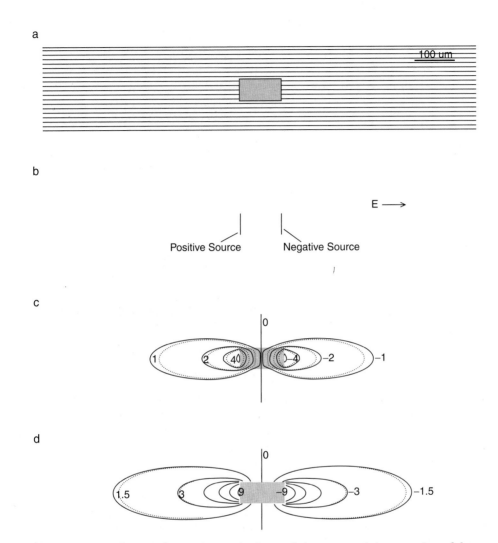

Figure 7: Field stimulation of an anisotropic sheet of tissue containing a region of depressed conductivity. (**a**) Geometry. Intracellular conductivity is depressed in the *shaded region* by a factor of 3 in both the longitudinal and transverse directions, and a 1 V/cm field is applied from left to right. (**b**) Generalized activating function. A positive source is produced along the left edge of the *shaded region*, and a negative source along the right edge. (**c**) Contours of induced v_{m} (in mV) for the approximate solution (*solid lines*) and the bidomain solution (*dashed lines*) when conductance in the *shaded region* is decreased by a factor of three. (**d**) Contours of the tissue response when conductance in the *shaded region* is zero (Sobie et al.)[24]

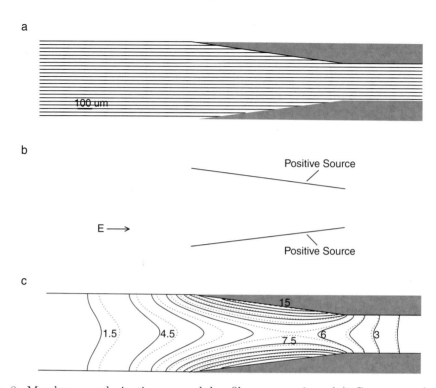

Figure 8: Membrane polarization caused by fiber narrowing. (**a**) Geometry. A $500\,\mu\mathrm{m}$ wide fiber narrows to $250\,\mu\mathrm{m}$ over $1\,\mathrm{mm}$, and a $1\,\mathrm{V/cm}$ field is applied along the fiber's longitudinal axis. (**b**) Generalized activating function. As the fiber narrows, positive sources are produced along the edges of the fiber. (**c**) Tissue response. Contours of the induced v_{m} (in mV) for the approximate (*solid lines*) and exact bidomain (*dashed lines*) solutions (Sobie et al.)[24]

Figure 9: Field stimulation of fibers curving around an obstacle. (**a**) Geometry. Intracellular conductivity is zero in the *shaded region*, the applied field is oriented from left to right, and the fibers curve around the obstacle as shown. Where the muscle fibers curve, the fiber angle θ is described by $\theta = -\tan^{-1}(x/y)$. (**b**) Generalized activating function. A hyperpolarizing source is produced along the edge of the obstacle, and distributed depolarizing sources arise owing to fiber curvature. Contours of the depolarizing sources are plotted, normalized to the function's peak value. (**c**) Tissue response. Contours of the induced v_{m} (in mV) for the approximate (*solid lines*) and exact bidomain (*dashed lines*) solutions. Contour values in the top half of the panel apply to the *solid lines*, while the values in the bottom half (*in italics*) apply to the *dashed lines*. The approximate solution assumes that Φ_{e} is in accordance with a uniform $1\,\mathrm{V/cm}$ applied field. (**d**) Tissue response with a more exact distribution of Φ_{e}. Contours of the induced v_{m} for the new approximate (*solid lines*) and bidomain (*dashed lines*) solutions. See text for details (Sobie et al.)[24]

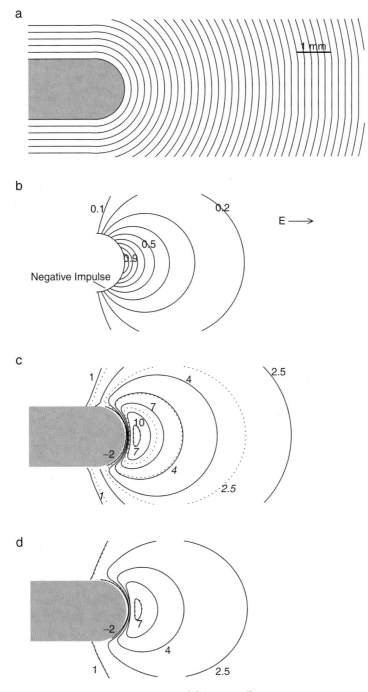

Figure 9: (*Continued*)

Changes in fiber cross-sectional area are yet another way to produce gradients in intracellular conductivity and have been proposed to be a mechanism for stimulation in the bulk myocardium.[6] For the case of fiber narrowing (Fig. 8a), the drop in intracellular conductance from left to right forces current to flow outward across the cell membrane, resulting in membrane depolarization. According to the generalized activating function, positive virtual sources are produced along the edges of the narrowing (Fig. 8b), resulting in the v_m responses shown in Fig. 8c. Here it is apparent that the approximate and exact solutions deviate from one another more than in the previous examples, but nonetheless they are still very similar.

A final example is instructive with respect to the influence of a more complex, heterogeneous tissue structure. Here a nominally uniform field is applied to fibers that are curved around an anatomical obstacle devoid of cardiac cells (Fig. 9a). By symmetry, only half of the tissue is shown. Extracellular current is uniformly applied at the left border and withdrawn at the right border of the tissue. Contours of S are shown in Fig. 9b under the assumption that the extracellular field is uniform across the tissue. A negative virtual source arises at the edge of the obstacle owing to the step change in intracellular conductivity. It is complemented by positive sources that arise because of fiber curvature, which are spatially distributed across the fibers and have a peak at the obstacle edge (Fig. 9b). In this example, however, it can be seen that the approximate and exact solutions are quite dissimilar (Fig. 9c), with a 42% difference in the peak amplitudes.[24] The reason for this discrepancy is that the heterogeneous structure represented by the curved fibers significantly perturbs the extracellular field and its gradient. If instead one treats the tissue as a monodomain having a bulk conductance equal to the sum of intracellular and extracellular conductances (i.e., their parallel combination) to solve for Φ_e and uses that Φ_e (which no longer has a constant gradient) in the computation of S, one obtains nearly identical approximate and exact distributions of v_m (Fig. 9d). Thus, this example serves to remind us that tissue conductivity and its gradient influence the generalized activating function not only by their direct contributions to the weighting functions of the extracellular field and its gradient (see (7)), but also in the spatial profile of the extracellular field itself (dashed pathway, Fig. 2).

Discussion

The concept of the generalized activating function[24] is a unifying concept that brings together various mechanisms that have been proposed to describe electrical stimulation of tissue, including discontinuities in fiber conductivity,[2] tissue anisotropy,[3] surface polarization,[4] fiber curvature,[4] fiber rotation,[5] heterogeneities in intracellular volume fraction,[6] and tissue clefts.[12] The notion of a polarization response in regions removed from the electrode has been previously described in terms of "virtual electrodes" or "secondary sources." The terms *virtual cathode* and *virtual anode* are accepted terms that refer to regions of positive or negative polarization in cardiac tissue that are produced during electrical stimulation[29] (i.e., the polarization response that would be expected in proximity to a physical cathode or anode placed at those regions). This definition makes sense from an experimental perspective, because the virtual sources driving the tissue response cannot be directly measured. However, as shown in the examples, the virtual sources are more properly related to the generalized activating function, which serves to define the locations and magnitudes of the virtual sources and mathematically is the forcing function for the transmembrane potential response (see (4)). The tissue response (at least, the passive component) is then the convolution of the generalized activating function with the tissue response to a point source under conditions of tissue homogeneity,[24] as has also been shown for the one-dimensional case (Fig. 1).[23,30,31] In general, because the point response decays monotonically with distance, the tissue response will appear as a low-pass filtered version of the generalized activation function.[24]

Additionally, the term *secondary source* has been used to describe the sources that drive the polarization changes at tissue boundaries or other discontinuities in tissue conductivity that occur secondary to primary field stimulation.[32] Again, the generalized activating function, through inclusion of the term G_i, accounts for secondary sources that accompany changes in tissue conductance at these discontinuities.

In much of the literature on defibrillation, the focus has been on the local extracellular potential gradient as the important parameter governing the shock response.[33] The generalized activating function (see (7)) shows that a constant potential gradient (electric field) does generate virtual sources provided that spatial variations exist in intracellular conductivity that can arise from cell–cell junctions, discrete fiber bundle sizes, fiber curvature, or tissue boundaries and inhomogeneities. The generalized activating function also shows that spatial gradients in extracellular potential gradient (i.e., nonuniform electric fields) can act as virtual sources and should be considered in discussions of defibrillation shock thresholds.

Limitations

Some comments are in order with respect to limitations of the activating function concept. The first limitation pertains to transverse field stimulation. It is known from cell culture experiments that fields that are perpendicular to the fiber axis can excite the fiber even when the fiber is isolated and decoupled from neighboring fibers,[34] yet the activating function would be zero. This is because fibers do not have a vanishingly small diameter and as such can polarize at diametrically opposing sides (a consequence of the microscopic discontinuity of intracellular conductivity in the transverse direction). Of course, because of the small diameter very large fields would need to be applied to produce an excitatory response. Thus, the activating function may not properly account for all of the polarization changes that may occur during transverse stimulation of cardiac fibers, particularly during high levels of shock of fibers that are relatively uncoupled, as may occur in the infarct border zone or in certain pathological conditions.

A second limitation is that the form shown here for the generalized activating function (see (5)) is not unique, and linear transformations of the bidomain equations can lead to alternative forms of the function that incorporate extracellular conductivities[35] or a combination of intra- and extracellular conductivities,[36] as described in the Appendix. However, the use of intracellular conductivities is appealing for the case of cardiac tissue, given that cell–cell coupling through gap junctions may be altered during pathological conditions such as ischemia, aging, or heart failure, and therefore may lead to altered tissue responses during electrical stimulation and defibrillation.

Validation

In experiments on rabbit hearts in which surface electrodes of different sizes were used to generate nonuniform or nominally uniform fields, optical recordings of the v_{m} responses were shown to depend primarily on the second derivative of Φ_{e} in both cases and to a lesser extent on the first derivative of Φ_{e} (the electric field).[35] Fiber orientation was found to have an influence, but primarily by modulating the spatial profile of Φ_{e} and affecting the nonuniformity of the gradient in Φ_{e} (much like the case in Fig. 9). Computer simulations using the bidomain model showed consistency between the experimental recordings and the components of the generalized activating function.[35]

In another experimental study using a surface electrode fabricated to generate uniform or nonuniform fields, optical recordings of v_{m} showed correlation between the signs of v_{m} and $\partial^2 \Phi_{\mathrm{e}}/\partial x^2$ under conditions of nonuniform fields, and the signs of v_{m} and $(\partial g_{\mathrm{i}}/\partial x)(\partial \Phi_{\mathrm{e}}/\partial x)$, as estimated from the gradient in heart width, with uniform fields.[37]

Conclusion

The generalized activating function acts as the forcing function for transmembrane potential responses arising from extracellular stimulation. It can serve to define the spatial pattern and magnitude of virtual electrodes that are distributed throughout the myocardium. It consists of two components, one proportional to the first derivative of extracellular potential (i.e., electric field) and the other to the second derivative of extracellular potential (i.e., gradient in electric field). Spatial variations in intracellular conductivity, as may arise from tissue boundaries, fiber curvature, or cellular or cell bundle structure, act as a weighting function for the first component and may also augment the nonuniformity of the electric field, thereby augmenting the contribution of the second component.

Appendix

The membrane current i_{m} contains two components: the capacitive current I_{C} and total ionic current I_{ion}.

$$i_{\mathrm{m}} = I_{\mathrm{C}} + I_{\mathrm{ion}} = C_{\mathrm{m}} \frac{\partial v_{\mathrm{m}}}{\partial t} + I_{\mathrm{ion}} \tag{8}$$

where C_{m} is the area-specific membrane capacitance (μF/cm^2). Along the intracellular pathway, intracellular current I_{i} is related to i_{m} and to intracellular potential Φ_{i} according to,

$$\frac{\partial I_{\mathrm{i}}}{\partial x} = -i_{\mathrm{m}} \tag{9}$$

$$r_{\mathrm{i}} I_{\mathrm{i}} = -\frac{\partial \Phi_{\mathrm{i}}}{\partial x} \tag{10}$$

where r_i is intracellular resistance per unit length. Combining (9) and (10), utilizing the relation $\Phi_i = v_m + \Phi_e$, where v_m is the change in transmembrane potential, and rearranging terms produces,

$$I_{ion} + C_m \frac{\partial v_m}{\partial t} - \frac{1}{r_i} \frac{\partial^2 v_m}{\partial x^2} = \frac{1}{r_i} f, \tag{11}$$

where f is the so-called activating function,[15] defined to be

$$f(x,t) = \frac{\partial^2 \Phi_e}{\partial x^2}. \tag{12}$$

Prior to the onset of the stimulus, v_m, its spatial derivatives and I_{ion} are zero. Thus, (11) reduces to,

$$C_m \frac{\partial v_m}{\partial t} = \frac{1}{r_i} f. \tag{13}$$

The polarity of the initial response of the fiber follows that of f and defines regions of virtual cathodes and anodes. Note, however, that over time, as charge diffuses through the tissue, the spatial polarity of v_m will no longer mirror that of f (compare Fig. 1c with 1e).

For the extracellular cathodal point source of Fig. 1a, Φ_e in the semi-infinite volume conductor is twice that for an infinite medium having conductivity σ_e:

$$\Phi_e = -\frac{I_e}{2\pi\sigma_e r} = -\frac{I_e}{2\pi\sigma_e \sqrt{x^2 + z_0^2}} \tag{14}$$

and the activating function is therefore,

$$f = \frac{\partial^2 \Phi_e}{\partial x^2} = -\frac{I_e}{2\pi\sigma_e} \frac{2x^2 - z_0^2}{(x^2 + z_0^2)^{5/2}}. \tag{15}$$

The activating function is greater than 0 in the region $|x| < \sqrt{2}z_0/2$, which from (13) leads to membrane depolarization, and is less than 0 for $|x| > \sqrt{2}z_0/2$, which leads to membrane hyperpolarization.

If the fiber possesses homogeneous properties, is infinitely long, and has a passive membrane with resistance R_m so that $I_{ion} = v_m/R_m$, (11) can be solved by convolving f with the response h of the fiber to a unitary point source of intracellular[§] current (i.e., the spatial impulse response),[23,30,31]

$$v_m(x) = \int \frac{1}{r_i} f(\xi) h(x - \xi) d\xi, \tag{16}$$

where h is well known[17] and in steady state has the form of an exponentially decaying function

$$h = \frac{r_i \lambda}{2} I_0 e^{-|x|/\lambda} \tag{17}$$

[§] The reason the source is intracellular rather than extracellular is because of the sign of f in (11), which dictates that f acts like an intracellular source.

with a space constant $\lambda = \sqrt{r_m/r_i}$, and $I_0 = 1$. Under transient conditions, the general time-varying response to a step input of current applied at $x = 0$ should be used instead of (17). Equations (17) and (16) are plotted in Fig. 1d and 1e, respectively, for the case where $z_0 = \lambda$.

Generalization of (11) to three dimensions involves the use of the bidomain equations

$$\nabla \cdot (\mathbf{G}_i \nabla \Phi_i) = \beta \left(I_{ion} + C_m \frac{\partial v_m}{\partial t} \right), \tag{18}$$

$$\nabla \cdot (\mathbf{G}_e \nabla \Phi_e) = -\beta \left(I_{ion} + C_m \frac{\partial v_m}{\partial t} \right), \tag{19}$$

where Φ_i, Φ_e, and v_m are the extracellular, intracellular, and transmembrane potentials, respectively, β is the surface membrane area-to-volume ratio, and I_{ion} and C_m are defined as in the one-dimensional fiber. Analogous to the case of the one-dimensional fiber, substituting the relation $\Phi_i = v_m + \Phi_e$ into (18) and rearranging terms produces,[24]

$$\beta \left(I_{ion} + C_m \frac{\partial v_m}{\partial t} \right) - \nabla \cdot (\mathbf{G}_i \nabla v_m) = S, \tag{20}$$

where $\mathbf{G}_i$ is the intracellular conductivity tensor relating currents in the x, y, and z directions to the potential gradients along those directions,

$$\mathbf{G}_i = \begin{vmatrix} g_x & g_{xy} & g_{xz} \\ g_{yx} & g_y & g_{yz} \\ g_{zx} & g_{zy} & g_z \end{vmatrix} \tag{21}$$

and S is the generalized activating function

$$S = \nabla \cdot (\mathbf{G}_i \nabla \Phi_e). \tag{22}$$

Equations (21) and (22) are written in their most general form, but can be understood more readily under some simplifying conditions. First, $\mathbf{G}_i$ is just a rotation of the conductivity tensor $\mathbf{G}_f$ in the fiber coordinate system

$$\mathbf{G}_i = \mathbf{A} \mathbf{G}_f \mathbf{A}^T, \tag{23}$$

where

$$\mathbf{G}_f = \begin{bmatrix} g_l & 0 & 0 \\ 0 & g_t & 0 \\ 0 & 0 & g_u \end{bmatrix}. \tag{24}$$

The parameters g_l, g_t, and g_u are the conductivities along the fiber axis and the two principal axes perpendicular to the fiber axis, respectively, and $\mathbf{A}$ is the rotation tensor.[24] Thus, $\mathbf{G}_i$ consists of the conductivities of a tissue having orthotropic anisotropy, adjusted for fiber angle in the tissue.

Next, S can be written as the sum of two components,[27]

$$S = -(\nabla \cdot \mathbf{G}_i) \cdot \mathbf{E} - \mathbf{G}_i : \nabla \mathbf{E}, \tag{25}$$

where the electric field $\mathbf{E} = -\nabla\Phi_e$. This equation tells us that sources can result either from the extracellular field weighted by spatial gradients of intracellular conductivity (the first term), or by spatial gradients of the extracellular field weighted by the intracellular conductivities (the second term). When fully expanded in component form for the two-dimensional case, (25) becomes,

$$
S = \left(
\begin{array}{l}
\dfrac{\partial g_x^i}{\partial x}\dfrac{\partial \Phi_e}{\partial x} + \dfrac{\partial g_{yx}^i}{\partial x}\dfrac{\partial \Phi_e}{\partial y} + \dfrac{\partial g_{xy}^i}{\partial y}\dfrac{\partial \Phi_e}{\partial x} + \dfrac{\partial g_y^i}{\partial y}\dfrac{\partial \Phi_e}{\partial y} \\[2mm]
+ g_x^i \dfrac{\partial^2 \Phi_e}{\partial x^2} + (g_{xy}^i + g_{yx}^i)\dfrac{\partial^2 \Phi_e}{\partial x \partial y} + g_y^i \dfrac{\partial^2 \Phi_e}{\partial y^2}
\end{array}
\right).
\tag{26}
$$

Other variants of (26) can be obtained starting with different combinations of the bidomain equations. Rewriting (19) as,

$$
-\beta\left(I_{\text{ion}} + C_m \frac{\partial v_m}{\partial t}\right) = S
\tag{27}
$$

gives for S terms that depend on extracellular conductivities,[35]

$$
S = \left(
\begin{array}{l}
\dfrac{\partial g_x^e}{\partial x}\dfrac{\partial \Phi_e}{\partial x} + \dfrac{\partial g_{xy}^e}{\partial x}\dfrac{\partial \Phi_e}{\partial y} + \dfrac{\partial g_{yx}^e}{\partial y}\dfrac{\partial \Phi_e}{\partial x} + \dfrac{\partial g_y^e}{\partial y}\dfrac{\partial \Phi_e}{\partial y} \\[2mm]
+ g_x^e \dfrac{\partial^2 \Phi_e}{\partial x^2} + (g_{xy}^e + g_{yx}^e)\dfrac{\partial^2 \Phi_e}{\partial x \partial y} + g_y^e \dfrac{\partial^2 \Phi_e}{\partial y^2}
\end{array}
\right).
\tag{28}
$$

Alternatively, combining (18) and (19) by multiplying (18) by $g_y^e/(g_y^i + g_y^e)$ and (19) by $g_y^i/(g_y^i + g_y^e)$, subtracting the latter from the former, and utilizing the relation $\Phi_i = v_m + \Phi_e$ yields,

$$
\beta\left(I_{\text{ion}} + C_m \frac{\partial v_m}{\partial t}\right) - \frac{g_y^i}{g_y^i + g_y^e}\nabla \cdot (\mathbf{G}_i \nabla v_m) = S
\tag{29}
$$

and gives for S terms that depend on both intra- and extracellular conductivities,[36]

$$
\begin{aligned}
S = \frac{1}{g_y^i + g_y^e}&\left(\left[g_y^e\left(\frac{\partial g_x^i}{\partial x} + \frac{\partial g_{yx}^i}{\partial y}\right) - g_y^i\left(\frac{\partial g_x^e}{\partial x} + \frac{\partial g_{yx}^e}{\partial y}\right)\right]\frac{\partial \Phi_e}{\partial x}\right. \\[2mm]
&+ \left.\left[g_y^e\left(\frac{\partial g_y^i}{\partial y} + \frac{\partial g_{xy}^i}{\partial x}\right) - g_y^i\left(\frac{\partial g_y^e}{\partial y} + \frac{\partial g_{xy}^e}{\partial x}\right)\right]\frac{\partial \Phi_e}{\partial y}\right) \\[2mm]
&+ \frac{g_x^i g_y^e - g_x^e g_y^i}{g_y^i + g_y^e}\frac{\partial^2 \Phi_e}{\partial x^2} + 2\frac{g_{xy}^i g_y^e - g_{xy}^e g_y^i}{g_y^i + g_y^e}\frac{\partial^2 \Phi_e}{\partial x \partial y}.
\end{aligned}
\tag{30}
$$

Just as with (26), S in (28) and (30) consists of the sum of terms containing first and second derivatives of Φ_e weighted by first derivatives of conductivities or conductivities, respectively.

According to (22), the generalized activating function is determined by the actual spatial distribution of extracellular potential, which as seen in the example of Fig. 9 is not necessarily determined solely by the applied electric field. To begin with, the presence of the cardiac fibers and their effect on the applied field need to be accounted for.[38] However, given that the fiber diameter is small compared with the typical distance to the electrode, such effects will be relatively minor.[23] More significantly, the extracellular potential distribution will be perturbed even further by the transmembrane currents that flow in response to the developing v_m (dashed pathway in Fig. 2). This is accounted for by (19). Rigorously speaking, the exact solution for v_m (and Φ_e) must satisfy both (20) and (19), whereas with the concept of the generalized activating function Φ_e is assumed to be known, and an approximate solution for v_m is obtained by using just (20) alone.

References

1. Roth BJ, Krassowska W. The induction of reentry in cardiac tissue. The missing link: how electric fields alter transmembrane potential. *Chaos* 1998;8(1):204–220
2. Plonsey R, Barr RC. Effect of microscopic and macroscopic discontinuities on the response of cardiac tissue to defibrillating (stimulating) currents. *Med Biol Eng Comput* 1986;24(2):130–136
3. Sepulveda NG, Roth BJ, Wikswo JP Jr. Current injection into a two-dimensional anisotropic bidomain. *Biophys J* 1989;55(5):987–999
4. Trayanova NA, Roth BJ, Malden LJ. The response of a spherical heart to a uniform electric field: a bidomain analysis of cardiac stimulation. *IEEE Trans Biomed Eng* 1993;40(9):899–908
5. Entcheva E, Trayanova NA, Claydon FJ. Patterns of and mechanisms for shock-induced polarization in the heart: a bidomain analysis. *IEEE Trans Biomed Eng* 1999;46(3):260–270
6. Fishler MG. Syncytial heterogeneity as a mechanism underlying cardiac far-field stimulation during defibrillation-level shocks. *J Cardiovasc Electrophysiol* 1998;9(4):384–394
7. Roth BJ. Mechanisms for electrical stimulation of excitable tissue. *Crit Rev Biomed Eng* 1994;22(3–4):253–305
8. Newton JC, Knisley SB, Zhou X, Pollard AE, Ideker RE. Review of mechanisms by which electrical stimulation alters the transmembrane potential. *J Cardiovasc Electrophysiol* 1999;10(2):234–243
9. Basser PJ, Roth BJ. New currents in electrical stimulation of excitable tissues. *Annu Rev Biomed Eng* 2000;2:377–397
10. Rohr S, Fluckiger-Labrada R, Kucera JP. Photolithographically defined deposition of attachment factors as a versatile method for patterning the growth of different cell types in culture. *Pflugers Arch* 2003;446(1):125–132
11. Gillis AM, Fast VG, Rohr S, Kleber AG. Spatial changes in transmembrane potential during extracellular electrical shocks in cultured monolayers of neonatal rat ventricular myocytes. *Circ Res* 1996;79(4):676–690
12. Fast VG, Rohr S, Gillis AM, Kleber AG. Activation of cardiac tissue by extracellular electrical shocks: formation of 'secondary sources' at intracellular clefts in monolayers of cultured myocytes. *Circ Res* 1998;82(3):375–385

13. Gillis AM, Fast VG, Rohr S, Kleber AG. Mechanism of ventricular defibrillation. The role of tissue geometry in the changes in transmembrane potential in patterned myocyte cultures. *Circulation* 2000;101(20):2438–2445

14. Tung L, Kleber AG. Virtual sources associated with linear and curved strands of cardiac cells. *Am J Physiol Heart Circ Physiol* 2000;279(4):H1579–H1590

15. Rattay F. Analysis of models for external stimulation of axons. *IEEE Trans Biomed Eng* 1986;33(10):974–977

16. McNeal DR. Analysis of a model for excitation of myelinated nerve. *IEEE Trans Biomed Eng* 1976;23(4):329–337

17. Barr RC, Plonsey R. *Bioelectricity: A Quantitative Approach*, 3rd edn. Berlin: Springer; 2007

18. Rattay F. Ways to approximate current-distance relations for electrically stimulated fibers. *J Theor Biol* 1987;125(3):339–349

19. Hoshi T, Matsuda K. Excitability cycle of cardiac muscle examined by intracellular stimulation. *Jpn J Physiol* 1962;12:433–446

20. Bonke FI. Passive electrical properties of atrial fibers of the rabbit heart. *Pflugers Arch* 1973;339(1):1–15

21. Henriquez CS. Simulating the electrical behavior of cardiac tissue using the bidomain model. *Crit Rev Biomed Eng* 1993;21(1):1–77

22. Rattay F. The basic mechanism for the electrical stimulation of the nervous system. *Neuroscience* 1999;89(2):335–346

23. Plonsey R, Barr RC. Electric field stimulation of excitable tissue. *IEEE Trans Biomed Eng* 1995;42(4):329–336

24. Sobie EA, Susil RC, Tung L. A generalized activating function for predicting virtual electrodes in cardiac tissue. *Biophys J* 1997;73(3):1410–1423

25. Roth BJ. How the anisotropy of the intracellular and extracellular conductivities influences stimulation of cardiac muscle. *J Math Biol* 1992;30(6):633–646

26. Weidmann S. Electrical constants of trabecular muscle from mammalian heart. *J Physiol* 1970;210(4):1041–1054

27. Susil RC, Sobie EA, Tung L. Separation between virtual sources modifies the response of cardiac tissue to field stimulation. *J Cardiovasc Electrophysiol* 1999;10(5):715–727

28. Krassowska W, Frazier DW, Pilkington TC, Ideker RE. Potential distribution in three-dimensional periodic myocardium – Part II: application to extracellular stimulation. *IEEE Trans Biomed Eng* 1990;37(3):267–284

29. Wikswo JP Jr, Lin SF, Abbas RA. Virtual electrodes in cardiac tissue: a common mechanism for anodal and cathodal stimulation. *Biophys J* 1995;69(6):2195–2210

30. Warman EN, Grill WM, Durand D. Modeling the effects of electric fields on nerve fibers: determination of excitation thresholds. *IEEE Trans Biomed Eng* 1992;39(12):1244–1254

31. Neunlist M, Tung L. Spatial distribution of cardiac transmembrane potentials around an extracellular electrode: dependence on fiber orientation. *Biophys J* 1995;68(6):2310–2322

32. Plonsey R. The nature of sources of bioelectric and biomagnetic fields. *Biophys J* 1982;39(3):309–312

33. Frazier DW, Krassowska W, Chen PS, Wolf PD, Dixon EG, Smith WM, Ideker RE. Extracellular field required for excitation in three-dimensional anisotropic canine myocardium. *Circ Res* 1988;63(1):147–164

34. Fast VG, Rohr S, Ideker RE. Nonlinear changes of transmembrane potential caused by defibrillation shocks in strands of cultured myocytes. *Am J Physiol Heart Circ Physiol* 2000;278(3):H688–H697

35. Knisley SB, Trayanova N, Aguel F. Roles of electric field and fiber structure in cardiac electric stimulation. *Biophys J* 1999;77(3):1404–1417

36. Trayanova N, Skouibine K, Aguel F. The role of cardiac tissue structure in defibrillation. *Chaos* 1998;8(1):221–233

37. Knisley SB. Evidence for roles of the activating function in electric stimulation. *IEEE Trans Biomed Eng* 2000;47(8):1114–1119

38. Altman KW, Plonsey R. Analysis of excitable cell activation: relative effects of external electrical stimuli. *Med Biol Eng Comput* 1990;28(6):574–580

Chapter 2.4

Theory of Electroporation

Wanda Krassowska Neu and John C. Neu

Concept of Electroporation

Experiments conducted on artificial bilayers, suspensions of vesicles or cells, and tissues have demonstrated that a large, externally induced transmembrane potential (V_m) causes an increase in the conductivity of the membrane by five to six orders of magnitude.[1–3] This effect is generally attributed to the creation of pores, which are the aqueous pathways in the lipid bilayer of the membrane, and whose creation and subsequent growth are facilitated by large V_m. This process, called electroporation, can be irreversible, leading to a mechanical rupture of the membrane,[2,4] or reversible, in which case pores reseal and the same membrane can experience multiple episodes of the high conductivity state.[1,3] Electroporation occurs as an undesirable side effect following the delivery of defibrillation shocks to the heart[5–10] and may be responsible for the late necrosis after accidental exposure to high voltage.[11] On the other hand, the transient state of high membrane permeability has important practical applications, allowing the fusion of cells and the introduction of biologically active substances (drugs or genetic material) into cells.[12–17]

Because of great interest in this method, studies use a variety of experimental techniques to provide insight into the processes taking place during electroporation. These techniques include measuring the time course of transmembrane voltage[1] or current though the membrane,[3,18] monitoring uptake or leakage of fluorescent molecules,[19–21] imaging the transmembrane potential,[8,10,22] measuring the tissue impedance,[23,24] and observing pores with rapid-freezing electron microscopy.[25] However, electroporation is difficult to observe directly because pores are very small (nanometers) and their creation and growth is very fast (microseconds), and many questions cannot be answered with available experimental techniques. Thus, there is a need to supplement experimental knowledge with a theoretical model.

This chapter provides an introduction to the theory of electroporation. The section "Physical Background of Electroporation" describes the physical mechanism involved in

Wanda Krassowska Neu

Department of Biomedical Engineering, Duke University, Durham, NC 27708, USA, wanda@eel-mail.bme.duke.edu

I. R. Efimov et al. (eds.), *Cardiac Bioelectric Therapy: Mechanisms and Practical Implications.*
© Springer Science+Business Media, LLC 2009

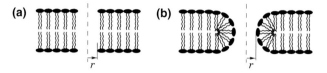

Figure 1: The structure of (**a**) hydrophobic and (**b**) hydrophilic pores. Pore radius is denoted by r. (From Abidor et al.,[2] Weaver,[30] and Glaser et al.[31])

creation, evolution, and resealing of pores, and "Mathematical Modeling of Electroporation" describes mathematical models of electroporation, including the advection-diffusion equation and its asymptotic approximation by a set of ordinary differential equations (ODEs). Theory is supplemented in the following section by an example of an electroporation process occurring in a uniformly polarized membrane, which is used to illustrate the distinct phases of electroporation: pore creation, evolution of their radii, postshock shrinkage of pores, and their resealing. Finally, the limitations of the current theory of electroporation and the usefulness of the models in studying electroporation in cardiac muscle are evaluated. Further information on the theory of electroporation can be found other reviews[10,16,26–29] and in the original literature referenced throughout this chapter.

Physical Background of Electroporation

Pore Energy

The theory assumes the existence of two types of pores.[2,30,31] The *hydrophobic* pores (Fig. 1a) are simply gaps in the lipid bilayer of the membrane, formed as a result of its thermal fluctuations. The *hydrophilic* or inverted pores (Fig. 1b) have their walls lined with the water-attracting heads of lipid molecules. Hydrophilic pores allow the passage of water-soluble substances, such as ions, and thus they conduct electric current while the hydrophobic pores do not. The models focus on the hydrophilic pores but some background on the hydrophobic pores is necessary to understand the creation and resealing of hydrophilic pores.

The creation and evolution of pores is strongly controlled by their contribution to the bilayer energy. First, we examine *pore energy*, which is the energy cost of introducing a *single pore* of radius r, with all other pores fixed. This pore energy consists of two curves, $U(r)$ for a hydrophobic pore and $E(r)$ for a hydrophilic pore. The hydrophobic pore energy $U(r)$ is given by the formula,

$$U(r) \approx E_* \left(\frac{r}{r_*}\right)^2 - \frac{1}{2h}(\varepsilon_\mathrm{w} - \varepsilon_\mathrm{m})V_\mathrm{m}^2\pi r^2, \tag{1}$$

where radius r_* and energy E_* are defined in Fig. 2, h is the membrane thickness, and ε_w and ε_m are permittivities of water and membrane, respectively. Values of all parameters are given in Appendix 1. The first term in (1) approximates the energy cost of creating a

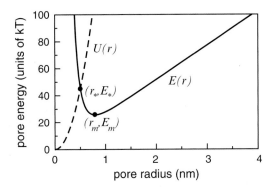

Figure 2: Energy of the hydrophobic pores ($U(r)$, *dashed line*) and the hydrophilic pores ($E(r)$, *solid line*) at $V_m = 0$. Energy of a pore is the lower of $U(r)$ and $E(r)$. It has a local maximum at r_* with energy E_* and a local minimum at r_m with energy E_m. Typical values of radii and energies are given in Appendix 1

cylindrical gap of radius r in the lipid bilayer.[32] The second term represents the effect of the transmembrane potential V_m.[2,33–35] Specifically, V_m decreases the energy by affecting the capacitive energy stored in the membrane; the second term is derived from the classical example of a dielectric slab sliding between the plates of a capacitor whose voltage is held constant.[36,37]

The hydrophilic pore energy $E(r)$ is given by the formula,

$$E(r) = \beta \left(\frac{r_*}{r}\right)^4 + 2\pi\gamma r - \sigma\pi r^2 - \int_{r_*}^{r} F(r', V_m)\, dr', \qquad (2)$$

where β and γ are constants, σ is the membrane tension, and F is the electric force, to be introduced below. The first term represents the steric repulsion between lipid heads lining the pore and is responsible for the increase in pore energy with shrinking radius, $r \to 0^+$.[32] The second term represents the energy required to bend the bilayer in order to form the pore perimeter.[33] The third term represents the decrease in the energy due to the effect of a pore on the tension of the membrane.[38] The fourth term represents the effect of V_m. It is different from the formulation used in (1) because a hydrophilic pore is conductive and cannot be approximated by a dielectric. Instead, the fourth term in (2) was derived by evaluating mechanical work required to deform a dielectric body in an ionic solution with steady-state electric current.[39] Thus, $F(r, V_m)$ is the electric force expanding the pore with toroidal inside surface,

$$F(r, V_m) = \frac{F_{max}}{1 + r_h/(r + r_t)} V_m^2, \qquad (3)$$

whose dependence on r is illustrated in Fig. 3; F_{max}, r_h, and r_t are constants.

As seen in Fig. 2, U and E intersect at radius $r_* \approx 0.5\,\text{nm}$. Pores spontaneously change configuration to minimize their energy,[31] so the energy of a pore of radius r is the lesser of U and E. Consequently, r_* is the threshold radius between hydrophobic and hydrophilic pores:

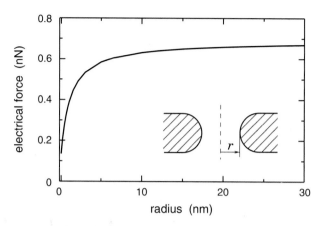

Figure 3: Electric force F (r, V_{m}) expanding a pore, given by (3) with $V_{\mathrm{m}} = 1\,\mathrm{V}$. *Inset*: Assumed geometry of a hydrophilic pore

pores with $r < r_*$ are hydrophobic, and pores with $r > r_*$ are hydrophilic. E_*, the value of pore energy at r_* can be considered an energy barrier against the creation of hydrophilic pores.

Pore Creation

The creation of pores is believed to be a two-step process.[2,27,30,31] All pores are initially created as hydrophobic. According to Barnett and Weaver[26] and Weaver and Mintzer,[34] hydrophobic pores with radii between r and $r + \mathrm{d}r$ are created at a rate

$$\nu_c h \frac{\partial}{\partial r} \left(\frac{U}{kT} \right) \mathrm{e}^{-U/kT} \mathrm{d}r \tag{4}$$

per unit area of the membrane. In (4), ν_c is the fluctuation rate of the bilayer per unit volume,[34] k is Boltzmann's constant, and T is absolute temperature. Since a hydrophobic pore created with radius $r > r_*$ spontaneously changes its configuration to hydrophilic, for $r > r_*$, (4) is effectively a creation rate density of hydrophilic pores (illustrated in Fig. 4b).

The increase in creation rate caused by the delivery of a strong electric shock, observed in experiments, is explained by the dependence of energy U on the square of the transmembrane potential V_{m} seen in (1). Figure 4a shows that a nonzero V_{m} decreases pore energy U. Near r_*, the decrease in U is small ($\approx 18\,kT$ for 1 V). However, because of an exponential dependence of creation rate on U, this small drop in energy translates in an increase in the creation rate by nearly eight orders of magnitude (Fig. 4b). Because the creation rate density (4) decreases like $\mathrm{e}^{-U/kT}$ and U grows quadratically with r (1), the inset in Fig. 4b shows that significant creation of hydrophilic pores is limited to a very narrow ($< 0.05\,\mathrm{nm}$) range of radii above r_*.[32] Consequently, we can assume that hydrophilic pores are created with the initial radius of r_*.

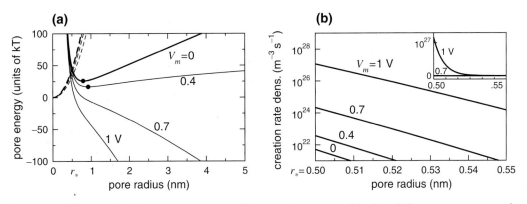

Figure 4: Change in the pore energy and in creation rate of hydrophilic pores as a result of V_{m}. (a) Dependence of pore energies U (*dashed lines*) and E (*solid lines*) on the transmembrane potential V_{m} (indicated by labels). *Filled circles* on plots for $V_{\mathrm{m}} = 0$ and $0.4\,\mathrm{V}$ indicate positions of the local energy minimum r_{m}. This panel assumes that only a single pore exists. (b) Increase in the creation rate density of hydrophilic pores ($r > r_*$) with V_{m}. Note that the ordinate in (b) is logarithmic; the *inset* shows the creation rate density for $V_{\mathrm{m}} = 0.7$ and $1\,\mathrm{V}$ on the linear scale. $V_{\mathrm{m}} = 1\,\mathrm{V}$ is the approximate threshold for pore creation

There is no sharp threshold for electroporation:[40] as expected from (4), any $V_{\mathrm{m}} > 0$ will create pores but weak shocks may require a very long time.[18,41] However, such weak shocks will not be recognized as electroporating in experiments, in which one sees an *apparently* sharp increase in pore formation as V_{m} increases through a narrow range about a "threshold" voltage. For the model parameters listed in Appendix 1, the apparent threshold for electroporation is approximately $1\,\mathrm{V}$.

Pore Evolution

Once created, hydrophilic pores expand or shrink in response to two factors: drift and diffusion. Drift (also called advection) refers to definite time rate of change of pore radius, leading to a decrease of the bilayer energy. Diffusion refers to random increases and decreases of pore radius induced by thermal fluctuations. Between these two factors, drift dominates by far: a pore radius r changes at the rate determined by the "drift velocity," with small random fluctuations added to it. Thus, to a leading order, the evolution of pores can be approximated by the movement of pore radius down the energy gradient.

In early theoretical works on electroporation,[26,27,33] a hydrophilic pore of radius r was assumed to evolve with the drift velocity u,

$$\frac{\mathrm{d}r}{\mathrm{d}t} = u = -\frac{1}{\zeta}\frac{\partial E}{\partial r} = -\frac{D}{kT}\frac{\partial E}{\partial r}, \tag{5}$$

where E is the pore energy (2) with the surface tension σ treated as a time-independent constant (usually assumed equal to the tension of the membrane without pores[26,33]). In (5), the drag coefficient ζ is expressed in terms of D, the diffusion coefficient associated with random fluctuation of pore radii, using the Einstein formula $\zeta = kT/D$.[42]

There exist two mechanisms that modify pore energy and thus affect drift velocity. The first mechanism is the transmembrane potential V_{m}. Assume that a membrane is charged to a voltage V_{m}. As seen in Fig. 4a, this voltage deforms E: for sufficiently large V_{m}, the local minimum at r_{m} disappears and E decreases monotonically for all $r > r_*$. Consequently, any pore created with $r \approx r_*$ increases its radius. As more pores are created and expand, the current through pores increases and V_{m} decreases. Lowering V_{m} restores the local minimum at r_{m}: the energy E looks like a plot for 0.4 V in Fig. 4b. Now, pores with $r > r_{\mathrm{m}}$ shrink until they reach $r_{\mathrm{m}} \approx 1$ nm, where the energy has a minimum.

The second mechanism affecting drift velocity is the decrease in membrane tension caused by creation of many pores and/or their expansion. According to (2), the decrease in σ increases the energy cost of expanding the pores, which slows down and eventually halts their further growth. Hence, the drift velocity of a pore is *coupled through membrane tension* to all other pores. This tension coupling is not included in our formula (5) for drift velocity, and thus, (5) is a good approximation only when a few small pores exist. The analysis of tension-coupled pores[43] yields the following modification of the drift velocity: (5) still applies but the constant membrane tension σ in the pore energy E is replaced by an *effective membrane tension* σ_{eff},

$$\sigma_{\mathrm{eff}}(A_{\mathrm{p}}) = 2\sigma' - \frac{2\sigma' - \sigma_0}{(1 - A_{\mathrm{p}}/A)^2}. \qquad (6)$$

Here σ' is the interfacial energy per area of the hydrocarbon–water interface, σ_0 is the surface tension of the membrane without pores, A_{p} is the total area of pores, and A is the area of the lipid bilayer. Hence, drift velocity of a single pore in the system of tension-coupled pores depends on pore radius r, transmembrane potential V_{m}, and total pore area A_{p} according to

$$u(r, V_{\mathrm{m}}, A_{\mathrm{p}}) = \frac{D}{kT}\left\{4\beta\left(\frac{r_*}{r}\right)^4 \frac{1}{r} - 2\pi\gamma + 2\pi\sigma_{\mathrm{eff}}(A_{\mathrm{p}})\,r + F(r, V_{\mathrm{m}})\right\}, \quad \text{in } r \geq r_*. \qquad (7)$$

Figure 5 combines the effect of both tension coupling and pore-induced decrease in V_{m}. At each time instant, σ_{eff} is computed from the current ensemble of pores, and tension σ in the individual pore energy (2) is set to the current value of σ_{eff}. We then plot E as a function of r. Figure 5a shows that the creation and growth of pores lifts the right side of the energy curve, producing a second energy minimum at $r_{\mathrm{s}} \gg r_{\mathrm{m}}$ (*diamonds* in Fig. 5a, plots labeled 100 µs and 1 ms). Thus, there exist simultaneously two energy minima: at $r_{\mathrm{m}} \approx 1$ nm and at $r_{\mathrm{s}} \gg r_{\mathrm{m}}$. We expect that in time, pores will divide themselves between two populations: "small" pores with $r \approx r_{\mathrm{m}}$ and "large" pores with $r \approx r_{\mathrm{s}}$. This prediction is confirmed by an example presented in the section "Pore Evolution Phase."

Postshock Pore Shrinkage and Coarsening

While initial stages of pore evolution are fairly rapid (microseconds), later evolution slows down considerably as parts of the energy E become nearly flat (plot labeled 1 ms in Fig. 5a),

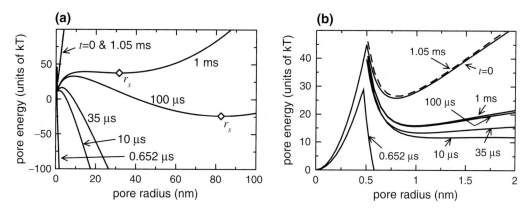

Figure 5: Change in the pore energy as a result of the creation of pores, evolution of their radii, and accompanying changes in V_m. Time instants are given by labels; *diamonds* in (**a**) indicate energy minimum r_s caused by creation and growth of pores. Electric shock of strength 3 V and duration 1 ms is applied to a membrane whose equivalent circuit is shown in Fig. 7. *Dashed line* labeled "1.05 ms" corresponds to pore energy 50 μs after the end of the shock. (**b**) Shows the same data as (**a**) but focuses on small radii to better visualize the existence of the energy minimum r_m

decreasing drift velocity u. Thus, reaching steady state can take a long time (milliseconds), and pore evolution is usually not complete at the end of the shock. Consequently, when the shock is terminated, there exist pores with radii from r_m to above r_s, although a majority of pores can be found near r_m and r_s.

When the external voltage is turned off, the membrane discharges. Because of the presence of pores, the discharge rate is very fast (under a microsecond) and the transmembrane potential V_m drops to near zero, even if the cell has a nonzero rest potential. At such small V_m, the minimum at r_s disappears and the pore energy increases monotonically for $r > r_m$ (Fig. 5, plot labeled 1.05 ms). Consequently, all pores shrink to r_m. This shrinkage is very fast because of the steepness of the energy curve.

Pore Resealing

Once hydrophilic pores shrink to the minimum energy radius r_m, they can reseal by first converting to a hydrophobic configuration and then by being destroyed by lipid fluctuations. Conversion to the hydrophobic configuration requires that a pore gains sufficient thermal energy to exceed difference in energy between the two types of pores, $E_* - E_m \approx 18\,kT$. Since this energy barrier is considerably larger than kT, it can be expected that conversion to the hydrophobic configuration will occur very slowly. In contrast, the destruction of hydrophobic pores is very fast: their lifetime is on the order of 10 ps.[31] In the physical model, hydrophobic pores with radii between r and $r + dr\,(r < r_*)$ are destroyed at a rate $(\nu_d n\,dr)$ per unit area of the membrane, where ν_d is the fluctuation rate per lipid molecule.

In experiments, resealing times vary from hundreds of microseconds to minutes.[18,31,44,45] This variability reflects differences in the energy barrier for different types of membrane.

Mathematical Modeling of Electroporation

Advection-Diffusion Equation

A population of pores existing at time t can be characterized by a pore density distribution, $n(r, t)$, such that the number of pores (per unit area) with radii between r and $r + dr$ is $n(r, t)dr$. All physics of pore creation, evolution, and resealing can be summed up in a single advection-diffusion partial differential equation (PDE)[43] that governs $n(r, t)$:

$$\frac{\partial n}{\partial t} = D \frac{\partial^2 n}{\partial r^2} - \frac{\partial}{\partial r}(u \, n) + \nu_c h \frac{\partial}{\partial r} \left(\frac{U}{kT} \right) e^{-U/kT} - \nu_d n H(r_* - r). \tag{8}$$

The four terms on the right-hand side of this PDE correspond to four mechanisms by which $n(r, t)$ is changed. First, the diffusion term describes random fluctuation of pore radii caused by thermal energy. Second, the drift term describes the changes in pore radii that are driven by minimization of the energy of the bilayer; u is the drift velocity. In $r > r_*$, u is given by (7); in $r < r_*$,

$$u = -\frac{D}{kT} \frac{\partial U}{\partial r},$$

where U is the energy of hydrophobic pores given by (1). Third, the creation term describes creation of pores according to (4). Fourth, the destruction term describes disappearance of pores; since only hydrophobic pores can be destroyed by lipid fluctuation, this term contains the Heaviside's step function $H(r)$. PDE (8) must be augmented by a governing equation for transmembrane potential V_m (see the section "Governing Equation for the Transmembrane Potential"), by the formula for current through the pores (see the section "Current–Voltage Relationship of a Pore") and by appropriate initial and boundary conditions. Initial conditions usually assume intact membrane at rest (i.e., $V_m(0) = V_{rest}$ and $n(r, 0) = 0$). Boundary conditions assume absorption of pores at $r = 0$ (i.e., pores disappear when their radii shrink to zero) and no-flux condition as $r \to \infty$ (i.e., pores do not grow without bounds).

Since the drift velocity u, appearing in the second term, contains the effective membrane tension σ_{eff}, PDE (8) is a nonlinear extension of the Smoluchowski equation that was first used to describe electroporation in 1979 by Pastushenko et al.[33] Further development of the theory of electroporation was undertaken by Weaver et al.[26,34,35,46] and by Neu et al.[32,39,43]

In principle, electroporation can be studied by discretizing the PDE (8) for $n(r, t)$ and the governing equation for V_m and solving them numerically. Although this approach has been used by some researchers,[26,46–48] it has a large computational cost. Because of the exponential dependence of the creation rate on the pore energy and the existence of disparate spatial and temporal scales, the numerical solution of (8) requires very small discretization steps. For example, Joshi and Schoenbach[48] used spatial and temporal discretization steps of 5 pm and 1 ps, respectively. Hence, the use of PDE (8) has been limited to investigating electroporation in a spatially clamped, uniformly polarized membrane patch,[26,46–48] or in a spherical cell, but the cell studies involved only very short shocks, up to a microsecond in duration.[49–51]

To avoid large computational cost associated with numerical solution of the PDE, Neu and Krassowska have developed an alternative approach of asymptotically reducing the PDE to a system of ODEs. By using two different scalings of the pore radius r in the PDE (8), they have extracted two distinct components of electroporation. The first component occurs for radii near $r_* = 0.5$ nm and describes creation and resealing of the hydrophilic pores.[32] It is governed by a single ODE for the density of hydrophilic pores. The second component occurs at radii above r_* and describes growth and shrinkage of pores. Here, they have obtained a set of ODEs governing the rate of change of the radius of each pore.[43] This *asymptotic model of electroporation* reduces discretization steps by up to five orders of magnitude and allows one to study the full spatiotemporal dynamics of electroporation over several milliseconds in membrane patches, single cells, one-dimensional fibers, and two-dimensional tissue.

Asymptotic Model of Electroporation

Creation and Resealing of Pores

Neu and Krassowska[32] have shown that under scaling of the radius r by $r_* = 0.5$ nm, PDE (8) reduces to an ODE,

$$\frac{\mathrm{d}N}{\mathrm{d}t} = \alpha \, e^{(V_m/V_{ep})^2} \left(1 - \frac{N}{N_{eq}(V_m)} \right), \tag{9}$$

where $N(t)$ is the density of hydrophilic pores defined as

$$N(t) = \int_{r_*}^{\infty} n(r,t)\mathrm{d}r, \tag{10}$$

and $N_{eq}(V_m)$ is the equilibrium pore density for a given voltage V_m,

$$N_{eq}(V_m) = N_0 e^{q(V_m/V_{ep})^2}. \tag{11}$$

Constants α, V_{ep}, N_0, q are defined in Appendix 1. ODE (9) is usually solved with the initial condition $N(0) = 0$ (no pores).

Equation (9) shows that hydrophilic pores appear at a rate that is exponentially dependent on the square of the transmembrane potential V_m. V_{ep} is the characteristic voltage of electroporation. Note that, just like the creation rate density (4), ODE (9) does not have a distinct threshold for pore creation. In this ODE, a sharp increase in pore creation occurs at approximately $4 V_{ep}$. The value of V_{ep} in Appendix 1 was chosen so that $V_m < 1$ V can be considered subthreshold for shocks up to 1 ms duration.

Equation (9) describes not only creation of pores but also their resealing: after the shock has created a certain number of pores, the pore density N becomes larger than N_0, the equilibrium pore density for $V_{\mathrm{m}} = 0$. Hence, if the shock is turned off and V_{m} drops near zero, the right-hand side of (9) becomes negative and the pore density N starts decreasing. With the parameters from Appendix 1, the time constant of resealing is approximately $3\,\mathrm{s}$.[31]

Note that the only pores that participate in resealing are those that have shrunk to a radius near r_{m}. If there exist any pores with $r \gg r_{\mathrm{m}}$, they cannot reseal by the mechanism represented in (9). The resealing of these macropores is beyond the scope of the present model because it involves such processes as a change in cell volume[52] or active, exocytotic rebuilding of the lipid bilayer.[53]

Evolution of Pore Radii

Neu and Krassowski[43] have shown that the diffusion term in the PDE (8) is at least two orders of magnitude smaller than the drift term and can be eliminated. Hence, (8) reduces to a first-order advection PDE, which can be further transformed using the method of characteristics.[54] This procedure leads to ODEs governing the time evolution of individual pore radii.

As discussed in sections "Pore Creation" and "Pore Evolution," hydrophilic pores are created with the initial radius of r_* and they subsequently change size to minimize the energy of the lipid bilayer. For a membrane with a total number of K pores, the rate of change of their radii, r_j, is determined by a set of ODEs:

$$\frac{\mathrm{d}r_j}{\mathrm{d}t} = u(r_j, V_{\mathrm{m}}, A_{\mathrm{p}}), \quad j = 1, 2, \ldots, K, \tag{12}$$

where u is the drift velocity given by (7).

Compared to the PDE (8), the ODEs (9) and (12) of the asymptotic model contain a smaller number of parameters and most of them are related in a straightforward way to experimental measurements.[31] The connection between the parameters of the ODE (9) and the molecular-level constants appearing in the PDE can be found in our previous publications.[32,55]

Current–Voltage Relationship of a Pore

In a membrane containing K pores, the total current I_{p} through these pores is computed by adding currents through all of them,

$$I_{\mathrm{p}}(t) = \sum_{j=1}^{K} i_{\mathrm{p}}(r_j, V_{\mathrm{m}}), \tag{13}$$

where i_{p} is the current–voltage relationship of an individual pore. The simplest representation of i_{p} is the ohmic approximation of the pore resistance that assumes a cylindrical pore,

$$R_{\mathrm{p}} = \frac{h}{s\pi r^2}, \tag{14}$$

where s is the conductivity of the solution filling the pore.

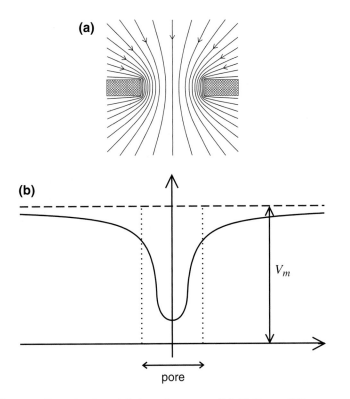

Figure 6: (**a**) Current lines in the vicinity of a pore. (**b**) Voltage difference across the pore (*solid line*) compared with the potential V_m across the membrane away from the pore (*dashed line*)

This approximation overestimates the current through large pores because such pores cannot maintain the same voltage drop V_m that develops across intact membrane (Fig. 6). To account for the decrease of the transpore voltage, the current–voltage relationship of a pore assumes that V_m occurs across the pore resistance, R_p, and the *input resistance*, $R_i = 1/(2sr)$, connected in series,[47,56]

$$i_p(r, V_m) = \frac{V_m}{R_p + R_i}.$$ (15)

Thus, (15) gives a nonlinear relationship between the pore area and the current through a pore.

Formula (15), which is used in the section "Example of the Electroporation Process," does not account for the interaction of ions with the pore walls. This interaction can be accounted for by introducing an energy barrier[31,57] or steric hindrance of ions.[47] In addition, (15) computes only the electric current, without specifying its ionic composition. Our group has developed another formula for i_p, in which the total current is computed as a sum of currents carried by Na^+, K^+, Ca^{2+}, and Cl^- ions.[58] A recent article by Vasilkoski et al.[41] contains a formula for i_p that combines all factors affecting current through pores: spreading resistance, energy barrier, steric hindrance, and the ionic composition of the current.

Example of the Electroporation Process

Governing Equation for the Transmembrane Potential

To determine the number and distribution of pores created by the shock, the time evolution of the transmembrane potential $V_m(t)$ must be given. V_m is a dynamical variable and its evolution depends on the experimental conditions. This example assumes the simplest experimental setup (Fig. 7): a uniformly polarized membrane of surface area A, represented by the capacitance C, resistance R, and an additional path for current I_p through electropores. Thus, V_m is governed by an ODE,

$$R_s C \frac{dV_m}{dt} = V_0 - V_m - \frac{R_s}{R}(V_m - V_{rest}) - R_s I_p, \tag{16}$$

where voltage V_0 represents external electric shock, V_{rest} is the rest potential, and R_s is the series resistance of the experimental setup.

This formulation includes two simplifications. First, the membrane capacitance C is assumed constant, although it is expected to decrease as a result of pore creation and growth.

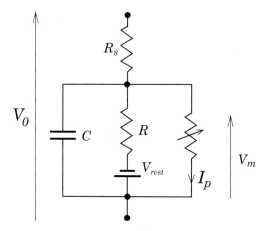

Figure 7: Circuit representation of a uniformly polarized membrane of the surface area A. The capacitor $C = C_m A$ represents the total capacitance of the membrane, the constant resistor $R = R_m/A$ accounts for the flow of current through channel proteins, and the battery represents the rest potential V_{rest}. The variable resistor accounts for the dynamically changing current through pores, I_p. The resistor R_s represents the series resistance of the experimental setup and V_0 is the external stimulus

However, the change in C measured experimentally was found to be below 2%,[3] which justifies this simplification. Second, the current through channel proteins is approximated by a constant resistance R. The model can be easily extended by incorporating equations describing the dynamics of excitable cardiac membrane.[59–62] However, the study by DeBruin and Krassowska[60] found that the current though active channels has only a second-order effect on the process of electroporation and thus can be neglected in studies that focus on electroporation.

Experimental and theoretical studies of electroporation reveal that it consists of a sequence of phases: membrane charging, pore creation, pore evolution, postshock pore shrinkage, and resealing. The remainder of this section will illustrate the individual phases for an example of a membrane exposed to a shock of strength 3 V for 1 ms. The membrane area A is assumed equal to the surface area of a spherical cell of a 50 μm radius. All parameters of the model are listed in Appendix 1; the numerical implementation is described in Appendix 2.

Membrane Charging Phase

Starting from an initial condition of an intact membrane at rest, an electroporating shock first charges the membrane, increasing V_m. Since the membrane does not yet contain any pores, the current I_p in (16) is zero, and the membrane charges like a parallel resistance and capacitance. This passive RC charging can be seen during the first 0.652 μs in Fig. 8a, when transmembrane potential increases in magnitude from its initial value of $V_{rest} = -0.08$ V according to the formula

$$V_m(t) = V_{rest} + \frac{V_0}{1 + R_s/R}(1 - e^{-t/\tau}), \quad \text{where } \tau = \frac{R_s C}{1 + R_s/R}. \tag{17}$$

If the shock strength V_0 is below the threshold voltage, then RC charging goes to completion with V_m approaching the steady-state value according to (17), and no significant pore creation occurs. For stronger V_0, the pure RC charging breaks down when V_m approaches threshold, signaling the ignition of significant pore creation. Here it is assumed that the charging phase ends with the creation of the first pore (i.e., when the density of pores N multiplied by the membrane area A reaches 1). The duration of the charging phase depends on the shock strength. For a 3-V shock, the charging phase ends and the creation phase starts at 0.652 μs.

Pore Creation Phase

When V_m exceeds a threshold value (≈ 1 V in this example), the membrane experiences a dramatic increase in the pore creation rate. The pores add pathways for current to cross the membrane and thus decrease its resistance. In consequence, V_m no longer follows the charging transient (17) that would be observed in a cell with a passive membrane. As seen in Fig. 8, the creation of the pores first slows down the increase and eventually decreases the transmembrane voltage V_m.

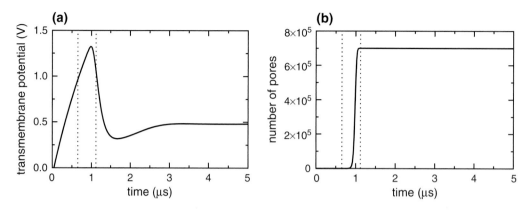

Figure 8: (a) Transmembrane potential and (b) number of pores as a function of time during the first 5 μs of a 3-V shock. The *dotted vertical lines* in (a) and (b) indicate the start and the end of the pore creation phase

Once V_m drops below the threshold value, the creation rate slows down dramatically. Here, it is assumed that the pore creation phase is completed when the relative increase in the total number of pores per time step drops below 10^{-6}. According to this definition, in the example of Fig. 8, creation ends at 1.119 μs. Although Table 1 shows that a few pores may be created after that time, the vast majority of pores are created within the time interval indicated by the dotted vertical lines in Fig. 8.

Pore Evolution Phase

Pore evolution is a considerably slower process than either pore creation or changes in V_m. Hydrophilic pores are created with a radius $r_* \approx 0.5$ nm; they immediately start growing but their radii are less than 4 nm by the end of the creation phase (Table 1, column labeled 1.119 μs). Most of the pore evolution occurs after the creation of new pores has ceased and

Table 1: Pore statistics at the end of creation (1.119 μs), end of shock (1 ms), after postshock shrinkage (1.05 ms), and 10 s after the shock

Time	1.119 μs	1 ms	1.05 ms	10 s
Number of all pores	700,311	700,314	700,291	1,719
Number of large pores	700,311	7,582	0	0
Radius of large pores[a] (nm)	1.50 ± 0.28	22.4 ± 4.3	–	–
Maximum radius (nm)	3.83	29.7	0.804	0.804
Fractional pore area ($\times 10^{-6}$)	162.2	460.4	45.2	0.11
Membrane conductivity[b] ($S\,m^{-2}$)	4.35×10^4	3.91×10^4	1.44×10^4	35.5
Transmembrane potential (V)	1.056	0.420	−0.024	−0.0796

[a]Mean ± standard deviation
[b]Includes conductivity of membrane without pores, $20\,S\,m^{-2}$

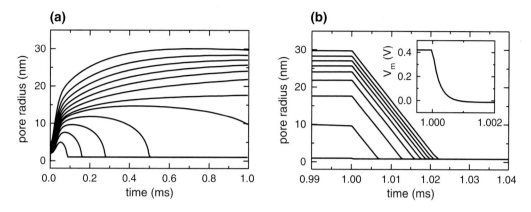

Figure 9: (a) Evolution of radii r_j of 12 selected pores during a 1-ms, 3-V shock. Note the different time scales in this panel and in Fig. 8. (b) Postshock shrinkage of the pores. The shock has been turned off at 1 ms. Inset shows the decrease of transmembrane potential from 0.42 V at the end of the shock to -0.024 V2 µs afterward. Main panel shows the decrease of radii r_j of 12 selected pores. This panel is a continuation of (a)

even after V_m has leveled off, both of which happen within microseconds. In contrast, some pore radii will not reach steady state by the end of a 1-ms, 3-V shock (Fig. 9a) and would have continued to evolve, although subsequent changes would have been relatively small.

All pores initially grow, but soon smaller pores start shrinking and eventually assume a radius of approximately 1 nm. Of the 12 pores illustrated in Fig. 9a, five have shrunk to the 1-nm radius by 1 ms. The remaining pores have their radii in the range of 15 to 30 nm. Thus, as predicted in the section "Pore Evolution," pores divide themselves into two distinct populations: "small" pores, with radii close to 1 nm, and "large" pores, with radii well above 1 nm.

The division of all pores into two populations is explained by examining the plots of pore energy shown in Fig. 5. At the beginning of the creation phase (0.652 µs plot in Fig. 5a), energy of the hydrophilic pores ($r > 0.5$ nm) decreases monotonically, causing all pores to grow. As pores grow, they relieve membrane tension, which decreases the effective membrane tension σ_{eff} and affects the shape of the pore energy. By 35 µs, the energy develops a local minimum near 1 nm (Fig. 5b), and by 100 µs, a second local minimum appears near 82 nm (Fig. 5a). The two minima are separated by a local maximum near 9 nm. Pores to the left of the maximum will shrink to 1 nm and form the population of small pores; pores to the right will grow toward the larger minimum energy radius and form the population of large pores. In time, the small pores greatly outnumber the large ones (Table 2). At 1 ms, 98.9% of all pores are small, and the remaining 1.1% are large. Despite their much greater numbers, small pores comprise only 14.3% of the total area of pores, and they contribute 51.6% to the increased conductivity of the membrane.

The evolution of radii within the large pore population is illustrated in Fig. 10. The number of large pores decreases with time (Table 1), while the distribution of pore radii

Table 2: Distribution of pores between small
and large pore populations at 1 ms

	Small	Large
Number of pores (%)	98.9	1.1
Average radius (nm)	≈ 1	22.4 ± 4.3
Maximum radius (nm)	≈ 1	29.7
Fractional pore area (%)	14.3	85.7
Membrane conductivity (%)	51.6	48.4

moves toward larger values, reaching 22.4 ± 4.3 nm (mean and standard deviation) at 1 ms, with 7,582 large pores.

Postshock Pore Shrinkage Phase

The electric shock is terminated at 1 ms. Immediately, the membrane starts discharging and $2\,\mu s$ later, V_m drops to -0.024 V (Table 1 and Fig. 9b, inset). The presence of pores does not allow the cell to maintain its normal rest potential of -0.08 V.

In response to the drop in V_m, pores start shrinking rapidly. Figure 9b shows the postshock evolution of pore radii (it is the continuation of pore evolution shown in Fig. 9a). The large pore population disappears when all large pores have shrunk to r_m. In this example, shrinkage lasts up to $22\,\mu s$, depending on the initial sizes of pores.

As a result of pore shrinkage, the fractional pore area decreases over tenfold and the membrane conductance decreases 2.7-fold (Table 1). This decrease in membrane conductance has been observed in experiments[31] and is sometimes interpreted as "rapid resealing"

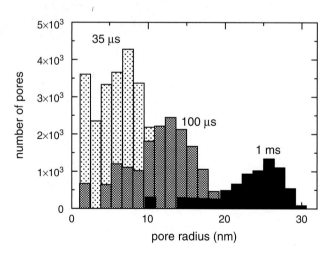

Figure 10: Distribution of pore radii at 35, $100\,\mu s$, and 1 ms. Only large pores are included in the distributions. The bin width = 1.4 nm

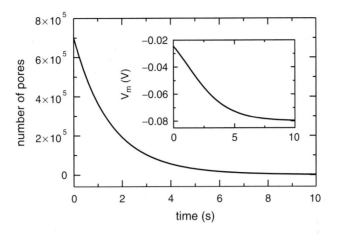

Figure 11: Resealing of the pores. Main panel shows the number of pores K as a function of time. K decreases from 700,291 immediately after the shock to 1,719 10 s later. This panel is a continuation of Fig. 8b. *Inset* shows the gradual restoration of the rest potential from -0.024 V 2 μs after the shock to -0.0796 V at 10 s. Note that the time scale in this figure is in seconds

of pores.[63] However, as seen in Table 1, a vast majority of the pores are still present 50 μs after the shock. This result is confirmed by the experimental observation that the permeable state is long lived for small, but not large, molecules.[64–66]

Pore Resealing Phase

The fast shrinkage of pores should not be confused with pore resealing, during which the pores disappear and the integrity of the lipid bilayer is restored. With parameters of Appendix 1, the resealing in the model proceeds with a time constant of 3 s (Fig. 11). As the pores reseal, the transmembrane potential gradually returns to rest (Fig. 11, inset).

Large difference in the durations of the shrinkage and resealing phases can be explained by energetics of each process. During shrinkage, the pore energy increases monotonically for radii above r_m (see *dashed line* labeled 1.05 ms in Fig. 5). Thus, it is energetically favorable for pores with radii $r > r_m$ to shrink, and the steep energy gradient translates into large drift velocity of pore shrinkage. In contrast, in order to reseal, pores must convert to hydrophobic: for example, hydrophilic pores with radii $r \approx r_m$ must surmount the energy barrier equal to $E_* - E_m \approx 18\,kT$ (Fig. 2).

Effects of Shock Strength

The pore number and distribution depend on the shock strength V_0 applied to the membrane, and the model is used to explore this dependence. Figure 12 illustrates the effect of

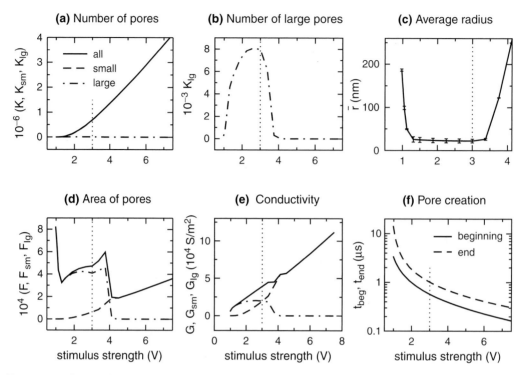

Figure 12: Dependence of electroporation on shock strength. (a) Number of all pores (K) and number of small (K_{sm}) and large (K_{lg}) pores. The lines corresponding to K and K_{sm} overlap. (b) Number of large pores (K_{lg}) shown on an expanded vertical scale. (c) Average radius ($\bar{r}$) of the large pore population. The *vertical bars* indicate standard deviation. The range of the shock strengths was truncated to 4.125 V because there are no large pores for stronger shocks. (d) Total area of pores reported as a fraction of the membrane surface area for all (F), small (F_{sm}), and large (F_{lg}) pores. (e) Conductivity of the membrane for all (G), small (G_{sm}), and large (G_{lg}) pores. (f) Beginning (t_{beg}) and end (t_{end}) of the pore creation phase. Note the logarithmic scale of the vertical axis. All results except those in (f) were collected at the end of a 1-ms shock. The legend in (a) applies also to (b), (d), and (e). The *dotted vertical lines* indicate the shock of 3 V, that is, the default shock strength used previously in this chapter

shock strength on the number of pores, their average radius, the area of pores, membrane conductivity, and the timing of the pore creation phase. The shock V_0 ranges from 0.975 V (below the apparent threshold) to 7.5 V, and all data except Fig. 12f were collected at the end of a 1-ms shock.

As expected, the number of pores increases with the shock strength but, except for very weak shocks, this increase is due to the creation of small pores. In Fig. 12a, curves representing all pores and small pores overlap and large pores appear to be a negligible fraction of all pores. As seen on the expanded vertical axis in Fig. 12b, the number of large pores initially increases, but above 4 V, large pores disappear altogether and only small pores are being created. This prediction was confirmed by experiments in which high-voltage, short pulses were shown to create a large number of pores with radii not substantially larger than 1 nm.[31,67,68] Additional confirmation came from the studies that observed decrease in the uptake of macromolecules (i.e., DNA) for strong pulses.[64,69]

The average radius of large pores decreases as the number of large pores grows but increases again once fewer large pores are created (Fig. 12c). Despite their relatively small number, large pores contribute significantly to the fractional pore area (Fig. 12d) and to the increase in membrane conductivity (Fig. 12e) for shocks below 4 V. As the shock strength increases, the contribution of small pores increases, and above 4 V, all pore area and all membrane conductance are due to small pores. Figure 12f shows that the pore creation phase begins earlier, and its duration is shorter for stronger shocks (note that the vertical axis is logarithmic).

Limitations

The theory described here uses a continuum representation of pore energetics, which is appropriate for large pores but is unlikely to remain valid as the size of the pore approaches the size of a lipid molecule. Studies of electroporation that use molecular dynamics (MD) simulations give us a fascinating picture of molecular-level events occurring during electroporation.[70,71] Unfortunately, MD simulations are so expensive computationally that at present these models are limited to very small pieces of the membrane (e.g., 256 lipid molecules) and very early stages of electroporation (up to 50 ns). Nevertheless, they confirm some of the assumptions of the theory presented here, such as that the pore creation occurs in two steps, starting with hydrophobic pores (called "water wires") that subsequently change conformation to hydrophilic.

Both experiments and MD simulations show that the electroporation process is probabilistic in nature, with the pore creation rate and the change in its radius subject to fluctuations. These fluctuations are of importance when one attempts to model a small number of pores, created very slowly in response to threshold-level shocks.[18,72] With stronger shocks, which create a large number of pores, individual variations in creation and expansion rates are of less significance, since they are not readily visible in the total current I_p. Hence, the theory presented here is an averaged, deterministic description of the electroporation process and its intended use is for above-threshold shocks.

The third limitation is the representation of the flow of matter through the pores. The present model is concerned only with the flow of electric current, which allows one to determine the decrease in the membrane resistance during electroporation. Previous studies have separated that current into currents carried by Na^+, K^+, Ca^{2+}, and Cl^- ions and examined the changes in intracellular ionic concentrations as a result of pore creation.[58,73] However, to date our group did not attempt to model flow of water through pores and the resulting change of cell surface area and volume: the cell geometry was assumed constant. In reality, the intracellular fluid will leak through the macropores, decreasing cell volume and reducing membrane tension.[52] This is an additional factor that can slow the growth and facilitate resealing of the pores, although cell swelling and growth of pores have also been observed.[25] Thus, future extension of the present theory should involve changes in cell volume. The coupling of pore evolution with a change in cell volume has been proposed before, although only in the case when one pore is present.[52,74] As a result of the constant cell volume assumption, the model presented here is valid for relatively short time intervals (milliseconds) before the flow of water through pores affects the cell volume. That is usually sufficient, as electroporation shocks are rarely longer than a few milliseconds.

The most significant limitation of all electroporation models is the lack of a consistent set of model parameters that would represent a specific tissue under study. This is because it is not possible to find in the literature all parameters required by the model for a single cell type. Typically, only the electroporation threshold is measured,[14,64,75] and sometimes the resealing time constant as well.[45,76,77] The most comprehensive parameter set is available for artificial lipid bilayers.[31] Although electroporation in cells is fundamentally the same as in artificial bilayers,[78] many parameters depend sensitively on the composition of the lipid bilayer.[79,80] There exist parameter sets that approximate electroporation in cardiac muscle[60] and in skeletal muscle,[81] but only for the earlier version of the asymptotic model that does not include the growth of pores. In the example included here, a "default" parameter set was used, which was developed from the measurements of Glaser et al.[31] on artificial lipid bilayers and then adjusted to match the study of Hibino et al.,[82] who used potentiometric dyes to visualize the evolution of transmembrane potential during electroporation of sea urchin eggs. Therefore, in interpreting the results given in the section "Example of the Electroporation Process," one needs to keep in mind that urchin eggs have a higher electroporation threshold than cardiac muscle: 1 V versus 0.4–0.5 V.[8,83]

Finally, electroporation presents considerable challenges to numerical simulations. Under conditions corresponding to most practical applications, the governing equations are stiff because of strong exponential dependence of the pore creation rate on the square of the transmembrane voltage. Even with the asymptotic approximations for pore creation and evolution, simulations of electroporation are expensive. This is because during an early part of the creation transient, the number of pores and their radii have to be tracked very accurately, which requires small time steps. Any errors in the number and distribution of pore radii would propagate to the transmembrane voltage. The data in Fig. 4b show that errors in V_m as small as 0.02 V can result in a threefold increase in the pore creation rate, and consequently, the number of pores would be predicted incorrectly. Recent research attempts to bypass this difficulty by using singular perturbation to "peel away" the strong exponential dependence of pore creation rate upon the transmembrane voltage V_m.[84] In particular, during the pore creation phase, the full system of ODEs (9) and (12) reduces to a single integrodifferential equation for the transmembrane voltage plus an expression for the pore density distribution. Hopefully, further progress in this direction will allow us to study both temporal and spatial aspects of electroporation in three-dimensional tissue without prohibitive computational costs.

Conclusion

The phases of electroporation, as seen in the section "Example of the Electroporation Process," closely resemble the steps of electropermeabilization identified by Teissié et al.[85] based on experimental observations. The "induction step" corresponds to the charging and pore creation phases of the model (Fig. 8), the "expansion step" corresponds to the pore evolution phase (Fig. 9a), the "stabilization step" corresponds to the postshock shrinkage of pores (Fig. 9b), and the "resealing step" corresponds to the resealing of small pores (Fig. 11). The only step not seen in the model is the "memory effect" that describes changes in the membrane and cell behavior persisting on the time scale of hours and that may be related to exchange of charged molecules between the two monolayers of the membrane.[86,87] Although some of the model's predictions still must be confirmed experimentally, the resemblance between the model's "phases" and "steps" of electroporation seen in experiments gives us reason to believe that the asymptotic model presented here is sufficiently accurate to provide theoretical support for real-life applications.

In particular, the asymptotic model can be very useful in assessing the effects of defibrillation shocks on cardiac muscle. Since the electroporation process is represented by a set of ODEs for $N(t)$ and $r_j(t)$, it can be naturally incorporated into any model of cardiac membrane by adding electroporation current I_p to the transmembrane current. In the past, such simulations were performed for cardiac membrane,[59,88] cardiac fibers,[60,89] and two- and three-dimensional myocardium.[61,62,90] These studies used an older version of the asymptotic model in which pores did not grow: their size was kept constant and equal to $r_m \approx 0.8\,\text{nm}$, the minimum-energy radius. The advantage of this simplification is a dramatic reduction in computational cost because only an ODE for $N(t)$ needs to be solved. This simplification is justified in studies that simulate only the increase of membrane conductance and changes in V_m caused by defibrillation shocks. If desired, the exchange of ions through pores can be added by replacing the current–voltage relationship (15) of a pore by the one that accounts for flow of distinct ions.[58,73] This extension will allow the use of the model with nongrowing pores to simulate shock-induced changes in ionic concentration that lead to postshock arrhythmias, as well as resealing of pores and restoration of normal concentrations. However, the model with nongrowing pores is not appropriate for the studies of cellular injury associated with the development of large-sized pores or for predicting the electroporation-mediated uptake of macromolecules such as DNA. Such studies need to use the full asymptotic model, which permits pores to expand and shrink, and thus give a complete picture of the electroporation process.

Acknowledgment

Supported in part by the National Science Foundation Grants BES-0401757 and DMS-0515616.

Appendix 1: Parameters of the Electroporation Model

Pore energy and drift velocity:

r_*	0.5×10^{-9} m	minimum radius of hydrophilic pores at $V_m = 0$[31]
E_*	$45\,kT$	energy barrier for creation of hydrophilic pores at $V_m = 0$[31]
r_m	0.8×10^{-9} m	minimum energy radius at $V_m = 0$[31]
E_m	$27\,kT$	energy at r_m with $V_m = 0$[32]
β	1.4×10^{-19} J	steric repulsion energy[32]
γ	1.8×10^{-11} J m^{-1}	edge energy[31,46]
σ_0	10^{-6} J m^{-2}	tension of the bilayer without pores[91]
σ'	2×10^{-2} J m^{-2}	tension of hydrocarbon–water interface[92]
D	5×10^{-14} m^2 s^{-1}	diffusion coefficient for pore radius[46]
T	310 K	absolute temperature (37°C)

Effect of V_m:

ε_0	8.85×10^{-12} F m^{-1}	permittivity of vacuum
ε_m	$2\varepsilon_0$	permittivity of the lipid bilayer[31,46]
ε_w	$80\varepsilon_0$	permittivity of the water filling the pores[31,46]
F_{max}	0.70×10^{-9} N V^{-2}	maximum electric force for $V_m = 1$ V[39]
r_h	0.97×10^{-9} m	characteristic length for electric force[39]
r_t	0.31×10^{-9} m	correction for toroidal pores[39]

Pore creation and resealing:

ν_c	2×10^{38} m^{-3} s^{-1}	fluctuation rate per unit volume[34]
ν_d	10^{11} s^{-1}	fluctuation rate per lipid molecule[31]
α	1×10^9 m^{-2} s^{-1}	creation rate coefficient[55]
V_{ep}	0.258 V	characteristic voltage of electroporation[55]
N_0	1.5×10^9 m^{-2}	equilibrium pore density at $V_m = 0$[55]
q	$\equiv (r_m/r_*)^2$	constant in (9) for pore creation rate[55]

Current–voltage relationship of a pore:

h	5×10^{-9} m	membrane thickness[31]
s	2 s m^{-1}	conductivity of the solution filling the pore[93]

Equation for V_m:

C_m	10^{-2} F m^{-2}	surface capacitance of the membrane[82]
R_m	$0.5\,\Omega\,$m^2	surface resistance of the membrane[82]
V_{rest}	-0.08 V	rest potential[94]
A	3.14×10^{-8} m^2	membrane area (of a 50-μm spherical cell[82])
R_s	$5 \times 10^3\,\Omega$	series resistance (chosen to give charging time constant of a 50-μm spherical cell[82])

Appendix 2: Numerical Implementation

The numerical implementation of the asymptotic model of electroporation[93] is based on an idea of "launching" individual pores as they are created and tracking the evolutions of their radii. Thus, it attempts to reproduce in silico the electroporation process occurring in a membrane. For a typical simulation, initial conditions assume an intact membrane at rest: transmembrane potential $V_m(0) = V_{rest}$, pore density $N(0) = 0$, and number of individual pores $K=0$. The time loop first solves the ODEs for V_m (16) and for N (9). If N holds more than one pore (i.e., $NA > 1$), these pores are "launched" and allowed to grow. To do so, K is increased by an integer number of pores, floor (NA), and N is decreased by a corresponding value. Next, radius r_j of each individual pore is updated according to (12). The updated values V_m, N, K, and r_j, $j = 1, \ldots, K$ are used to compute the current through pores I_p (13) and the effective membrane tension σ_{eff} (6). I_p is used in the next time step to determine V_m. All ODEs are solved using the midpoint implicit method.

The run time depends on the number of large pores created by the shock. Stronger shocks, which create more than 10^4 pores, result in unacceptably long runs. Hence, three features of implementation aim at increasing computational efficiency. First, pores created at the same time step are launched as a group rather than individually, which limits the number of pore radii that need to be updated by solving (12). Second, the solution uses adaptive time stepping. Initially, $\Delta t = 1.5\,\text{ns}$ is used to resolve very fast transients associated with the creation of pores. Once pore creation ends and the dependent variables change less rapidly, Δt is gradually increased to $0.1\,\mu\text{s}$. The above initial and final Δt yield mean errors in voltage and maximum pore radius below 0.1%, and in pore density, below 4%.

The third feature takes advantage of the fact that as pores evolve, they naturally divide themselves into two distinct populations (Fig. 9a): small pores, with radii near $r_m \approx 1\,\text{nm}$, and large pores, with radii larger than r_m. The model keeps track of these two populations. Because all small pores have approximately the same radius, they are accounted for by the pore density N and radius r_m, which evolves according to (12) with r_j replaced by r_m. Large pores are represented individually: the radius r_j of each pore evolves according to (12). With two pore populations, the number of ODEs governing the pores radii decreases from K (total number of pores) to $K_{lg} + 1$ (number of large pores plus an ODE for r_m). Since for large shocks $K \gg K_{lg}$ (Table 2), this method significantly limits the number of independently evolving pore radii.

The exchange of pores between the small and large pore populations proceeds as follows. As described above, pores created according to (9) are all initially treated as large. Pores remain in the large pore population throughout the initial phase of creation and rapid expansion of pores. Afterward, pore growth slows down and eventually some pores start to shrink (Fig. 9a). If any large pore shrinks to within $1\,\text{pm}$ of r_m, it is "absorbed" into the small pore population, thereby increasing N and decreasing the number of large pores, K_{lg}. To ensure that the absorption of pores does not introduce artifacts, key simulations have been repeated without pore absorption. The simulation of a 1-ms, 3-V shock takes approximately

0.5 s (model implemented in C and running on a 3.4 GHz Pentium 4 processor under CentOS 4.0).

References

1. Benz R, Beckers F, Zimmermann U. Reversible electrical breakdown of lipid bilayer membranes: a charge-pulse relaxation study. *Memb Biol* 1979;48:181–204

2. Abidor IG, Arakelyan VB, Chernomordik LV, Chizmadzhev YA, Pastushenko VF, Tarasevich MR. Electric breakdown of bilayer lipid membranes: I. Main experimental facts and their qualitative discussion. *Bioelectrochem Bioenerg* 1979;6:37–52

3. Chernomordik LV, Sukharev SI, Abidor IG, Chizmadzhev YA. Breakdown of lipid bilayer membranes in an electric field. *Biochim Biophys Acta* 1983;736:203–213

4. Diederich A, Bahr G, Winterhalter M. Influence of surface charges on the rupture of black lipid membranes. *Phys Rev E* 1998;58:4883–4889

5. Jones JL, Jones RE, Balasky G. Microlesion formation in myocardial cells by high-intensity electric field stimulation. *Am J Physiol* 1987;253:H480–H486

6. Tung L, Tovar O, Neunlist M, Jain SK, O'Neil RJ. Effects of strong electric shock on cardiac muscle tissue. *Ann N Y Acad Sci* 1994;720:160–175

7. Kodama I, Sakuma I, Mitsui K, Iida M, Suzuki R, Fukui Y, Hosoda S, Toyama J. Aftereffects of high-intensity DC stimulation on the electromechanical performance of ventricular muscle. *Am J Physiol* 1994;267:H248–H258

8. Knisley SB, Grant AO. Asymmetrical electrically induced injury of rabbit ventricular myocytes. *J Mol Cell Cardiol* 1995;27:1111–1122

9. Fast VG, Cheek ER. Nonlinear changes of transmembrane potential during electrical shocks: role of membrane electroporation. *Circ Res* 2004;94:208–214

10. Nikolski VP, Efimov IR. Electroporation of the heart. *Europace* 2005;7[Suppl 2]:S146–S154

11. Lee RC, Kolodney MS. Electrical injury mechanisms: electrical breakdown of cell membranes. *Plast Reconst Surg* 1987;80:672–679

12. Potter H. Electroporation in biology: methods, applications, and instrumentation. *Anal Biochem* 1988;174:361–373

13. Hofmann GA, Dev SB, Nanda GS. Electrochemotherapy: transition from laboratory to the clinic. *IEEE Eng Med Biol Mag* 1996;15:124–132

14. Sukharev SI, Klenchin VA, Serov SM, Chernomordik LV, Chizmadzhev YA. Electroporation and electrophoretic DNA transfer into cells. The effect of DNA interaction with electropores. *Biophys J* 1992;63:1320–1327

15. Dev SB, Rabussay DP, Widera G, Hofmann GA. Medical applications of electroporation. *IEEE Trans Plasma Sci* 2000;28:206–223

16. Gehl J. Electroporation: theory and methods, perspectives for drug delivery, gene therapy and research. *Acta Physiol Scand* 2003;117:437–447

17. Andrè F, Mir LM. DNA electrotransfer: its principles and an updated review to its therapeutic applications. *Gene Ther* 2004;11:S33–S42

18. Melikov KC, Frolov VA, Ahcherbakov A, Samsonov AV, Chizmadzhev YA. Voltage-induced nonconductive and metastable pores in unmodified lipid bilayers. *Biophys J* 2001;80:1829–1836

19. Teissié J, Tsong TY. Electric field induced transient pores in phospholipid bilayer vesicles. *Biochemistry* 1981;20:1548–1554

20. Tekle E, Astumian RD, Chock PB. Selective and asymmetric molecular transport across electroporated cell membranes. *Proc Natl Acad Sci* 1994;91:11512–11516

21. Gabriel B, Teissié J. Direct observation in the millisecond time range of fluorescent molecule asymmetrical interaction with the electropermeabilized cell membrane. *Biophys J* 1997;73:2630–2637

22. Hibino M, Shigemori M, Itoh H, Nagayama K, Kinosita K Jr. Membrane conductance of an electroporated cell analyzed by submicrosecond imaging of transmembrane potential. *Biophys J* 1991;59:209–220

23. Ghosh PM, Keese CR, Giaver I. Monitoring electropermeabilization in the plasma membrane of adherent mammalian cells. *Biophys J* 1993;64:1602–1609

24. Huang Y, Sekhon NS, Borninski J, Chen N, Rubinsky B. Instantaneous, quantitative single-cell viability assessment by electrical evaluation of cell membrane integrity with microfabricated devices. *Sens Actuators A* 2003;105:31–39

25. Chang DC, Reese TS. Changes in membrane structure induced by electroporation as revealed by rapid-freezing electron microscopy. *Biophys J* 1990;58:1–12

26. Barnett A, Weaver JC. Electroporation: a unified, quantitative theory of reversible electrical breakdown and mechanical rupture in artificial planar bilayer membranes. *Bioelectrochem Bioenerg* 1991;25:163–182

27. Weaver JC, Chizmadzhev YA. Theory of electroporation: a review. *Bioelectrochem Bioenerg* 1996;41:135–160

28. Weaver JC. Electroporation of biological membranes from multicellular to nano scales. *IEEE Trans Dielectr Electr Insul* 2003;10:754–768

29. Chen C, Smye SW, Robinson MP, Evans JA. Membrane electroporation theories: a review. *Med Biol Eng Comput* 2006;44:5–14

30. Weaver JC. Molecular basis for cell membrane electroporation. *Ann N Y Acad Sci* 1994;720:141–152

31. Glaser RW, Leikin SL, Chernomordik LV, Pastushenko VF, Sokirko AI. Reversible electrical breakdown of lipid bilayers: formation and evolution of pores. *Biochim Biophys Acta* 1988;940:275–287

32. Neu JC, Krassowska W. Asymptotic model of electroporation. *Phys Rev E* 1999;59:3471–3482

33. Pastushenko VF, Chizmadzhev YA, Arakelyan VB. Electric breakdown of bilayer lipid membranes: II. Calculations of the membrane lifetime in the steady-state diffusion approximation. *Bioelectrochem Bioenerg* 1979;6:53–62

34. Weaver JC, Mintzer RA. Decreased bilayer stability due to transmembrane potential. *Phys Lett A* 1981;86A:57–59

35. Powell KT, Weaver JC. Transient aqueous pores in bilayer membranes: a statistical theory. *Bioelectrochem Bioenerg* 1986;15:211–227

36. Feynman RP, Leighton RB, Sands M. *The Feynman Lectures on Physics*, Vol. II. Reading, MA: Addison-Wesley; 1963

37. Plonsey R, Collin RE. *Principles and Applications of Electromagnetic Fields.* New York: McGraw-Hill; 1961

38. Krassowska W, Neu JC. Post-shock evolution of pores. *Ann Biomed Eng* 2001;29:S101

39. Neu JC, Smith KC, Krassowska W. Electrical energy required to form large conducting pores. *Bioelectrochem Bioenerg* 2003;60:107–114

40. Glaser RW. Appearance of a "critical voltage" in reversible electric breakdown. *Studia Biophysica* 1986;16:77–86

41. Vasilkoski Z, Esser AT, Gowrishankar TR, Weaver JC. Membrane electroporation: the absolute rate equation and nanosecond time scale pore creation. *Phys Rev E* 2006;74(021904):1–12

42. Plonsey R, Barr RC. *Bioelectricity. A Quantitative Approach.* New York: Plenum; 1988

43. Neu JC, Krassowska W. Modeling postshock evolution of large electropores. *Phys Rev E* 2003;67(021915):1–12

44. Saulis G, Venslauskas MS, Naktinis J. Kinetics of pore resealing in cell membranes after electroporation. *Bioelectrochem Bioenerg* 1991;26:1–13

45. Bier M, Hammer SM, Canaday DJ, Lee RC. Kinetics of sealing for transient electropores in isolated mammalian skeletal muscle cells. *Bioelectromagnetics* 1999;20:194–201

46. Freeman SA, Wang MA, Weaver JC. Theory of electroporation of planar bilayer membranes: predictions of the aqueous area, change in capacitance, and pore–pore separation. *Biophys J* 1994;67:42–56

47. Powell KT, Derrick EG, Weaver JC. A quantitative theory of reversible electrical breakdown of bilayer membranes. *Bioelectrochem Bioenerg* 1986;15:243–255

48. Joshi RP, Schoenbach KH. Electroporation dynamics in biological cells subjected to ultrafast electrical pulses: a numerical simulation study. *Phys Rev E* 2000;62:1025–1033

49. Joshi RP, Hu Q, Schoenbach KH, Bebe SJ. Simulations of electroporation dynamics and shape deformations in biological cells subjected to high voltage pulses. *IEEE Trans Plasma Sci* 2002;30:1536–1546

50. Joshi RP, Hu Q, Schoenbach KH. Modeling studies of cell response to ultrashort, high-intensity electric fields – implications for intracellular manipulation. *IEEE Trans Plasma Sci* 2004;32:1677–1686

51. Hu Q, Viswanadham S, Joshi RP, Schoenbach KH, Beebe SJ, Blackmore PF. Simulations of transient membrane behavior in cells subjected to a high-intensity ultrashort electric pulse. *Phys Rev E* 2005;71:031914

52. Sandre O, Moreaux L, Brochard-Wyart F. Dynamics of transient pores in stretched vesicles. *Proc Natl Acad Sci* 1999;96:10591–10596

53. McNeil PL, Steinhardt RA. Loss, restoration and maintenance of plasma membrane integrity. *J Cell Biol* 1997;137:1–4

54. Zauderer E. *Partial Differential Equations of Applied Mathematics.* New York: Wiley; 1983

55. DeBruin KA, Krassowska W. Modeling electroporation in a single cell. I: effects of field strength and rest potential. *Biophys J* 1999;77:1213–1224

56. Newman J. Resistance for flow of current to a disk. *J Electrochem Soc* 1966;113:501–502
57. Barnett A. The current-voltage relation of an aqueous pore in a lipid bilayer membrane. *Biochim Biophys Acta* 1990;1025:10–14
58. DeBruin KA, Krassowska W. Modeling electroporation in a single cell. II: effects of ionic concentrations. *Biophys J* 1999;77:1225–1233
59. Sakuma I, Haraguchi T, Ohuchi K, Fukui Y, Kodama I, Toyama J, Shibata N, Hosoda S. A model analysis of aftereffects of high-intensity DC stimulation on action potential of ventricular muscle. *IEEE Trans Biomed Eng* 1998;45:258–267
60. DeBruin KA, Krassowska W. Electroporation and shock-induced transmembrane potential in a cardiac fiber during defibrillation strength shocks. *Ann Biomed Eng* 1998;26:584–596
61. Ashihara T, Trayanova NA. Asymmetry in membrane responses to electric shocks: insights from bidomain simulations. *Biophys J* 2004;87:2271–2282
62. Sambelashvili AT, Nikolski VP, Efimov IR. Virtual electrode theory explains pacing threshold increase caused by cardiac tissue damage. *Am J Physiol* 2004;286:H2183–H2194
63. Bier M, Chen W, Gowrishankar TR, Astumian RD, Lee RC. Resealing dynamics of a cell after electroporation. *Phys Rev E* 2002;66(062905):1–4
64. Wolf H, Rols M-P, Boldt E, Neumann E, Teissié J. Control by pulse parameters of electric field-mediated gene transfer in mammalian cells. *Biophys J* 1994;66:524–531
65. Rols M-P, Teissié J. Electropermeabilization of mammalian cells to macro-molecules: control by pulse duration. *Biophys J* 1998;74:1415–1423
66. Satkauskas S, Bureau MF, Puc M, Mahfoudi A, Scherman D, Miklavčič D, Mir LM. Mechanisms of in vivo DNA electrotransfer: respective contributions of cell electroper-meabilization and DNA electrophoresis. *Mol Ther* 2002;5:133–140
67. Kakorin S, Neumann E. Ionic conductivity of electroporated lipid bilayer membranes. *Bioelectrochem* 2002;56:163–166
68. Schwister K, Deuticke B. Formation and properties of aqueous leaks induced in human erythrocytes by electrical breakdown. *Biochim Biophys Acta* 1985;816:332–348
69. Tekle E, Astumian RD, Chock PB. Electroporation by using bipolar oscillating electric field: an improved method for DNA transfection of NIH 3T3 cells. *Proc Natl Acad Sci* 1991;88:4230–4234
70. Tieleman DP, Leontiadou H, Mark AE, Marrink S-J. Simulation of pore formation in lipid bilayers by mechanical stress and electric fields. *J Am Chem Soc* 2003;125:6382–6383
71. Tarek M. Membrane electroporation: a molecular dynamics simulation. *Biophys J* 2005;88:4045–4053
72. Kotulska M, Koronkiewicz S, Kalinowski S. Self-similar process and flicker noise from a fluctuating nanopore in a lipid membrane. *Phys Rev E* 2004;69(031920):1–10
73. Cranford J, Krassowska W. Effects of ionic concentrations on density and size of pores created by electric pulses. In: *Proceedings of the 2006 Annual Fall Meeting of the BMES*, vol. 418, 2006
74. Brochard-Wyart F, de Gennes PG, Sandre O. Transient pores in stretched vesicles: role of leak-out. *Physica A* 2000;278:32–51

75. Teissié J, Rols M-P. An experimental evaluation of the critical potential difference inducing cell membrane electropermeabilization. *Biophys J* 1993;65:409–413

76. Hama-Inaba H, Takahashi M, Kasai M, Shiomi T, Ito A, Hanaoka F, Sato K. Optimum conditions for electric pulse mediated gene transfer to mammalian cells in suspension. *Cell Struct Funct* 1987;12:173–180

77. Golzio M, Mora M-P, Raynaud C, Delteil C, Teissié J, Rols M-P. Control by osmotic pressure of voltage-induced permeabilization and gene transfer in mammalian cells. *Biophys J* 1998;74:3015–3022

78. Chernomordik LV, Sukharev SI, Popov SV, Pastushenko VF, Sokirko AV, Abidor IG, Chizmadzhev YA. The electrical breakdown of cells and lipid membranes: the similarity of phenomenologies. *Biochim Biophys Acta* 1987;902:360–373

79. Genco I, Gliozzi A, Relini A, Robello M, Scalas E. Electroporation in symmetric and asymmetric membranes. *Biochim Biophys Acta* 1993;1149:10–18

80. Kotulska M, Koronkiewicz S, Kalinowski S. Cholesterol induced changes in the characteristics of the time series from planar lipid bilayer membrane during electroporation. *Acta Physica Polonica B* 2002;1115–1129

81. Stewart DA, Gowrishankar TR, Weaver JC. Transport lattice approach to describing cell electroporation: use of a local asymptotic model. *IEEE Trans Plasma Sci* 2004;32:1696–1708

82. Hibino M, Itoh H, Kinosita K Jr. Time courses of cell electroporation as revealed by submicroscopic imaging of transmembrane potential. *Biophys J* 1993;64:1789–1800

83. Tovar OH, Tung L. Electroporation of cardiac cell membranes with monophasic or biphasic rectangular pulses. *PACE* 1991;14:1887–1892

84. Neu JC, Krassowska W. Singular perturbation analysis of the pore creation transient. *Phys Rev E* 2006;74(031917):1–9

85. Teissié J, Golzio M, Rols M-P. Mechanisms of cell membrane electropermeabilization: a minireview of our present (lack of?) knowledge. *Biochim Biophys Acta* 2005;1724:270–280

86. Haest CWM, Kamp D, Deuticke B. Transbilayer reorientation of phospholopid probes in the human erythrocyte membrane. Lessons from studies on electroporated and resealed cells. *Biochim Biophys Acta* 1997;1325:17–33

87. Vernier PT, Sun Y, Marcu L, Craft CM, Gundersen MA. Nanopulse-induced phosphatidylserine translocation. *Biophys J* 2004;86:4040–4048

88. Ohuchi K, Fukui Y, Sakuma I, Shibata N, Honjo H, Kodama I. A dynamic action potential model analysis of shock-induced aftereffects in ventricular muscle by reversible breakdown of cell membrane. *IEEE Trans Biomed Eng* 2002;49:18–30

89. Krassowska W. Effects of electroporation on transmembrane potential induced by defibrillation shocks. *PACE* 1995;18:1644–1660

90. Aguel F, DeBruin KA, Krassowska W, Trayanova N. Effects of electroporation on the transmembrane potential distribution in a two-dimensional bidomain model of cardiac tissue. *J Cardiovasc Electrophysiol* 1999;10:701–714

91. Hénon S, Lenormand G, Richert A, Gallet F. A new determination of the shear modulus of the human erythrocyte membrane using optical tweezers. *Biophys J* 1999;76:1145–1151

92. Israelachvili J. *Intermolecular and Surface Forces*, 2nd ed. London: Academic; 1992

93. Smith KC, Neu JC, Krassowska W. Model of creation and evolution of stable macropores for DNA delivery. *Biophys J* 2004;86:2813–2826

94. Chambers EL, de Armendi J. Membrane potential, action potential and activation potential of eggs of the sea urchin, *Lytechinus variegates*. *Exp Cell Res* 1979;122:203–218

Part III

Electrode Mapping of Defibrillation

Chapter 3.1

Critical Points and the Upper Limit of Vulnerability for Defibrillation

Raymond E. Ideker and Derek J. Dosdall

Introduction

Electric shocks delivered to the heart are like a double-edged sword. Depending on the circumstances, they can either halt an arrhythmia or initiate one. Except for very large shocks that are so strong that their damaging effects cause immediate refibrillation, there is a range of shock strengths, below which shocks almost always fail to defibrillate and above which they usually successfully defibrillate. Throughout this range, the probability of successful defibrillation increases as the shock strength increases. The defibrillation threshold (DFT) is a single shock strength within this range whose mean value depends on the method used to estimate it.[1] For example, one method gave a mean DFT value that was at the 71% probability of success point (DF71), meaning that this shock strength would be expected to succeed 71% of the time.[2]

There is a different range of shock strengths in which ventricular fibrillation (VF) is induced when the shock is given during cardiac repolarization (i.e., the vulnerable period). The lower limit of this range, the ventricular fibrillation threshold (VFT), is considerably lower than the range of shock strengths that defibrillate. However, the upper limit of this range, the upper limit of vulnerability (ULV), is typically within the range of shock strengths that successfully defibrillate.[3,4] If the ULV did not exist, then it might not be possible to defibrillate with a shock of any strength because VF is so complex that some cardiac regions are probably in the vulnerable period at any time during VF. Thus, if the ULV did not exist, a shock larger than the VFT, even if it halted all the VF wavefronts, would immediately reinitiate VF in the regions in the vulnerable period. Just as for defibrillation, the ULV is also not a single value, but is a probability function in which the odds of not inducing VF increase with increasing shock strength.[5]

Raymond E. Ideker

Departments of Medicine, Biomedical Engineering and Physiology, University of Alabama–Birmingham, Birmingham, AL 35294-0019, USA, rei@crml.uab.edu

I. R. Efimov et al. (eds.), *Cardiac Bioelectric Therapy: Mechanisms and Practical Implications.*
© Springer Science+Business Media, LLC 2009

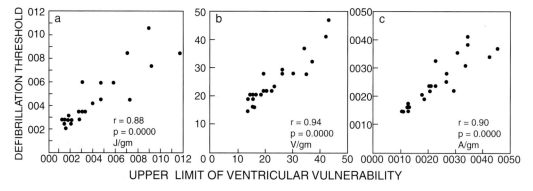

Figure 1: Correlation of the defibrillation threshold (DFT) and upper limit of vulnerability (ULV) for defibrillation electrodes on the right atrium (anode) and the left ventricular apex (cathode) for a monophasic waveform in 22 dogs. Results are expressed per gram of heart weight in units of energy (**a**), voltage (**b**), and current (**c**). (Chen et al. 1986)[4]

Multiple studies have shown that the ULV and DFT are correlated and similar in magnitude (Fig. 1).[3,4] Because of this similarity Swerdlow et al.[6] have recommended that the ULV, instead of the DFT, be determined during the implantation of internal cardiovertor/defibrillators since it avoids the possible detrimental effects of inducing VF multiple times. The correlation of the ULV and DFT also led to the development of the ULV hypothesis for the mechanism of defibrillation.[4,7] This hypothesis states that there are two requirements for defibrillation. First, the shock must halt the activation wavefronts present during VF. Second, the shock must not stimulate new wavefronts that reinitiate VF. Because the second criterion requires a larger shock strength than the first,[7] the second criterion determines the DFT, which explains why the ULV and DFT are correlated.

The ULV hypothesis does not require that the DFT during VF be identical with the ULV determined by scanning the vulnerable period of the T wave during paced or regular rhythm. During ULV determination, the vulnerable period is scanned to find the time point in which the cardiac region in which the shock field has its weakest effect on the tissue is most susceptible to VF initiation by the shock, although during VF the shock is not timed to be given when this region is in its vulnerable period. Therefore, it would be expected that a particular point on the ULV probability of success curve such as ULV50 would be a higher voltage than that for the same point on the defibrillation probability of success curve (i.e., DF50). However, during VF, the heart geometry may be different than during regular rhythm,[8] so that the shock electric field may be different. Also during VF, the activation rate is much faster, and the catecholamine levels are higher than during regular rhythm or pacing.[9,10] Therefore, the action potential duration and refractory period are shorter during VF,[11,12] which might affect the induction of VF by a shock. Such geometrical and functional differences between VF and regular rhythm would also be expected to cause the DFT and ULV to differ. These considerations suggest that if the ULV is determined while pacing at a rapid rate to mimic the electrical and geometrical effects of VF, then the ULV should correspond to a point high on the defibrillation probability of success curve. Malkin

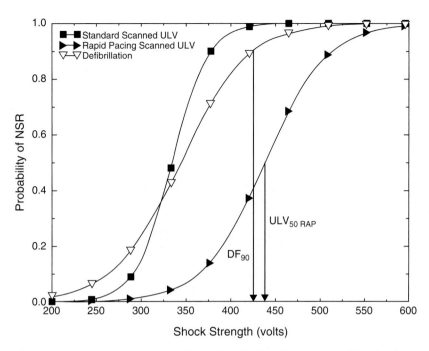

Figure 2: Probability of success curves for defibrillation (*open triangle*), the upper limit of vulnerability (ULV) determined by pacing at 80% of the intrinsic sinus rhythm cycle length (*closed square*), and the ULV determined at a pacing rate so rapid that an abrupt drop in arterial pressure occurred (*closed triangle*). The rapid pacing ULV curve is shifted to the right so that ULV50 is greater than DF90. NSR indicates normal sinus rhythm. (Malkin et al. 1995)[5]

et al.[5] verified that this prediction is true. They found that the ULV50 determined during rapid pacing is higher than the DF90 (Fig. 2).

Mechanisms by which Shocks Induce VF

An implication of the ULV hypothesis is that to understand the mechanisms of defibrillation one must also understand the mechanisms by which a shock initiates VF. Before the development of electrical and optical mapping techniques, it was thought that the induction of VF by a premature electrical stimulus was caused by a nonuniform dispersion of refractoriness.[13] According to this hypothesized mechanism, an activation wavefront was launched at the site of the electric stimulus, which then propagated away from the stimulus site until it encountered one or more regions that were still refractory (Fig. 3). Because of the nonuniform dispersion of refractoriness, other regions had already passed out of their refractory period by this time and served as conduits through which the wavefronts could propagate. During this time, the regions where block had occurred earlier had time to

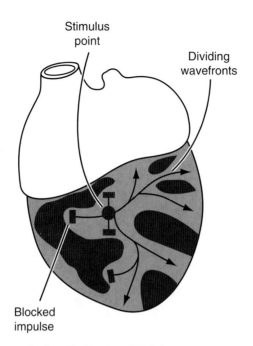

Figure 3: Initiation of ventricular fibrillation (VF) by a premature stimulus caused by the nonuniform dispersion of refractoriness. The refractory regions are shown in *black*. (Guyton and Hall 2000)[14]

recover so that these wavefronts could return through these regions and then reenter the tissue that it first activated proximal to the blocked region to initiate a reentrant circuit.

Although nonuniform dispersion of refractoriness coupled with restitution may be the mechanism by which a burst of rapid stimuli that are a few times stronger than the diastolic threshold induce VF,[15] electrical and optical mapping studies have revealed that somewhat stronger electrical stimuli initiate reentry and VF by different mechanisms than this. Instead of the stimulus initiating a wavefront that blocks some time period after the stimulus, electrical and optical mapping studies indicate that the electrical stimulus itself creates a block, which causes unidirectional propagation immediately after the stimulus, which leads to reentry and VF. These mechanisms involve the creation of a critical point in the tissue by the stimulus. The term *critical point* refers to the location of critical values in the spatial distribution of different electrophysiological variables through the tissue. As explained below, one of these critical points is created at the intersection of a critical level of refractoriness with a critical level of the extracellular potential gradient field generated in the tissue by the stimulus as predicted by Winfree (field-recovery critical point).[16] The other critical point occurs where the spatial rate of change of the trans-membrane potential caused by the shock reaches a critical level (virtual electrode critical point).[17]

The Field-Recovery Critical Point

The field-recovery critical point was observed during an attempt to record the entire strength-interval curve from a single electrical stimulus.[18] Classically, the strength-interval curve is determined by sequentially giving shocks of different strengths at a number of different coupling intervals to determine the excitation threshold throughout the relative refractory period (Fig. 4). To determine the entire strength-interval relationship from a single stimulus, Frazier et al.[18] recorded simultaneously from 117 electrodes covering approximately $10 \, cm^2$ of the right ventricular epicardium of dogs. They launched a linear activation wavefront during S_1 pacing by stimulating simultaneously from a row of pacing electrodes on the right side of the array of recording electrodes (Fig. 5a). The recovery times to a local 2 mA 3 ms stimulus following the S_1 stimulus were determined at 24–44 recordings

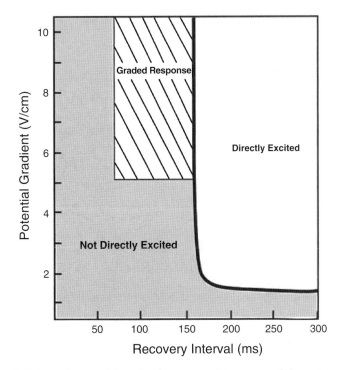

Figure 4: Strength-interval curve (*dark line*) expressed in terms of the extracellular potential gradient and of the degree of refractoriness of the tissue as indicated by the recovery interval from the previous excitation until the time of the stimulus. Three types of responses are indicated. The region to the right of the strength-interval curve is directly excited by the stimulus (*clear region*). The region below and some of the region to the left of the strength-interval curve is not directly excited by the stimulus (*shaded region*). The region immediately to the left of the upper portion of the strength-interval curve undergoes a graded response to the stimulus (*hatched region*).

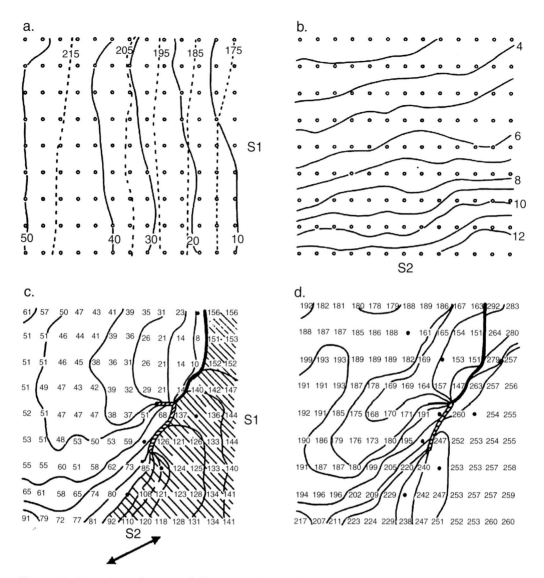

Figure 5: Initiation of reentry following orthogonal interaction of myocardial refractoriness and the extracellular potential gradient field created by a large stimulus. (a) Distribution of activation times following the last S_1 stimulus (*solid lines*) and recovery times following the time of the S_1 stimulus (*dashed lines*) in milliseconds. (b) Potential gradient magnitude in $V\,cm^{-1}$ for a 3 ms, 150 V S_2 stimulus. (c, d) First two cycles of activation following the S_2 stimulus demonstrating reentry. The S_1–S_2 interval was 191 ms. The *numbers* represent the activation time in milliseconds following the beginning of the 3 ms S_2 stimulus at each mapping electrode. *Dots* represent inadequate recordings. The isochronal lines are spaced 10 ms apart. The *solid line* represents the transition between successive activation maps. The *hatched line* represents a line of conduction block. The *hatched region* in (c) indicates the region thought to have undergone direct excitation or a graded response induced by the S_2 stimulus. The *double-headed arrow* (*bottom* of (c)) indicates the direction of the long axis of the myofibers in the mapped region. Reentry occurs around a critical point formed by the intersection of a potential gradient of $5.8\,V/cm^{-1}$ with tissue that is within 2 ms of passing out of its refractory period (the 191 ms recovery interval) at the time the S_2 stimulus is given. (Modified from Frazier et al. 1989)[18]

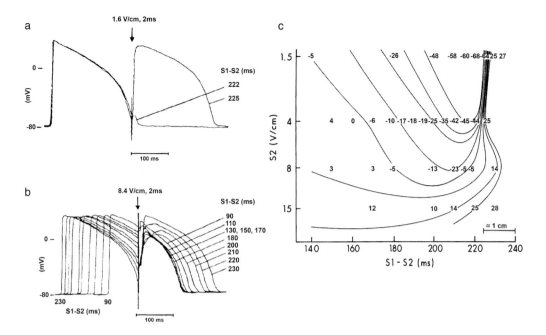

Figure 6: Use of microelectrode recordings to show an all-or-none response for an S_2 electric field less than $5-6\,\mathrm{V/cm^{-1}}$ (a), to show a graded response for a larger S_2 field (b), and to estimate the transmembrane potential $10\,\mathrm{ms}$ after the S_2 stimulus (c). In (a) and (b), the S_1–S_2 stimulus interval for each response is indicated to the right of the recording. The recordings were all made from the same impalement and are aligned with the time of the S_2 stimulus, which is indicated by the *arrow*. The complex to the left of the *arrow* was produced by the last S_1 stimulus. (a) For a $1.8\,\mathrm{V/cm^{-1}}$ S_2 potential gradient, the responses are markedly different, even though the change in S_1–S_2 timing is only $3\,\mathrm{ms}$. Although almost no response occurred following an S_1–S_2 interval of $222\,\mathrm{ms}$, a new action potential was generated following an S_1–S_2 interval of $225\,\mathrm{ms}$. (b) For an S_2 potential gradient of $8.4\,\mathrm{V/cm^{-1}}$, a range of graded responses was observed as the S_1–S_2 interval was varied. The longest and shortest S_1–S_2 intervals tested, 230 and $90\,\mathrm{ms}$, are indicated beneath phase zero of their respective last S_1 activations. In (c), the recordings of the type shown in (a) and (b) for four S_2 field strengths at a number of S_1–S_2 intervals were used to estimate the transmembrane potential in mV $10\,\mathrm{ms}$ after the S_2 stimulus for the experiment shown in Fig. 5. The isopotential *contour lines* represent transmembrane potentials from -45 to $25\,\mathrm{mV}$ in $10\,\mathrm{mV}$ increments. Contours more negative than $-45\,\mathrm{mV}$ in the upper right portion of (c) are not shown because of uncertainty in interpolation. In the region where the S_2 field strength is 1.5–$4\,\mathrm{V/cm^{-1}}$, an abrupt boundary (*upper right*) is present between tissue to the right that is directly excited by the S_2 field, and tissue to the left that is not directly excited. A large gradient in transmembrane potential at this boundary probably accounts for the propagation from right to left in this region observed in Fig. 5c. In the region where the S_2 field is 8–$15\,\mathrm{V/cm^{-1}}$, there is no abrupt boundary between high and low transmembrane potentials. Also, the transmembrane potentials in this region are in the range in which the sodium current is inactivated. The absence of a large transmembrane potential gradient and the presence of sodium channel inactivation probably explain the absence of propagation in this region where the S_2 field strength is high. (Knisley et al. 1992)

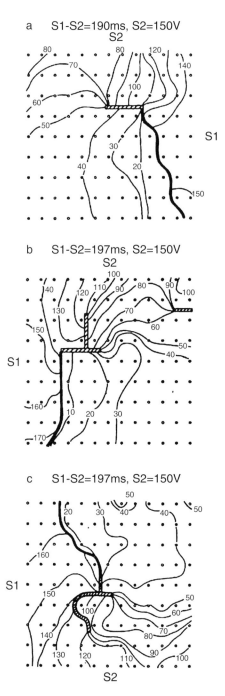

Figure 7:

sites throughout the mapped region (dashed lines in Fig. 5a). Because the refractory period was approximately the same throughout the mapped region, the tissue recovered from its refractory period in roughly the same sequence as the activation sequence. After the last of ten S_1 stimuli, a 3 ms premature S_2 stimulus was given from a mesh electrode that spanned the bottom of the mapped region to a return electrode that was off the heart. The S_2 stimulus generated an extracellular potential gradient field that was strongest next to the mesh electrode and that decreased with distance from it (Fig. 5b). This configuration of S_1 and S_2 electrodes created isolines of the stimulus potential gradient that were orthogonal to the isolines of tissue refractoriness expressed as isorecovery lines. In this way, the entire strength-interval region (shown in Fig. 4) was created throughout the mapped region.

When different S_2 strength stimuli were given or when the same S_2 stimulus was given with a different S_1–S_2 interval, the strength-interval curve separating the directly excited

---

Figure 7 (*Continued*): Effect of different S_1 and S_2 electrode locations on the chirality and phase of reentry. (**a**) The first postshock cycle of reentry is shown following a 150 V S_2 stimulus at an S_1–S_2 interval of 190 ms, with the S_2 electrode at the top of the mapped region and the S_1 electrode to the right. Earliest activation after the S_2 stimulus occurs distant from the S_2 electrode, with the ensuing wavefront forming a clockwise reentrant circuit, as opposed to the counterclockwise circuit when the S_2 electrode was at the bottom of the mapped region (Fig. 5). In addition, earliest post-S_2 activation was at the bottom of the mapped region with this circuit, opposite to the circuit in Fig. 5, where earliest activation occurred at the top of the mapped region. Reentry circulated about a critical point where the S_2 potential gradient was 5.4 V/cm^{-1} and the tissue was within 4 ms of its recovery period at the time of the S_2 stimulus. (**b**) The first postshock cycle of reentry is shown following a 150 V S_2 stimulus at an S_1–S_2 interval of 197 ms, with the S_2 electrode at the top of the mapped region and the S_1 electrode to the left. Earliest activation after the S_2 stimulus occurred distant from the S_2 electrode, with the ensuing wavefront forming a counterclockwise reentrant circuit, similar to the counterclockwise circuit when the S_2 electrode was at the bottom of the mapped region (Fig. 5). Again, earliest post-S_2 activation was recorded at the bottom of the mapped region for this reentrant circuit, opposite that of the circuit in Fig. 5, where earliest activation occurred at the top of the mapped region. Reentry circulated about a critical point where the S_2 potential gradient was 5.2 V/cm^{-1} and the tissue was within 2 ms of its recovery period at the time of the S_2 stimulus. (**c**) The first postshock cycle of reentry is shown following a 150 V S_2 stimulus at an S_1–S_2 interval of 197 ms, with the S_2 electrode at the bottom of the mapped region and the S_1 electrode to the left. Earliest activation after the S_2 stimulus occurred distant from the S_2 electrode, with the ensuing wavefront forming a counterclockwise reentrant circuit, as opposed to the counterclockwise circuit when the S_2 electrode was at the bottom of the mapped region (Fig. 5). However, earliest post-S_2 activation for this circuit was at the top of the mapped region similar to the circuit in Fig. 5. Reentry circulated about a critical point where the S_2 potential gradient was 5.9 V/cm^{-1} and the tissue was within 1 ms of its recovery period at the time of the S_2 stimulus. (Frazier et al. 1989)[18]

region from the nonexcited region in the mapped tissue moved in the direction that would be expected. In some cases, however, reentry was initiated (Fig. 5c, d) that usually was present for at least ten cycles and then degenerated into VF. Earliest activation following the 150 V S_2 stimulus did not appear adjacent to the S_2 electrode and then propagate away from it as occurs following stimuli only slightly greater than the pacing threshold (Fig. 3). Instead, following the large S_2 stimulus, activation first appeared where the potential gradient generated by the shock was less than 5 or $6 \, V/cm^{-1}$ and then propagated almost at a right angle to the S_2 electrode into the less recovered tissue (Fig. 5c). This finding suggests that the tissue to the right of the solid black line in Fig. 5c was directly excited during the shock by the shock electric field, and an activation wavefront was launched at the boundary of this directly excited region at the solid black line where the tissue was still too refractory to be directly excited by the shock field.[19] When this activation pattern was first observed, it was puzzling why propagation did not occur from right to left in the region where the shock field was greater than 5 or $6 \, V/cm^{-1}$, because this larger shock field should have had a greater ability to stimulate the myocardium than the weaker field above it where propagation did occur. Later studies indicated that a shock field greater than 5 or $6 \, V/cm^{-1}$, but not a weaker shock field, induced a graded response in partially recovered tissue (Fig. 6).[19,20] This finding suggests that the region around the hatched line of block and the tissue between it and the S_2 electrode in Fig. 5c experienced a graded response caused by the shock. Although these graded responses prolonged the refractory period in the tissue, they were not able to launch an activation wavefront after the shock that could propagate to the left of this region. Therefore, unidirectional block probably occurred in this region, allowing the wavefront in the top part of the mapped region to circle into the bottom part of the mapped region. By the time this wavefront reached the region of graded response, the tissue may have had time to recover so that this wavefront propagated through it to establish a reentrant circuit.

Frasier et al.[18] tested the hypothesis that the location of the reentrant circuit was not significantly affected in their study by differences in tissue properties in different portions of the mapped area, but was primarily determined by the creation of a critical point formed by the intersection of a critical shock field strength and a critical stage of recovery of the tissue. They tested this hypothesis by varying the S_1 and S_2 electrode locations, the S_2 strength, and the S_1–S_2 interval, and determining the location and direction of propagation of the reentrant circuits that were created (Figs. 7–9). Changing the S_1 or S_2 electrode locations changed the site of earliest post-S_2 activation and changed the direction of rotation of the reentrant circuit (Fig. 7). Increasing the S_2 strength moved the reentrant circuit away from the S_2 electrode, while decreasing the S_2 strength moved the reentrant circuit nearer to the S_2 electrode (Fig. 8a). Increasing the S_1–S_2 interval moved the reentrant circuit away from the S_1 electrode, while decreasing it moved the reentrant circuit closer to the S_1 electrode (Fig. 8b). In all cases, reentry centered about a critical point where, for a 3 ms monophasic waveform, the critical S_2 potential gradient was a mean of $5.1 \, V/cm^{-1}$ and the critical stage of recovery was within a few ms of the refractory period for a local 2 mA stimulus (Fig. 9). In a later study, the critical point was found to differ for different monophasic and biphasic waveforms and for different waveform durations (Fig. 10).[21]

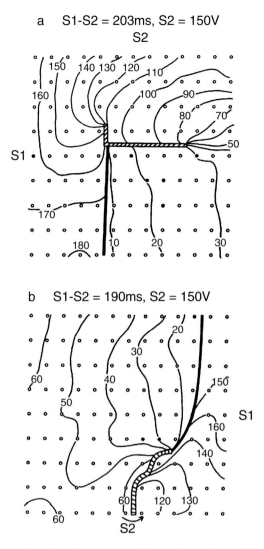

Figure 8: Effects of changing S_1–S_2 interval (**a**) or S_2 voltage (**b**) on the location of the reentrant circuit. (**a**) Because the critical point about which reentry occurs is in a region where the tissue is just passing out of its refractory period, increases and decreases in the S_1–S_2 interval moved the reentrant site away from and toward the S_1 site, respectively. The reentrant pattern in (**a**) followed a 150 V S_2 at an S_1–S_2 interval of 203 ms and should be compared with the pattern following a 150 V S_2 at an S_1–S_2 interval of 197 ms, as shown in Fig. 7b. The increase in the S_1–S_2 interval by 6 ms caused the critical point about which the reentrant circuit formed to move 5.5 mm to the right, away from the S_1 electrode, to the region that was passing out of its refractory interval at the time of the S_2 stimulus. (**b**) A change in the S_2 voltage produced changes in the potential gradient field, with an increase in S_2 voltage increasing the gradient at all sites and a decrease in voltage decreasing the gradient at all sites. The reentrant pattern in (**b**) followed a 100 V S_2 at an S_1–S_2 interval of 190 ms and should be compared to the pattern in Fig. 5c following a 150 V S_2 stimulus with identical S_1 and S_2 locations and almost the same S_1–S_2 interval (190 ms vs. 191 ms). Decreasing the S_2 voltage moved the reentrant circuit toward the S_2 site. The potential gradient at the critical point, following the 100 V S_2, 5.6 V/cm^{-1}, remained approximately the same as that following the 150 V S_2, 5.8 V/cm−1 (Fig. 5c), even though the locations of the critical points differed by 5.5 mm. (Frazier et al. 1989)[18]

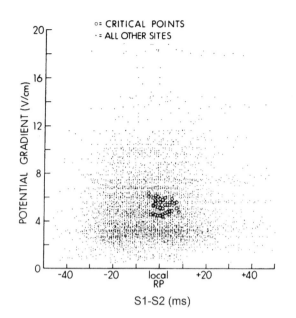

Figure 9: S_1–S_2 intervals in relation to the refractory period and S_2 potential gradients at the critical points for all dogs. Values for critical points about which reentry circulated are shown as *circles*. Values for all other recording electrodes are designated as *dots*. The S_1–S_2 intervals are shown on the X axis referenced to the refractory period (RP) of the site of the critical point. Although the mean refractory periods differed widely among the 11 dogs (129–179 ms), the S_1–S_2 intervals at the critical points approximately equaled the refractory periods for all cases. For the critical points, the mean preshock interval is 1 ± 3 ms longer than the refractory period. The S_2 potential gradients are shown on the Y axis. Although the S_2 voltages that initiated reentry within the mapped region varied from 75 to 175 V, the mean potential gradient at the critical point is relatively constant, 5.1 ± 0.6 V/cm^{-1}. (Frazier et al. 1989)[18]

Figure 10: Plot of mean internal (**a**) and external (**b**) defibrillation thresholds (DFTs) versus mean critical point location for eight waveforms in dogs. M indicates monophasic waveforms, B indicates biphasic waveforms. The number preceding M gives the duration in milliseconds of the monophasic waveform and the number preceding B indicates each phase of the biphasic waveform in milliseconds. The recovery interval between the time of activation at the critical point for the last S_1 stimulated activation until the time of the S_2 is plotted on the X axis. The larger this number, the lower is the refractoriness, because the site had more time to recover before the S_2 stimulus. The potential gradient at the critical point is shown on the Y axis. The mean DFT voltage is shown on the Z axis. The DFT decreases significantly with a decrease in potential gradient as well as with a decrease in refractoriness (increase in recovery interval of the critical point). The 8 ms biphasic waveform ($8B$), whose critical point was at the intersection of a low potential gradient as well as more recovered tissue, has the lowest DFT voltage. (Ideker et al. 2001)[21]

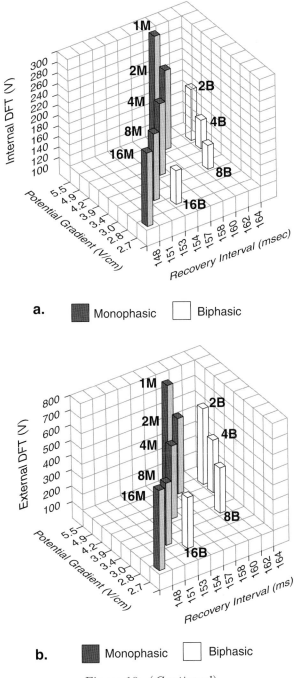

a. 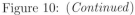 Monophasic   □ Biphasic

b. ■ Monophasic   □ Biphasic

Figure 10: (*Continued*)

Table 1: Mean base-to-apex location of earliest recorded site of postshock activation for all animals

	Shock energy (J)								
	0.01	0.02	0.05	0.1	0.2	0.5	1	2	5
Location of earliest postshock site	3.6±1.2	3.1±0.8	3.8±0.8	3.9±0.8	4.4±0.8	5.2±0.4	5.2±0.4	5.8±0.2	5.8±0.2

Values are mean±SD. Apex = 1, base = 6, as shown in Fig. 11a

Reentry consistent with the creation of a critical point is observed, not only within a few centimeters of the S_2 electrode, as in Fig. 5, but also distant from the S_2 electrode with shocks given with defibrillation-type electrodes (Fig. 11).[22] As the S_2 strength increased, the site of earliest recorded post-S_2 activation moved farther from the S_2 electrode (Table 1), consistent with the critical level of potential gradient moving away from the S_2 electrode as the S_2 strength increased. With S_2 shocks of 1 J given through the electrode configuration shown in Fig. 11a, earliest recorded post-S_2 activation was at the base of the ventricles, many centimeters away from the apical and right atrial S_2 electrodes (Fig. 11c–j). As predicted by theory,[16] the combination of S_1 activation sequence and the S_2 shock field distribution in this study should have produced two critical points, each of which would create a reentrant circuit where the critical potential gradient intersected the critical degree of refractoriness (Fig. 12). Other findings consistent with critical point theory were that the reentrant circuits moved progressively farther away from the S_1 pacing site as the S_1–S_2 interval increased (Fig. 11f–i), and that the direction of rotation of the reentrant circuits reversed with reversal of the S_1 activation (and hence recovery) sequence by moving the S_1 pacing site to the opposite side of the ventricles (Fig. 11j).[22]

According to critical point theory, the ULV occurs when the shock is so strong that the critical potential gradient is exceeded everywhere throughout the ventricles. The ULV hypothesis for defibrillation combined with critical point theory leads to the following predictions. Defibrillation will occur 100% of the time when the critical potential gradient is exceeded everywhere throughout the ventricles. With a slightly weaker shock, so that the critical potential gradient is present in a region of the ventricles, the shock will fail to defibrillate when the critical degree of refractoriness is present within this region. As the shock is made progressively smaller, the size of the region containing the critical potential gradient increases for most defibrillation electrode configurations so that the odds of the region containing tissue in the critical stage of refractoriness, and hence the odds of the shocks failing to defibrillate, increase. This phenomenon is one cause of the probability of success curve for defibrillation.

Other predictions of the ULV hypothesis for defibrillation combined with critical point theory have been verified experimentally. For shocks just below the ULV, as well as for shocks just below the DFT, earliest postshock activation occurs in the same region (i.e., the region where the shock potential gradient is weakest) (Fig. 13).[7] The potential gradient in this region is approximately the same for ULV and DFT shocks, and this potential gradient

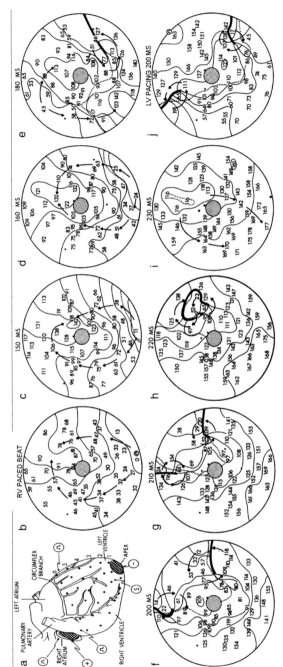

Figure 11: Effect of S_1–S_2 interval on the site of earliest postshock activation for monophasic S_2 shocks slightly weaker than the defibrillation threshold (DFT). (a) Location of shock electrodes (cross-hatched regions) and recording electrodes (black dots). The anode (+) was on the right atrium and the cathode (−) was on the apex of the left ventricle. Epicardial recording electrodes were distributed in six rows from apex to base (indicated by numbers 1–6). The locations of ventricular S_1 pacing electrodes are indicated by square pulses within circles. (b) Isochronal map of S_1 beat while pacing from the right ventricle. The square wave within a circle indicates the pacing site. A polar projection of the ventricles is shown with the apical shocking electrode in the center (stippled region) and with the atrioventricular groove circumferentially at the periphery. The numbers represent the locations of the recording electrodes with satisfactory recordings and give the time of activation with the earliest activation taken as time zero. Black dots represent electrodes where satisfactory recordings were not obtained. The isochronal lines are spaced 20 ms apart. The arrows indicate the direction of the spread of activation. (c–i) Isochronal maps of the first post-S_2 cycle for S_1–S_2 intervals of 150–230 ms (given above the maps), with S_1 pacing from the right ventricle. Time zero is the onset of the 5 ms 1 J monophasic S_2 stimuli. The dotted line is the location of tissue that last activated 145 ms before the S_2 stimulus. If all of the myocardium had a refractory period of 145 ms, this line would represent the border between myocardium that is still refractory on the side of the dotted line away from the S_1 pacing electrode and myocardium that is recovered on the side of the dotted line closer to the pacing electrode. The wide black line in (d–h) represents the transition between the first and second post-S_2 cycles. After the shortest and the longest S_1–S_2 intervals (c, i), only a single cycle occurred, and it spread in a focal pattern on the epicardium. After all other S_1–S_2 intervals (d–h), reentry was initiated that degenerated into ventricular fibrillation (VF). In (g) and (h), a pair of oppositely rotating reentrant cycles was formed. In (i), the two circuits were so close together that they fused to form a figure-of-eight reentrant circuit. The center of the reentrant circuits moved progressively around the base of the heart, becoming farther away from the pacing site as the S_1–S_2 interval lengthened, but always remaining near the dotted line. The time of earliest post-S_2 activation increased as the S_1–S_2 interval increased. (j) Isochronal map of the first post-S_2 cycle of reentry after a 1 J S_2 stimulus was given following a 200 ms S_1–S_2 interval with the S_1 pacing electrode in the left ventricle (square wave in circle). This map is almost a mirror image of the map of the first post-S_2 cycle with S_1 pacing from the right ventricle (f), with the reentrant circuits rotating in opposite directions. (Shibata et al. 1988)[22]

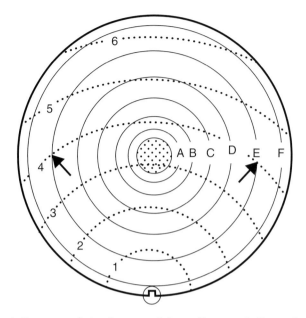

Figure 12: Idealized diagram of shock potential gradient and dispersion of refractoriness, demonstrating that there are two critical points where a critical potential gradient and a critical stage of refractoriness intersect in the experiment of Fig. 11. The apical S_2 electrode is indicated by the stippled region in the center. The *solid lines* indicate different levels of shock potential gradient with A representing the highest gradient and F the lowest gradient. The *square wave* indicates the right ventricular S_1 pacing electrode. The *dotted lines* represent different stages of refractoriness after the S_1 stimulus with 1 representing least refractoriness and 6 representing most refractoriness. If the critical potential gradient is E and the critical degree of refractoriness is 4, then two critical points are produced at the intersection of these lines (*arrows*). (Shibata et al. 1988)[22]

is approximately the critical potential gradient about which reentry occurs.[23] The lower the critical potential gradient for a particular waveform, the lower the DFT for that waveform (Fig. 10).[21] These findings are all consistent with the hypothesis that, to defibrillate, field-recovery critical points must not be present in the myocardium.

Inconsistencies with the Field-Recovery Critical Hypothesis for Defibrillation

There are several findings, however, that are not in total agreement with this hypothesis. One finding is that one or two rapid postshock cycles can appear following a defibrillation shock, yet the shock can still succeed (i.e., a type B successful defibrillation).[24] This phenomenon may be similar to that of repetitive responses after shocks given during the

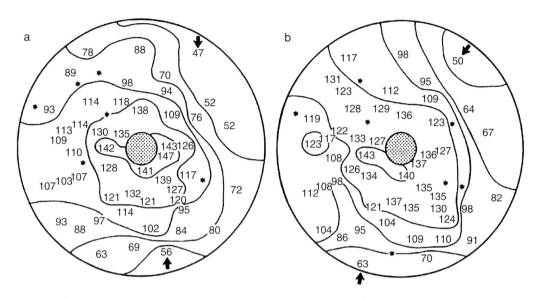

Figure 13: Example of the similarity of isochronal maps of the first postshock cycle after (a) the largest shock that induced ventricular fibrillation (VF) (2 J) and (b) the largest shock that failed to defibrillate (2 J) in the same animal. The display is similar to those in Fig. 11. Earliest postshock activation (*arrows*) was in the basal third of the ventricles for the shock given during the vulnerable period of paced rhythm (a) as well as for the failed defibrillation shock given during VF (b). The interval from the shock until earliest recorded activation for the first postshock cycle was 47 ms for the shock given during the vulnerable period and 50 ms for the shock given during VF. (Shibata et al. 1988)[7]

vulnerable period of regular rhythm. It may be in both of these cases that, even though a critical point is formed, activation propagates around it so quickly that the tissue that was directly excited by the shock field is still refractory when the postshock wavefront circles around to encounter it, causing the wavefront to block. This explanation is supported by the finding that waveforms that cause critical points to form in more recovered tissue, where the conduction velocity should be faster than in refractory tissue, have lower DFTs than waveforms with a similar critical potential gradient but a more refractory critical degree of recovery (Fig. 10).[21]

Another finding not in complete agreement with the refractory potential gradient critical point hypothesis for defibrillation is that earliest postshock activation, even when mapped with intramural electrodes, does not always appear immediately after the shock and appears to arise focally instead of immediately forming a reentrant circuit.[25] However, this finding is consistent with the ULV hypothesis for the mechanism of defibrillation, because shocks given during the vulnerable period of regular rhythm can appear after an interval of tens of milliseconds and can appear focal (Figs. 11i and 13a).

Other findings not in agreement with the refractory potential gradient critical point hypothesis for defibrillation are that the critical potential gradient appears to increase as the distance from the S_2 electrode to the critical point is increased by increasing shock strength,[26] and that the ULV is not a single value but is a probability function. The DFT probability function can be explained by the fact that the state of the heart is different for each shock, so that a critical degree of refractoriness may or may not intersect the critical potential gradient at the time of the shock. The ULV shocks, however, are timed to occur at the same point in the vulnerable period, yet a probability function is still present, although with shocks given to scan the entire T wave, the ULV probability curve is steeper than that for the DFT.[5] The existence of a ULV probability curve may indicate that the response to the shock is very sensitive to small variations in the electrophysiological state of the heart between one shock and the next.

A major limitation of the refractory potential gradient critical point hypothesis for defibrillation is that it does not explicitly consider the effects of the shock field and of the polarity of the shock electrodes on the transmembrane potential. One reason for this is that little was known about these effects at the time the hypothesis was put forward, and it was thought that the primary effect of the shock was to hyperpolarize the portion of each cell or each bundle of cells closer to the anode and depolarize the portion of each cell or each bundle of cells closer to the cathode, creating a "sawtooth" pattern.[27]

The Virtual Electrode Critical Point

The development of bidomain theory and optical mapping led to simulations and experiments that showed the importance of large regions of depolarization or hyperpolarization called virtual electrodes in the response of the myocardium to an electrical stimulus.[17,28–31] When the S_2 stimulus is given during the plateau phase of the action potential, a critical point can be formed by the virtual electrodes around which reentry circles (Fig. 14). The hyperpolarized region, which is depolarized in its plateau phase at the time of the shock, undergoes deexcitation by the shock so that excitability is restored. Where the spatial change in the transmembrane potential between the depolarized and hyperpolarized regions is large and occurs over a short distance so that the spatial gradient of the transmembrane potential is larger than a critical value, postshock activation arises by break excitation of the hyperpolarized tissue by the adjacent depolarized region, as seen in the bottom half of Fig. 14c. Where the spatial change in the transmembrane potential between the depolarized and hyperpolarized regions is small, so that the spatial gradient of the transmembrane potential is less than a critical value, break excitation and propagation into the hyperpolarized region does not occur, as shown in the top half of Fig. 14c, so that unidirectional block occurs.[17] These findings are discussed in more detail in the chapter by Ripplenger and Efimov.

The membrane polarization critical point hypothesis for the induction of reentry is probably not responsible for the reentry observed in Figs. 5, 7, and 8 because (1) the reentry was induced by S_2 stimulation during the repolarization phase, not the plateau

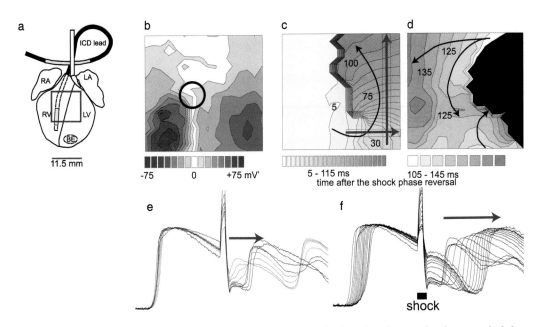

Figure 14: Creation of a membrane polarization critical point by a shock recorded by optical mapping. (**a**) Representation of an isolated, Langendorff perfused rabbit heart. S_1 pacing was performed from bipolar electrodes at the site marked *BE*. The S_2 stimulus was biphasic, with the first phase 100 V and the second phase 200 V. It was delivered between the electrodes shown in gray along the implantable cardioverter-defibrillator (ICD) lead. Optical recordings were made from the square outlined region with a 16 by 16 photodiode array. (**b**) The transmembrane potential at the end of the S_2 stimulus. The region overlying the RV electrode, which was a cathode during the second phase of the biphasic stimulus, was depolarized, while the region to the right was hyperpolarized. The circle encloses the critical point. (**c**) Isochrones spaced 5 ms apart, illustrating the activation sequence during the first postshock cycle. (**d**) Isochrones during the second postshock cycle. The wavefront reentered the area that was directly excited by the S_2 stimulus. Reentry terminated during the second cycle when the wavefront encountered refractory tissue in the lower right-hand corner of the mapped region. (**e**) Optical recordings from the rectangle containing the *horizontal arrow* in (**c**). (**f**) Optical recordings from the rectangle containing the *vertical arrow* in (**c**). RA, right atrium; LA, left atrium; RV, right ventricle; LV, left ventricle. (Efimov et al. 1998)[17]

phase of the action potential, and (2) optical recordings indicate that the tissue in the mapped region when the S_2 stimulus is given from a long strip electrode parallel to the long axis of the myocardial fibers as in Figs. 5, 7, and 8 is all of the same polarity so that no large gradient between depolarized and hyperpolarized regions is present within the mapped region (Fig. 15).[32]

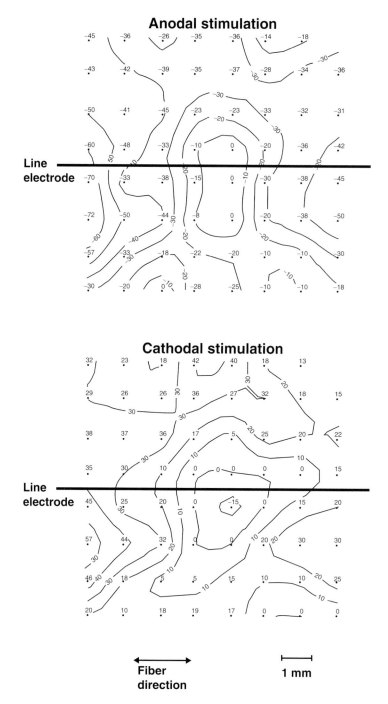

Figure 15: Changes in the transmembrane potential caused by stimulation with a line electrode that is parallel to the long axis of the myocardial fibers in rabbits. The change in transmembrane potential at each of 64 optical recordings is indicated as a percentage of the action potential amplitude during pacing. (a) Anodal stimulation produced hyperpolarization (negative percentages) throughout most of the mapped region. (b) Cathodal stimulation produced depolarization (positive percentages) throughout most of the mapped region. (Knisley and Baynham 1997)[33]

Other Possible Mechanisms for Defibrillation

Recent studies have presented evidence that other mechanisms may also contribute to the success of defibrillation besides the creation of critical points. Trayanova et al.[30] have shown by simulation studies the possible importance of propagating graded responses in defibrillation. Dosdall et al.[12] have recently reported that Purkinje fibers are active early during the first postshock cycle following a defibrillation cycle. However, it is not known if they are important in determining the outcome of a defibrillation shock.

The effects of high potential gradients such as electroporation also may affect defibrillation outcome.[33] In addition, small areas of hyperpolarization in larger areas that are predominantly depolarized and vice versa have recently been reported.[34,35] These small areas of hundreds of microns or less are missed when optical mapping is performed in which the pixel size is 1 mm or larger. These results suggest that the different mechanisms of defibrillation and their relative importance in determining the success or failure of a shock are still not completely understood. It is hoped that as our knowledge improves, improved methods to defibrillate with less shock voltage and energy will become apparent that cause less damage and discomfort.

Acknowledgment

This work was supported in part by National Health Institutes, Heart, Lung and Blood Institute Research Grants HL 28429, HL 66256, and HL 85370.

References

1. Singer I, Lang D. Defibrillation threshold: clinical utility and therapeutic implications. *PACE* 1992;15:932–949
2. Davy JM, Fain ES, Dorian P, Winkle RA. The relationship between successful defibrillation and delivered energy in open-chest dogs: reappraisal of the "defibrillation threshold" concept. *Am Heart J* 1987;113(1):77–84
3. Lesigne C, Levy B, Saumont R, Birkui P, Bardou A, Rubin B. An energy-time analysis of ventricular fibrillation and defibrillation thresholds with internal electrodes. *Med Biol Eng* 1976;14(6):617–622
4. Chen PS, Shibata N, Dixon EG, Martin RO, Ideker RE. Comparison of the defibrillation threshold and the upper limit of ventricular vulnerability. *Circulation* 1986;73(5):1022–1028
5. Malkin RA, Idriss SF, Walker RG, Ideker RE. Effect of rapid pacing and T-wave scanning on the relation between the defibrillation and upper-limit-of-vulnerability dose-response curves. *Circulation* 1995;92(5):1291–1299
6. Swerdlow CD, Shehata M, Chen PS. Using the upper limit of vulnerability to assess defibrillation efficacy at implantation of ICDs. *Pacing Clin Electrophysiol* 2007;30(2):258–270

7. Shibata N, Chen PS, Dixon EG, Wolf PD, Danieley ND, Smith WM, Ideker RE. Epicardial activation after unsuccessful defibrillation shocks in dogs. *Am J Physiol* 1988;255(4 Pt 2):H902–H909

8. De Piccoli B, Rigo F, Raviele A, Piccolo E, Maggiolo C, Milanesi A, Simone M. Transesophageal echocardiographic evaluation of the morphologic and hemodynamic cardiac changes during ventricular fibrillation. *J Am Soc Echocardiogr* 1996;9(1):71–78

9. Foley PJ, Tacker WA, Wortsman J, Frank S, Cryer PE. Plasma catecholamine and serum cortisol responses to experimental cardiac arrest in dogs. *Am J Physiol* 1987;253(3 Pt 1):E283–E289

10. Kern KB, Elchisak MA, Sanders AB, Badylak SF, Tacker WA, Ewy GA. Plasma catecholamines and resuscitation from prolonged cardiac arrest. *Crit Care Med* 1989;17(8):786–791

11. Tovar OH, Jones JL. Electrophysiological deterioration during long-duration ventricular fibrillation. *Circulation* 2000;102(23):2886–2891

12. Dosdall DJ, Cheng KA, Huang J, Allison JS, Allred JD, Smith WM, Ideker RE. Transmural and endocardial Purkinje activation in pigs before local myocardial activation after defibrillation shocks. *Heart Rhythm* 2007;4(6):758–765

13. Han J, Moe GK. Nonuniform recovery of excitability in ventricular muscle. *Circ Res* 1964;14:44–60

14. Guyton AC, Hall JE. Cardiac arrhythmias and their electrocardiographic interpretation. *Textbook of Medical Physiology*, 10th edn. Philadelphia: W.B. Saunders; 2000:134–142

15. Cao JM, Qu Z, Kim YH, Wu TJ, Garfinkel A, Weiss JN, Karagueuzian HS, Chen PS. Spatiotemporal heterogeneity in the induction of ventricular fibrillation by rapid pacing: importance of cardiac restitution properties. *Circ Res* 1999;84(11):1318–1331

16. Winfree AT. Time encircles a singularity. *When Time Breaks Down: The Three-Dimensional Dynamics of Electrochemical Waves and Cardiac Arrhythmias*. Princeton, NJ: Princeton University Press; 1987:125–153

17. Efimov IR, Cheng Y, Van Wagoner DR, Mazgalev T, Tchou PJ. Virtual electrode-induced phase singularity: a basic mechanism of defibrillation failure. *Circ Res* 1998;82(8):918–925

18. Frazier DW, Wolf PD, Wharton JM, Tang AS, Smith WM, Ideker RE. Stimulus-induced critical point. Mechanism for electrical initiation of reentry in normal canine myocardium. *J Clin Invest* 1989;83(3):1039–1052

19. Daubert JP, Frazier DW, Wolf PD, Franz MR, Smith WM, Ideker RE. Response of relatively refractory canine myocardium to monophasic and biphasic shocks. *Circulation* 1991;84(6):2522–2538

20. Knisley SB, Smith WM, Ideker RE. Effect of field stimulation on cellular repolarization in rabbit myocardium. Implications for reentry induction. *Circ Res* 1992;70(4):707–715

21. Ideker RE, Alferness C, Melnick S, Sreenan KM, Johnson E, Smith WM. Reentry site during fibrillation induction in relation to defibrillation efficacy for different shock waveforms. *J Cardiovasc Electrophysiol* 2001;12(5):581–591

22. Shibata N, Chen PS, Dixon EG, Wolf PD, Danieley ND, Smith WM, Ideker RE. Influence of shock strength and timing on induction of ventricular arrhythmias in dogs. *Am J Physiol* 1988;255(4 Pt 2):H891–H901

23. Idriss SF, Wolf PD, Smith WM, Ideker RE. Effect of pacing site on ventricular fibrillation initiation by shocks during the vulnerable period. *AJP* 1999;277(Heart Circ Physiol 46):H2065–H2082

24. Chen PS, Shibata N, Dixon EG, Wolf PD, Danieley ND, Sweeney MB, Smith WM, Ideker RE. Activation during ventricular defibrillation in open-chest dogs. Evidence of complete cessation and regeneration of ventricular fibrillation after unsuccessful shocks. *J Clin Invest* 1986;77(3):810–823

25. Chattipakorn N, Ideker RE. Delayed afterdepolarization inhibitor: a potential pharmacologic intervention to improve defibrillation efficacy. *J Cardiovasc Electrophysiol* 2003;14(1):72–75

26. Idriss SF, Wolf PD, Smith WM, Ideker RE. Effect of pacing site on ventricular fibrillation initiation by shocks during the vulnerable period. *Am J Physiol* 1999;277(5 Pt 2):H2065–H2082

27. Krassowska W, Frazier DW, Pilkington TC, Ideker RE. Potential distribution in three-dimensional periodic myocardium – Part II: application to extracellular stimulation. *IEEE Trans Biomed Eng* 1990;37(3):267–284

28. Lin SF, Roth BJ, Wikswo JP Jr. Quatrefoil reentry in myocardium: an optical imaging study of the induction mechanism. *J Cardiovasc Electrophysiol* 1999;10(4):574–586

29. Cheng Y, Mowrey KA, Van Wagoner DR, Tchou PJ, Efimov IR. Virtual electrode-induced reexcitation: a mechanism of defibrillation. *Circ Res* 1999;85(11):1056–1066

30. Trayanova NA, Gray RA, Bourn DW, Eason JC. Virtual electrode-induced positive and negative graded responses: new insights into fibrillation induction and defibrillation. *J Cardiovasc Electrophysiol* 2003;14(7):756–763

31. Efimov IR, Gray RA, Roth BJ. Virtual electrodes and deexcitation: new insights into fibrillation induction and defibrillation. *J Cardiovasc Electrophysiol* 2000;11(3):339–353

32. Knisley SB, Baynham TC. Line stimulation parallel to myofibers enhances regional uniformity of transmembrane voltage changes in rabbit hearts. *Circ Res* 1997;81(2):229–241

33. Nikolski VP, Efimov IR. Electroporation of the heart. *Europace* 2005;7(Suppl 2):146–154

34. Sharifov OF, Fast VG. Role of intramural virtual electrodes in shock-induced activation of left ventricle: optical measurements from the intact epicardial surface. *Heart Rhythm* 2006;3(9):1063–1073

35. Windisch H, Platzer D, Bilgici E. Quantification of shock-induced microscopic virtual electrodes assessed by subcellular resolution optical potential mapping in guinea pig papillary muscle. *J Cardiovasc Electrophysiol* 2007;18(10):1086–1094

Chapter 3.2

The Role of Shock-Induced Nonregenerative Depolarizations in Ventricular Fibrillation and Defibrillation: The Graded Response Hypothesis

Hrayr S. Karagueuzian

Brief Historical Perspectives

The link between death and cardiac arrest was perhaps first recorded in the epic of Gilgamesh, the "oldest" written story on Earth (circa 2700 BC). "I touched his heart, but it beat no longer," lamented Gilgamesh, the Babylonian hero-king in the Mesopotamian epic of Gilgamesh, as he witnessed the death of his best friend, Enkidu.[1] Perhaps the earliest pictorial and informative description of the sudden cardiac death was discovered on the relief sculpture of the tomb of an Egyptian nobleman in the sixth dynasty (2625–2475 BC) at Sakkara. The scene, titled "Sudden Death" by the German egyptologist von Bissing, is described by a sequence of pictorial events that lead to the sudden collapse of the Egyptian nobleman[2] (Fig. 1). The later discovery of Egyptian writings on papyri (circa 1534 BC) directly linked heart beat irregularities to death: "If the heart trembles, has little power and sinks, the disease is advancing...and death is near."[3] Heartbeat irregularities as a marker of disease were also recognized and described in ancient China as can be deduced from a conversation between the "Golden Emperor" Huang Ti and his physician Ch'i Pai (circa 2600 BC) "When the pulse beats are long the constitution of the pulse is well regulated.... When the pulse is quick, and contain six beats to 1 cycle of respiration, it indicates heart trouble...and the disease becomes grave."[4]

Department of Medicine, Division of Cardiology, David Geffen School of Medicine at UCLA, Los Angeles, CA, USA,
hkaragueuzian@mednet.ucla.edu

I. R. Efimov et al. (eds.), *Cardiac Bioelectric Therapy: Mechanisms and Practical Implications.*

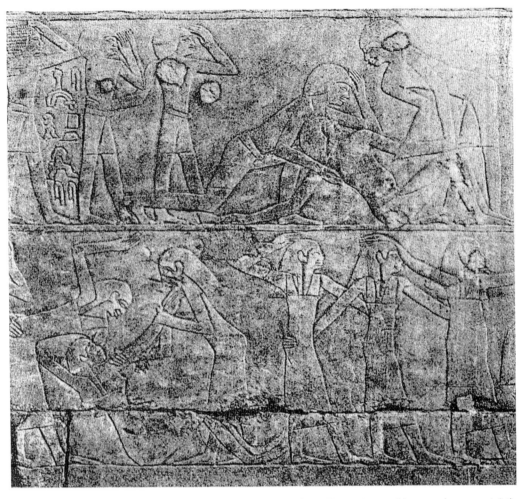

Figure 1: Tomb relief depicting the sudden death of an Egyptian nobleman (*upper right*), who collapses in the midst of his family. Two servants busy themselves with the dead noble, while others show their utter grief with the characteristic gesture–hands to the foreheads–expressing sorrow in ancient (and present) Egypt. Below, the wife, overcome by emotion, has fainted and sunk to the floor. She is being attended by two women who are trying to revive her. To the right, the wife, holding on to two servants, is led from the scene. Tomb of Sesi of Sakkara (sixth dynasty 2625–2475 BC). (Bruetsch 1959)[2]

Aristotle (384–322 BC) had already recognized in 340 BC the efficacy of electrical therapy in pain management using torpedo (electric) fish,[5] a presumed replica of present transcutaneous electric nerve stimulation. Aristotle, however, knew little if any, of the flow of electrical current (shock) in pain management. It was two millennia later, and in 1752, when Benjamin Franklin (AD 1706–1790) discovered that it was the electricity in lightning that was capable of causing sudden death. The discovery of the link between sudden death and electricity motivated the erudite of the date to determine if in fact electrical shocks can cause death. Perhaps the first curious mind to unravel the interaction of electricity with living animals was Peter Christian Abildgaard. This Danish eighteenth-century physician succeeded to render a fowl "lifeless" by an electrical shock stored in a Leyden jar (primitive capacitor) and then "revived" it with a second electrical shock.[6] In his words: "With a shock the animal was rendered lifeless, and arose with a second shock to the chest...then the hen walked with some difficulty...then later it was very well and even laid an egg."[6] Ventricular fibrillation (VF) and defibrillation were unknown phenomena in those days, but Abildgaard's observations and descriptions on the fowl unmistakably demonstrate that he had already accomplished these goals in 1775.

It was in 1850 when Hoffa and Ludwig[7] first recorded in animals the irregular contractions patterns, reflecting irregular electrical activity during VF that was induced by electrical shocks using Ludwig's 1848 "kymographion."[8] Since 1850 and henceforth some 20 different terms were used to describe what we now call "ventricular fibrillation." For example, MacWilliam[9] in his 1887 studies coined the term "fibrillar contractions" to describe "the rapid succession of inco-ordinated peristaltic contractions" induced by faradic stimulation of the ventricles in open-chest anesthetized animals. He was perhaps the first to describe the "feeling" of the fibrillating waves as they propagated under his fingers: "The excitation of the muscular fibers travels peristaltically, producing the characteristic movement; the inco-ordianted contractions of the various fibers may be most distinctly realized when the ventricles are held between the forefingers and thumb; there is a sort of wriggling sensation to be felt as the individual muscle bundles become hard and wiry while the contraction is passing over them in succession."[9]

Relevant to the current writing, MacWilliam was able to induce VF with point electrical stimulation applied to a small region of the heart. "I have on several occasions introduced a fine platinum wire electrode through the chest wall so as to come in contact with the ventricles and have then faradized...the fibrillar contraction was at once induced."[9]

In 1899 Battelli[10] provided a dramatic leap in our understanding of the critical role played by the intensity of the electrical current to cause "paralysis of the heart" in man in 1899. This Swiss investigator collected mortality data in man that resulted from accidental electrical shocks in industrial workers (four cases) and death after the electrocution of criminals (nine cases) in the United States and compared these data to the large body of data that he had amassed on a host of animal models. Battelli concluded and described in no uncertain terms a major concept that is frequently used and appreciated in the current practice of cardiology. In his words "in order for the current to produce paralysis of the heart (*trémulations fibrillaires*) in man, the current strength needs to be neither too low, because in this case we do not obtain any deleterious effect, nor too high because the heart no longer gets paralyzed, as we previously have seen in animals."[10] Battelli thus appears poised to claim being the first ever to introduce the concept of "lower" and "upper limits of vulnerability" to VF in man. Battelli, however, was unable to provide a satisfactory answer as to why currents with *similar* intensities, while causing death in some individuals, did not induce any deleterious effects in others. For him, the concept of the "vulnerable phase" of the cardiac cycle was still 31 years away, awaiting King's discovery of the window of vulnerability in the cardiac cycle.

With the turn of the century and the advent of reasonably accurate recording instruments of the electrical activity of the heart, the nature of the "fibrillar contractions" and "*trémulations fibrillaire*" during VF was refined at a mechanistic level and with the introduction of fundamental and characteristic electrophysiological variables, including refractoriness, cycle length, and conduction block. The "demonstration" of reentrant waves of excitation during ventricular tachycardia (VT) or VF using a handful of recording electrodes by Mines[11,12] in 1913–1914, Garrey[13] in 1914, and Lewis[14] in 1924 provided reasonably accurate electrophysiological basis to describe the "fibrillar" waves. The original contributions of Louis N. Katz's insightful and integrated interpretation of wave dynamics during VF are as remarkable as they are valid today.[15] In his paper with Bram, Katz emphasized: "The relative differences between excitability and conductivity in an area may act like areas of block. The areas of block may shift in location at time or remain or recur at the same points. Such areas of obstruction would cause the impulse to assume circuitous path and would act to break up the initial single impulse into several 'daughter' impulses, each shuttling and weaving among the areas of block."[15]

Carl Wiggers et al.[16] in 1930 provided a surface electrocardiographic (ECG) account of the alterations of ventricular activation pattern in situ for canine hearts as VF progressed in time unperturbed by an outside intervention. This investigator, simultaneously recording surface ECG and taking moving pictures, observed that the process of fibrillation evolves over time into four distinct ECG phenotypes (see Fig. 2). The duration of VF induced by an electrical shock in otherwise normal hearts, could last between 15 and 55 min before the heart became electrically quiescent. Given the frequent citation of VF stages in the current literature and their importance in clinical practice, for example, implantable cardioverter-defibrillators (ICDs) deliver shock during stage II VF, we provide Wiggers's original description of the four stages of VF in its entirety:

> *Stage I.* "The initial stage of tachysytole lasts less than one second and is characterized by the spread of rapidly recurring but coordinated contraction waves, by large electrocardiographic deflections with steep gradients and by definite if small intraventricular pressure variations."

> *Stage II.* "The second stage of convulsive incoordination ordinarily lasts fifteen to forty seconds and is characterized by rapid irregular localized contractions which spread short and variable distances over the heart. They are accompanied by large electrical deflections, 600 or more per minute, which vary considerably in size, amplitude and contour."

> *Stage III.* "The third stage of tremulous incoordination ordinarily continues two or three minutes and is characterized by multitudes of irregular yet forceful shivering or trembling motions, each spreading over different surface regions. They give rise to small irregular electrocardiographic oscillations having frequencies between 1100 and 1700 per min, and are capable of increasing intraventricular pressure level slightly."

> *Stage IV.* "The fourth stage of atonic incoordination is characterized by feeble wavelets of contraction spreading irregularly and at sloe rates over small areas until more areas become quiescent and finally the very slightest movements remain in a few areas only. The electrical deflections perhaps become slightly more regular in contour and spacing, but their amplitude becomes progressively smaller, and their frequency is gradually reduced to 400 per minutes or less."[16] (Fig. 2)

A fundamental principle of success for VF induction by an electrical shock was described by King,[17] who in 1934 introduced and systematically described the concept and the

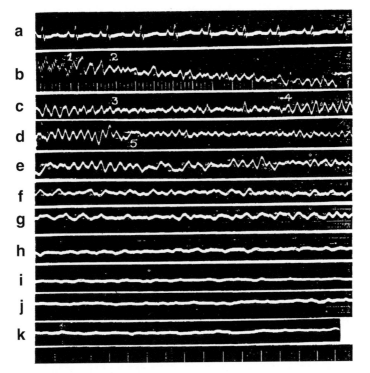

Figure 2: Segments of electrocardiogram (lead II) taken at various stages of VF induced by an electrical shock in the dog: (**a**) preshock sinus rhythm; (**b, c**) immediate postshock rhythm; (**d**) after 30 s; (**e**) 1 min; (**f**) after 1.5 min; (**g**) after 2 min; (**h**) after 5.5 min; (**i**) after 16 min; (**j**) after 20 min; (**k**) after 21 min. Time scale 40 and 200 ms. (Wiggers et al. 1930)[16]

arrhythmic consequences of the "vulnerable phase" of the cardiac cycle. King et al., from Columbia University's College of Physicians and Surgeons, provided for the first time a clear and detailed description of the vulnerable period of the cardiac cycle. Using their words: "The heart is most sensitive to fibrillation for shocks occurring during the partial refractory period of its cycle, which is about 20 per cent of the whole and which occurs simultaneously within the T wave of the electrocardiogram. With shocks of durations of about 0.1 second or less, it is practically impossible to produce ventricular fibrillation, unless such shocks coincide in part at least with these sensitive phase of the cardiac cycle. The middle of the partial refractory phase is more sensitive than its beginning or end."[18]

During the period just after World War II, biomedical research underwent a period of relative stagnation and hiatus, but it resumed again in the early 1960s. A seminal experimental work on cardiac defibrillation was reported by the Philip Coumel's group in France in 1967, which most remarkably equated the upper limit of vulnerability (ULV) for the induction of VF by a shock on the T wave to the defibrillation threshold (DFT).[19] The concept that the ULV is close to the DFT greatly helped to estimate the DFT during ICD implantation without recourse to multiple fibrillation/defibrillation trials. Given the historic importance of this finding, the original relevant text of French with its translation is provided.

> Il y a indentité entre le seuil de disparition de la fibrillation ventriculaire par choc dans la période vulnéerable (D.F.V.) et de la valeur optimal des chocs de defibrillation (V.O.C.D.)

> The threshold of disappearance of ventricular fibrillation by countershock in the vulnerable period (V.P.D.) [i.e., ULV] and the optimal value of the defibrillation countershock (D.C.O.V.) [i.e., DFT] were identical.[19]

The Era of Computerized Cardiac Mapping: New Insights

The mid-1980s witnessed the advent of high-resolution computerized electrode, and subsequently fluorescent mapping techniques provided insights on wavefront activation patterns of VF seen before, during, and after delivery of electrical shocks. Particular attention was focused on comparative wavefront dynamics between successful and unsuccessful shocks of similar strengths applied to the same heart. Although much was learned, it is however somewhat disconcerting that the remarkable advances achieved in imaging of VF wavefronts, the mechanism(s) by which an electrical shock terminates VF still remains elusive. Perhaps more important, the current advances did not result in improved electrotherapy (i.e., reduction in energy level for a successful defibrillation). Most of the current reports on defibrillation are observational in nature, and the attempts aimed at improving defibrillation efficacy remain an exercise in trial and errors. In fact it can successfully be argued that most of the current mechanistic and conceptual insights of VF and defibrillation are derived and based on fundamental concepts developed over a span of more than 100 years. Only few innovations and discoveries were added over the existing discoveries that can be embodied in seven fundamental concepts: (1) the ability of an electrical shock to cause VF ("cardiac death") and a subsequent shock causing resuscitation (VF and defibrillation);[6] (2) a finite range of shock strengths needed to cause cardiac death, as shocks too low or too high fail to promote the desired event, thus establishing the principle of lower and upper limits of vulnerability (LLV and ULV, respectively) to VF[10]; (3) electrical stimulation to a very small region of the heart (i.e., <1 mm), known as point stimulation, can induce VF;[9] (4) VF induced by an electrical shock is preceded by a periodic activation (VT), which degenerates to irregular ECG patterns within 30 s, characteristic of VF;[16] (5) in order for a shock to induce VF it must fall within the vulnerable period of the cardiac cycle (shock on T wave);[17,18] (6) wave breaks and generation of multiple eaves during fibrillation result from functional cardiac conduction block that vary in site and timing;[15] (7) the strength of the current at the ULV is very close to the strength of the current for successful defibrillation.[19]

During the past 40 years or so five orders of innovative contributions provided a greater insight into the defibrillation process. However, no breakthroughs were made that allowed use of reduced shock energy for successful defibrillation. First, single cell recordings with glass microelectrodes identified in a systematic manner the cellular basis of the interaction between electrical stimuli of different strengths, with cardiac cells at different levels of recovery (i.e., repolarization, or "membrane responsiveness"). Second, biphasic shocks were found to be more effective in terminating VF than monophasic shocks.[20–22] Third, optical mapping studies identified the phenomenon of "virtual electrode" polarization, whereby a shock induces membrane polarization (depolarization and hyperpolarization) at sites located outside the physical dimensions of the current passing electrodes.[23,24] Fourth, simulation of reasonably realistic models of excitable media provided new insights into possible mechanisms of defibrillation scenarios.[25–27] Fifth, the similarity of ventricular ULV to DFT, first observed in the dog model,[19] was extended to humans, a contribution of considerable clinical impact in the practice of ICD implantation in humans (reduction in the number of VF induction).[24,28]

Initiation of VF by Electrical Stimuli

VF has been shown to be reproducibly inducible in normal ventricles by a single, critically timed point electrical stimulation with an appropriate strength.[16,18,29] Although extremely strong shocks may induce VF during any period of the cardiac cycle,[9] criticality of the shock, both in terms of timing and strength, is crucial for VF induction.[18,29] Three-dimentional computerized mapping studies of intact canine ventricles have shown that shock-induced VF in the normal ventricles is initiated by the immediate formation of figure-8 functional reentrant wavefront of excitation (scroll wave in three dimensions and spiral wave, or figure-8 in two dimensions). This first postshock reentry actually characterizes stage I VF.[30] After two to four beats, in the case of a point S_2 stimulus,[30] or up to ten rotations, in the case of a multiple linear array of S_2 electrodes,[31] the single scroll wave breaks down into multiple irregular wavefronts, signaling the onset of VF, or stage II VF.[16]

The ability of a point premature stimulation at the site of the reentry to terminate the reentrant wavefront and the VF[32] provides convincing evidence that the reentrant wavefront seen at the onset of stage I VF is causally related to the stage I VF, and it is not an epiphenomenon.[16,32] Using epicardial surface electrode mapping, Chen et al.[33] speculated that the mechanism of unidirectional block at the site of the electrical stimulus resulted from refractory period prolongation by the "graded responses." It was speculated that the graded responses could have traveled slowly away from the S_2 stimulus site to initiate activation at distant recovered site. Reentry, single arm, or a figure-8 was then formed when the front rotated around the site of the stimulus-induced block to reenter and excite it when it recovers its excitability. This speculation was based on earlier glass microelectrode studies by Van Dam et al.[34] on isolated canine Purkinje-muscle preparations. These authors have shown that strong electrical currents applied prior to the cellular recovery of excitability evoke nonregenerative cellular depolarizations (graded responses) that not only propagate, albeit decrementally, but also are capable of initiating regenerative responses in more fully recovered cells at some distance from the stimulus site.

Electrical shocks and termination of VF. Shocks there are otherwise successful often fail to terminate fibrillation on repeat trials. This characteristic property of VF indicates that defibrillation is a probabilistic phenomenon.[35–37] Detailed computerized studies suggest that failed defibrillation shocks, while terminating many of the reentrant and nonreentrant wave

fronts of the VF, induce reentry (phase singularity)[24] at one or more "vulnerable" sites
that degenerate to VF, causing failure of defibrillation.[38] This phenomenon might appear
counterintuitive. How is it possible to induce VF when in VF? The answer lies in the
criticality of the timing and the strength of the shock relative to available sites with partial
or relative recovery in the fibrillating ventricles. Should a shock of a critical strength (i.e.,
between the LLV and ULV) find a site (or sites) in the fibrillating ventricle in its relative
refractory period (vulnerable period), reentry may then be induced (phase singularity), as
is the case of shocks on T wave.[24] During the ensuing rotations of the induced reentrant
wavefront typical at a cycle length of around 100 ms, the from becomes subject to increased
likelihood of breakup by the phenomenon known as fibrillatory conduction, which leads to
recommencement of VF and failure of defibrillation.[39,40] The phraseology used to describe
the shock outcome then depends on the nature of the preshock rhythm. If the shock induces
reentry during VF, then the phenomenon is described as *failed defibrillation shock*; however,
when reentry and VF are induced during sinus or regularly paced rhythm, the phenomenon
is known as *vulnerability to VF*. It is clear that a relationship, however implicit, does exist
between a shock that fails to defibrillate a fibrillating ventricle and a shock that induces VF
during regular rhythm. The common link between failed defibrillation and induction of VF
by a strong electrical stimulus in normal ventricles is then reduced to a precise mechanistic
understanding of how an electrical stimulus induces reentry in recovering normal ventricular
cells. This subject will be dealt with in greater detail later in the chapter.

Virtual electrode polarization. Taking advantage of the immunity of optical signals to
shock-induced artifacts, it was shown that both cathodal and anodal electrical shocks
produce hitherto unrecognized patterns of cardiac muscle polarization, dubbed as *virtual
electrode polarization*, which is characterized by the juxtaposition of depolarized and hyperpolarized myocardial regions observed on the surface of the ventricles beyond the physical
dimensions of the current passing electrodes.[24,41,42]

It is apparent then that an understanding of the cellular basis of shock-induced reentry
in normal ventricular myocardium could provide an insight into the cellular basis of
defibrillation. According to the VF/defibrillation paradigms, it is not surprising to expect
that increasing shock strengths applied during regular rhythms should also decrease the
vulnerability to reentry and VF. This inferred paradigm has not only been demonstrated
experimentally, but it also has shown that a close numerical similarity exists between the
DFT and the ULV in animals[19,43] and man.[28,44]

Different Proposed Hypotheses of Defibrillation

There are five proposed hypotheses of defibrillation mechanism, which while seemingly
different, are interrelated and complementary to one another. The first hypothesis, the
critical point hypothesis, was proposed by Frazier et al.[31] in Ideker's laboratory using
epicardial electrode mapping system. These authors have show that reentry induced by
a strong electrical stimulus develops at the intersection of critical tissue refractoriness with
a critical electrical field strength. According to this hypothesis VF is initiated by a single-
loop reentry when a specific voltage gradient ($5\,\mathrm{V/cm^{-1}}$) interacts with the recovering

tissue.[31] Such states are presumed to underlie the mechanism of defibrillation failure because critical points lead to the formation of reentry and subsequent regeneration of fibrillation.[31] The *critical point hypothesis* explains the mechanisms by which the coupling interval and increasing shock strength move the location where reentry is formed (away from the shock electrode and pacing electrode, respectively).[45] With sufficiently high shock strength, the critical point is pushed outside of the heart, resulting in failure of reinducing VF (successful defibrillation). No clear cellular electrophysiological descriptors are provided to explain the mechanism of the functional block that develops to produce single-loop reentry. Rather, it is proposed that block occurs "when a line corresponding to one of the excitatory states intersects a line corresponding to one of the critical recovery states, (the critical point) excitation wave front occurs on one side of the critical point [block] and then pivots around the critical point."[46] This proposal is based on the postulate "that critical states of each of the excitatory and recovery processes occur when a stimulus of an appropriate strength is given at an appropriate time during the recovery."[31,46] This hypothesis is based on Winfree's[47] theoretical proposal of rotor formation in excitable media. Winfree anticipated that paired mirror-image vortices (rotors) organized around phase singularities "arise in the myocardium near the intersection of a moving critical contour of phase in the normal cycle of excitation and recovery with a momentary critical contour of local stimulus strength."[47] Such intersections, and the corresponding aftermath of paired rotors, should only occur following certain combinations of stimulus size and stimulus timing.

The second hypothesis was proposed by Witkowski et al.,[48] who suggested that defibrillation shocks fail because certain regions of the fibrillating ventricles remain unaffected by the shock. Fibrillation will thus continue, provided the unaffected fibrillating region is of a critical mass to sustain the VF. Since the earlier work of Zipes et al.,[49] who for the first time extended Garrey's[13] in vitro observations of the "critical mass" hypothesis of fibrillation to in situ ventricles, variants of the critical mass hypothesis of defibrillation have been formulated. Upon induction of a progressively larger mass of myocardial tissue inexcitable by regional hyperkalemic depolarization, they concluded that VF could be terminated when "the remaining number of excitable cells represented a critical mass insufficient to maintain fibrillation." The concept of critical mass was extended to explain electrical defibrillation. Witkowski et al.[48] maintained that for a shock to be successful, it must extinguish wavefronts only in a portion of the fibrillating ventricles, as postshock "residual fibrillating activity" in a mass smaller then the critical mass "can either go on to reinitiate global VF or not," depending on the surrounding tissue excitability. The probabilistic nature of defibrillation success argues against this tenet. The fact that a successful shock may fail to defibrillate on a subsequent trial in the same heart argues against the failed shock being unable to interact with more than a critical mass of myocardium. This is so because similar shock strengths, when successful, are claimed to interfere with all wavefronts in both ventricles without "leaving out" some regions of the ventricle (i.e., critical mass) that remain unaffected by the shock. No cellular descriptors of shock-induced block were proposed by Witkowski et al.[48]

The third hypothesis was proposed by Dillon and Kwaku,[50] who, by using optical mapping system, suggested that defibrillation success is related to the ability of the shock to increase refractoriness at the border of shock-depolarized areas so as to prevent initiation of propagating new wavefronts from the depolarized areas by the shock. This hypothesis suggests that "the shock always produces a propagating impulse," and that the likelihood of the induced propagating wavefront "to run the risk of breaking down into fibrillation" (failed defibrillation) will depend on how much myocardium is depolarized by the shock. Analysis of activation maps showed that postshock propagating activity arose from areas depolarized by the shock that were found to be inversely related to refractoriness, as indexed by coupling interval (CI) or the optical takeoff potential (Vm). These authors concluded that shock-induced depolarization of the effectively refractory myocardium (i.e., depolarized to $\geq 60\%$ optical action potential amplitude) is required to guarantee the cessation of continued wavefront propagation in defibrillation. Stronger shocks, it is argued, are less likely to be followed by fibrillation because the stronger shocks "progressively prolong and synchronize repolarization in an increasing fashion of the ventricle to antagonize the arrhythmic propagation of wave fronts present after the shock."[50] One caveat with this proposal is that stronger shocks also increase the probability of inducing activation from partially recovered sites according to the strength–interval relationship that otherwise could not have been initiated with weaker shocks. In addition, the increased number of wavefronts in a setting of increased prolongation and synchronization of refractoriness increases the probability of wave breaks and causes electrical defibrillation to fail. This indicates that the shock must be associated with a state of total depolarization everywhere in the heart (i.e., ULV) so that no new waves can be launched. This proposal, as will be seen later, is compatible with the graded response hypothesis that proposes shock-induced bidirectional conduction block as a mechanism for ULV and defibrillation. It must also be mentioned that Kwaku and Dillon[51] failed to observe "critical points" in more than 95% of the failed defibrillation shocks. As in previous hypotheses no specific single cellular descriptors of vulnerability to reentry or reentry termination by an electrical shock were provided in this study.

The fourth hypothesis, virtual electrode-induced phase singularity, was proposed by Efimov et al.[24,52] According to this hypothesis, defibrillation fails when shock-induced virtual electrode polarization leads to reentry (phase singularity), and successful defibrillation results when shocks fail to induce phase singularity (reentry).[24] In support of this mechanism these authors have demonstrated that biphasic shocks are more effective than monophasic shock because the opposite polarity of the shock cancels virtual electrode polarization and prevents formation of phase singularity (reentry) resulting in VF termination.[24,52] Biphasic waveforms are therefore likely to prevent formation of unidirectional conduction block and reentry (phase singularity) because the second phase of the shock will remove or abbreviate the graded response-induced prolongation of refractoriness of the first phase, thus causing faster recovery of excitability and prevention of block. Although this scenario is speculative, the demonstration of reduced probability of phase singularity formation with biphasic shock[24,52] and the absence of net effective refractory period (ERP) prolongation with successful biphasic shocks[53] lend some support to the proposed scenario. Biphasic waveforms with intermediate second-phase voltages (20–70% of first-phase voltage) produced no virtual electrode polarization, because of an asymmetric reversal of the first-phase polarization, therefore preventing the creation of a substrate for postshock dispersion of repolarization and reentry (phase singularity).

The Graded Response Hypothesis of Fibrillation and Defibrillation

The fifth hypothesis is the graded response hypothesis, which was proposed a decade ago.[54] This hypothesis, developed with the use of combined single cell microelectrode and extracellular electrode mapping of thin epicardial ventricular myocardium in vitro, not only mimics the sequence of events leading to VF in the in situ open-chest anesthetized dogs but also provides step-by-step cellular events leading to either reentry or failure to reentry after a strong electrical stimulus. Figure 3 is a diagram that describes our methods of recording and stimulating in the isolated thin epicardial tissue blocks. The cellular mechanisms by which a strong electrical stimulus leads to reentry/VF, or failure to form reentry, is compatible with the four proposed mechanisms of vulnerability to fibrillation and defibrillation with strong electrical shocks. Specifically, the graded response hypothesis provides insight into eight major characteristics of vulnerability and defibrillation by electrical shocks described in the literature: (1) The hypothesis describes in a stepwise manner the chain of cellular events through which a critical electrical shock leads to reentry formation in a normal uniformly anisotropic myocardium. (2) It elucidates the mechanism for the need of critical shock strength for the induction of reentry (i.e., the shock strength must fall between the LLV and ULV). (3) It explains the need for a critical timing of the shock (i.e., the vulnerable period) for the induction of reentry by a stimulus. (4) It provides a cellular mechanism for the phenomenon of break excitation (i.e., excitation occurring some time *after* the end of the stimulus). (5) It elucidates the mechanism by which the earliest activation after a stimulus arises from a low voltage gradient area away from the site of the stimulating electrode. (6) It is compatible with virtual electrode polarization-mediated failure or success for initiating reentry. (7) It provides cellular insight into the numerical similarity between ULV and DFT. (8) It suggests a plausible mechanistic scenario for the greater efficacy of biphasic shocks over monophasic shocks in terminating VF.

The subsequent sections discuss these eight characteristic properties of the graded responses and provide experimental evidence in support of the cellular graded response hypothesis of vulnerability to reentry or failure to reentry.

Graded Response Characteristics

Graded response or progressive cellular depolarization develops when electrical stimuli of progressively increasing intensity are applied during the relative refractory period, when the regenerative inward currents (I_{Na} and ICa_{L-type}) have not yet recovered from inactivation. The term graded or progressive indicates that the response is not an all-or-none type (i.e., regenerative), but it is rather a function of the stimulus strength. For a given coupling interval, a progressive increase in the strength of the stimulating current and a progressive increase in the amplitude and duration of the depolarizing responses develop. Similarly, for a given stimulus current intensity, the more negative the transmembrane potential the higher the amplitude and duration of the graded response. Figure 4 illustrates an example. The graded depolarizations that are induced during the repolarization lengthen the refractory period in proportion to the duration of the graded response duration. Figure 5

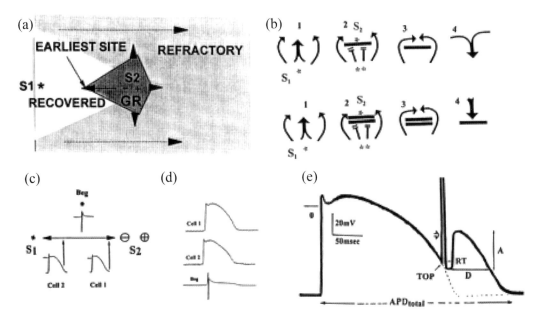

Figure 3: Diagram of graded-response hypothesis (**a**, **b**) and methods of recording and measurement (**c**–**e**). (**a**) *Dark-shaded* polygon is area of graded responses (GR) spread by an S_2. Note spread of GR for longer distances along the fiber (*horizontal arrow-headed doted lines*) and toward cathode side ($-$) than anode ($+$) of S_2. *White area* represents area of recovering tissue after S_1, with most recovered area located near S_1 site (*single asterisk*), and *light-shaded area* represents refractory (less recovered) tissue. The two *arrow-headed dotted lines* point to direction of wave front propagation during S_1 pacing. (**b**) Initiation of figure-8 reentry according to GR hypothesis. Fiber orientation is north–south. Numbers 1 in both rows show wavefront propagation during regular S_1 pacing (*single asterisk*). Number 2 in upper row shows response after S_2 stimulus (*single asterisk*), with earliest site of activity arising between S_1 and S_2 (*double asterisk*). Front then blocks at S_2 site (B2, *horizontal line*), rotates around area of block (B3), then reenters (B4) when this area recovers its excitability as first figure-8 reentry cycle. Lower row of (**b**) shows same scenario but with an S_2 strength above the ULV. In this case, excess prolongation of refractory period (*double horizontal lines* in 2 and 3) prevents reentry (frame 4). (**c**) Locations of two microelectrodes and bipolar (Beg) recordings. *Double-headed arrow* is fiber orientation. (**d**) shows simultaneous recordings during S_1 pacing. (**e**) shows the method of measurement of graded-response properties induced by an S_2. TOP is the takeoff potential in mV; D, A, and RT are duration (ms), amplitude (mV), and rise time (ms) of graded response, respectively. APD total is total APD (100% repolarization). *Dashed line* shows time course of repolarization of regular action potential without interruption by an S_2. *Horizontal white arrow* points to S_2 stimulus artifact, and horizontal line near action potential upstroke is 0 reference potential. (Gotoh et al. 1997)[54]

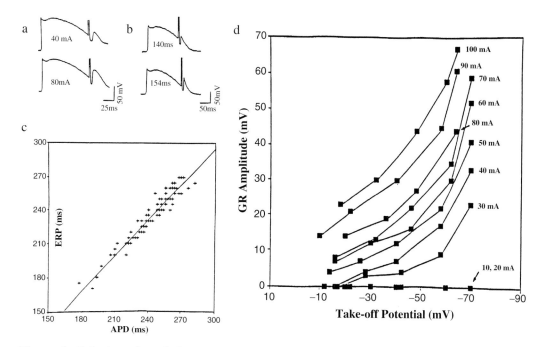

Figure 4: Relation of graded-response properties to S_2 stimulus characteristics. (a) effects of increasing S_2 current strength from 40 to 80 mA. (b) effects of increasing S_2 coupling intervals from 140 to 154 ms in a different tissue. In both cases an increase in the amplitude (c) and duration (d) of the graded responses occur

illustrates an example of graded-response induced prolongation of the refractory period. Depolarizing graded responses have the ability to propagate, albeit slowly and poorly (decremental conduction). Slow conduction of the graded responses is illustrated in Fig. 6. An important consequence of propagating graded responses is the initiation of a regenerative response in recovered cells when the propagated wave of depolarization enters a tissue with recovered excitability. Figure 6 illustrates an example of graded response induced action potential in a recovered cell some 5 mm away from the S_2 source. The onset of a regenerative action potential some 20 ms after the shock provides a cellular explanation of the phenomenon of break excitation. The conduction time needed for the depolarizing wave of the graded responses to travel from the S_2 electrode site to recovered cells and evoke a regenerative action potential unambiguously explains this delay in excitation after a critical S_2. This delay forms the basis of break excitation that is often present after a critical S_2 induces reentry in normal myocardium.[55,56] A delay (i.e., a period of about 60 ms electrical quiescence, or *isoelectric window*) in the first postshock activation is also present after a failed defibrillation shock, as shown in isolated tissues[57] and also in the in situ hearts using three-dimentional mapping studies.[38] The graded responses propagate at a velocity that is 50–80% slower than the regenerative responses supported by fast sodium transient current. Figure 7a illustrates an example. The distally initiated activity by the propagating graded

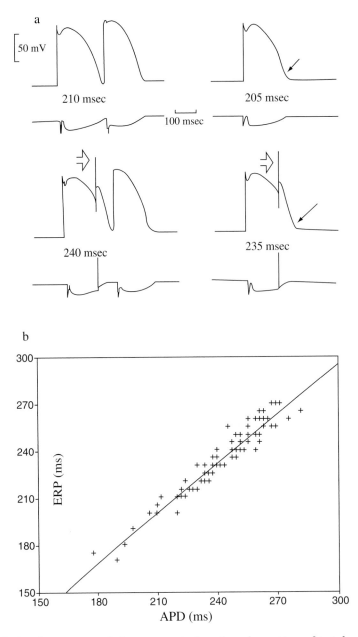

Figure 5: Relation between graded response-induced prolongation of total action potential duration (APD) (i.e., 100% repolarization) and the resultant effective refractory period (ERP). (a) Action potentials from an isolated thin canine epicardial slices (*top*) and a bipolar electrogram (*bottom*). Note that without additional prolongation of the APD, the ERP is 205 ms (*downward pointing arrow*). However, the ERP lengthens to 235 ms when the APD is prolonged by a graded response (*open arrows*). (b) A plot of ERP (ordinate) versus APD prolonged by additional repolarization time caused by a graded response

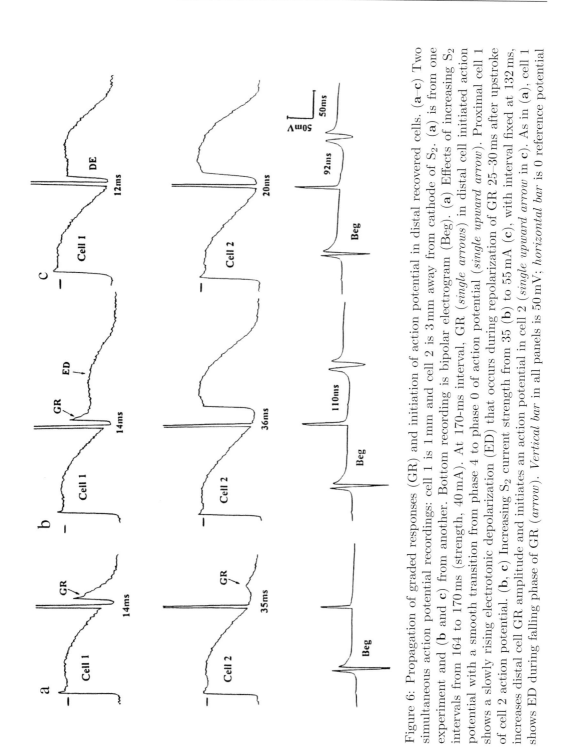

Figure 6: Propagation of graded responses (GR) and initiation of action potential in distal recovered cells. (a–c) Two simultaneous action potential recordings: cell 1 is 1 mm and cell 2 is 3 mm away from cathode of S₂. (a) is from one experiment and (b and c) from another. Bottom recording is bipolar electrogram (Beg). (a) Effects of increasing S₂ intervals from 164 to 170 ms (strength, 40 mA). At 170-ms interval, GR (single arrows) in distal cell initiated action potential with a smooth transition from phase 4 to phase 0 of action potential (single upward arrow). Proximal cell 1 shows a slowly rising electrotonic depolarization (ED) that occurs during repolarization of GR 25–30 ms after upstroke of cell 2 action potential. (b, c) Increasing S₂ current strength from 35 (b) to 55 mA (c), with interval fixed at 132 ms, increases distal cell GR amplitude and initiates an action potential in cell 2 (single upward arrow in c). As in (a), cell 1 shows ED during falling phase of GR (arrow). Vertical bar in all panels is 50 mV; horizontal bar is 0 reference potential

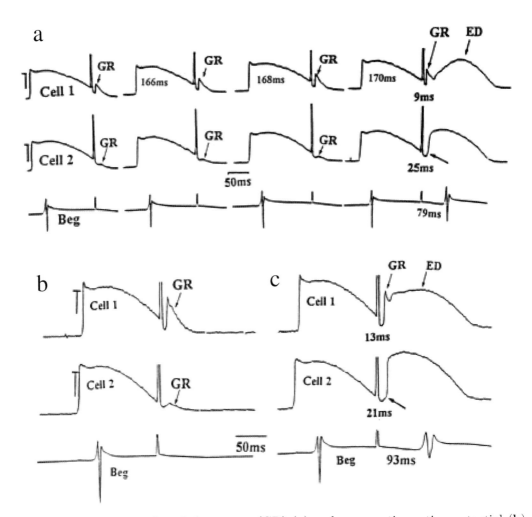

Figure 7: Comparison of graded response (GR) (a) and regenerative action potential (b) propagation in an isolated canine thin epicardial slice. Recording arrangement same as in Fig. 3 Note the longer delay (56 ms) of the GR from cell 1 near S_2 to cell 2 (1 cm away from S_2) relative to a regenerative response (30 ms) (b). (c) Initiation of action potential in cell 2 in another tissue induced by the propagating GR (*first small downward arrow*; S_2 is 40 mA, with 154 ms coupling interval). The GR induces in cell 2 an action potential that blocks in cell 1 near the S_2 site (*upward arrow*), causing an electrotonic depolarization (ED) in cell 1. However, following 239 ms delay after the upstroke of the cell 2 action potential, cell 1 initiates an action potential (*double downward arrows*), which then excites cell 2 (*second downward arrow*) as the first reentrant action potential. Excitation of the same distal cell 2 by a regenerative action potential is evoked by direct excitation (DE) of cell 1 after full recovery. Note the faster distal cell activation (19 vs. 53 ms) reflecting slower conduction of the GR to the distal cell 1. Cell 1 is 1 mm and cell 2 12 mm away from the cathodal pole of the bipolar S_2 stimulating electrode. (Gotoh et al. 1997)[54]

response appears to initiate a reentrant activation as suggested in Fig. 7b. To determine if reentry occurs in this in vitro model, we have done sequential electrode mapping first with 56 electrodes and then with 456 electrodes. The results in the in vitro studies show figure-8 or single arm reentry induced by the S_2 that is similar to the reentry induced in the is situ open-chest anesthetized dogs. Figure 8 illustrates an example of reentry induced by an S_2 in vitro. This sequence of events recorded in isolated canine epicardial slices demonstrates step by step how an S_2 stimulus induces reentry by the propagating "wave" of graded responses. Since similar stimulation protocols, stimulation sites and electrode configurations also induce similar functional reentrant activations (which precede VF) in the in situ normal canine hearts, the graded response hypothesis of vulnerability to reentry (precursor of VF) may also be operative in the intact heart.

The spread of the wave of the graded responses is anisotropic, being faster along the fibers than across it. Figure 9 illustrates the anisotropic nature of the graded response propagation in the epicardium.

Criticality of the electrical stimulus strength and timing. Reentry could be induced only when the current strength of the S_2 is within the LLV and the ULV. Current strengths falling outside this range cannot induce reentry even if the current is applied during the vulnerable period (Fig. 10). These findings are similar to in situ observation using similar electrode configurations and stimulation protocols.[30]

Earliest site of activation arises in low voltage gradient areas. In our in vitro model of reentry the earliest activation after a premature S_2 stimulus always arose away from the S_2 stimulus site and close to more recovered cells. Since the voltage gradient at the source of the stimulating electrical current is the highest and diminishes at distances away from the S_2 source,[58] the site of the earliest postshock activation therefore arises from a low voltage area. The graded response hypothesis of vulnerability to reentry is therefore compatible with the reported findings that the earliest postshock activation in normal in situ canine hearts arises away from current source located in low voltage gradient areas.[31,58]

Virtual electrode effect and vulnerability to reentry. Unipolar stimulation in bidomain models[42,59] have shown that under a cathode, the contours of transmembrane potential form a "dog bone" of depolarization, with two areas of hyperpolarization on both sides of the dog bone shape. These areas of depolarization and hyperpolarization that form away and at some distance from the physical dimension of the stimulating electrode are known as *virtual electrodes polarization.*[59] Using optical mapping it was found that bipolar stimulation, as was done in the graded response studies, also induces virtual electrode polarization that is quite analogous to the virtual electrode polarization observed during unipolar stimulation.[60] Adjacent to each real electrode polarization (depolarization at the cathode side of the bipole and hyperpolarization at the anode side of the bipole), virtual electrode polarization of opposite polarity develops. A question may then arise if the proposed graded response hypothesis of reentry formation is compatible with the development of virtual electrode polarization. The answer to this question is yes. The virtual anode that develops near the real cathode of the bipole accelerates cellular repolarization and provides a greater opportunity for the depolarizing wave of graded responses induced by the real cathode to encounter recovered cells and initiate regenerative activation. Recent simulation studies using a two-dimentional bidomain model and unipolar stimulation with juxtaposition of

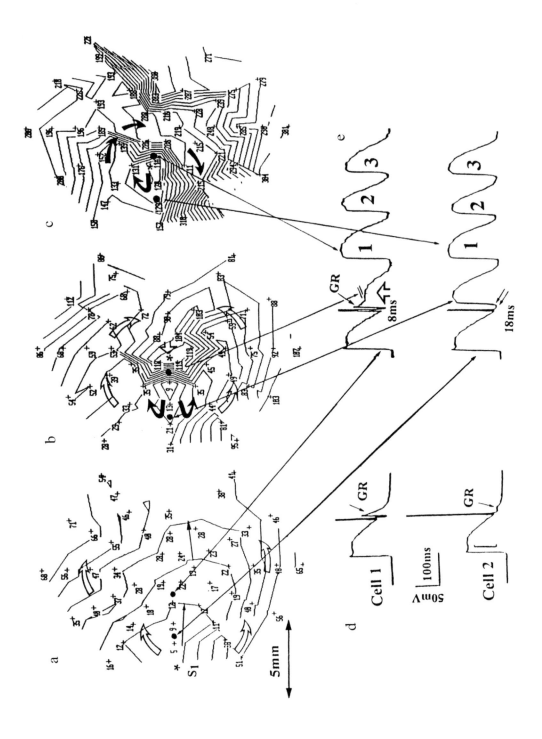

Figure 8: Isochronal activation map and two simultaneous action potential recordings in an isolated thin canine epicardial slice. A 56-channel bipolar electrode array was used in this study to map 3×3 cm tissue. (**a**) shows isochronal activation map (10 ms isochronal interval) during regular S_1–S_1 pacing at 600 ms cycle length (*asterisk*). The *crosses* represent electrode locations and the numbers give the time of activation, with the onset of S_1 as time zero. The *two dots* represent the two sites from which subsequent simultaneous action potentials are recorded. The *arrows* in (**a**–**c**) point to the direction of wave front propagation. The *horizontal double-headed arrow* indicates the fiber orientation and also serves as length scale. (**b**) is an isochronal activation map of an S_2 stimulus (40 mA at 136-ms interval) applied in the center of the tissue (*asterisk*; pointed to by an *open arrow*). The site of earliest activation is located 3 mm away from the S_1 site toward the S_1 site (isochrone encircling 9-ms site). The S_2-initiated wavefront first propagates toward the S_1 site then rotates (*double curved arrows*) around the site of block and reaches proximal to the site of block in 104 ms, forming a figure-8. (**c**) shows the activation reentering through the initial site of block near the S_2 stimulus site. (**d**) shows two simultaneous action potential recordings from sites indicated in (**a**). An S_2 stimulus (40 mA, 122-ms interval) induces a graded response in cell 1 (*arrow*) that propagates to cell 2 with decrement in amplitude (35–5 mV) (*single arrows*). (**e**) shows that an S_2 (40 mA and 136-ms interval) initiates a graded response from the graded response in cell 1 with an 8-ms delay and an action potential in cell 2 with an 18-ms delay that arises from the graded response (*double arrows*). The action potential initiated in cell 2 blocks at the site of cell 1 (*large open arrow* with *double horizontal lines* in cell 1) with an electrotonic depolarization. The reentrant wavefront in (**c**) excites cell 1 then cell 2 as shown in (**e**) with action potential 1. Two subsequent reentrant action potentials are also shown (**2** and **3**). (Gotoh et al. 1997)[54]

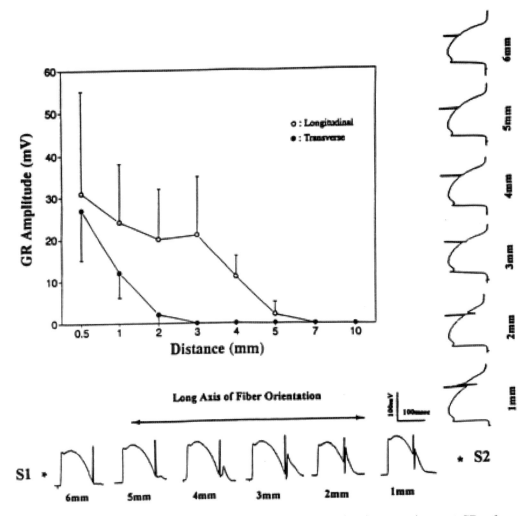

Figure 9: Anisotropic propagation of graded responses (GR). Plot (mean ± SD of ten tissue samples) shows effects of distance from cathodal pole of S$_2$ source (abscissa) on GR (ordinate). *Open circles*, GR amplitude along fiber; *solid circles*, across it. S$_2$ current strength was 50 mA and coupling interval 140 ms. Recordings below *double-headed arrow* (fiber orientation) are sequential action potential recordings along fiber from cells at increasing distances (1–6 mm) from S$_2$ stimulus site (*asterisk*). Vertical recordings are from cells across fiber orientation toward top of tissue

real electrode depolarization and virtual electrode hyperpolarization replicated the figure-8 reentry that was observed with bipolar stimulation in isolated canine epicardial tissue slices.[56] Furthermore, these findings demonstrate that the graded response hypothesis of reentry, first formulated using bipolar stimulation, is also operative for unipolar stimulation.[56]

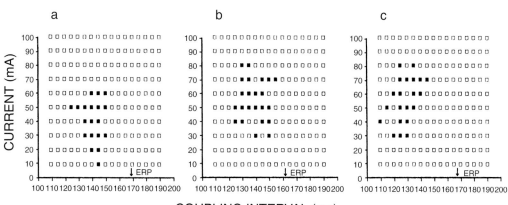

Figure 10: Strength-interval plots for reentry induction in three epicardial tissue slices (**a**–**c**) during pacing at a cycle length of 600 ms. *Solid squares* indicate S_2 trials that induced reentry, and the *open squares* indicate the S_2 trials that failed to induce reentry. Ordinate, in milliamperes, is S_2 current strengths; abscissa is coupling intervals in milliseconds. ERP is effective refractory period (*downward arrow*) measured with twice diastolic current threshold during 600-ms cycle length

ULV and DFT numeric similarities. Based on the observation that defibrillation shocks fail because shock induces reentry formation, it could then be inferred that for a defibrillation shock to be successful, the shock must fail to induce reentry. Our in vitro mapping studies show that shock strengths just above the ULV (Fig. 10) fail to produce reentry during regular pacing, and that the graded response hypothesis of vulnerability to reentry can adequately explain the failure to produce reentry. Super-strong S_2 electrical currents are associated with longer duration graded responses and refractoriness, which when above a critical duration fail to recover when the distally originated activation wavefront arrives at the S_2 site. This will cause conduction block and failure to reentry by converting unidirectional block to bidirectional block. Figure 11 shows two simultaneous cell recordings with an S_2 below the ULV, causing reentry and a super-strong (above the ULV) S_2 that fails to induce reentry because of the conversion of unidirectional to bidirectional block. A high-resolution electrode activation map verified the presence of bidirectional block with super-strong S_2 current strength.[54] Strong currents capable of converting unidirectional to bidirectional block can prevent the formation of reentry during regular rhythm (ULV) or during VF (successful defibrillation). It is apparent then how the ULV is similar to the DFT.

Monophasic versus biphasic shocks. It is now common knowledge that biphasic shocks are more effective than monophasic shocks in terminating VF.[20,21,53] Although the precise mechanism of such an effect still remains somewhat elusive, the graded response hypothesis might tentatively provide a plausible explanation for such an effect. Focusing on the phenomenon of conversion from unidirectional to bidirectional block by super-strong currents, the hyperpolarizing effect induced by the real electrode effect of the

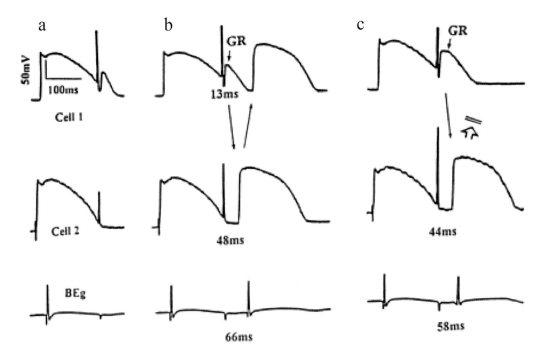

Figure 11: Super-strong S_2 stimulus prevents reentry. Recording arrangements are as in Fig. 3. Cell 1 is 1 mm and cell 2 is 6 mm away from the cathode of the S_2. Increasing the S_2 current strength from 40 mA at a coupling interval of 170 ms (**a**) to 50 mA (**b**) initiates an action potential in the distal cell 2 (*arrow pointing downward*) with a delay of 58 ms. Activation at cell 2 reenters and excites cell 1 (*upward pointing arrow* in **b**) (see also Fig. 8 for activation map). (**c**) shows that when the S_2 current strength is further increased to 70 mA (10 mA above the upper limit of vulnerability [ULV]), the graded response (GR) duration increases from 58 ms (**b**) to 102 ms (**c**). With such prolongation of repolarization time in cell 1, the distally originated action potential in cell 2 fails to excite cell 1 (*open arrow* intercepted by *double horizontal lines*)

biphasic shock accelerates repolarization of cells in their plateau phase where no graded or only a short duration graded response could be induced. The induced acceleration of repolarization by the hyperpolarizing phase of the biphasic shock can then be followed by depolarizing graded responses from adjoining real and virtual depolarized areas, causing lengthening of the total repolarization time and a net increase in refractoriness. This net increase in refractoriness that otherwise might be absent with a monophasic shock might prevent propagation of an induced reentrant wavefront by converting unidirectional block to bidirectional block. This scenario, however plausible, still remains speculative, as the greater efficacy of biphasic shocks may not necessarily be associated with a net ERP lengthening.[53]

Ionic mechanisms, channel block, and DFT. The ionic mechanism(s) of the graded response remains undefined. It is possible that both passive and active ionic mechanisms may participate in the depolarizing process after a strong premature electrical stimulus.[61] Passive capacitative currents may be present during the slowly rising phase of the graded response because it is unlikely that the impedance during such slow dv/dt is purely ohmic. However, two properties of the graded responses argue against an exclusively passive mechanism. One is the voltage dependence of the graded response amplitude and duration (i.e., the increase in amplitude and duration with increasing voltage negativity and the decrease at positive transmembrane voltages).[41,54] The second property is the incompatibility of the voltage decay pattern of the graded response amplitude along the fiber with the measured space constants (0.9–1.2 mm).[62] Although the nature of the active currents involved in the generation of the graded response remains undefined, it is possible that some sodium and/or calcium ions may be "forced" to cross the membrane by strong depolarizing currents.

Limitations. There are two limitations to the graded response hypothesis of vulnerability. The lack of greater ERP prolongation with biphasic shocks over monophasic shocks, while increasing the success rate of defibrillation, is not compatible with the graded response hypothesis.[53] However, the ULV hypothesis can be accounted for by the mechanism of graded response-induced conversion of unidirectional block to directional block to prevent reentry. Although there may in absolute terms be a greater ERP prolongation with monophasic shocks, areas that were not prolonged or only minimally prolonged with monophasic shocks may manifest a net increase in their ERP with biphasic shocks, leading to bidirectional block and prevention of reentry. More studies are needed to clarify this issue. The second limitation is that strong electrical stimuli fail to terminate VF not because of bidirectional block but because of the phenomenon of depolarization-induced automaticity by ventricular myocardial cells,[63,64] which is independent of the graded responses.[65] Perhaps equally important is the fact that the Purkinje fibers appear to manifest greater sensitivity to transient postshock triggered activity, while the ventricular myocardial cells remain quiescent with intermittent activation by the rapidly firing PF. Such postshock effect, if present in intact fibrillating hearts, may actually cause failure of defibrillation.[66] The rapid triggered activity initially propagates as a single wavefront, which may undergo wave breaks, producing multiple irregular wavefronts and resumption of fibrillation.[67,68] It however still remains unclear if biphasic shocks, which are the preferred shock waveform in patients with ICD,[69,70] could also promote triggered activity. It is reported that shocks can cause reduction of intracellular calcium ions (Ca_i^{2+}) uptake by the sarcoplasmic reticulum,[71] an event that may lead to elevation of Ca_i^{2+},[72] leading to afterpotentials and triggered activity[73] and causing failure of defibrillation.

Conclusions and Future Directions

The graded response hypothesis of vulnerability to reentry explains step by step how a critical electrical stimulus interacts with an activation wave to either succeed or fail to induce reentry. The demonstration that reentry can be induced by a critical shock during regular pacing *and* during VF supports the notion that the origin of the wavefront (sinus or VF) is of no consequence in reentry formation. Given the ability of the graded response hypothesis to adequately explain the cellular basis of reentry formation for both in vitro and in vivo settings, it is highly likely that reentry (phase singularity) formation by a failed defibrillation shock may also be explained by graded responses. Because failed shocks may induce propagating graded responses, reentry leading to VF is strongly suggested by the presence of a period of "electrical quiescence" after a failed shock just before the VF resumes.[38] Our recent optical mapping studies confirmed that the period of quiescence after a failed shock is unrelated to amplifier saturation and reflects a true tissue characteristic.[57] This period of quiescence is compatible with the presence of a subthreshold wave of propagating supported by the graded responses. More work is needed to verify this claim. The ability of postshock activation wavefronts to either evolve to more complex patterns (breakup) or undergo extinction signals failure or success of defibrillation, respectively.

A word must be mentioned on type-B successful defibrillation, where two to three postshock beats precede VF termination, unlike type-A successful defibrillation where no postshock activity is present. Type-B defibrillation may result when the cycle length of the postshock activations is slower than the postshock cycle length of failed defibrillation.[38] Slower rotation periods are less likely to destabilize the wavefront to cause wave break[40] and thus fail to induce VF.[67] It is highly likely that shocks causing type-B successful defibrillation may actually involve larger areas of block and therefore larger reentry core size, causing longer cycle lengths of rotations.[74,75]

Recently changes in Ca_i^{2+} dynamics were found to play a key role in the induction of VF in different experimental models[76–78] and in simulation studies.[79] Whether Ca_i^{2+} dynamics play a role in defibrillation remains to be elucidated. We recently have demonstrated that the first postactivation after failed defibrillation arises from a site where Ca_i^{2+} has returned to normal diastolic level but was still surrounded with cells that had elevated Ca_i^{2+} (calcium sink hole).[80] Although we do not know the mechanisms by which the calcium sink holes promotes early postshock activation, it nevertheless stresses the fact that Ca_i^{2+} dynamics could have a role in defibrillation outcome and as such needs to be taken into account in designing new strategies for effective defibrillation therapy.

Acknowledgment

This work was supported by the University of California Tobacco-Related Diseases Research Program, the American Heart Association, the National Institutes of Health, and Laubisch Endowment.

References

1. The Epic of Gilgamesh (Table VIII). Available at URL: http://www.ancienttexts.org/library/msopotamian/gilgamesh/tab8.htm. Accessed February 22, 2007

2. Bruetsch WL. The earliest record of sudden death possibly due to atherosclerotic coronary occlusion. *Circulation* 1959;20:438–441
3. Breasted JH. *The Edwin Smith Surgical Papyrus*. Chicago: University of Chicago Press; 1930
4. Veith I (Trans). *The Yellow Emperor's Classic of Internal Medicine*. Berkeley: University of California Press; 1972
5. Kane K, Taub, A. A history of local electric analgesia. *Pain* 1975;1:125–138
6. Driscol TE, Ratnoff ODNOF. The remarkable Dr. Abildgaard and countershock. The bicentennial of his electrical experiments on animals. *Ann Int Med* 1975;83: 878–882
7. Hoffa A, Ludwig C. Einnige neue Versuche uber Herzewegung. *Zeitschrift Rationelle Medizin* 1850;9:107–144
8. Ludwig C. Über die Herznerven des Frosches. *Arch Anat Physiol* 1848;139
9. MacWilliam JA. Fibrillar contraction of the heart. *J Physiol* 1887;8:296–310
10. Battelli F. Le mécanisme de la mort par les courants électriques chez l'homme. *Rev Méd Suisse Romande* 1899;19:605–618
11. Mines GR. On circulating excitation in heart muscles and their possible relation to tachycardia and fibrillation. *Trans R Soc Can* 1914;4:43–53
12. Mines GR. On dynamic equilibrium in the heart. *J Physiol (Lond)* 1913;46:349–383
13. Garrey WE. The nature of fibrillatory contraction of the heart-its relation to tissue mass and form. *Am J Physiol* 1914;33:397–414
14. Lewis T. *Mechanism and Graphic Registration of the Heart Beat*, 3rd ed. Chicago: Chicago Book; 1924
15. Brams WA, Katz LN. The nature of experimental flutter and fibrillation of the heart. *Am Heart J* 1931;7:249–261
16. Wiggers CJ, Bell JR, Paine M. Studies of ventricular fibrillation caused by electric shock. II. Cinematographic and electrocardiographic observation of the natural process in the dog's heart. Its inhibition by potassium and the revival of coordinated beats by calcium. *Am Heart J* 1930;5:351–365
17. King BG. *The Effect of Electric Shock on Heart Action with Special Reference to Varying Susceptibility in Different Parts of the Cardiac Cycle* (Ph.D. thesis). New York: Aberdeen Press, Columbia University; 1934
18. Ferris LP, King BG, Spence PW, Williams HB. Effect of electric shock on the heart. *Electrical Eng* 1936;55:498–515
19. Fabiato PA, Coumel P, Gourgon R, Saumont R. Le seuil de résponse synchrone des fibres myocardiques. Application à la comparaison expérimentale de l'efficacité des différentes formes de chocs électriques de défibrillation. *Arch Mal Coeur Vaiss* 1967;60:527–544
20. Jones JL, Jones RE. Improved defibrillator waveform safety factor with biphasic waveforms. *Am J Physiol* 1983;245:H60–H65
21. Dixon EG, Tang ASL, Wolf PD, Meador JT, Fine MJ, Calfee RV, Ideker RE. Improved defibrillation thresholds with large contoured epicardial electrodes and biphasic waveforms. *Circulation* 1987;76:1176–1184
22. Liquori CL, Ricker K, Moseley ML, Jacobsen JF, Kress W, Naylor SL, Day JW, Ranum LP. Myotonic dystrophy type 2 caused by a CCTG expansion in intron 1 of ZNF9. *Science* 2001;293(5531):864–867

23. Block M, Hammel D, Isbruch F, Borggrefe M, Wietholt D, Hachenberg T, Scheld HH, Breithardt G. Results and realistic expectations with transvenous lead systems. *PACE* 1992;15:665–670

24. Efimov IR, Cheng Y, Van Wagoner DR, Mazgalev T, Tchou PJ. Virtual electrode-induced phase singularity: a basic mechanism of defibrillation failure. *Circ Res* 1998;82:918–925

25. Efimov IR, Aguel F, Cheng Y, Wollenzier B, Trayanova N. Virtual electrode polarization in the far field: implications for external defibrillation. *Am J Physiol Heart Circ Physiol* 2000;279(3):H1055–H1070

26. Hildebrandt MC, Roth BJ. Simulation of protective zones during quatrefoil reentry in cardiac tissue. *J Cardiovasc Electrophysiol* 2001;12(9):1062–1067

27. Trayanova N. Defibrillation of the heart: insights into mechanisms from modelling studies. *Exp Physiol* 2006;91:323–337

28. Hwang C, Swerdlow CD, Kass RM, Gang ES, Mandel WJ, Peter CT, Chen P-S. Upper limit of vulnerability reliably predicts the defibrillation threshold in humans. *Circulation* 1994;90(5):2308–2314

29. Wiggers CJ, Wegria R. Ventricular fibrillation due to single, localized induction and condenser shocks applied during the vulnerable phase of ventricular systole. *Am J Physiol* 1940;128:500–505

30. Chen P-S, Wolf PD, Dixon EG, Danieley ND, Frazier DW, Smith WM, Ideker RE. Mechanism of ventricular vulnerability to single premature stimuli in open-chest dogs. *Circ Res* 1988;62:1191–1209

31. Frazier DW, Wolf PD, Wharton JM, Tang ASL, Smith WM, Ideker RE. Stimulus-induced critical point: mechanism for electrical initiation of reentry in normal canine myocardium. *J Clin Invest* 1989;83:1039–1052

32. Bonometti C, Hwang C, Hough D, Lee JJ, Fishbein MC, Karagueuzian HS, Chen P-S. Interaction between strong electrical stimulation and reentrant wavefronts in canine ventricular fibrillation. *Circ Res* 1995;77:407–416

33. Chen P-S, Cha Y-M, Peters BB, Chen LS. Effects of myocardial fiber orientation on the electrical induction of ventricular fibrillation. *Am J Physiol* 1993;264:H1760–H1773

34. Van Dam RT, Moore NE, Hoffman BF. Initiation and conduction of impulses in partially depolarized cardiac fibers. *Am J Physiol* 1963;204:1133–1144

35. Schuder JC, Rahmoeller GA, Stoeckle H. Transthoracic ventricular defibrillation with triangular and trapezoidal waveforms. *Circ Res* 1966;19:689–694

36. Yashima M, Kim Y-H, Armin S, Wu T-J, Miyauchi Y, Mandel WJ, Chen P-S, Karagueuzian HS. On the mechanism of the probabilistic nature of ventricular defibrillation threshold. *Am J Physiol Heart Circ Physiol* 2003;284(1):H249–H255

37. Hamzei A, Ohara T, Kim Y-H, Lee M-H, Voroshilovsky O, Lin S-F, Weiss JN, Chen P-S, Karagueuzian HS. The role of approximate entropy in predicting ventricular defibrillation threshold. *J Cardiovasc Pharmacol Ther* 2002;7(1):45–52

38. Chen P-S, Shibata N, Dixon EG, Wolf PD, Danieley ND, Sweeney MB, Smith WM, Ideker RE. Activation during ventricular defibrillation in open-chest dogs. Evidence of complete cessation and regeneration of ventricular fibrillation after unsuccessful shocks. *J Clin Invest* 1986;77(3):810–823

39. Weiss JN, Garfinkel A, Karagueuzian HS, Qu Z, Chen P-S. Chaos and the transition to ventricular fibrillation: a new approach to antiarrhythmic drug evaluation. *Circulation* 1999;99:2819–2826

40. Weiss JN, Chen P-S, Qu Z, Karagueuzian HS, Garfinkel A. Ventricular fibrillation: how do we stop the waves from breaking? *Circ Res* 2000;87:1103–1107

41. Knisley SB, Hill BC, Ideker RE. Virtual electrode effects in myocardial fibers. *Biophys J* 1994;66:719–728

42. Wikswo JP Jr, Wisialowski TA, Altemeier WA, Balser JR, Kopelman HA, Roden DM. Virtual cathode effects during stimulation of cardiac muscle. Two-dimensional in vivo experiments. *Circ Res* 1991;68:513–530

43. Chen P-S, Shibata N, Dixon EG, Martin RO, Ideker RE. Comparison of the defibrillation threshold and the upper limit of ventricular vulnerability. *Circulation* 1986;73(5):1022–1028

44. Chen P-S, Swerdlow CD, Hwang C, Karagueuzian HS. Current concepts of ventricular defibrillation. *J Cardiovasc Electrophysiol* 1998;9:553–562

45. Banville I, Gray RA, Ideker RE, Smith WM. Shock-induced figure-of-eight reentry in the isolated rabbit heart. *Circ Res* 1999;85:742–752

46. Knisley SB, Smith WM, Ideker RE. Effect of field stimulation on cellular repolarization in rabbit myocardium. Implication for reentry induction. *Circ Res* 1992;70:707–715

47. Winfree AT. Electrical instability in cardiac muscle: phase singularities and rotors. *J Theor Biol* 1989;138(3):353–405

48. Witkowski FX, Penkoske PA, Plonsey R. Mechanism of cardiac defibrillation in open-chest dogs with unipolar DC-coupled simultaneous activation and shock potential recordings. *Circulation* 1990;82(1):244–260

49. Zipes DP, Fischer J, King RM, Nicoll AD, Jolly WW. Termination of ventricular fibrillation in dogs by depolarizing a critical amount of myocardium. *Am J Cardiol* 1975;36:37–44

50. Dillon SM, Kwaku KF. Progressive depolarization: a unified hypothesis for defibrillation and fibrillation induction by shocks. *J Cardiovasc Electrophysiol* 1998;9:529–552

51. Kwaku KF, Dillon SM. Shock-induced depolarization of refractory myocardium prevents wave-front propagation in defibrillation. *Circ Res* 1996;79:957–973

52. Cheng Y, Mowrey KA, Van Wagoner DR, Tchou PJ, Efimov IR. Virtual electrode-induced reexcitation: a mechanism of defibrillation. *Circ Res* 1999;85:1056–1066

53. Zhou X, Daubert JP, Wolf PD, Smith WM, Ideker RE. Epicardial mapping of ventricular defibrillation with monophasic and biphasic shocks in dogs. *Circ Res* 1993;72: 145–160

54. Gotoh M, Uchida T, Mandel WJ, Fishbein MC, Chen P-S, Karagueuzian HS. Cellular graded responses and ventricular vulnerability to reentry by a premature stimulus in isolated canine ventricle. *Circulation* 1997;95:2141–2154

55. Roth BJ, Krassowska W. The induction of reentry in cardiac tissue. The missing link: how electric fields alter transmembrane potential. *Chaos* 1998;8:204–220

56. Lindblom AE, Roth BJ, Trayanova NA. Role of virtual electrodes in arrhythmogenesis: pinwheel experiment revisited. *J Cardiovasc Electrophysiol* 2000;11:274–285

57. Wang NC, Lee M-H, Ohara T, Okuyama Y, Fishbein GA, Lin S-F, Karagueuzian HS, Chen P-S. Optical mapping of ventricular defibrillation in isolated swine right ventricles:

demonstration of a postshock isoelectric window after near-threshold defibrillation shocks. *Circulation* 2001;104(2):227–233

58. Chen P-S, Wolf PD, Claydon FJ, Dixon EG, Vidaillet HJ Jr, Danieley ND, Pilkington TC, Ideker RE. The potential gradient field created by epicardial defibrillation electrodes in dogs. *Circulation* 1986;74(3):626–636

59. Wikswo JP Jr, Lin S-F, Abbas RA. Virtual electrodes in cardiac tissue: a common mechanism for anodal and cathodal stimulation. *Biophys J* 1995;69:2195–2210

60. Nikolski V, Efimov IR. Virtual electrode polarization of ventricular epicardium during bipolar stimulation. *J Cardiovasc Electrophysiol* 2000;11:605

61. Kao CY, Hoffman BF. Graded and decremental response in heart muscle fibers. *Am J Physiol* 1958;194:187–196

62. Weidmann S. Effects of current flow on the membrane potential of cardiac muscle. *J Physiol* 1951;115:227–236

63. Karagueuzian HS, Katzung BG. Relative inotropic and arrhythmogenic effects of five cardiac steroids in ventricular myocardium: oscillatory afterpotentials and the role of endogenous catecholamines. *J Pharmacol Exp Ther* 1981;218:348–356

64. Karagueuzian HS, Katzung BG. Voltage-clamp studies of transient inward current and mechanical oscillations induced by ouabain in ferret papillary muscle. *J Physiol* 1982;327:255–271

65. Jones JL, Lepeschkin E, Jones RE, Rush S. Response of cultured myocardial cells to countershock-type electric field stimulation. *Am J Physiol* 1978;235(2):H214–H222

66. Li HG, Jones DL, Yee R, Klein GJ. Defibrillation shocks produce different effects on Purkinje fibers and ventricular muscle: implications for successful defibrillation, refibrillation and postshock arrhythmia. *J Am Coll Cardiol* 1993;22(2): 607–614

67. Cao J-M, Qu Z, Kim Y-H, Wu T-J, Garfinkel A, Weiss JN, Karagueuzian HS, Chen P-S. Spatiotemporal heterogeneity in the induction of ventricular fibrillation by rapid pacing: importance of cardiac restitution properties. *Circ Res* 1999;84:1318–1331

68. MacLeod DP, Hunter EG. The pharmacology of the cardiac muscle of the great veins of the rat. *Can J Physiol Pharmacol* 1967;45(3):463–473

69. Swerdlow CD, Kass RM, O'Connor ME, Chen P-S. Effect of shock waveform on relationship between upper limit of vulnerability and defibrillation threshold. *J Cardiovasc Electrophysiol* 1998;9:339–349

70. Walcott GP, Walker RG, Cates AW, Krassowska W, Smith WM, Ideker RE. Choosing the optimal monophasic and biphasic waveforms for ventricular defibrillation. *J Cardiovasc Electrophysiol* 1995;6:737–750

71. Jones DL, Narayanan N. Defibrillation depresses heart sarcoplasmic reticulum calcium pump: a mechanism of postshock dysfunction 1. *Am J Physiol* 1998;274(1 Pt 2):H98–H105

72. Eisner DA, Diaz ME, Li Y, O'Neill SC, Trafford AW. Stability and instability of regulation of intracellular calcium. *Exp Physiol* 2005;90(1):3–12

73. Schlotthauer K, Bers DM. Sarcoplasmic reticulum Ca(2+) release causes myocyte depolarization. Underlying mechanism and threshold for triggered action potentials. *Circ Res* 2000;87(9):774–780

74. Uchida T, Yashima M, Gotoh M, Qu Z, Garfinkel A, Weiss JN, Fishbein MC, Mandel WJ, Chen P-S, Karagueuzian HS. Mechanism of acceleration of functional reentry in the ventricle: effects of ATP-sensitive potassium channel opener. *Circulation* 1999;99:704–712

75. Mandapati R, Asano Y, Baxter WT, Gray R, Davidenko J, Jalife J. Quantification of effects of global ischemia on dynamics of ventricular fibrillation in isolated rabbit heart. *Circulation* 1998;98:1688–1696

76. Omichi C, Lamp ST, Lin SF, Yang J, Baher A, Zhou S, Attin M, Lee MH, Karagueuzian HS, Kogan B, Qu Z, Garfinkel A, Chen PS, Weiss JN. Intracellular Ca dynamics in ventricular fibrillation. *Am J Physiol Heart Circ Physiol* 2004;286:H1836–H1844

77. Pruvot EJ, Katra RP, Rosenbaum DS, Laurita KR. Role of calcium cycling versus restitution in the mechanism of repolarization alternans. *Circ Res* 2004;94(8):1083–1090

78. choi BR, Burton F, Salama G. Cytosolic Ca2+triggers early after depolarizations and Torsade de Pointes in rabbit hearts with type 2 long QT syndrome. *J Physiol* 2002;543(Pt 2):615–631

79. Chudin E, Garfinkel A, Weiss J, Karplus W, Kogan B. Wave propagation in cardiac tissue and effects of intracellular calcium dynamics (computer simulation study). *Prog Biophys Mol Biol* 1998;69:225–236

80. Hwang GS, Hayashi H, Tang L, Ogawa M, Hernandez H, Tan AY, Karagueuzian HS, Weiss JN, Lin SF, Chen PS. Intracellular calcium and vulnerability to fibrillation and defibrillation in Langendorff-perfused rabbit ventricles. *Circulation* 2006;114:2595–2603

Part IV

Optical Mapping of Stimulation and Defibrillation

Chapter 4.1

Mechanisms of Isolated Cell Stimulation

Vinod Sharma

Introduction

It is a common practice in several fields of modern science to reduce a complex system to its simplest unit to gain fundamental insights into phenomena of interest. Field stimulation of cardiac cell is no different. Understanding the effects of an electrical shock at the simplest unit of cardiac tissue, an isolated cardiac cell, can lend valuable insights into mechanisms of field stimulation, especially those involved in phenomena such as fibrillation and defibrillation. These mechanisms have remained largely unresolved despite defibrillation having been applied clinically for over 60 years[1] and become the mainstay of clinical medicine with the advent of implantable cardioverter-defibrillators (ICDs)[2-4] and automatic external defibrillators (AED).[5] Taking a reductionism approach, this chapter discusses the field-induced responses of single cardiac cells to electric field stimulation. Transmembrane voltage (V_m) is widely acknowledged as the most important parameter during electric field stimulation of cardiac tissue, and hence we spend a significant portion of the chapter discussing the interaction between an externally applied field and isolated cell. Building on this we then discuss a slightly more complex system of a cell-pair. A coupled cell-pair is the simplest system in which the effects of intercellular gap junction on field-induced V_m responses can be studied. Finally, we briefly discuss the effects of externally applied fields on intracellular Ca^{2+} dynamics since Ca^{2+} is intimately linked to V_m via voltage-dependent responsiveness of L-type Ca^{2+} channels.

New Therapies and Diagnostics, Medtronic, Inc., 8200 Coral Sea Street N.E.,
Minneapolis, MN 55112, USA, vinod.sharma@medtronic.com

I. R. Efimov et al. (eds.), *Cardiac Bioelectric Therapy: Mechanisms and Practical Implications.*
© Springer Science+Business Media, LLC 2009

Transmembrane Potential (V_m) Responses of an Isolated Cell

In this section we first start with theoretical investigation of the electric field–induced responses of a passive cell. Unlike the more complex system of a cardiac cell, a passive cell is devoid of any time- and voltage-dependent ion channels, and hence is a simple system to consider. This is then followed by the discussion of a cardiac-type active cell. Finally, we present the experimental data on field-induced responses of a ventricular myocyte and discuss them in the context of our theoretical framework.

Theoretical Framework of Field Stimulation

V_m Responses of a Passive Cell

The transmembrane potential (V_m) responses of spheroidal passive cells have been well studied theoretically.[6,7] The most general solution for a cell stimulated along its major axis ($+x$) with a uniform electric field E_o is given by,

$$V_m = f E_o x g(t), \tag{1}$$

where origin ($x = 0$) is at the cell center, $f(1 < f < 1.5)$ is a cell-shape dependent form factor, and $g(t)[g(t = 0) = 0$ and $g(t \to \infty) = 1]$ is a cell-shape dependent function that describes the transient behavior of V_m at the field onset. For example, for a spherical cell of radius a,

$$V_m = 1.5 E_o x [1 - \exp(-t/\tau)], \tag{2a}$$

$$= 1.5 E_o a \cos \theta [1 - \exp(-t/\tau)], \tag{2b}$$

$$\tau = a C_m (r_i + r_e/2), \tag{3}$$

where, θ is the angle between the field direction and the position vector from the cell center to the measurement point on the cell surface, C_m is the membrane specific capacitance, and r_i and r_e are the specific resistances of the intracellular and extracellular media, respectively. For physiological values of r_i and r_e the time constant (τ) is estimated to be $\sim 1 - 10\,\mu s$ for a cell of $\sim 100\,\mu m$ in diameter. Indeed, the early experiments to study field-induced changes in transmembrane potential were performed in passive spherical cells, and a sinusoidal variation in V_m consistent with (2b) was confirmed.[8,9] The time constant (τ) for polarization was close to the theoretically predicted value and changed predictably with changes in the ionic strength of the extracellular medium.[10]

For a cylindrical cell with large length to diameter ratio (approximate geometry of a cardiac cell) the form factor f is ~ 1, and therefore in the steady-state (2a) reduces to

$$V_m = E_o x. \tag{4}$$

Equation (4) predicts V_m to vary linearly along the cell length, with the cell end facing the anode to be negatively polarized and the cell end facing the cathode to be positively polarized.

To understand the physical basis of nonuniform cell polarization, consider a cell of length L stimulated with field E_o (Fig 1a). Since the field is spatially uniform, the extracellular potential ($\phi_e = -E_o x$) varies linearly along the cell length (Fig. 1b, top subpanel). Moreover, since the intracellular space is small and highly conductive, the intracellular potential (ϕ_i) remains isopotential at zero (Fig. 1b, top subpanel). Thus, the transmembrane potential, which is the difference between the ϕ_i and ϕ_e ($V_m = \phi_i - \phi_e$), is as shown in Fig. 1b, bottom subpanel. V_m varies linearly along the cell length with a slope (dV_m/dx) that is equal to the applied field E_o. In the above analysis we assumed that ϕ_e is symmetric about the cell center. For an asymmetric ϕ_e, the ϕ_i is offset by a constant value from zero that is equal to the average potential around the cell,[6] but V_m does not change. As a hypothetical experiment, let the cell be stimulated with a uniform electric field pulse of amplitude E_o (Fig. 1c, top row) and responses recorded from three sites (represented by overlaid circles) along the cell length. The resulting responses should have amplitude and polarity that are position dependent (Fig. 1c, bottom 3 rows), and the responses should stay constant with time during the field pulse.

V_m Responses of an Active Cell

When an active cell is field stimulated, the ion channels all along the cell length activate and inactivate to varying degrees as the cell is polarized. As a result, different regions of the cell have different membrane resistance (R_m). Moreover, as the channels gate, R_m dynamically changes with time. Therefore, R_m is a function of space and time, that is, $R_m = R_m(x, t)$. Consequently the transmembrane current ($i_m = V_m/R_m$) integrated over the entire cell can have a time-varying nonzero value, that is,

$$I_m = \int\int i_m ds \neq 0, \tag{5}$$

where ds is the elemental membrane area. Note that in the case of a passive cell I_m is always zero since either the i_m is zero, or $i_m s$ in the regions symmetrically located about the cell center are equal and opposite. A nonzero I_m for an active cell results in a net charge transfer from or into the cell and causes a change in ϕ_i, and hence a change in V_m. However, because the intracellular space is small and highly conductive, any such change in ϕ_i (and V_m) is uniform along the cell length (i.e., ϕ_i is only a function of t). Thus, V_m for an active cell is given by

$$V_m = E_o x + \phi_i(t). \tag{6}$$

Figure 2 presents two possible situations during field stimulation. Figure 2a presents the case of a cell in which the inward current in the negatively polarized regions exceeds the outward current in the positively polarized regions. The I_m is inward, and therefore the ϕ_i increases with time. Consequently, the V_m from the various sites show a parallel positive

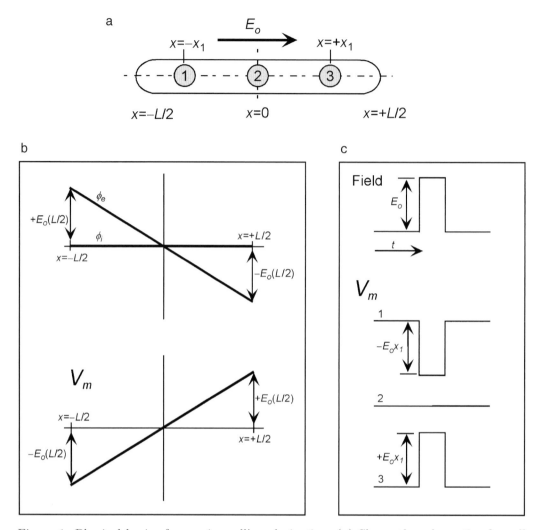

Figure 1: Physical basis of a passive cell's polarization. (a) Shows the schematic of a cell of length L with origin at $x = 0$. The cell is stimulated with a uniform electric field E_o in the indicated direction, and the steady-state extracellular potential (ϕ_e) and intracellular potential (ϕ_i) are shown in (b), *top subpanel*. The ϕ_e varies linearly along the cell length, and the ϕ_i stays isopotential at zero. The resulting transmembrane potential ($V_m = \phi_i - \phi_e$) is shown in (b), *bottom subpanel*. (c) Shows the result of a hypothetical experiment in which the cell shown in (a) is stimulated with a field pulse shown in (c), *top row*. The responses corresponding to three sites on the cell (overlaid circles; $x = -x1$, 0 and $+x1$) are shown in (c), *bottom three rows*

shift during the field pulse. Figure 2b depicts a situation in which the I_m is outward, and therefore V_m shows a negative shift with time.

In the next section we will turn to experimental examination of V_m responses during field stimulation of a cardiac cell and attempt to understand them in the context of theoretical framework described above.

Experimental Responses During Field Stimulation

Electric field stimulation of cardiac tissue, as during defibrillation, involves interaction of the applied field with the tissue during different phases of the action potential.[11] Thus, it is instructive to understand the field-cell interaction for at least two contrasting action potential phases: at rest when a cell is most excitable and during the action potential plateau when it is refractory. But first, let us briefly review the technology that enables recording of V_m responses from a specimen as small as a cardiac cell (a typical cardiac cell is approximately 120 μm in length and 20 μm in diameter).[12]

Optical Mapping Technology for Recording Membrane Potential

High-resolution spatiotemporal V_m measurements from an isolated cell are typically accomplished using a custom designed optical mapping setup.[13–17] Optical recording of membrane potentials employs voltage-sensitive dyes that undergo spectral shifts with change in transmembrane potential. The dye molecules are designed to localize in the cell membrane and, when excited with an intense light source, emit fluorescence whose intensity changes linearly with field-induced changes in $V_m(\Delta V_m)$.

A typical setup for recording V_m responses is shown in Fig. 3. Isolated cardiac cells obtained by standard techniques of enzymatic dissociation[16] are stained with a voltage sensitive dye such as pyridinium, 4-[2-[6[(dioctylamino)-2-naphthalenyl]ethenyl]-1-(sulfopropyl)-,inner salt (di-8-ANEPPS) and placed in the specimen plane of an inverted microscope. The cell is then excited using an intense green light ($\lambda = 460$–570 nm) via microscope's epifluorescence pathway. The emitted fluorescence is collected by microscope's objective, filtered ($\lambda > 570$), and projected onto image plane with sensing elements. Several different options are available for configuring the sensing elements, including photodiode array, charge-coupled device (CCD) camera, and optical-fiber bundle (which then carry signals to discrete photodiodes). All the recordings presented in this chapter were obtained using a custom-built fiber-bundle system in which each 1 mm diameter optical fiber corresponds to a circular site of 25 μm in the microscope's image plane at 40× magnification. The rise time of this system to a step response is ~0.3 ms. The overall signal quality for a given system, however, depends not just on the type of sensing element, but also on other factors such as excitation light intensity, magnification, numerical aperture of the optics, and dye staining methodology (e.g., concentration and time). A limitation of optical mapping methodology utilizing voltage sensitive dyes is that absolute measurements of membrane potential are not readily available. Thus, the field-induced change in V_m is indirectly estimated by normalizing the observed fluorescence change to a known potential

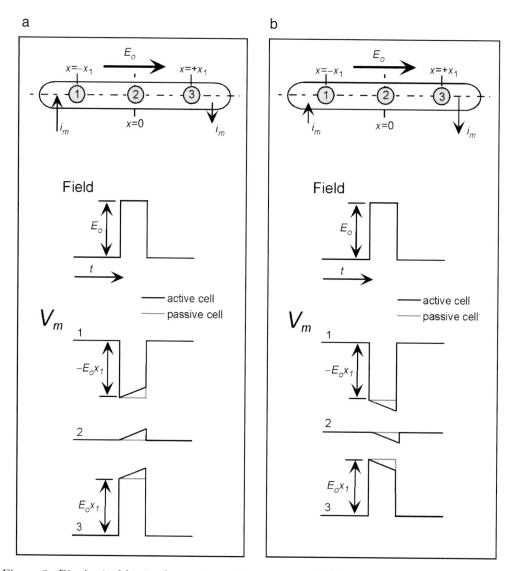

Figure 2: Biophysical basis of an active cell's response. (a) Depicts a situation in which the inward current in the hyperpolarized regions of the cell is larger than the outward current in the depolarized regions. The net charge injected into the cell raises the ϕ_i. The hypothetical V_m responses from three sites on the cell are shown in (a), *bottom three rows*. (b) Depicts a situation in which the inward current in the hyperpolarized regions of the cell is smaller than the outward current in the depolarized regions. The net charge ejected out of the cell depresses the ϕ_i. The V_m responses from the three sites are shown in (b), *bottom three rows*

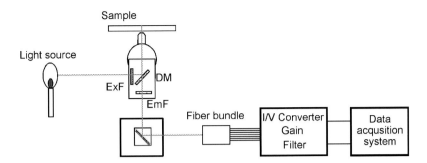

Figure 3: Experimental setup for recording V_m responses from a single cardiac cell. The light (*gray line*) from an intense light source is filtered using an excitation filter (ExF) and deflected onto the dye-stained cells using a dichroic mirror (DM). The fluorescence light from the cells is collected by the microscope objective, long pass filtered, and projected onto the face of an optical fiber bundle. The signals carried by individual fibers are fed into signal detection, sensing and conditioning circuits, and then digitized and acquired into a computer

change (e.g., fluorescence change corresponding to the action potential amplitude, which is ~ 100–$120\,mV$ for the cardiac tissue).

Field-Induced Responses at Rest

When a cell is stimulated at rest with field pulses of increasing amplitude, it elicits an action potential once the pulse amplitude exceeds a threshold.[16,18] Figure 4 shows the response of a cell stimulated at rest with a $2\,ms$ duration pulse of suprathreshold amplitude (labeled as S1). The cell polarizes rapidly at the onset of the field pulse with the speed of polarization limited by the bandwidth of the setup electronics (rise time of $\sim 0.3\,ms$). The cell end facing the anode (site 1) undergoes maximum negative polarization, the cell end facing the cathode undergoes maximum positive polarization (Fig. 4b), and polarization varies linearly along the cell length (Fig. 4c). During the pulse the polarization is not constant, but exhibits a gradual positive shift. This spatially linear pattern for the field-induced ΔV_m with a nonconstant value during the field pulse is reminiscent of theoretical responses of an active cell (Fig. 2). The positive shift in V_m responses is indicative of the fact that there is a net inward current during the field pulse that facilitates cell excitation by elevating membrane potential toward the excitation threshold. We will examine the source of this net current in more detail below. In the above example the cell fired an action potential following the termination of the pulse. However, this is not a typical scenario, and often the excitation occurs during the S1 pulses (e.g., refer to Figs. 7 and 8). Several factors intrinsic (e.g., cell length and excitability) and extrinsic (e.g., pulse parameters) to the cell seem to play a role in determining the early (during S1) versus late (after S1) pattern of excitation.

The excitation of an isolated cell at rest exhibits an interesting pattern when stimulated with a field pulse of short duration and increasing amplitude.[19] For a pulse $\leq 1\,ms$ in duration, the cell is excited normally at lower amplitudes once above a lower threshold for

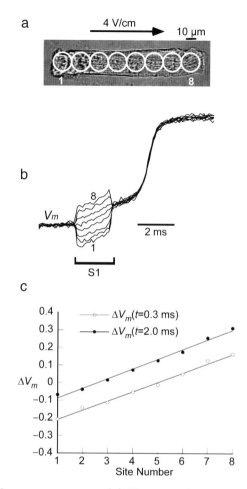

Figure 4: Field-induced responses at rest. (**a**) Shows a cell stimulated with a 2 ms, 4.1 V/cm S1 pulse. (**b**) Shows the field-induced change in V_m (ΔV_m) normalized to action potential amplitude from eight sites on the cell. (**c**) plots the ΔV_m responses measured 0.3 and 2 ms [$\Delta V_m(t = 0.3)$ and $\Delta V_m(t = 2.0)$, respectively] from the onset of S1 pulse along the cell length. ΔV_m has been normalized to the action potential amplitude

excitation. However, as the field amplitude is gradually raised, it reaches a threshold at which the excitation is suppressed (Fig. 5). This loss of excitation is reversible and hence not associated with cell damage (e.g., resulting from membrane electroporation).[20,21] The excitation is restored upon lowering the pulse amplitude or increasing the pulse duration while maintaining the pulse amplitude at the level of paradoxical unexcitation.

One approach to understand the mechanism of paradoxical unexcitation at higher amplitudes is to resort to computer modeling. A convenient model to use is phase 1 Luo-Rudy model[22] with description of six major cardiac membrane currents. Although there

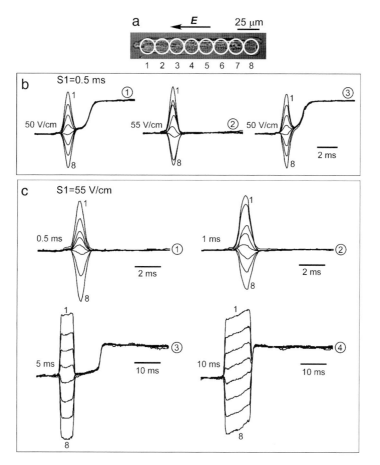

Figure 5: Paradoxical loss of excitation at rest with short-duration high amplitude pulses. (a) Shows a cell stimulated successively with three S1 pulses of 50, 55, and 50 V/cm. (b) Shows the responses corresponding to the three S1 pulses. (c) Shows the pattern of excitation with S1 amplitude fixed at 55 V/cm, and the S1 duration increased from 0.5 to 1, 5, and 10 ms. The circled numbers next to each set of traces indicate sequence of stimulation. The recordings corresponding to sites 1 and 8 have also been numbered

are a number of sophisticated membrane models available,[23] the simple phase-1 Luo-Rudy model would suffice for our purposes. Figure 6a shows the responses of a model cell with Luo-Rudy phase-1 membrane kinetics that is stimulated with a field pulse of ~6.3 V/cm. The pattern of V_m for various patches along the cell length is similar to that observed experimentally (e.g., Fig. 4). In addition the modeling experiments also reveal flow of ionic currents along the cell length. There is a large inward sodium current (I_{Na}) at the cathode facing regions of the cell that experience depolarization during the field pulse. I_{Na} gradually diminishes moving toward the anodal end of the cell and is negligible in the cell half facing

a　　　　　　　　b

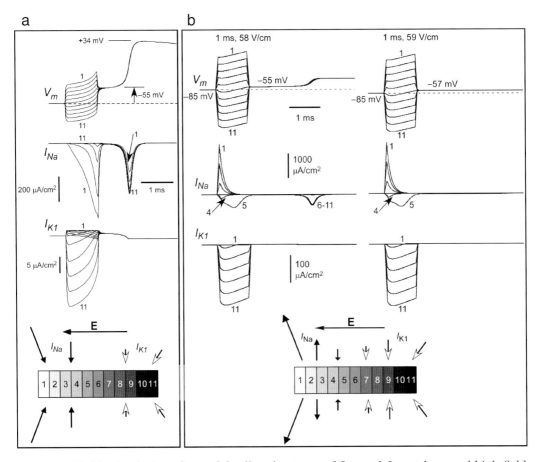

Figure 6: Field-stimulation of a model cell and pattern of I_{Na} and I_{K1} at low- and high-field amplitudes. (**a**) Shows V_m, I_{Na}, and I_{K1} for a Luo-Rudy phase I model cell stimulated with 5 ms, 6.3 V/cm pulse in the indicated direction. (**b**) Shows V_m, I_{Na}, and I_{K1} for the model cell stimulated with two 1 ms duration pulses. The first pulse (58 V/cm) is just below the threshold for paradoxical unexcitation, and the second pulse is at threshold for unexcitation. Also shown in each panel is the schematic of the cell along with the flow of I_{Na} and I_{K1}, where the lengths of various *arrows* signify the relative amplitudes of the corresponding currents. Note that the time bar in each panel is applicable to all sets of traces

the anode. This is consistent with the fact that any hyperpolarization of the membrane will maintain the sodium channels in an inactivated state and limit I_{Na}. In contrast to I_{Na}, inward rectifying potassium current (I_{K1}) is maximal in the hyperpolarized regions of the cell and diminishes moving toward the opposite end of the cell. I_{K1} eventually reverses direction in the maximally depolarized regions, albeit it much lower in amplitude. This pattern is consistent with inward rectifying characteristics of I_{K1} exhibiting large inward current for membrane potentials below $\sim -85\,\mathrm{mV}$, which is close to the resting potential around which the cell's V_{m} is perturbed spatially. Since both I_{Na} and I_{K1} are largely inward, they work synergistically at lower field amplitudes to bring a net inward current and depolarize the cell to its excitation threshold.[24]

As the pulse amplitude is increased, the positive depolarization in the cathodal regions of the cell can exceed the reversal potential of I_{Na}. Consequently, I_{Na} now counters the inward I_{K1} rather than working synergistically with it. Thus, the net inward current begins to diminish with increasing field strength and is not sufficient to raise the membrane potential to the excitation threshold. The return of excitation with increasing pulse duration can occur because even at threshold amplitude for paradoxical unexcitation the cell exhibits a slow depolarizing drift during the pulse.[19] Consequently, as the pulse duration is extended the portions of the cell away from the cathode that remained below I_{Na} threshold can now be triggered, bringing in net inward current and aiding in the cell depolarization. This in turn excites neighboring regions and a miniwave of I_{Na} is set in that proceeds toward the hyperpolarized regions of the cell. This additional inward current via I_{Na} is presumably sufficient to overcome paradoxical unexcitation observed with shorter duration pulses.

Responses During Action Potential Plateau

Field stimulation of cardiac cells during plateau phase has been studied extensively.[13,14,16,25,26] The responses during the plateau phase are typically studied by using a S1–S2 pulse protocol (Fig. 7), wherein the first pulse (S1) is suprathreshold and excites the cell, and the second pulse (S2) is applied during the plateau phase of the action potential. Figure 7b shows the responses of an isolated guinea pig ventricular cell to such an S1–S2 pulse pair. Note that unlike the case of the cell in Fig. 4 for which the excitation occurred after the S1 termination, the excitation in Fig. 7 occurs immediately following the onset of the S1 pulse because the pulse amplitude is presumably much higher than the excitation threshold.

An examination of responses in Fig. 7 reveals that the initial responses immediately after the S2 onset are similar to the S1 responses. The cell end facing the cathode undergoes positive polarization, the cell end facing the anode undergoes negative polarization, and polarization varies monotonically along the cell length. The superimposed responses (Fig. 7b) show that after the initial step change in polarization, the recordings from various sites exhibit a parallel shift reminiscent of the behavior for S1 pulse (Fig. 4) except that now the shift is in the negative direction. When field-induced ΔV_{m} is plotted along the cell length, it is found to be linear both during an early time point ($t = 0.3\,\mathrm{ms}$) and a late time point ($t = 9.0\,\mathrm{ms}$) during the S2 pulse. The parallel time courses of the responses from the various sites are reflected as the parallel shift in the spatially linear responses.

Figure 8 shows the example of another cell that was stimulated sequentially with two S1–S2 pair of pulses, first in left-to-right direction and then in right-to-left direction. The pattern of responses is similar to that depicted in Fig. 7 for both field directions except that the reversal in responses with field of opposite polarity is now evident. For example, the site 1 that exhibited positive response with first S2 pulse changed to negative response with the second S2 pulse of opposite polarity. The opposite trend was observed for signals from site 5.

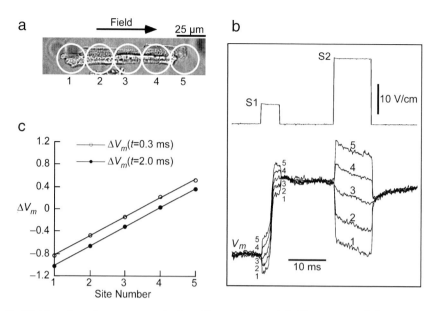

Figure 7: Field-induced responses during the plateau. (**a**) Shows an adult guinea pig cell that was stimulated with an S1–S2 pulse pair (S1 = 5.9 V/cm and S2 = 22.0 V/cm). $V_{\mathrm{m}}s$ from the five sites are shown superimposed in (**b**) along with the S1–S2 pair. (**c**) Shows the spatial plots of field-induced change in V_{m} (ΔV_{m}) measured 0.3 and 9 ms [$\Delta V_{\mathrm{m}}(t = 0.3)$ and $\Delta V_{\mathrm{m}}(t = 9.0)$ respectively] after the S2 onset and normalized to the action potential amplitude

However, a close examination of signals from the central site 3 reveals that these signals remain unchanged with the reversal in field direction. If the central signal is subtracted from the signals for the other sites, we obtain the result of Fig. 8d. A comparison of these responses with those discussed earlier in the context of Fig. 1 reveals that they are similar to those expected from a passive cell. Thus, fairly complex spatiotemporal responses of a cardiac cell can be decomposed into simpler components: a passive component (V_{mp}) that is a function of space (x) only, varies linearly along the cell length, and switches polarity with the reversal in field direction; and an active component (V_{ma}) that is a function of time (t) only, uniform along the cell length, and is independent of field direction.[25] Thus

$$V_{\mathrm{m}}(x, t) = V_{\mathrm{mp}}(x) + V_{\mathrm{ma}}(t). \tag{7}$$

Comparing (6) and (7), it is clear that $V_{\mathrm{mp}}(x) = E_{\mathrm{o}}x$ and $V_{\mathrm{ma}}(t) = \phi_{\mathrm{i}}(t)$.

One point that we have not yet discussed is concerning the slope (dV_{m}/dx) of the V_{m} response. As discussed above, the slope of the total response (which is in essence the slope of V_{mp}) should be equal to the applied field E_{o}. Figure 9 shows the result of such measurements in 50 cells. The slope of ΔV_{m} was calculated by transforming the relative fluorescence recordings to millivolt units, assuming an action potential amplitude of 128 mV.[12] The

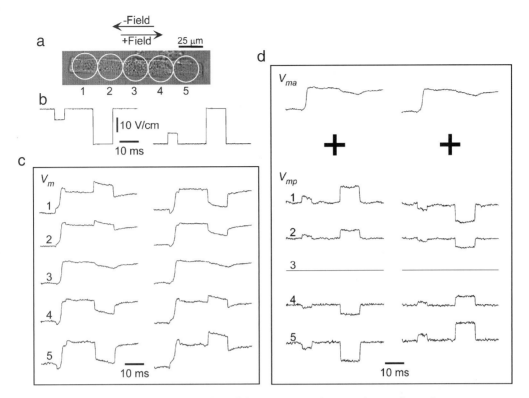

Figure 8: Decomposition of field-induced V_m responses into active and passive components. (a) Shows a cardiac cell stimulated with negative and positive field pulses shown in (b). The V_m responses recorded from the five sites along the cell length are shown in (c). The *left column* shows the responses for the negative field pulses and *right column* shows responses for the positive field pulses. (d) *Top row* shows the active component, V_{ma}, which is the response from the cell center. (b) *Bottom rows* show responses corresponding to the passive component, V_{mp}, that were obtained by subtracting the respective $V_{ma}s$ from the total V_m responses

ΔV_m slope is approximately equal to the applied field over a wide range of field amplitudes extending up to 45 V/cm.

Although responses during the S2 maintain a negative drift for all amplitudes, the temporal details of the response change with the increasing S2 amplitude (Fig. 10). This temporal behavior of the S2 response is captured in the active component (V_{ma}), and hence for brevity only V_{ma} is shown in Fig. 10a (note that V_{md} stays constant during the S2 pulse). For a low amplitude pulse, V_{ma} is negligible (type I response). With an increase in field amplitude, the V_{ma} begins to show a slow negative drift throughout the S2 duration (type II response). A further increase in S2 amplitude results in a response showing an initial sharp negative deflection followed by constant response during the S2 duration (type III response). Finally, upon further increasing the amplitude, initial negative deflection is

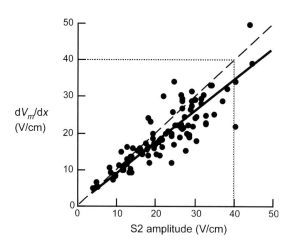

Figure 9: Relationship between the slope of field-induced V_m (dV_m/dx) and applied field. The dV_m/dx is shown for 105 S2 stimuli applied to 50 cells. The linear fit has a slope of ~0.860 ($r = 0.67, p < .001$). The *dashed line* is the line of identity with slope equal to 1

followed by a positive deflection (type IV response). Although in Fig. 10 the S2 amplitude is labeled in the units of V cm, a better metric would include V_m since it is the V_m that drives active response of a cell by influencing the ion channel gating. One useful metric is maximum V_m experienced by a cell, which is the V_m developed at cell ends.[13] This maximum $V_m(V_{mo})$ is equal to $E_o(L/2)$. Figure 10b summarizes frequency of occurrences of various response types as a function of V_{mo}.

Unlike the case of field stimulation at rest, the actual ionic currents involved in the responses during the plateau phase are less amenable to being dissected using computational modeling. The difficulty arises because even the fairly advanced updated Luo-Rudy model[27,28] of a cardiac cell is unable to reproduce experimentally observed responses with negative drift.[13] In contrast, the model predicts responses with slight positive drift. This discrepancy can be corrected by incorporating a hypothetical outwardly rectifying current, I_a, in the model.[13] Nevertheless, the true identity of I_a is under debate. One approach to unravel identity of I_a is to perform experiments using selective ion channel blockers. In a series of experiments specific ion channel blockers for I_{Kr}, I_{Ks}, I_{to}, I_{Cl}, Na-Ca exchanger (NCX), and I_{CaL} failed to modify the plateau responses in isolated cells.[29] However, at considerably higher concentration (1 mM) of Ba^{2+}, which is known to produce a nonspecific block of sustained plateau K^+ current (I_{Kp}), the negative drift during plateau responses was ablated (Fig. 11). This hints that I_{Kp} may in fact be the molecular correlate of hypothetical I_a. Indeed the current–voltage relation of I_{Kp} has an outwardly rectifying behavior, although it has not been fully characterized outside physiological range of $V_m s$.[27] However, these experiments are not conclusive since such high levels of extracellular K^+ also depolarize the cell and diminish the action potential amplitude (Fig. 11b, c). Thus, ablation of negative drift may simply be caused by the S2 pulse being applied against a different background of resting membrane potential and action potential morphology.

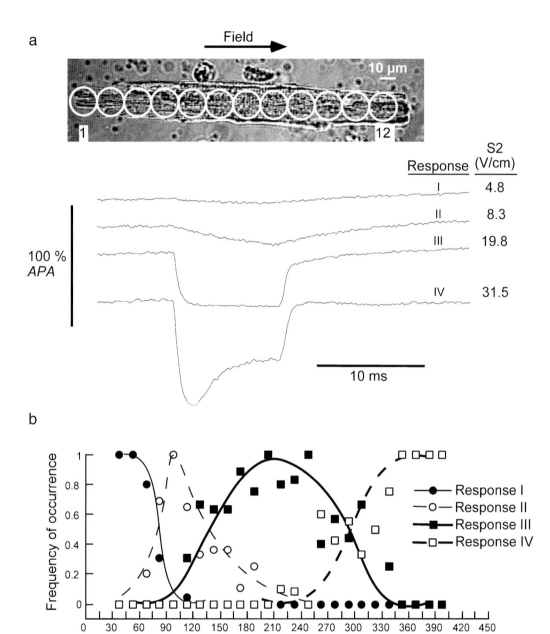

Figure 10: Effect of increasing field and maximum developed V_m (V_{mo}) on S2 responses. (a) Shows the four type (I–IV) of responses for a cell that is stimulated with four successive stimuli of increasing S2 amplitude. (b) Shows the frequency of various response types as a function of maximum $V_m(V_{mo})$ developed at the cell end

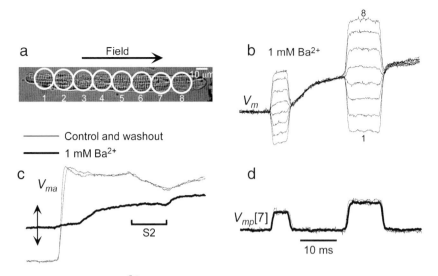

Figure 11: Effect of $1\,\mathrm{mM}$ Ba^{2+} on asymmetry of V_m responses during the plateau stimulation. The V_m responses recorded from eight sites for the cell shown in (**a**) upon stimulation with an S1–S2(S1 = $10\,\mathrm{V/cm}$, S2 = $15\,\mathrm{V/cm}$) pair are shown in (**b**). The symmetric looking V_m responses were decomposed, and the V_{ma}s and V_{mp}s from a representative site (#7) are shown in (**c**, **d**) (*thick traces*) along with the V_{ma} and V_{mp} for the control and washout recordings. V_{ma} components in (**c**) show the extent of action potential amplitude depression with $1\,\mathrm{mM}$ Ba^{2+}. As the amount of depolarization cannot be quantified using voltage sensitive dyes, the baseline for action potential in the presence of Ba^{2+} could not be ascertained accurately. This uncertainty is indicated by the *double-headed vertical arrow* in (**c**)

In a separate series of experiments in monolayers of neonatal rat myocytes, I_{CaL} has been implicated to be a contributing current for negative drift in the plateau responses.[30] However, even in these experiments the response asymmetry was not completely eliminated, thus suggesting that I_{CaL} may just be a piece of the puzzle and not the complete answer to asymmetric responses during the plateau phase. Recently, K^+ component of $I_{CaL}(I_{CaL,K})$ has been suggested as a likely candidate for I_a.[31] $I_{CaL,K}$ becomes large and positive for $V_m > 56\,\mathrm{mV}$, which is the reversal potential of L-type Ca^{2+} channels, and hence would have current–voltage characteristic matching that of I_a. Although the computational data and supporting arguments in support of $I_{CaL,K}$ stand on their own, they still fall short of definitive experimental evidence.

Single Cells Versus Tissue Responses: Similarities and Differences

As is almost always true, although a reductionism approach helps simplify aspects of a phenomenon for mechanistic understanding, it never completely captures system level complexities. Although there are numerous examples in which the field responses of isolated cells qualitatively resemble those from the tissue, several quantitative differences exist. For example, V_m signals recorded from tissue preparations stimulated at rest show a positive trend,[32,33] and V_m signals recorded during the plateau stimulation show a negative trend.[34-36] This hints that the primary mechanisms responsible for shaping the field-induced responses might be similar in isolated cells and tissue. However, polarization in a single cell is ultrarapid, with a time constant of several microseconds, whereas in tissue the polarization is relatively slower and occurs at milliseconds time scale.[37,38] The experiments in cultured monolayer further reveal that the speed of polarization decreases with the increasing size (e.g., strand width) of the system.[39] This is consistent with modeling studies[40] that predict speed of polarization to decrease with increasing tissue size, owing to the increased separation between the field-induced virtual sources (refer to next section below). Finally, the responses from tissue and equivalent multicellular preparations contain additional complexities not found in single cells. For example, the responses of cultured neonatal myocytes have markedly nonparallel time courses at moderate field strengths.[39,41] One explanation for this is that unlike isolated cells in which intracellular stays isopotential, in multicellular structures a time-dependent intracellular potential gradient might be present during field stimulation.[16]

Field-Induced Responses of an Isolated Cell-Pair: Sawtooth Effect

As noted at the beginning of this chapter, the mechanisms of defibrillation are not well understood. However, it is well accepted that for a shock to be successful in terminating an arrhythmia, it must affect tissue far (several centimeters away) from the electrodes. The mechanism(s) by which such distant effect of a shock is mediated is the missing link[42] in our understanding of defibrillation. If the heart is assumed to be a homogeneous continuum medium, then the resulting polarization should decay within a few millimeters.[42] However, it is now known that the heart is not a homogeneous structure and instead is replete with heterogeneities at various length scales,[43] including those arising from fiber branching, changes in fiber direction, intercellular clefts, vasculature, and intercellular gap junctions.[42-45] These discontinuities can perturb the flow of electric current in the intracellular and extracellular spaces, giving rise to tissue polarization that can be conceptually thought to arise from virtual sources, which are elegantly captured by the activating function concept (refer to Chapter 2.3 by Tung). In this section we specifically focus on microscopic discontinuities and resulting polarization arising from the intercellular gap junctions.

Intercellular gap junctions consist of an arrangement of pipe-like structures known as *connexons*, which are embedded in the lipid matrix separating the adjacent cells.[46] Each connexon is composed of six protein subunits called connexins arranged in a hexagonal array. Several types of connexins have been identified in the cardiac muscle, the predominant one being a 43 kDa molecule known as connexin-43. Although gap junctions allow free flow of ions between the neighboring cells, their resistance is relatively higher than that of the cytoplasm.[47-49] Consequently, intercellular junctions are a source of discontinuities in the intracellular domain and are the sites of virtual sources during field stimulation. Because of the spatial periodicity of gap junctions, the resulting polarization is also periodic and has a "sawtooth"-like pattern. In this polarization pattern every cell in the bulk of the myocardium undergoes simultaneous depolarization (positive response) and hyperpolarization (negative response).

Theoretical Treatment of Sawtooth Effect

To understand the physical basis of the sawtooth effect, consider several single uncoupled cells, each of length L, arranged end-to-end in a single row (Fig. 12a). If such a system is stimulated with a uniform field E_o, the ϕ_e and ϕ_i are as shown in Fig. 12b. Although the ϕ_e is linear, the ϕ_i has a staircase-like pattern because each cell is raised to a different offset potential (recall that ϕ_i is the average of extracellular potential all around a cell). Thus, V_m has a sawtooth pattern when viewed over the length scale of several cells (Fig. 12c), and the sawtooth amplitude (STA) is equal to $E_o L$. If the cells are coupled to one another via intercellular junctions of finite resistance comparable to the total cytoplasmic resistance, then the intracellular potential drop along the cell length becomes comparable to the potential drop at the junction. Thus, ϕ_i can now have a finite slope over the extent of

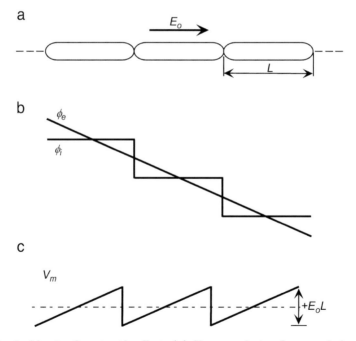

Figure 12: Physical basis of sawtooth effect. (**a**) Shows a chain of uncoupled cells stimulated with a uniform field E_o. The ϕ_i and ϕ_e for this system are shown in (**b**). The resulting V_m is shown in (**c**). The sawtooth amplitude (STA) is equal to $E_o L$

each cell, and the discrete change in ϕ_i at the intercellular junction is smaller than the case of completely uncoupled cells. Consequently, the STA is diminished.

For a more quantitative analysis of the sawtooth concept, it is useful to consider the limiting case of two cells coupled with a variable resistance, R_j, and stimulated with electric field, E_o (e.g., refer to Fig. 13a, b). The V_m for such a system can be obtained by solving the following differential equation subject to appropriate boundary conditions:[50]

$$\lambda^2 \frac{d^2 V_m}{dx^2} - V_m = 0. \tag{8}$$

In (8), λ is the space constant, which is a function of extracellular and intracellular resistivities and membrane-specific resistance. The STA can be computed by solving V_m for the two cells at the position of intercellular junction, and taking the difference. For two cells of lengths $L1$ and $L2$, STA is given by

$$\text{STA} = \frac{4 R_j E_o}{\kappa r_i} \sinh\left(\frac{L1}{2\lambda}\right) \sinh\left(\frac{L2}{2\lambda}\right) \sinh\left(\frac{L1 + L2}{2\lambda}\right), \tag{9}$$

$$\text{where } \kappa = \sinh\left(\frac{L1 + L2}{\lambda}\right) + \frac{R_j}{\lambda r_i} \sinh\left(\frac{L1}{\lambda}\right) \sinh\left(\frac{L2}{\lambda}\right). \tag{10}$$

An important implication of (9) is that V_m always reverses polarity when the two cells are of equal lengths (Fig. 13a). However, a reversal in V_m polarity is not necessary when the two cells are of unequal lengths, and the sawtooth effect in this case can be manifested merely as discontinuity in V_m (Fig. 13b). As the R_j is increased, a threshold is reached above which STA is accompanied by a change in polarity and is given by

$$R_j > \frac{\lambda r_i \sinh\left(\frac{L1 + L2}{2\lambda}\right) \sinh\left(\frac{L1 - L2}{2\lambda}\right)}{\sinh\left(\frac{L1}{\lambda}\right) \sinh^2\left(\frac{L2}{2\lambda}\right)}. \tag{11}$$

Figure 13c shows STA for a range of R_j for a field of $E_o = 10\,\text{V/cm}$ applied to a cell-pair with the first cell of fixed length ($L1 = 120\,\mu\text{m}$) and the second cell of variable length ($L2 = 90, 120$ and $150\,\mu\text{m}$).

Experimental Measurement of Sawtooth Effect

Experiments to verify the sawtooth hypothesis were first undertaken almost 10 years after the effect was first predicted.[51–53] This is because such experiments are technically challenging and require recording of transmembrane potential responses at subcellular spatial resolution with sufficient signal-to-noise ratio. Fluorescence microscopy is one of the few techniques available that provides such a capability. In the two studies investigating sawtooth effect in multicellular preparations, the first[35] using a fluorescence technique and the second[36] using a novel double-barrel microelectrode technique, the authors were unable to detect a measurable sawtooth effect. In multicellular preparations the cells are coupled not only end to end, but also via lateral connections, which allow for a more dispersed intracellular current path. A number of modeling studies using one-dimensional (chain of cells), two-dimensional (sheet of cells), and three-dimensional networks of cells have

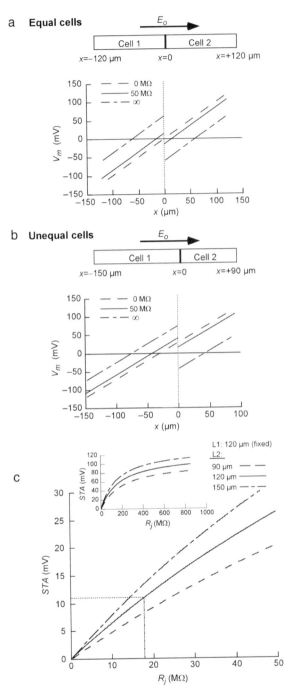

Figure 13:

shown that although the STA is depressed with increasing order of the system,[54,55] it is not completely obliterated. Thus, the anxiously awaited experimental results seemed to refute the theory. Why was the sawtooth effect, which is based on the fundamental physical concept of Ohm's law and has been predicted consistently by numerous modeling studies, not found experimentally? To probe this question we again turn to the simple system of a coupled cell-pair. The preceding theoretical analysis provides a convenient backdrop against which the experimental results can be compared.

Functionally coupled cell-pairs can be obtained by slight modification of enzymatic methods for dissociating cells from a whole heart.[16,50] The standard cell isolation procedure using Langendorff perfused hearts involve a phase in which the heart is perfused with Ca^{2+}-free solution. This facilitates break down of the extracellular matrix and dissociation of cells. Elevating the Ca^{2+} concentration to $\sim 15\,\mu M$ during this perfusion phase has been shown to preserve cell connections and produce cell-pairs with functionally intact gap junctions.[56]

Figure 14a shows a cell-pair obtained using above described technique. The intercellular junction can be clearly seen in the fluorescence image (right pictograph in Fig. 14a). Upon stimulation of the cell-pair with an S1–S2 pulse pair (S1 = 6 V/cm, S2 = 20 V/cm), the transmembrane potential responses shown in Fig. 14b are obtained. When these responses are measured at a fixed time point following the S2 onset and plotted against the cell-pair's length (Fig. 14c), a discontinuity in slope of linear fits is observed at the intercellular junction. This discontinuity is the STA and is $\sim 27\,mV$, which corresponds to $R_j = 23\,M\Omega$ computed using (9). The threshold R_j for polarity reversal using (11) is computed to be $27\,M\Omega$. Thus, the nonreversal of V_m at the junction in Fig. 14c is consistent with the theoretical expectation. Figure 14d presents the summary of similar experiments performed in 14 cell-pairs for a range of S2 amplitudes. Scaling the STA for various cell-pairs by a factor of 10/(S2 amplitude) provides an estimate for the mean STA for a nominal 10 V/cm field and yields a value of $11 \pm 4\,mV$. Using (9), an 11 mV STA corresponds to an R_j of $18.9\,M\Omega$.

Sawtooth Effect's Role in Tissue: "Fact or Fantasy"

Although the sawtooth effect is undoubtedly a "fact" in single cells and coupled cell-pairs, whether it is present in tissue and plays a significant role during field stimulation of

---

Figure 13: Theoretical estimation of sawtooth effect. (**a**) Shows the steady state V_m for two passive cells of equal length, stimulated longitudinally with a uniform electric field stimulus (E_o) of 10 V/cm, for three different values of intercellular resistance (R_j)–0 MΩ (perfect coupling), 50 MΩ (intermediate coupling), and completely uncoupled cells. (**b**) Shows V_m for the two cells of unequal length for a field of 10 V/cm and R_j values of 0, 50, and ∞ MΩ. (**c**) Shows the sawtooth amplitude (STA) as a function of R_j for a cell-pair with fixed length of the first cell ($L1 = 120\,\mu m$) and variable length of the second cell ($L2 = 90, 120,$ and $150\,\mu m$). The inset shows the same plot over a wider range of R_j. *Gray lines* indicate $R_j(= 18.9\,M\Omega)$ corresponding to an STA of ~ 11 mV, which is the average STA for a nominal field of 10 V/cm (see text for details and refer to Fig. 14d)

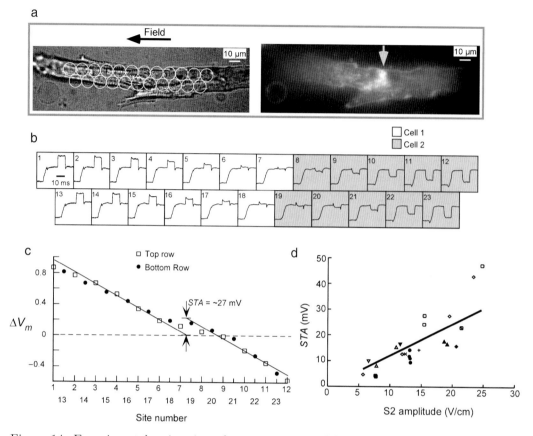

Figure 14: Experimental estimation of sawtooth effect. (**a**) Shows the brightfield and fluorescence images of a cell-pair stimulated with an S1–S2 pair (S1 $=$ 6 V/cm, S2 $=$ 20 V/cm) in the direction indicated by the *arrow*. (**b**) Shows V_m responses recorded from the cell-pair corresponding to the two rows of sites on the cell-pair. (**c**) Shows the response to the S2 pulse plotted along the cell-pair's length by merging the data from the two rows of sites. The V_m is linear over the extent of each individual cell (*fitted lines*) and shows a discontinuity near the junction that is equal to the sawtooth amplitude (STA). (**d**) Shows the STA estimated in 12 cell-pairs using the method illustrated in (**c**). STA increased monotonically with the S2 amplitude with a slope of 1.3 mV/V/cm ($R = 0.77, P < .001$)

cardiac tissue are legitimate questions.[57] In phenomenon such as reentry induction requiring relatively low field strengths ($\sim$5 V/cm),[58,59] the sawtooth effect may not be important.[60] However, during defibrillation in which a significant portion of the heart presumably experiences relatively high electric fields so that a minimum threshold electric field is achieved in the regions least affected by the shock,[61] the sawtooth effect may begin to play an important role. After decades of efforts to unravel mechanisms of defibrillation, it is now becoming clear that there is probably no single dominant mechanism that is the missing link to explain far-field effect of a shock.[42] Instead, it may be a combination of all the factors mentioned above (i.e., fiber branching, changes in fiber direction, intercellular clefts, etc.) working together synergistically that might be an answer to the elusive missing link.[62] The contribution of the sawtooth effect to net field-induced polarization might be expected to be particularly important under pathophysiological conditions such as ischemia,[63] when the cells become relatively uncoupled and intercellular resistance is elevated. An unequivocal demonstration of the sawtooth effect would require tissue level experiments. However, current techniques do not measure up to the task. Conventional optical mapping averages signal from a depth of 300 μm to 1 mm.[64] More advanced optical techniques (e.g., confocal and two-photon microscopy)[65] may run into signal-to-noise, temporal resolution, and other technical issues (e.g., phototoxicity, photobleaching, etc.). Multiple-electrode impalements in tissue are hard to maintain especially at the subcellular resolution. The various techniques are easier to apply in the neonatal rat monolayer system because of their two-dimensional nature, but this system differs from the adult myocardium in several ways. For example, neonatal cell are ~50–70 μm long[66] and their gap junctions are distributed uniformly around the cell edges.[35] These differences could impact amplitude of sawtooth effect. Thus, further advancements in recording techniques and cellular preparations may be needed before the sawtooth effect can be measured in tissue or an appropriate multicellular preparation. Until then verifying sawtooth effect in tissue remains a major challenge.

Effect of Electric Fields on Intracellular Calcium

Calcium (Ca^{2+}) serves as a vital link between depolarization and many cellular processes such as muscle contraction, enzyme regulation, and neurotransmitter secretion.[67,68] In cardiac cells the calcium varies from a resting concentration of 0.1 μM to a peak concentration of ~1 μM during every action potential.[69] Molecular machinery involved in this remarkably fine-tuned regulation consists of several proteins in the sarcolemma (cell membrane) and sarcoplasmic reticulum (SR). Upon membrane depolarization the Ca^{2+} enters mainly via L-type Ca^{2+} channels. The voltage dependence of L-type Ca^{2+} current has a bell-shaped relationship with peak influx of Ca^{2+} occurring at V_m of ~10 mV and falling off for more positive and negative $V_m s$. The Ca^{2+} influx via L-type channels induces further Ca^{2+} release from the SR via a mechanism of Ca^{2+}-induced Ca^{2+} release.[70] The Ca^{2+} release from the SR varies monotonically with the L-type Ca^{2+} current, although the exact relationship between them is unclear as slightly different relationships have been reported by various investigators (e.g., Callewaert et al.[71] have shown a linear relation whereas Santana et al.[72] and Cannell et al.[73] have reported a more complex relationship). During the action potential the intracellular Ca^{2+} reaches a peak within 10–30 ms after the upstroke, and thereafter begins to decline. The majority of the Ca^{2+} is pumped by a SR pump (SR-adenosine triphosphatase [ATPase]) back into the SR, while some is extruded out of the cell by a sodium–calcium exchanger. The cardiac cells also have sarcolemmal calcium pump (Ca^{2+}-ATPase), but they appear to play an unimportant role in removing Ca^{2+} from the cytoplasm under physiological conditions.[74] Obviously, for a fixed pacing rate (and contractility) all Ca^{2+} fluxes are balanced so that no net build up or decline in intracellular Ca^{2+} occurs over time.

As we discussed above an externally applied field induces spatially varying V_m along the length of a cardiac cell. Since L-type Ca^{2+} channels are V_m dependent, and Ca^{2+} release from the SR in turn depends on the L-type Ca^{2+} current, it is not unreasonable to hypothesize that intracellular Ca^{2+} concentration might be affected by external fields. Below we present experiments investigating the effect of applied fields on intracellular Ca^{2+} transients.[75] The observed results are then discussed in the context of known electrophysiology of Ca^{2+} transients and current–voltage relationship of L-type Ca^{2+} channels.

Measurement of Intracellular Ca^{2+} Transients Using Fluorescent Probes

Optical techniques similar to those used for recording V_m can be used for recording intracellular Ca^{2+} as well. In fact, the optical mapping setup described in Fig. 3 can be used for Ca^{2+} measurements except that now we must use a Ca^{2+}-sensitive dye along with appropriate optical filters. Among a diverse array of Ca^{2+} indicator dyes available,[76] one of the most commonly used dyes is fluo-3 (and its newer version fluo-4). The fluorescence intensity of fluo-3 increases manyfold ($\sim$40) upon binding calcium. The dye loading into the cell is performed using acetoxymethyl ester (AM) derivatives of fluo-3 (fluo-3/AM) in which each –COO-group is replaced with –COOCH$_2$OAc (where Ac means –OCOCH$_3$). The fluo-3/AM is membrane permeable, but once inside the cell the AM portion is cleaved by cellular esterase, thus rendering the molecule membrane impermeable. Similar to voltage-sensitive dyes, fluo-3 does not measure absolute intracellular calcium. However, when only relative changes in Ca^{2+} are of interest (e.g., Ca^{2+} with and without a field stimulus) fluo-3 is an attractive option because of a large fluorescence change and simplicity of use.

Effect of Field Stimulation on Intracellular Ca^{2+} Transients at Rest

Figure 15 shows the typical effect of applied field on intracellular Ca^{2+}($[Ca^{2+}]_i$) transients at rest recorded from a cell loaded with fluo-3. The $[Ca^{2+}]_i$ transients are shown for eight sites along the cell length and for two S1 field pulses of opposite polarity (S1 = +10 V/cm and S1 = −11 V/cm). For both field directions the $[Ca^{2+}]_i$ transients from the various sites are asynchronous. For positive S1 pulses the $[Ca^{2+}]_i$ signal from site 1 is the fastest, and $[Ca^{2+}]_i$ signal from site 8 is the slowest (Fig. 15b, middle row). On field reversal this trend is reversed, and now the signal from site 8 is the fastest (Fig. 15b, bottom row). Thus, for both field directions the $[Ca^{2+}]_i$ transients in the anode-facing regions of the cell are faster. These asynchronous signals imply that the $[Ca^{2+}]_i$ is nonuniform along the cell length during the rising phase of the transients, and that a spatial gradient in $[Ca^{2+}]_i$ ($\nabla[Ca^{2+}]_i$) is developed. An estimate of $\nabla[Ca^{2+}]_i$ can be obtained at a given time point during the rising phase of the transients (e.g., time point corresponding to the thick vertical line in Fig. 15b) by plotting $[Ca^{2+}]_i$ along the cell length (Fig. 15c). The $[Ca^{2+}]_i$ in Fig. 15c has been normalized to the peak of the $[Ca^{2+}]_i$ transient, which is $\sim$980 nM for a typical guinea pig cell.[69] The $\nabla[Ca^{2+}]_i s$ in the anodal half of the cell in Fig. 14a are 4.2 and 6.3 nM μm^{-1}

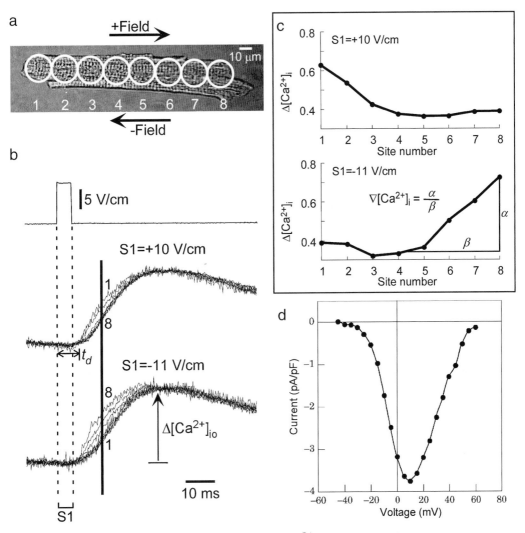

Figure 15: Effect of field stimulation at rest on Ca^{2+} transients. (a) Shows a cell that is stimulated with positive and negative S1 pulses, and (b) shows the corresponding $[Ca^{2+}]_i$ transients superimposed from all eight sites. (b) *Top row* shows the positive S1 pulse, and the *bottom two rows* show the $[Ca^{2+}]_i$ transients for the two field directions. The vertical *dashed lines* mark the duration of S_1 pulse to help discern temporal relationship between the S1 pulse and $[Ca^{2+}]_i$ transients. The onset of $[Ca^{2+}]_i$ transients is delayed from the make of the S1 pulse by a duration t_d (~ 7.5 ms for both positive and negative S1 pulses). The change in $[Ca^{2+}]_i$ relative to the resting level ($\Delta[Ca^{2+}]_i$) was measured during the rising phase of the transients at the time indicated by the *thick line* in (b). $\Delta[Ca^{2+}]_i$ is normalized to its peak value ($\Delta[Ca^{2+}]_{io}$ in (b), *bottom row*), and the resulting normalized change in $\Delta[Ca^{2+}]_i$ is plotted in (c) for positive S_1 pulse (*top plot*) and negative S1 pulse (*bottom plot*). The gradient in $[Ca^{2+}]_i$ ($\nabla[Ca^{2+}]_i = \alpha/\beta$) in the anodal half of the cell can be computed as illustrated in (c), *bottom plot*, and is estimated to be 4.2 and 6.3 nM/μm for the positive and negative S1 pulses, respectively. (d) Shows the current–voltage relationship for the L-type Ca^{2+} current. (Mukherjee and Spinole 1998)[82]

for the positive and negative S1 pulses, respectively. Performing additional experiments (26 cells and 114 S1 stimuli) like the one described in Fig. 15, the $\nabla[Ca^{2+}]_i$ in the anodal half of the cell is found to increase monotonically with the S1 amplitude, and is $\sim 3.4\,\text{nM}\,\mu\text{m}^{-1}$ for a nominal field of $\sim 10\,\text{V/cm}$. No measurable $\nabla[Ca^{2+}]_i$ exists in the cathode facing half of the cell.

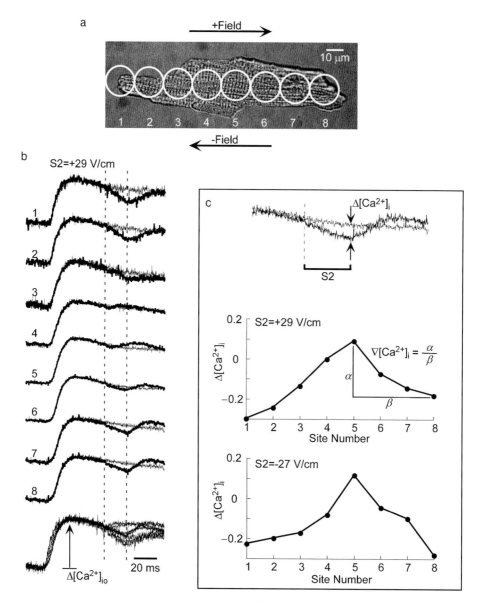

Figure 16:

Recall that a field pulse applied at rest hyperpolarizes the anodal and depolarizes the cathodal end of the cell (Fig. 4). The resting potential ($\sim -90\,$mV) is situated at the leftmost extreme of the bell-shaped I–V relation of the L-type Ca^{2+} current (Fig. 15d). Thus, the observed behavior of fastest $[Ca^{2+}]_i$ transients in the anodal regions of the cell counters what would be predicted from a larger activation of Ca^{2+} current in the cathodal (depolarized) regions of the cell and negligible Ca^{2+} current in the anodal (hyperpolarized) regions. This paradoxical behavior can be resolved by noting that onset of $[Ca^{2+}]_i$ transients occurs after the S1 pulse and not during the pulse. The typical delay (t_d; Fig. 14b) is $\sim$7 ms from the S1 onset for a 10 V/cm pulse. Thus, a possible explanation for the faster $[Ca^{2+}]_i$ transients in the anodal regions may involve voltage-dependent inactivation of the L-type Ca^{2+} channels, which exists to some extent in guinea pig ventricular cells.[77,78] The S1-induced hyperpolarization would diminish the inactivation of the Ca^{2+} channels compared with the cathodal end, so that upon S1 termination a larger influx of Ca^{2+} would occur at the anodal end. A second possible explanation involves Ca^{2+}-dependent inactivation of the L-type Ca^{2+} channels.[79] During the S1 pulse calcium is brought into the cell in the depolarized regions and extruded from the hyperpolarized regions of the cell via electrogenic sodium–calcium exchanger.[80] This would result in a graded calcium concentration along the cell length in the restricted dyadic subspace, which is the region between the cell membrane and SR membrane.[81] The net effect would be to accentuate inactivation of Ca^{2+} channels in the depolarized regions and to relieve inactivation in the hyperpolarized regions of the cell (assuming Ca^{2+} conductance was partially inactivated at rest via calcium-dependent inactivation). Thus, there would be a spatially varying calcium conductance along the cell length that could explain the observed S1-induced pattern of calcium transients.

Figure 16: Effect of field stimulation during the plateau phase on Ca^{2+} transients. (a) Shows a cell that is first stimulated with a S1 pulse only, and then with a pair of S1–S2 pulses. The $[Ca^{2+}]_i$ recordings obtained from eight sites in response to the S1 pulse and S1–S2 pair are shown superimposed for each site in (b). (b) *Bottommost row* shows the $[Ca^{2+}]_i$ transients superimposed from all sites in response to the S1–S2 pair. The pair of *vertical dashed lines* represents the duration of the S2 pulse. The perturbation of the $[Ca^{2+}]_i$ transients is measured at the end of the S2 pulse with respect to the $[Ca^{2+}]_i$ recorded with the S1 pulse only as illustrated in the inset of (c). The change is normalized to the peak change in $[Ca^{2+}]_i (\Delta[Ca^{2+}]_{io})$ and is plotted against the site number in (c), *top plot*. (c) *Bottom plot* shows the normalized change $\Delta[Ca^{2+}]_i$ for the same cell in response to an S1–S2 pair applied in the negative direction (S2 $= -27$ V/cm). For both field directions $\Delta[Ca^{2+}]_i$ was smallest at the cell center and increased in either direction implying that $[Ca^{2+}]_i$ gradients ($\nabla[Ca^{2+}]_i$) developed directed from the cell center to both cell ends. For $+29$ V cm^{-1} S2 pulse (c, *top plot*) $\nabla[Ca^{2+}]_i s$ are 5.6 and 5.2 nM μm^{-1} for the anodal and cathodal halves of the cell, respectively. For -27 V cm^{-1} S2 pulse (c, *bottom plot*) $\nabla[Ca^{2+}]_i s$ are 7.7 and 5.0 nM μm^{-1}, respectively

Effect of Field Stimulation on Intracellular Ca^{2+} Transients During Plateau

The effect of externally applied electric field on Ca^{2+} transients during the plateau phase of the action potential is illustrated in Fig. 16. For this experiment the cell is stimulated with an S1–S2 pulse protocol with an interpulse duration of 50 ms. The recordings from eight sites on the cell are shown in Fig. 16b. Also shown superimposed in the same figure are the Ca^{2+} transients for a S1 pulse with no S2 pulse applied. The nonoverlapping behavior of these recordings suggest that the S2 pulse induced $[Ca^{2+}]_i$ nonuniformity along the cell length. The S2-induced change in $[Ca^{2+}]_i$ ($\Delta[Ca^{2+}]_i$) was measured at the end of S2 pulse relative to the $[Ca^{2+}]_i$ at the same time recorded with S1 pulse only (Fig. 16c inset). Similar to the case of the S1 pulse above, $\Delta[Ca^{2+}]_i$ is normalized to the peak of the $[Ca^{2+}]_i$ transients and the result is plotted in Fig. 16c. On field reversal a similar behavior of $\Delta[Ca^{2+}]_i$ along the cell length is observed (Fig. 16c, bottom plot). These results suggest that electric field applied during the plateau phase of the action potential induces intracellular Ca^{2+} gradients ($\nabla[Ca^{2+}]_i$) from the center to either end of the cell. In Fig. 16c the $\nabla[Ca^{2+}]_i s$ in the anodal and cathodal halves of the cell are 5.6 and 5.2 nM/μm, respectively, for the positive fields, and 7.7 and 5.0 nM/μm, respectively, for the negative fields. From similar results in 12 cells (24 S1–S2 stimuli; S2 = 25 ± 6 V/cm), the $\nabla[Ca^{2+}]_i$ in the anodal half (4.2 ± 2.2 nM/μm) of the cell is found to be higher than in the cathodal half (2.8 ± 1.6 nM/μm).

Similar to the S1 pulse, the S2 pulse also causes hyperpolarization at the anode-facing end and depolarization at the cathode-facing end of the cell. However, unlike S1 this perturbation occurs about the center ($\sim$10 mV) of the I–V relation for Ca^{2+} current (Fig. 15d). Thus, Ca^{2+} current and $[Ca^{2+}]_i$ should decrease at both ends of the cell compared with the center, and experimental data are consistent with this theoretical expectation (Fig. 16b). Upon S2 termination the transmembrane potential returns close to the prepulse plateau level, resulting in a large inward Ca^{2+} current and surge in $[Ca^{2+}]_i$ at both ends of the cell as observed experimentally. The deactivation of Ca^{2+} channels at the anodal end and associated reduction in the channel conductance as described above may explain the smaller amplitude of $[Ca^{2+}]_i$ surge in the anodal regions. Recently, these results have been replicated and extended in neonatal cell culture system by studying the field-induced changed in $[Ca^{2+}]_i$ over a broader range of coupling intervals. Although $[Ca^{2+}]_i$ is depressed at the cathodal and anodal ends during the early plateau stimulation, the pattern of field-induced changes in $[Ca^{2+}]_i$ varies as the coupling interval between S1 and S2 is changed and the shock applied during various phases of repolarization.[83]

Implications of Field-Induced Ca^{2+} Gradients

Although the finding about perturbation in intracellular Ca^{2+} and induction of spatially gradients in $[Ca^{2+}]_i$ by external electric fields is of fundamental biophysical interest, whether it is of any real consequence during defibrillation or other phenomenon involving application of high electric fields needs further investigation.[84–86] Perhaps accounting for $[Ca^{2+}]_i$ gradients is necessary to accurately predict the shock outcome during defibrillation.

Considering that Ca^{2+} is a ubiquitous second messenger and voltage-gated Ca^{2+} channels are present in several different cell types, the field-induced changes in $[Ca^{2+}]_i$ could have implications beyond the cardiac system. For phenomena involving applications of long-lasting (pulsed) electric fields, one must consider the possibility that field-induced changes in $[Ca^{2+}]_i$ may in fact be able to alter cellular signaling and impact cellular function, perhaps by design in some situations.

Conclusion

In this chapter we reviewed the effects of external fields on voltage and Ca^{2+} responses of isolated cardiac cells and cell-pairs. Although the focus of our discussion has been cardiac cell, the concepts and framework presented should have broader applications for other excitable cell systems as well. For example, decomposition of responses into active and passive components should be applicable to any excitable cell except that the details of the active component, which depend on ion channel mix and their current–voltage characteristics, could vary among cells. The effect of intercellular junction on field-induced responses and sawtooth effect also has fundamental biophysical underpinning, and hence should have applications in other cell systems containing gap junctions, which are known to express in almost every tissue type in the body.[87] The only requirement is that gap junction should be the site of resistive discontinuity. Finally, because Ca^{2+} is such an important ion for the various cellular signaling and functions, and voltage-dependent Ca^{2+} is an important player via which exquisite regulation of Ca^{2+} is accomplished, the field-induced gradients in intracellular Ca^{2+} may be a phenomenon that is not just restricted to a cardiac cell, but instead may be universal to all cell types when stimulated with electric fields of appropriate strengths.

References

1. Beck CS. Resuscitation for cardiac standstill and ventricular fibrillation occurring during operation. *Am J Surg* 1941;54:273–279
2. Cesario DA, Dec GW. Implantable cardioverter-defibrillator therapy in clinical practice. *J Am Coll Cardiol* 2006;47:1507–1517
3. DiMarco JP. Implantable cardioverter-defibrillators. *N Engl J Med* 2003;349:1836–1847
4. Goldberger Z, Lampert R. Implantable cardioverter-defibrillators: expanding indications and technologies. *JAMA* 2006;295:809–818
5. Marenco JP, Wang PJ, Link MS, Homoud MK, Estes NA III. Improving survival from sudden cardiac arrest: the role of the automated external defibrillator. *JAMA* 2001;285:1193–1200
6. Klee M, Plonsey R. Stimulation of spheroidal cells – the role of cell shape. *IEEE Trans Biomed Eng* 1976;23:347–354
7. Jeltsch E, Zimmerman U. Particles in a homogeneous field: a model for the electrical breakdown of living cells in a Coulter counter. *Bioelectrochem Bioenerg* 1979;6:349–384

8. Gross D, Loew LM, Webb WW. Optical imaging of cell membrane potential changes induced by applied electric fields. *Biophys J* 1986;50:339–348

9. Hibino M, Shigemori M, Itoh H, Nagayama K, Kinosita K Jr. Membrane conductance of an electroporated cell analyzed by submicrosecond imaging of transmembrane potential. *Biophys J* 1991;59:209–220

10. Ehrenberg B, Farkas DL, Fluhler EN, Lojewska Z, Loew LM. Membrane potential induced by external electric field pulses can be followed with a potentiometric dye. *Biophys J* 1987;51:833–837 [published erratum appears in *Biophys. J* 1987 Jul;52(1):following 141]

11. Kwaku KF, Dillon SM. Shock-induced depolarization of refractory myocardium prevents wave-front propagation in defibrillation. *Circ Res* 1996;79:957–973

12. Watanabe T, Rautaharju PM, McDonald TF. Ventricular action potentials, ventricular extracellular potentials, and the ECG of guinea pig. *Circ Res* 1985;57:362–373

13. Cheng DKL, Tung L, Sobie EA. Nonuniform responses of transmembrane potential during electric field stimulation of single cardiac cells. *Am J Physiol* 1999;277 (*Heart Circ Physiol* 46):H351–H362

14. Knisley SB, Blitchington TF, Hill BC, Grant AO, Smith WM, Pilkington TC, Ideker RE. Optical measurements of transmembrane potential changes during electric field stimulation of ventricular cells. *Circ Res* 1993;72:255–270

15. Windisch H, Ahammer H, Schaffer P, Muller W, Platzer D. Optical multisite monitoring of cell excitation phenomena in isolated cardiomyocytes. *Pflugers Arch* 1995;430:508–518

16. Sharma V, Tung L. Spatial heterogeneity of transmembrane potential responses of single guinea-pig cardiac cells during electric field stimulation. *J Physiol* 2002;542:477–492

17. Rohr S, Kucera JP. Optical recording system based on a fiber optic image conduit: assessment of microscopic activation patterns in cardiac tissue. *Biophys J* 1998;75:1062–1075

18. Windisch H, Ahammer H, Schaffer P, Muller W, Platzer D. Optical multisite monitoring of cell excitation phenomena in isolated cardiomyocytes. *Pflugers Arch* 1995;430:508–518

19. Sharma V, Susil RC, Tung L. Paradoxical loss of excitation with high intensity pulses during electric field stimulation of single cardiac cells. *Biophys J* 2005;88:3038–3049

20. Koning G, Veefkind AH, Schneider H. Cardiac damage caused by direct application of defibrillator shocks to isolated Langendorff-perfused rabbit heart. *Am Heart J* 1980;100:473–482

21. O'Neill RJ, Tung L. Cell-attached patch clamp study of the electropermeabilization of amphibian cardiac cells. *Biophys J* 1991;59:1028–1039

22. Luo CH, Rudy Y. A model of the ventricular cardiac action potential. Depolarization, repolarization, and their interaction. *Circ Res* 1991;68:1501–1526

23. Puglisi JL, Wang F, Bers DM. Modeling the isolated cardiac myocyte. *Prog Biophys Mol Biol* 2004;85:163–178

24. Tung L, Borderies JR. Analysis of electric field stimulation of single cardiac muscle cells. *Biophys J* 1992;63:371–386

25. Sharma V, Lu SN, Tung L. Decomposition of field-induced transmembrane potential responses of single cardiac cells. *IEEE Trans Biomed Eng* 2002;49:1031–1037

26. Sharma V, Tung L. Transmembrane responses of single guinea pig ventricular cell to uniform electric field stimulus. *J Cardiovasc Electrophysiol* 1999;10:1296

27. Luo CH, Rudy Y. A dynamic model of the cardiac ventricular action potential. I. Simulations of ionic currents and concentration changes. *Circ Res* 1994;74:1071–1096

28. Zeng J, Laurita KR, Rosenbaum DS, Rudy Y. Two components of the delayed rectifier K+ current in ventricular myocytes of the guinea pig type. Theoretical formulation and their role in repolarization. *Circ Res* 1995;77:140–152

29. Sharma V, Tung L. Ionic currents involved in shock-induced nonlinear changes in transmembrane potential responses of single cardiac cells. *Pflugers Arch* 2004;449:248–256

30. Cheek ER, Ideker RE, Fast VG. Nonlinear changes of transmembrane potential during defibrillation shocks: role of Ca^{2+} current. *Circ Res* 2000;87:453–459

31. Ashihara T, Trayanova NA. Cell and tissue responses to electric shocks. *Europace* 2005;7:155–165

32. Neunlist M, Tung L. Optical recordings of ventricular excitability of frog heart by an extracellular stimulating point electrode. *Pacing Clin Electrophysiol* 1994;17:1641–1654

33. Tung L, Neunlist M, Sobie EA. Near-field and far-field stimulation of cardiac muscle. *Clin Appl Mod Imaging Technol II* 1994;2132:367–374

34. Neunlist M, Tung L. Spatial distribution of cardiac transmembrane potentials around an extracellular electrode: dependence on fiber orientation. *Biophys J* 1995;68:2310–2322

35. Gillis AM, Fast VG, Rohr S, Kleber AG. Spatial changes in transmembrane potential during extracellular electrical shocks in cultured monolayers of neonatal rat ventricular myocytes. *Circ Res* 1996;79:676–690

36. Zhou X, Knisley SB, Smith WM, Rollins D, Pollard AE, Idekar RE. Spatial changes in the transmembrane potential during extracellular electric stimulation. *Circ Res* 1998;83:1003–1014

37. Mowrey KA, Cheng Y, Tchou PJ, Efimov R. Kinetics of defibrillation shock-induced response: design implications for the optimal defibrillation waveform. *Europace* 2002;4:27–39

38. Sharma V, Qu F, Nikolski VP, DeGroot P, Efimov IR. Direct measurements of membrane time constant during defibrillation strength shocks. *Heart Rhythm* 2007;4:478–486

39. Fast VG, Rohr S, Ideker RE. Nonlinear changes of transmembrane potential caused by defibrillation shocks in strands of cultured myocytes. *Am J Physiol Heart Circ Physiol* 2000;278:H688–H697

40. Susil RC, Sobie EA, Tung L. Separation between virtual sources modifies the response of cardiac tissue to field stimulation. *J Cardiovasc Electrophysiol* 1999;10:715–727

41. Tung L, Kleber AG. Virtual sources associated with linear and curved strands of cardiac cells. *Am J Physiol Heart Circ Physiol* 2000;279:H1579–H1590

42. Roth BJ, Krassowska W. The induction of reentry in cardiac tissue. The missing link: how electric fields alter transmembrane potential. *Chaos* 1998;8:204–220

43. Dorri F, Niederer PF, Redmann K, Lunkenheimer PP, Cryer CW, Anderson RH. An analysis of the spatial arrangement of the myocardial aggregates making up the wall of the left ventricle. *Eur J Cardiothorac Surg* 2007;31:430–437

44. LeGrice IJ, Smaill BH, Chai LZ, Edgar SG, Gavin JB, Hunter PJ. Laminar structure of the heart: ventricular myocyte arrangement and connective tissue architecture in the dog. *Am J Physiol* 1995;269:H571–H582

45. White JB, Walcott GP, Pollard AE, Ideker RE. Myocardial discontinuities: a substrate for producing virtual electrodes that directly excite the myocardium by shocks. *Circulation* 1998;97:1738–1745

46. Makowski L, Caspar DL, Phillips WC, Goodenough DA. Gap junction structures. II. Analysis of the X-ray diffraction data. *J Cell Biol* 1977;74:629–645

47. White RL, Spray DC, Campos de Carvalho AC, Wittenberg BA, Bennett MV. Some electrical and pharmacological properties of gap junctions between adult ventricular myocytes. *Am J Physiol* 1985;249:C447–455

48. Weingart R, Maurer P. Action potential transfer in cell pairs isolated from adult rat and guinea pig ventricles. *Circ Res* 1988;63:72–80

49. Kieval RS, Spear JF, Moore EN. Gap junctional conductance in ventricular myocyte pairs isolated from postischemic rabbit myocardium. *Circ Res* 1992;71:127–136

50. Sharma V, Tung L. Theoretical and experimental study of sawtooth effect in isolated cardiac cell-pairs. *J Cardiovasc Electrophysiol* 2001;12:1164–1173

51. Plonsey R, Barr RC. Inclusion of junction elements in a linear cardiac model through secondary sources: application to defibrillation. *Med Biol Eng Comput* 1986;24:137–144

52. Plonsey R, Barr RC. Effect of junctional resistance on source-strength in a linear cable. *Ann Biomed Eng* 1985;13:95–100

53. Plonsey R, Barr RC. Inclusion of junction elements in a linear cardiac model through secondary sources: application to defibrillation. *Med Biol Eng Comput* 1986;24:137–144

54. Krinsky V, Pumir A. Models of defibrillation of cardiac tissue. *Chaos* 1988;8:188–203

55. Juhlin SP, Pormann JB. Dimensional comparison of the sawtooth pattern in transmembrane potential. *Comput Cardiol* 1994;413–416

56. Wittenberg BA, White RL, Ginzberg RD, Spray DC. Effect of calcium on the dissociation of the mature rat heart into individual and paired myocytes: electrical properties of cell pairs. *Circ Res* 1986;59:143–150

57. Roth BJ. Sawtooth effect: fact or fancy? *J Cardiovasc Electrophysiol* 2001;12:1174–1175

58. Knisley SB, Smith WM, Ideker RE. Effect of field stimulation on cellular repolarization in rabbit myocardium. Implications for reentry induction. *Circ Res* 1992;70:707–715

59. Frazier DW, Wolf PD, Wharton JM, Tang AS, Smith WM, Ideker RE. Stimulus-induced critical point. Mechanism for electrical initiation of reentry in normal canine myocardium. *J Clin Invest* 1989;83:1039–1052

60. Krassowska W, Kumar MS. The role of spatial interactions in creating the dispersion of transmembrane potential by premature electric shocks. *Ann Biomed Eng* 1997;25:949–963

61. Ideker RE, Wolf PD, Tang AS. *Mechanisms of Defibrillation* St. Louis: Mosby; 1994

62. Trayanova N, Skouibine K, Aguel F. The role of cardiac tissue structure in defibrillation. *Chaos* 1998;8:221–233

63. Huang X, Sandusky GE, Zipes DP. Heterogeneous loss of connexin43 protein in ischemia dog hearts. *J Cardiovasc Electrophysiol* 1999;10:79–91

64. Gray RA. What exactly are optically recorded "action potentials"? *J Cardiovasc Electrophysiol* 1999;10:1463–1466

65. Rubart M. Two-photon microscopy of cells and tissue. *Circ Res* 2004;95:1154–1166

66. Rohr S, Scholly DM, Kleber AG. Patterned growth of neonatal rat heart cells in culture. Morphological and electrophysiological characterization. *Circ Res* 1991;68:114–130

67. Berridge MJ, Bootman MD, Lipp P. Calcium – a life and death signal. *Nature* 1998;395:645–648

68. Berridge MJ, Lipp P, Bootman MD. The versatility and universality of calcium signalling. *Nat Rev Mol Cell Biol* 2000;1:11–21

69. Beuckelmann DJ, Wier WG. Mechanism of release of calcium from sarcoplasmic reticulum of guinea- pig cardiac cells. *J Physiol (Lond)* 1988;405:233–255

70. Fabiato A. Simulated calcium current can both cause calcium loading in and trigger calcium release from the sarcoplasmic reticulum of a skinned canine cardiac Purkinje cell. *J Gen Physiol* 1985;85:291–320

71. Callewaert G, Cleemann L, Morad M. Epinephrine enhances Ca^{2+} current-regulated Ca^{2+} release and Ca^{2+} reuptake in rat ventricular myocytes. *Proc Natl Acad Sci USA.* 1988;85:2009–2013

72. Santana LF, Cheng H, Gomez AM, Cannell MB, Lederer WJ. Relation between the sarcolemmal Ca^{2+} current and Ca^{2+} sparks and local control theories for cardiac excitation-contraction coupling. *Circ Res* 1996;78:166–171

73. Cannell MB, Berlin JR, Lederer WJ. Effect of membrane potential changes on the calcium transient in single rat cardiac muscle cells. *Science* 1987;238:1419–1423

74. Sipido KR, Wier WG. Flux of Ca^{2+} across the sacroplasmic reticulum of guinea pig cardiac cells during excitation contraction coupling. *J Physiol* 1991;435:605–630

75. Sharma V, Tung L. Effects of uniform electric fields on intracellular calcium transients in single cardiac cells. *Am J Physiol Heart Circ Physiol* 2002;282:H72–H79

76. Simpson AW. Fluorescent measurement of $[Ca^{2+}]_c$: basic practical considerations. *Methods Mol Biol* 2006;312:3–36

77. Hadley RW, Lederer WJ. Ca^{2+} and voltage inactivate Ca^{2+} channels in guinea-pig ventricular myocytes through independent mechanisms. *J Physiol* 1991;444:257–268

78. White E, Terrar DA. Inactivation of Ca current during the action potential in guinea-pig ventricular myocytes. *Exp Physiol* 1992;77:153–164

79. Eckert R, Chad JE. Inactivation of Ca channels. *Prog Biophys Mol Biol* 1984;44:215–267

80. Grantham CJ, Cannell MB. Ca^{2+} influx during the cardiac action potential in guinea pig ventricular myocytes. *Circ Res* 1996;79:194–200

81. Langer GA, Peskoff A. Role of the diadic cleft in myocardial contractile control. *Circulation* 1997;96:3761–3765

82. Mukherjee R, Spinale FG. L-type calcium channel abundance and function with cardiac hypertrophy and failure: a review. *J Mol Cell Cardiol* 1998;30:1899–1916

83. Raman V, Pollard AE, Fast VG. Shock-induced changes of Ca_i^{2+} and Vm in myocyte cultures and computer model: dependence on the timing of shock application. *Cardiovasc Res* 2007;73:101–110

84. Heida T. Electric field-induced effects on neuronal cell biology accompanying dielectrophoretic trapping. *Adv Anat Embryol Cell Biol* 2003;173:3–9
85. Lee RC, Zhang D, Hannig J. Biophysical injury mechanisms in electrical shock trauma. *Annu Rev Biomed Eng* 2000;2:477–509
86. Trollet C, Bloquel C, Scherman D, Bigey P. Electrotransfer into skeletal muscle for protein expression. *Curr Gene Ther* 2006;6:561–578
87. Goodenough DA, Goliger JA, Paul DL. Connexins, connexons, and intercellular communication. *Annu Rev Biochem* 1996;65:475–502

Chapter 4.2

The Role of Microscopic Tissue Structure in Defibrillation

Vladimir G. Fast

Introduction

Ventricular fibrillation is the most important immediate cause of sudden cardiac death, which is the main source of mortality in developed countries. Currently, the only practical method for treating ventricular fibrillation is electrical defibrillation. External defibrillators accessible to public and implantable devices are becoming more widespread, reducing the risk of sudden cardiac death. Nevertheless, current defibrillation techniques have significant drawbacks. Shocks can be detrimental by causing pain, tissue damage, and reinducing arrhythmias.[1] In addition, shocks may fail, which requires multiple shock application,[2] or fibrillation can be terminated but normal heartbeat and blood circulation not restored.[3,4] Therefore, there is a need to increase defibrillation efficacy and reduce its side effects, which underlies the continuing search for better defibrillation techniques. This search would have higher chances for success if it were guided by the exact knowledge of the defibrillation mechanism. Significant advances in understanding defibrillation were made in recent years using sophisticated electrical and optical mapping techniques as well as advanced mathematical models of cardiac excitation that provided a wealth of new information about the effects of electrical fields on cardiac tissue. Despite these efforts the defibrillation mechanism still remains a mystery. One of the main unresolved questions is why an electrical shock causes any significant effect on the heart at all; the other question is how exactly the shock affects the heart and stops abnormal electrical activity. Fibrillation is generally considered a distributed process, which is maintained by multiple reentrant circuits or randomly wandering wavelets in various parts of the heart.[5–7] To interrupt such fibrillation, all reentrant wavefronts have to be extinguished. According to the "excitatory" hypothesis of defibrillation, this is achieved by simultaneous activation of cardiac tissue in the excitable and relatively refractory states.[8,9] The newly depolarized tissue presents

Department of Biomedical Engineering, University of Alabama at Birmingham, Birmingham, AL, USA,
fast@crml.uab.edu

I. R. Efimov et al. (eds.), *Cardiac Bioelectric Therapy: Mechanisms and Practical Implications.*
© Springer Science+Business Media, LLC 2009

functional obstacles to excitation waves, blocking their propagation and, therefore, arresting fibrillation. An important requirement of defibrillation is that abnormal activity must be stopped in a critical mass of ventricular myocardium estimated at 80–90% of the total mass.[9,10] This means that the shock must change membrane potential (V_m) of nearly all cardiac cells across the ventricular wall. How this global shock effect is achieved is not presently known. The classical cable model of cardiac muscle indicates that shock-induced V_m changes should be restricted only to the tissue near shock electrodes or muscle surface,[11] leaving the intramural bulk of the myocardium unaffected by the shock. This model's prediction about the locality of shock effects is in stark contradiction with the distributed nature of fibrillation. This contradiction was recognized about 20 years ago.[12–14] To resolve it, a so-called secondary source hypothesis was proposed, which linked shock effects with the microscopic tissue structure. More specifically, it was postulated that shocks cause widespread changes of V_m due to numerous microscopic discontinuities in the tissue structure, such as cell boundaries.[12–14]

The hypothesis of microscopic secondary sources still remains unproven. Direct experimental verification of this hypothesis in the heart faces several obstacles. First, it requires measurement of V_m in the intramural myocardium with microscopic resolution, but such methods are not currently available. Second, even if microscopic V_m measurements were possible, interpretation of such data would be difficult because of the structural complexity of cardiac muscle, which contains discontinuities at different spatial scales. To circumvent these limitations, we adopted an indirect approach consisting of two main elements. The first element of this approach is to determine the effects of shocks on V_m in two-dimensional monolayers of cultured myocytes. The use of cell cultures allows for optical mapping of V_m with microscopic resolution. In addition, the structure of cell cultures can be controlled and modified using the techniques of patterned cell growth, which makes possible investigation of the contributions of individual structural elements into the shock effects. The second element of this approach is to measure the effects of shocks on intramural V_m at macroscopic resolution in isolated wedge preparations of left ventricular muscle. These measurements are then compared with the spatially averaged data obtained in microscopic studies of shock effects in cell cultures. This chapter describes results of experiments of both types and analyzes their similarities and differences. This analysis supports the important role of tissue structure in defibrillation and provides evidence that intramural secondary sources are caused by tissue discontinuities with microscopic dimensions.

Possible Mechanisms of Intramural Shock-Induced V_m Changes

Analysis of the classical cable model indicates that in structurally continuous tissue V_m changes induced by a uniform extracellular field should be limited to a very small tissue area near the shock electrodes.[11–14] With increasing distance from the electrodes, changes

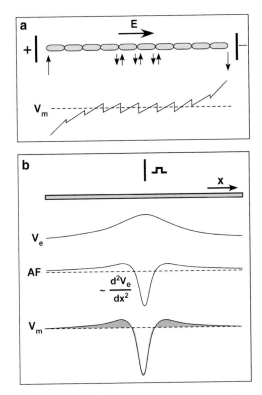

Figure 1: Possible mechanisms of intramural shock-induced V_m changes. (a) Mechanism associated with nonuniform tissue structure. E, uniform shock field. *Vertical arrows* depict current flow across cell membrane at intercellular boundaries. (b) Mechanism associated with nonuniform shock field. V_e, extracellular potential; AF, "activating function" proportional to the second spatial derivative of V_e

in V_m decay exponentially, approaching zero beyond 1–2 mm from the shock electrodes. To induce V_m changes in the tissue far from the shock electrodes, a redistribution of shock current between intracellular and extracellular spaces has to take place, which can occur via two main mechanisms (Fig. 1). In the first mechanism, known as the *mechanism of secondary sources*, V_m changes are produced by variations in resistive tissue properties. One example of this mechanism is the "saw-tooth" pattern of ΔV_m formed at cell boundaries that present microscopic resistive barriers to current flow (Fig. 1a).[12–14] In a similar fashion, ΔV_m can be caused by larger resistive barriers associated with the vasculature, intercellular clefts, or connective tissue sheets separating cell bundles and cell layers. Other structure-dependent mechanisms relate V_m changes to rotation of anisotropy axes in space[15] or to variation of the ratio between intracellular and extracellular volume fractions.[16] The second main mechanism relates V_m changes to nonuniformities of the shock field. In this case, V_m changes are caused by so-called virtual electrodes produced at sites with significant spatial derivative of the extracellular field called *activating function* (Fig. 1b).[17–19] Combination of both structural factors (tissue anisotropy) and the nonuniform shock field can produce V_m changes via the "dog-bone" effect.[18,20]

The Role of Microscopic Tissue Structure in the Shock Effects: Experiments in Cell Cultures

Until recently, the effects of microscopic tissue structure on defibrillation were investigated almost exclusively in computer models.[12–15,21] Experimental studies of structural effects in the heart are hampered by the inability to measure V_m at the microscopic level and by the three-dimensional complexity of cardiac muscle that prevents precise correlation of V_m changes with the tissue structure. Also, because cardiac muscle contains structural discontinuities of multiple types, separating the effects of one individual structure from another as well as from effects of other structure-independent factors is extremely difficult. These obstacles can be overcome using cultures of cardiac cells. The main advantage of cell cultures is that they grow as two-dimensional monolayers that allow precise microscopic measurements of both the tissue structure and electrophysiological parameters and their correlation. In addition, the monolayer structure can be modified in a desired way using techniques for patterned cell growth, which greatly facilitates structure-function studies. Electrophysiological parameters of cell cultures such as the maximal upstroke rate of rise and the conduction velocity are quite similar to those measured in adult ventricular tissue.[22]

The use of cell cultures allows V_m measurements at microscopic resolution using the optical mapping technique. This method involves staining of tissue with a voltage-sensitive dye and measurement of either dye absorption or, more often, dye fluorescence, using an array of photodetectors. This method has been widely used for multisite recordings of V_m from brain and cardiac tissue. It has several important advantages over conventional recordings that use electrodes. One of the main advantages is that optical mapping allows simultaneous measurements of V_m at hundreds or thousands of locations, whereas electrical V_m recordings are limited to just a few sites. Another advantage is that optical signals are devoid of stimulation artifacts, which is especially important in defibrillation studies where strong artifacts created by defibrillation shocks interfere with electrical measurements of V_m during shocks and 20–50 ms after the shocks. A disadvantage of optical mapping is that the optical signals reflect only relative changes of membrane potential. The absolute value of optical signals depends on multiple factors, including the density of dye staining, degree of dye internalization, uniformity of excitation light intensity, and others. Combination of these factors results in a significant variability of fluorescence intensity throughout a preparation, independently of the underlying variation of V_m. The V_m-independent variability of optical signals can be somewhat reduced by measuring the fractional changes in fluorescence relative to the background fluorescence level. This does not, however, eliminate the signal variability completely, because the fractional change of fluorescence itself may vary throughout the preparation (mainly due to nonuniform dye internalization).

In defibrillation studies, the V_m-independent variability can be eliminated by normalization of optical signals relative to their respective action potential amplitudes (APA).[23] This procedure is especially useful in measuring shock-induced V_m changes (ΔV_m) that are typically normalized by the APA values. Such signal normalization is based on the assumption that APA does not change across the imaged area, which is likely to be true in healthy, well-coupled tissue. The validity of this condition is even more likelier in microscopic measurements, when the size of an imaged area is comparable to the length of the electrotonic constant, which in cell monolayers is about $360\,\mu m$.[24] This assumption might not hold true on a larger spatial scale in pathologic conditions, such as ischemia, which leads to nonuniform distribution of APA.

The Role of Cell Boundaries in Shock Effects

Cell cultures were used to evaluate contributions of several microscopic tissue structures into shock effects. One of the most intriguing possibilities is that V_m changes can be caused by the boundaries of individual cells. This idea was proposed based on theoretical studies using a one-dimensional cable model with periodic resistive barriers.[12-14] In this model, changes in V_m appear as periodic (saw-tooth) oscillations with hyperpolarization on one side of a resistive barrier and depolarization on the other side. The idea that cell boundaries account for defibrillation is very attractive because this type of structural discontinuity is the most universal feature of biological tissue. However, the hypothesis that cell boundaries induce major changes in V_m was not confirmed experimentally.

The effect of cell boundaries on shock-induced ΔV_m was investigated in cultured cell strands.[23] Strands were narrow, accommodating only four to six cells across their width. In such strands, because of the aligning influence of the strand edges, cells were oriented along the strand axis, mimicking anisotropic cell arrangement in the intact tissue. Uniform-field shocks were applied along the strand axis and shock-induced V_m changes (ΔV_m) were measured optically with microscopic resolution. Figure 2 illustrates a typical example of ΔV_m measurements with resolution of $6\,\mu m$ per diode during application of a shock in the action potential plateau. At all mapping sites, the cell membrane was hyperpolarized during the shock. There was no abrupt transition from hyperpolarization to depolarization, as expected from secondary sources. In addition, no significant changes in ΔV_m magnitudes between sites located across cell membranes were found. These data indicate a complete absence of secondary sources at intercellular junctions.

This finding is at odds with the prediction of discontinuous cable model with cellular structure. A likely explanation for this discrepancy is the effect of "lateral averaging" in two- and three-dimensional tissues described for microscopic conduction,[22] which is absent in one-dimensional models representing cardiac tissue as a single cell chain. In cell chains, strong secondary sources are formed because all axial current generated by a shock is forced to flow through every intercellular junction, which results in a large voltage drop across the junction. Such secondary sources at intercellular junctions were observed using optical mapping in isolated cell pairs.[25] In a two- or three-dimensional tissue, however, a portion of

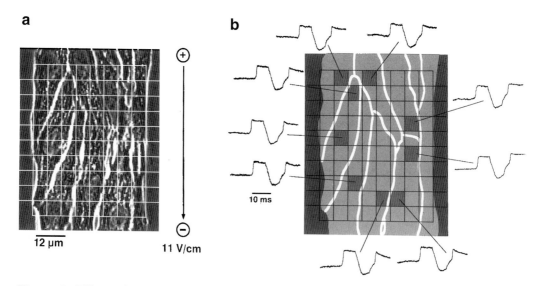

Figure 2: Effect of cell boundaries on shock-induced ΔV_{m} in cultured cell monolayers. (a) Phase-contrast image of cells in a strand (magnification ×100). The grid illustrates the region monitored by each photodiode. The area of each square is $6 \times 6\,\mu\mathrm{m}^2$. (b) Drawing of the cell strand with outlined borders of individual cells. Traces show selected action potentials demonstrating the ΔV_{m} measured at sites within individual cells and across cell borders during a shock with a field strength of $11\,\mathrm{V\,cm}^{-1}$ delivered in the longitudinal direction of the strand (from Ref. 23)

axial current can bypass a given junction and flow through other junctions offered by lateral cell contacts. In cell cultures, this averaging effect might be especially prominent because of the relatively uniform distribution of gap junctions along the cell perimeter.[26] In the adult cardiac tissue in vivo, competing factors can alter the contributions of cell junctions to ΔV_{m}. On one hand, adult myocytes are longer than the cultured neonatal cells, and gap junctions in the ventricular myocardium tend to concentrate at cell ends,[27] thus favoring the formation of secondary sources. On the other hand, cells in the intact tissue are arranged in a three-dimensional structure, where each cell has connections with an average of 11.3 cells.[28] Such cell arrangement increases the degree of intercellular connectivity, which should reduce the effects of individual resistive barriers on V_{m}. How these opposing influences affect ΔV_{m} in the intact adult myocardium is not presently known. However, measurements of shock-induced ΔV_{m} in rabbit papillary muscle using a roving microelectrode moved at microscopic steps[29] or high-resolution optical mapping[30] did not reveal a pattern of alternating positive and negative polarization changes on a subcellular scale. These data support the conclusion drawn from cell culture studies about the lack of secondary sources at intercellular junctions.

The Role of Intercellular Clefts in the Shock Effects

After it was found that cell boundaries do not produce significant changes in V_m, the search for secondary sources shifted to larger anatomical discontinuities. One example of such discontinuities is represented by inclusions of connective tissue into the myocardial structure that interrupt the continuity of the intracellular space on a scale of several cell lengths or more. To investigate the effect of such structures on V_m, we produced cell monolayers with intercellular clefts of variable dimensions.[31] Uniform-field shocks were applied across clefts, and the V_m changes were measured as a function of the cleft length.

Figure 3a, b demonstrate the effect of electrical shocks applied during action potential (AP) plateau on V_m near an intercellular cleft with a length of approximately 240 μm. The isopotential ΔV_m map of selected V_m traces shows that the pattern of ΔV_m distribution was consistent with the mechanism of secondary sources. The shock depolarized cells on the anodal side of the cleft and hyperpolarized cells on the cathodal side. With the reversed shock polarity (not shown), the regions of depolarization and hyperpolarization were interchanged. Similar ΔV_m patterns were observed in other cell cultures. The strength of secondary sources, defined as the ΔV_m difference measured across the middle of an obstacle, depends on both field strength and cleft length. Within the range of cleft lengths of 45–270 μm, the relation between the obstacle length and the secondary source strength could be closely approximated by a linear fit. These data can be used to estimate the cleft length required for direct cell stimulation. Assuming that the cell activation threshold is $\sim$25 mV, the estimated critical obstacle length was approximately 85 ± 8 μm for a shock strength of 18.0 $V\,cm^{-1}$ and 171 ± 7 μm for a shock strength of 8.5 V/cm^{-1}.

To test the prediction that resistive discontinuities cause direct excitation of cardiac tissue during application of extracellular shocks, shocks were delivered during diastole. Figure 3c, d show an isochronal map of activation spread and selected V_m recordings from the sites surrounding the cleft. The shock directly activated a small cell region on the right side of the cleft, which corresponded to the region of maximal depolarization produced by the shock during AP plateau. Cells on the other side of the cleft were transiently hyperpolarized by the shock. This initial hyperpolarization was followed by depolarization, which resulted from the propagating wave. An almost symmetrically reversed activation pattern was observed when the shock polarity was reversed (not shown). The stimulating efficacy of secondary sources depended on shock strength and obstacle length. With an average shock strength of 8.2 V/cm^{-1}, shocks of both polarities directly excited cells when the obstacle length was 196 ± 53 μm, and no direct activation was observed at obstacles with length of 84 ± 23 μm. Thus, the critical cleft length necessary for the direct cell activation with shocks of 8.2 V/cm^{-1} was between 84 and 196 μm. The estimate of critical length of 171 ± 7 μm obtained from shock-induced changes of V_m during the plateau phase of action potential falls within this range. Discontinuities with dimensions of several hundred micrometers and larger are common in ventricular myocardium. In human pectinate muscle, connective tissue septa with such dimensions were found in ventricular tissue from young individuals, and much larger (up to 1 mm) septa were found in the aging myocardium.[32] Experiments in

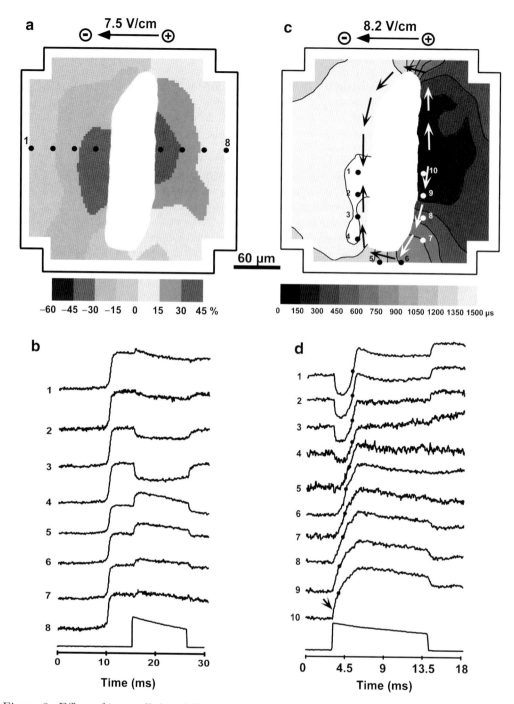

Figure 3: Effect of intercellular clefts on shock-induced ΔV_m and activation in cell cultures. (a) Isopotential map of ΔV_m produced by a shock applied during action potential plateau. Gray area depicts an intercellular cleft (length $= 240\,\mu\mathrm{m}$). (b) Selected V_m traces from locations indicated in (a). (c) Isochronal map of activation spread (interval $0.15\,\mathrm{ms}$) initiated by a shock. Activation was started by a secondary source on the anodal side of the cleft. (d) Selected V_m traces from locations indicated in (c). *Arrow* indicates the direct membrane depolarization produced by the shock (from Ref. 31)

cell cultures suggest that such unexcitable obstacles may contribute to tissue excitation and defibrillation during the application of extracellular electrical shocks in the whole heart.

Shock-Induced ΔV_m in Cell Strands

Cell bundles and cell layers represent another common type of structural tissue organization at the microscopic level. The laminar structure might be especially important because it is present in the intramural bulk of ventricular myocardium where cardiac cells are organized into layers with thickness varying from tens to hundreds of microns.[21,33] Boundaries of cell layers form resistive barriers to current flow and, therefore, may provide substrates for secondary sources during shock application. Similar to cell borders, the magnitude of laminar secondary sources and their relevance for defibrillation depend on multiple factors, including layer thickness, density of interlayer connections, electrotonic space constant, and so forth. The direct experimental observation of microscopic secondary sources in the intact tissue is not currently feasible. Therefore, to estimate their role in defibrillation, researchers mimicked the laminar type of structure in cell cultures, using linear cell strands of variable width, and measured their filed responses, using optical mapping.

Optical measurements of shock-induced ΔV_m were performed in cell strands with width varying between 0.2 and 2 mm.[34–36] As expected, shocks applied during AP plateau depolarized cells facing the cathode and hyperpolarized cells facing the anode (Fig. 4). Similar to the predictions of the linear cable model, weak shocks applied to narrow strands produced linear V_m responses with equal magnitudes of positive and negative ΔV_m (Fig. 4a). The symmetry of V_m response was maintained for ΔV_m below approximately 40% APA.[34] Increasing the shock strength and/or the strand width resulted in an increase of ΔV_m magnitude and a loss of ΔV_m linearity. One such change was that polarizations became asymmetric where negative ΔV_m significantly exceeded positive ΔV_m (Fig. 4b, thin black traces). When the shock strength was further increased, another change in ΔV_m shape was observed. In these cases, ΔV_m became nonmonotonic, with negative ΔV_m exhibiting shift to more positive levels, which reduced the degree of negative ΔV_m asymmetry (Fig. 4b, thick black traces). Besides changes in ΔV_m shapes, both positive and negative ΔV_m exhibited saturation at high shock strength. The saturation level depended on the ΔV_m polarity: positive ΔV_m reached saturation at a relatively low level of $\sim 100\%$ APA, whereas negative ΔV_m saturated above 200% APA.

The nonlinear features of V_m responses described above, including ΔV_m asymmetry, nonmonotonic ΔV_m shape, and saturation, were also observed in the intact myocardium.[37–40] These effects may have important implications for defibrillation. For instance, since during fibrillation most of the myocardium is in the depolarized state, the effects of electrical shocks on V_m are predicted to be asymmetric, with a larger portion of myocardium undergoing negative rather than positive polarizations. It was shown that an interaction between areas of hyper- and depolarization might determine the success or the failure of defibrillation.[41,42] Therefore, ΔV_m asymmetry affects the outcome of a defibrillation shock. The knowledge of ionic mechanisms involved in shock-induced ΔV_m might provide an opportunity

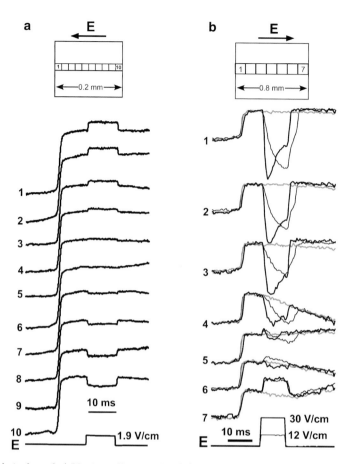

Figure 4: Shock-induced ΔV_{m} in cell strands. (**a**) Linear ΔV_{m} produced by weak shocks in narrow cell strands. Strand width equals $200\,\mu\mathrm{m}$; shock strength $E = 1.9\,\mathrm{V/cm}^{-1}$. Insert shows schematics of a cell strand with photodiode locations. (**b**) Nonlinear asymmetric (*thin black traces*) and nonmonotonic (*thick traces*) ΔV_{m}. *Gray traces* show V_{m} recordings without shocks (from Refs. 34,36)

for pharmacological modulation of ΔV_{m} asymmetry and, therefore, of defibrillation efficacy.

Until now ionic mechanisms of nonlinear V_{m} responses were investigated only in cell cultures[34,35,43–45] and isolated single cells.[46] The ΔV_{m} asymmetry with larger $\Delta V_{\mathrm{m}}^{-}$ than $\Delta V_{\mathrm{m}}^{+}$ reflects an increase in the net outward current. Inhibition of potassium currents in cell cultures using barium chloride (blocker of inward rectifier current), dofetilide (delayed rectifier current), and 4-AP (transient outward current) did not change ΔV_{m} significantly,[34,35] indicating that none of these outward currents was responsible for the ΔV_{m} asymmetry. In contrast, it was found that the asymmetric behavior of ΔV_{m} was partially reversed by inhibition L-type calcium current.[35] As shown in Fig. 5, application of nifedipine in cell strands increased positive ΔV_{m} while leaving negative ΔV_{m} unaffected, thus reducing the degree of ΔV_{m} asymmetry. These findings indicate that ΔV_{m} asymmetry is caused by the outward flow of $I_{\mathrm{Ca,L}}$ in the depolarized portions of strands. Normally, $I_{\mathrm{Ca,L}}$ is inward but it changes the direction when V_{m} exceeds the $I_{\mathrm{Ca,L}}$ reversal potential. According to patch clamp studies, the $I_{\mathrm{Ca,L}}$ reversal potential in rat and rabbit myocytes is 45–50 mV.[47,48] Therefore, positive ΔV_{m} with magnitudes larger than $\sim$50 mV should be reduced by the outward flow of $I_{\mathrm{Ca,L}}$, which explains why blocking of $I_{\mathrm{Ca,L}}$ with nifedipine increases $\Delta V_{\mathrm{m}}^{+}$.

The important role of $I_{\mathrm{Ca,L}}$ in ΔV_{m} asymmetry was corroborated by measurements of shock-induced Ca_i^{2+} changes.[44] According to this mechanism, shocks should decrease Ca_i^{2+} in the area of positive ΔV_{m} due to the outward flow of Ca^{2+} ions through of L-type channels. To test this prediction, shock-induced ΔCa_i^{2+} were measured in cultured cell strands. As shown in Fig. 6, shocks applied during AP plateau transiently decreased Ca_i^{2+} in areas of both positive and negative ΔV_{m}. Inhibition of $I_{\mathrm{Ca,L}}$ by nifedipine eliminated shock-induced Ca_i^{2+} decrease at sites of positive ΔV_{m} (not shown). On the other side, inhibition of sarcoplasmic reticulum by either caffeine or thapsigargin had no effect on ΔCa_i^{2+}.

Computer simulations in an ionic model of rat ventricular myocytes further supported these experimental findings.[44,45] Similar to experiments, application of shocks in the model during the early AP produced (1) negatively asymmetric ΔV_{m} and (2) decrease of Ca_i^{2+} in areas of both $\Delta V_{\mathrm{m}}^{+}$ and $\Delta V_{\mathrm{m}}^{-}$. Selective inhibition of sarcoplasmic reticulum had no effect on ΔCa_i^{2+}. In contrast, inhibition of $I_{\mathrm{Ca,L}}$ increased $\Delta V_{\mathrm{m}}^{+}$, reduced ΔV_{m} asymmetry, and eliminated shock-induced Ca_i^{2+} decrease in the $\Delta V_{\mathrm{m}}^{+}$ area. Thus, both experiments and computer simulations support the hypothesis about the role of $I_{\mathrm{Ca,L}}$ in negative ΔV_{m} asymmetry and shock-induced Ca_i^{2+} decrease.

The second type of nonlinear V_{m} response in cell cultures characterized by nonmonotonic negative ΔV_{m} can be due to an inward ionic current activated at negative V_{m} or due to a nonspecific leakage current caused by membrane electroporation. The occurrence of such nonmonotonic ΔV_{m} in cell cultures was paralleled with diastolic elevation of V_{m} as well as with induction of postshock arrhythmias.[36] The polarization threshold for nonmonotonic $\Delta V_{\mathrm{m}}^{-}$ was approximately 200% APA, which corresponds to a V_{m} level of approximately -180 mV. There are two inward currents that are open at such V_{m} levels: "funny" current (I_{f}) and inward rectifier current (I_{K1}). Their role in nonlinear ΔV_{m} was examined using channel blockers. It was found that inhibition of I_{K1} by barium chloride and of I_{f} by cesium chloride caused no effect on ΔV_{m} shape,[43] indicating that these currents were not responsible for nonmonotonic ΔV_{m}. The role of membrane electroporation was examined by measuring shock-induced uptake of a cell impermeable dye, propidium iodide, which becomes fluorescent after entering cells and binding to nucleic acids. It was found that application of a series of shocks with strength similar to the one inducing nonmonotonic $\Delta V_{\mathrm{m}}^{-}$ caused cell uptake of propidium iodide at the anodal side of cell strands where negative ΔV_{m} were induced but not on the cathodal side (Fig. 7).[43] Shock-induced dye uptake paralleled with nonmonotonic ΔV_{m} and diastolic V_{m} elevation were also observed

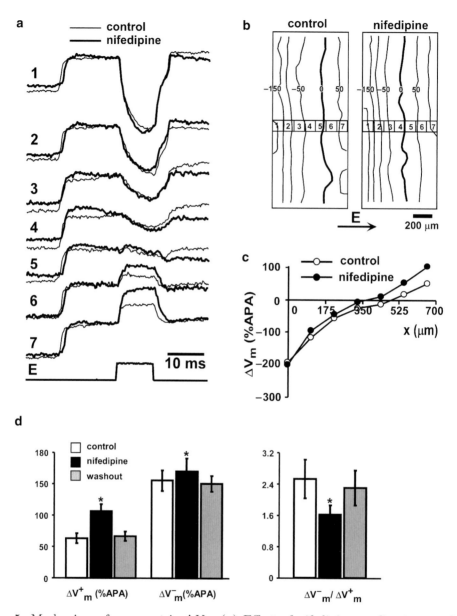

Figure 5: Mechanism of asymmetric ΔV_m. (a) Effect of nifedipine application on shock-induced ΔV_m. Shock strength was $\sim 10.7\,\mathrm{V/cm^{-1}}$. (b) Isopotential maps of ΔV_m distribution. (c) Spatial profiles of ΔV_m across the strand. (d) Effect of nifedipine on magnitudes of ΔV_m^+, ΔV_m^-, and asymmetry ratio $\Delta V_m^-/\Delta V_m^+$. Shock strength was $9.3 \pm 0.8\,\mathrm{V/cm^{-1}}$. *Statistically significant difference from control value ($p < .05$) (from Ref. 35)

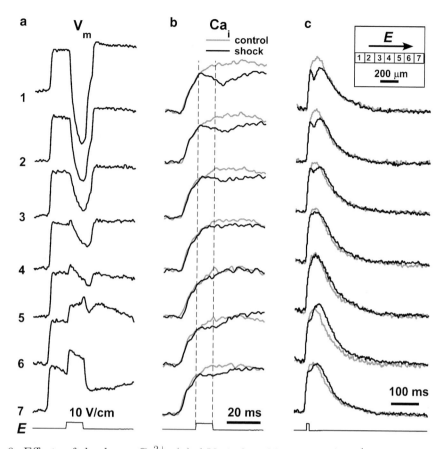

Figure 6: Effects of shocks on Ca_i^{2+}. (a) ΔV_m induced by a 10-V/cm^{-1} shock in a cultured cell strand (width = 0.8 mm). Locations of recordings are shown in the inset in (c). (b) Changes in Ca_i^{2+} during the shock in comparison to control recordings. (c) Longer recordings of Ca_i^{2+} transients (from Ref. 44)

on epicardial surface of rabbit hearts.[49] These data in combination with the results of experiments with ionic channel blockers indicate that nonmonotonic negative ΔV_m were due to membrane electroporation.

Strong shocks may induce arrhythmias,[50–53] which can explain the reduced defibrillation efficacy of very strong shocks.[54] The field threshold for postshock arrhythmias in cell cultures was very close to the thresholds for nonmonotonic negative ΔV_m and electroporation.[36] Optical mapping in cell strands with local expansions demonstrated that postshock arrhythmias were focal, and that the arrhythmia source was located in the hyperpolarized area of strands (Fig. 8),[36] indicating that postshock arrhythmias were caused by membrane electroporation.

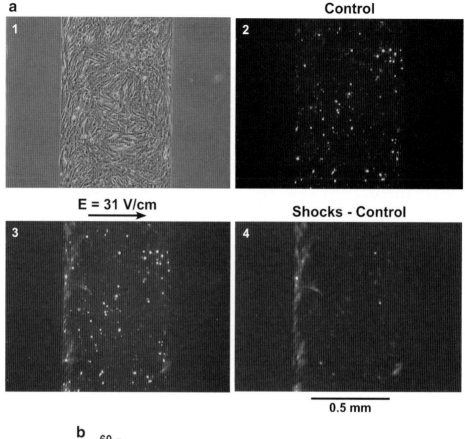

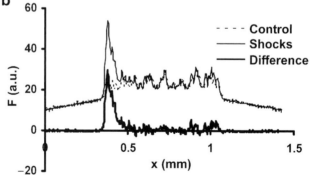

Figure 7: Mechanism of nonmonotonic ΔV_m: shock-induced uptake of cell-impermeable dye propidium iodide. (**a1**) Phase contrast image of a cell strand (width = 0.7 mm). (**a2**) Image of dye fluorescence after control dye application for 4 min (no shocks). (**a3**) Image of dye fluorescence after application of a series of shocks with a strength of 31 V/cm^{-1} and interval of 2 s. (**a4**) Difference between images in (**a2**) and (**a3**). The resulting image was filtered with a median filter. (**b**) Average horizontal profiles of fluorescent intensity (in arbitrary units) from images in (**a2**) (control), (**a3**) (shocks), and (**a4**) (difference) (from Ref. 43)

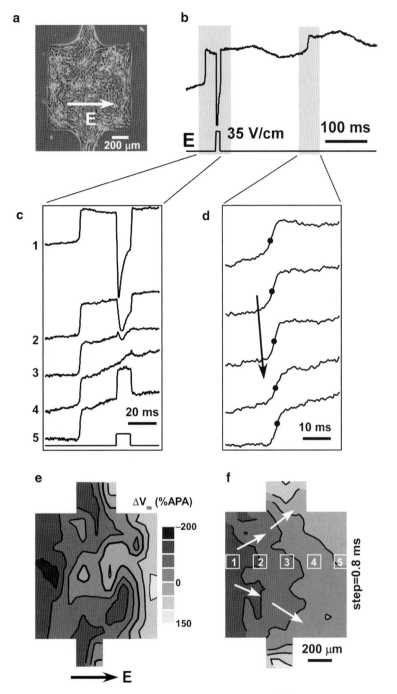

Figure 8: Localization of the shock-induced arrhythmias. (**a**) Phase contrast image of a narrow cell strand with an area of local expansion. (**b**) Recordings of V_m during application of $35\,\mathrm{V/cm}^{-1}$ shock. (**c**, **d**) V_m recordings at selected sites during shock application and during the postshock extrabeat. The *arrow* in (**d**) depicts the direction of activation spread. (**e**) Isopotential map of shock-induced ΔV_m distribution 5 ms after the shock onset. (**f**) Isochronal map of activation spread during the extra beat (from Ref. 36)

Measurements of Intramural Shock-Induced ΔV_m in Wedge Preparations

Experiments in cell cultures provided information about the effects of shocks on V_m at the microscopic level. However, cell cultures are structurally and electrophysiologically different from the intact myocardium. Therefore, results obtained in cell cultures cannot be directly applied to the whole myocardium, which necessitates measurements of the shock effects in the whole tissue. Since no experimental methods to measure intramural V_m in the intact heart are currently available, an approach based on optical mapping of V_m on the cut transmural surface in isolated wedge preparations of left ventricular was used. Such a preparation consists of a portion of left ventricular (LV) wall maintained viable via perfusion through a branch of coronary artery. Uniform-field shocks were applied parallel to the cut surface in order to avoid formation of ΔV_m due to the boundary conditions on this surface. Several optical mapping studies were carried out in these preparations to characterize the effects of shocks on transmural V_m.

In the first study,[39] the whole transmural surface was mapped at a spatial resolution of ~ 1.2 mm per diode. Shocks of variable strength (2–50 V/cm^{-1}) were applied in the early phase of AP. It was found that effects of shocks on transmural V_m strongly depended on the shock strength. Relatively weak shocks (~ 2 V/cm^{-1}) induced positive and negative polarizations at the tissue edges facing the cathode and the anode, respectively (Fig. 9a). Changing the shock polarity reversed the polarization pattern. For shocks of both polarities, maximal ΔV_m^+ and ΔV_m^- were achieved at the wall edges, and there was a relatively gradual transition of ΔV_m magnitude between the edges with relatively small ($< 6\%$ APA) local V_m changes in the wall middle. Shocks caused prolongation of action potential duration (APD)$_{50}$ at sites of maximal ΔV_m^+, whereas at sites of maximal ΔV_m^- the APD$_{50}$ was either not changed or slightly prolonged.

Increasing shock strength above ~ 4 V/cm^{-1} produced several important changes in polarization patterns. First, such shocks produced localized positive and negative ΔV_m inside the wall (Fig. 9b). Such isolated polarizations, as well as the overall nonuniform distribution of ΔV_m across the wall, indicated the presence of intramural virtual electrodes. Second, shock-induced polarizations became strongly asymmetric, with negative ΔV_m exceeding positive ΔV_m measured at the same sites at the opposite shock polarity. This is similar to the ΔV_m behavior observed in cell cultures. Third, negative ΔV_m extended toward the cathodal side of the preparation. This was different from measurements in cell cultures where only positive polarizations were observed at the cathodal edge of cell strands. Fourth, shocks prolonged APD everywhere across the wall, including sites with both positive and negative ΔV_m and ΔV_m. This finding was also surprising because APD was expected to decrease at the sites of negative ΔV_m where positive charges are removed from the intracellular space.

Increasing the shock strength further caused even more drastic changes in polarization patterns. Shocks with a strength of ~ 20 V/cm^{-1} and larger of both polarities produced predominantly negative ΔV_m across the whole transmural wall (Fig. 9c). In addition, shocks prolonged APD everywhere in the wall. The degree of APD prolongation was

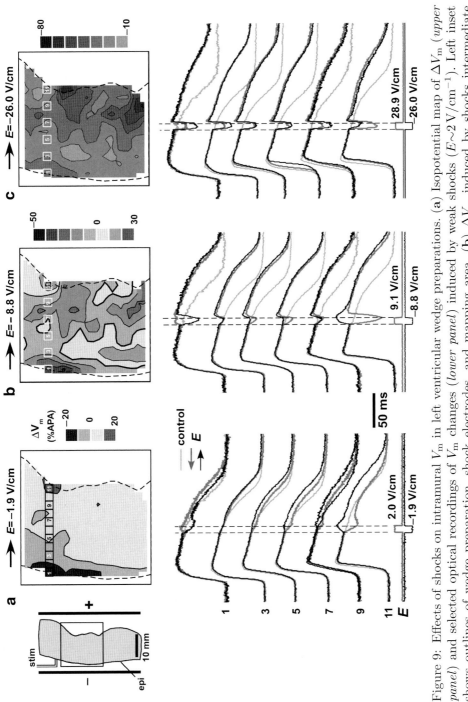
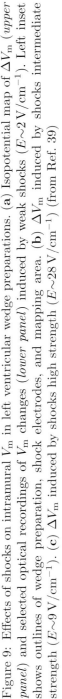

Figure 9: Effects of shocks on intramural V_{m} in left ventricular wedge preparations. (a) Isopotential map of ΔV_{m} (*upper panel*) and selected optical recordings of V_{m} changes (*lower panel*) induced by weak shocks ($E{\sim}2\,\mathrm{V/cm}$). Left inset shows outlines of wedge preparation, shock electrodes, and mapping area. (b) ΔV_{m} induced by shocks intermediate strength ($E{\sim}9\,\mathrm{V/cm^{-1}}$). (c) ΔV_{m} induced by shocks high strength ($E{\sim}28\,\mathrm{V/cm^{-1}}$) (from Ref. 39)

similar for shocks of both polarities, and it was not dependent on the local ΔV_m value. Again, these findings are at odds with observations in cell cultures as well as with basic biophysical principles postulating that (1) shocks should induce both positive and negative polarizations, reflecting inflow of shock current into intracellular space at some locations and outflow at other locations and (2) shocks should shorten APD at sites of negative ΔV_m where charges are removed from the cell interior.

A limitation of the wedge preparation is that boundary conditions at the cut transmural surface are different from those in the intact myocardium. Since boundary conditions play a critical role in shock-induced ΔV_m, it may be asked whether or not intramural polarizations are an artifact of the boundary conditions. To prove that this is not the case, intramural polarizations have to be demonstrated in the intact myocardium. Experiments in the wedge preparations showed that negatively biased intramural polarizations induced by strong shocks may extend to the wall surface facing the cathode electrode. It is well known that optical measurements from a surface reflect V_m changes spatially averaged over a certain tissue depth.[55,56] Therefore, it is hypothesized that negative ΔV_m could be measured on the epicardial surface when this surface is facing the cathode. Because only positive polarizations can be produced on the cathodal wall surface, registration of negative ΔV_m on this surface would unequivocally prove the existence of intramural virtual electrodes.

This hypothesis was tested by measuring ΔV_m on the intact epicardial surface in LV preparations stained with a V_m-sensitive dye using two methods: (1) staining via surface dye application (surface staining), and (2) staining via coronary perfusion (global staining).[57,58] With the first method, a surface tissue layer with a thickness of approximately 0.25 mm was stained. In the second case, tissue was stained uniformly across the whole LV wall. Shocks (2–50 V/cm^{-1}) were applied in the epicardial-to-endocardial direction via transparent mesh electrodes. Shock-induced ΔV_m were mapped through the epicardial electrode from the same locations after both surface and global staining. Optical recordings revealed significant differences between ΔV_m measured in two staining conditions, and these differences were especially prominent for cathodal shocks (Fig. 10). Relatively weak cathodal shocks produced positive ΔV_m in both staining conditions. However, ΔV_m measured in the surface-stained tissue were much larger than those measured in the globally stained tissue (Fig. 10c, d). At higher shock strength, cathodal ΔV_m measured in globally stained tissue became uniformly negative, whereas in surface-stained tissue they remained positive (Fig. 10a, b, black traces). These differences in the magnitude and polarity of ΔV_m induced by cathodal shocks in surface- and globally stained tissue can be explained by the presence of intramural virtual electrodes in the subepicardial tissue layers.

The most important finding from these experiments is that shocks cause widespread polarizations in intramural myocardium. The mechanism of these polarizations, however, remains uncertain. It is unlikely that they were due to nonuniform shock field because the electrical field in the bath was uniform without preparations. Therefore, it is more likely that intramural ΔV_m were due to nonuniform tissue structure. It is also likely that two different types of ΔV_m were due to different structural properties. The isolated areas of positive or negative ΔV_m induced by shocks of moderate strength were probably caused by relatively large-scale nonuniformities such as fiber rotation, variation in the intracellular

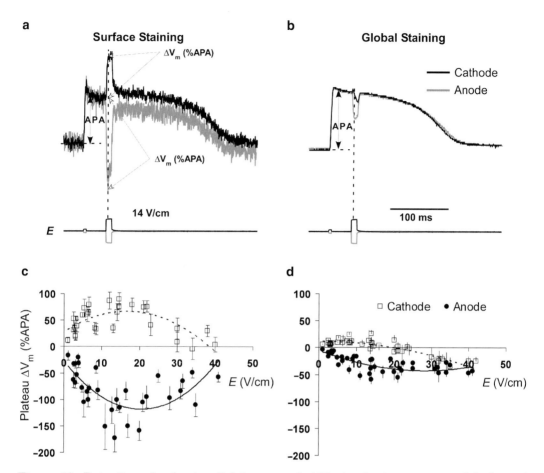

Figure 10: Detection of subepicardial intramural ΔV_{m} in the intact tissue. (**a**) Optical recordings of epicardial V_{m} during application of cathodal (*black trace*) and anodal (*gray trace*) shocks with $E \approx 14\,\mathrm{V/cm}^{-1}$ in a surface-stained preparation. Measurements were performed through an opening in epicardial mesh electrode. (**b**) Corresponding V_{m} recordings in a globally stained preparation. (**c, d**) Dependences of corresponding averaged ΔV_{m} magnitudes on the shock strength. Curves are second order polynomial fits of data (from Ref. 58)

volume fraction, or blood vessels. As expected from ΔV_{m} produced by large nonuniformities, they changed their sign with a change in the shock polarity.

Intramural polarizations of the second type, which remained negative for shocks of both polarities, are likely to have a different anatomic substrate. It is hypothesized that these ΔV_{m} are due to microscopic discontinuities in the tissue structure associated with collagen septa that are present in the LV wall at a high density.[39] Such layers have microscopic thickness. Therefore, their V_{m} response to electrical shocks should be similar to the behavior of microscopic cultured cell strands. Particularly, shocks are expected to induce both positive and negative ΔV_{m} on the opposite sides of cell layers. However, because these polarizations were measured on a macroscopic scale (1.2 mm), negative and positive polarizations should be averaged out. When cardiac tissue has a linear V_{m} response to electrical field, the net result should be zero or a negligible macroscopic polarization. This explains the absence of intramural ΔV_{m} during weak shocks when V_{m} response is linear. Stronger shocks, however, induce nonlinear ΔV_{m} with a strong negative bias ($\Delta V_{\mathrm{m}}^{-} > \Delta V_{\mathrm{m}}^{+}$) during AP plateau. Because of this asymmetry, macroscopic measurements should yield only negative ΔV_{m}. This can potentially explain globally negative polarizations observed in wedge preparations.

The logical test of the hypothesis postulating the existence of microscopic polarizations is mapping of ΔV_{m} at a high spatial resolution. Therefore, transmural ΔV_{m} was mapped at a tenfold higher optical magnification ($0.11 \, \mathrm{mm/diode}^{-1}$ vs. $1.2 \, \mathrm{mm/diode}^{-1}$).[59] As shown previously, in low-magnification recordings ΔV_{m} produced by strong shocks were globally negative, extending to the wall edge for both anodal and cathodal shocks (Fig. 11a, b). In contrast, high-magnification recordings at the wall edge revealed positive ΔV_{m} for cathodal shocks (Fig. 11d) and negative ΔV_{m} for anodal shocks (Fig. 11c) for all shock strengths. Positive ΔV_{m} were also observed at high magnification in the middle of the wall (not shown). However, alternation of positive and negative ΔV_{m}, expected from microscopic secondary sources, was not found. This can be explained by the fact that optical resolution does not scale up with increasing optical magnification. Indeed, it was shown in a mathematical model of light propagation that, due to light scattering in three-dimensional cardiac tissue, an increase in optical magnification leads only to a modest increase in resolution.[55] Even when the size of the imaged area becomes negligible, dimensions of the interrogated tissue volume remain relatively above several hundred microns.

The excitatory hypothesis of defibrillation mechanism postulates that shocks cause direct and simultaneous activation of the majority of excitable or partially excitable tissue. To test this hypothesis, transmural activation patterns induced by shocks applied during diastolic phase of cardiac cycle in wedge preparations were measured.[40] It was found that during the weakest shocks ($\sim$1–4 V/cm^{-1}) applied in diastole, earliest activation occurred predominantly (but not exclusively) on the cathodal side of preparations. The time of transmural spread (several milliseconds) was significantly shorter than the activation time after local epicardial stimulation, indicating that transmural activation was the result of the direct tissue activation by a shock of some areas as well as of impulse propagation from these directly excited areas. During shocks of intermediate strength ($\sim$4–23 V/cm^{-1}), activation was initiated at multiple transmural sites from where it rapidly (within ¡1 ms) spread across the whole LV wall. Very strong shocks ($\sim$23–44 V/cm^{-1}) could cause discontinuous activation, where some areas were activated immediately on the shock onset and other areas were activated with a large delay. In all cases, the sites of the earliest activation corresponded to the areas of largest ΔV_{m} measured during AP plateau; the sites of delayed activation observed during the strongest shocks corresponded to the areas of minimal plateau ΔV_{m}. Thus, diastolic shocks with a strength varying over a wide range cause direct and nearly simultaneous activation of the whole LV wall. Sites of earliest and latest activation correspond to areas of maximal and minimal ΔV_{m} measured during shocks applied in AP plateau. These findings support the excitatory hypothesis of defibrillation.

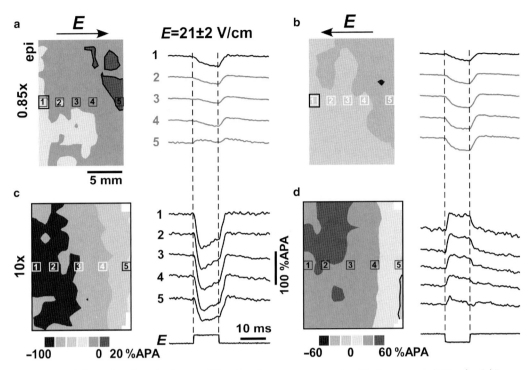

Figure 11: The role of optical magnification in measurements of intramural ΔV_{m}. (a, b)Low-magnification (0.85×) measurements of ΔV_{m} in the subepicardial transmural region of LV wall during action potential plateau. Resolution equals $1.2\,\mathrm{mm/diode^{-1}}$. Shock strength $E \approx 21\,\mathrm{V/cm^{-1}}$. (c, d) High-magnification (10×) measurements of ΔV_{m} from the area shown in (a) and (b) by the *thick rectangle*. *Thin rectangles* correspond to individual photodiodes. *Thick lines* in maps depict boundaries between areas of positive and negative ΔV_{m}. *Black and gray traces* display plateau ΔV_{m} inside and outside of the high-magnification mapping area (from Ref. 59)

They also indicate that shock-induced activation is caused by formation of microscopic intramural secondary sources.

Comparison between Microscopic and Macroscopic ΔV_{m} Measurements

Optical measurements of V_{m} changes in wedge preparations support the hypothesis of microscopic intramural secondary sources. However, the origin of these sources, their anatomic substrate, and their dimensions remain unknown. To obtain an estimate of their dimensions, we compared spatially averaged microscopic V_{m} responses measured in patterned cell cultures with macroscopic intramural V_{m} changes measured in wedge preparations.[60]

Microscopic measurements were performed in cultured cell strands with widths of 0.1 and 0.8 mm. Shocks applied during AP plateau produced ΔV_m similar to those shown in Fig. 4. Figure 12a shows the effects of spatial averaging of microscopic polarizations induced by shocks applied either during AP plateau or diastole in cell strands. For weak shocks $(4.4\,\text{V/cm}^{-1})$ applied in narrow strands during AP plateau (gray traces), spatial averaging

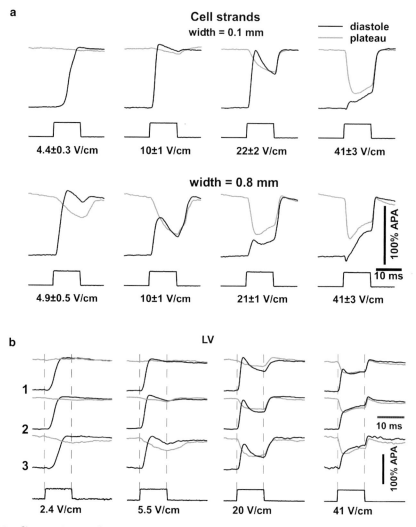

Figure 12: Comparison of microscopic and macroscopic measurements of shock-induced V_m changes. (a) Spatially averaged optical V_m measurements in cultured cell strands with width of 0.1 mm (*upper panel*) and 0.8 mm (*lower panel*). Shocks of various strength were applied either during action plateau (*gray traces*) or during diastole (*black traces*). (b) Measurements of shock effects on intramural V_m in wedge preparations of porcine left ventricular (from Ref. 60)

resulted in negligible ΔV_m. This was because positive and negative microscopic polarizations had nearly equal magnitudes, canceling each other after averaging. Negligible polarizations were also observed in macroscopic intramural measurements in LV wedge preparations during weak shocks (Fig. 12b, shock strengths 2.4 and 5.5 V/cm^{-1}). In contrast, in wider 0.8-mm strands, averaged plateau ΔV_m were negative for all shock strengths, reflecting the fact that microscopic polarizations became negatively asymmetric. Increasing shock strength caused an increase of negative ΔV_m in strands of both widths and a change of the ΔV_m shape from monotonic to nonmonotonic (Fig. 12a). Similar ΔV_m changes were also observed in LV tissue (Fig. 12b). The transition from monotonic to nonmonotonic ΔV_m in narrow strands occurred between 20 and 40 V/cm^{-1}, which was similar to the same transition in LV tissue. In wide cell strands, this transition was at a lower shock strength, between 10 and 20 V/cm^{-1}. Thus, changes in the magnitude and shape of ΔV_m in LV tissue were better approximated by ΔV_m changes in narrow cell strands than in wide strands. This was also the case with regard to the shape of AP upstrokes induced by shocks in diastole (black traces). These data indicate that structures responsible for intramural V_m changes in LV tissue have dimensions on the order of a hundred microns. It should be mentioned that the correspondence between averaged microscopic and macroscopic V_m measurements was not complete. In particular, the magnitude of average polarizations in cell strands (Fig. 12a) was larger than that in LV tissue (Fig. 12b). This difference could be due to different ionic membrane properties of neonatal cultured cells and adult intact myocardium.

Conclusion

Experiments in wedge preparations demonstrate that electrical shocks induce intramural polarizations and directly excite tissue far from the wall surfaces due to formation of secondary sources with submillimeter dimensions. Experiments in cell cultures indicate that the smallest resistive discontinuities related to individual cell boundaries produce negligible polarizations that play no role in defibrillation. These experiments also demonstrate that larger structures such as intercellular clefts and cell strands lead to significant shock-induced polarizations. Comparison of optical measurements in cell cultures and wedge preparations revealed significant similarities between the shapes of macroscopic polarizations measured in whole tissue and of spatially averaged microscopic polarizations measured in cultured cell strands with the width of approximately a hundred microns. These findings indicate that intramural cell layers with such dimensions may be responsible for defibrillation.

References

1. Tung L. Detrimental effects of electrical fields on cardiac muscle. *Proc IEEE* 1996;84:366–378
2. Valenzuela TD, Roe DJ, Cretin S, Spaite DW, Larsen MP. Estimating effectiveness of cardiac arrest interventions: a logistic regression survival model. *Circulation* 1997;96:3308–3313

3. Garcia LA, Allan JJ, Kerber RE. Interactions between CPR and defibrillation wave-forms: effect on resumption of a perfusing rhythm after defibrillation. *Resuscitation* 2000;47:301–305

4. Geddes LA, Roeder RA, Kemeny A, Otlewski M. The duration of ventricular fibrillation required to produce pulseless electrical activity. *Am J Emerg Med* 2005;23:138–141

5. Kléber AG, Janse MJ, Fast VG. Normal and abnormal conduction in the heart. *Handbook of Physiology. Section 2: The Cardiovascular System*. Oxford: Oxford University Press; 2001:455–530

6. Chen PS, Wu TJ, Ting CT, Karagueuzian HS, Garfinkel A, Lin SF, Weiss JN. A tale of two fibrillations. *Circulation* 2003;108:2298–2303

7. Weiss JN, Chen PS, Wu TJ, Siegerman C, Garfinkel A. Ventricular fibrillation: new insights into mechanisms. *Ann N Y Acad Sci* 2004;1015:122–132

8. Gurvich NL, Yuneiv GS. Restoration of regular rhythm in the mammalian fibrillating heart. *Am Rev Sov Med* 1946;3:236–239

9. Zipes DP, Fisher J, King RM, Nicoll AB, Jolly WW. Termination of ventricular fibrillation in dogs by depolarizing a critical amount of myocardium. *Am J Cardiol* 1975;36:37–44

10. Zhou XH, Daubert JP, Wolf PD, Smith WM, Ideker RE. Epicardial mapping of ventricular defibrillation with monophasic and biphasic shocks in dogs. *Circ Res* 1993;72:145–160

11. Weidmann S. Electrical constants of trabecular muscle from mammalian heart. *J Physiol* 1970;210:1041–1054

12. Plonsey R, Barr RC. Effect of microscopic and macroscopic discontinuities on the response of cardiac tissue to defibrillating (stimulating) currents. *Med Biol Eng Comput* 1986;24:130–136

13. Plonsey R, Barr RC. Inclusion of junction elements in a linear cardiac model through secondary sources: application to defibrillation. *Med Biol Eng Comput* 1986;24:137–144

14. Krassowska W, Pilkington T, Ideker RE. Periodic conductivity as a mechanism for cardiac stimulation and defibrillation. *IEEE Trans Biomed Eng* 1987;34:555–560

15. Trayanova N, Plank G, Rodriguez B. What have we learned from mathematical models of defibrillation and postshock arrhythmogenesis? Application of bidomain simulations. *Heart Rhythm* 2006;3:1232–1235

16. Fishler MG. Syncytial heterogeneity as a mechanism underlying cardiac far-field stimulation during defibrillation-level shocks. *J Cardiovasc Electrophysiol* 1998;9:384–394

17. Rattay F. Analysis of models for extracellular fiber stimulation. *IEEE Trans Biomed Eng* 1989;36:676–682

18. Wikswo JP, Lin S-F, Abbas RA. Virtual electrode effect in cardiac tissue: a common mechanism for anodal and cathodal stimulation. *Biophys J* 1995;69:2195–2210

19. Sobie E, Susil R, Tung L. A generalized activating function for predicting virtual electrodes in cardiac tissue. *Biophys J* 1997;73:1410–1423

20. Sepulveda NG, Roth BJ, Wikswo JP. Current injection into a two-dimensional anisotropic bidomain. *Biophys J* 1989;55:987–999

21. Hooks DA, Tomlinson KA, Marsden SG, LeGrice IJ, Smaill BH, Pullan AJ, Hunter PJ. Cardiac microstructure: implications for electrical propagation and defibrillation in the heart. *Circ Res* 2002;91:331–338

22. Fast VG, Kléber AG. Microscopic conduction in cultured strands of neonatal rat heart cells measured with voltage-sensitive dyes. *Circ Res* 1993;73:914–925

23. Gillis AM, Fast VG, Rohr S, Kléber AG. Effects of defibrillation shocks on the spatial distribution of the transmembrane potential in strands and monolayers of cultured neonatal rat ventricular myocytes. *Circ Res* 1996;79:676–690

24. Jongsma HJ, van Rijn HE. Electrotonic spread of current in monolayer cultures of neonatal rat heart cells. *J Membr Biol* 1972;9:341–360

25. Sharma V, Tung L. Theoretical and experimental study of sawtooth effect in isolated cardiac cell-pairs. *J Cardiovasc Electrophysiol* 2001;12:1164–1173

26. Darrow BJ, Laing JG, Lampe PD, Saffitz JE, Beyer EC. Expression of multiple connexins in cultured neonatal rat ventricular myocytes. *Circ Res* 1995;76:381–387

27. Hoyt RH, Cihen ML, Saffitz JE. Distribution and three-dimensional structure of inter-cellular junctions in canine myocardium. *Circ Res* 1989;64:563–574

28. Luke RA, Beyer EC, Hoyt RH, Saffitz JE. Quantitative analysis of intercellular connections by immunohistochemistry of the cardiac gap junction protein Connexin43. *Circ Res* 1989;95:1450–1457

29. Zhou X, Knisley SB, Smith WM, Rollins D, Pollard AE, Ideker RE. Spatial changes in the transmembrane potential during extracellular electric stimulation. *Circ Res* 1998;83:1003–1014

30. Windisch H, Platzer D, Bilgici E. Quantification of shock-induced microscopic virtual electrodes assessed by subcellular resolution optical potential mapping in guinea pig papillary muscle. *J Cardiovasc Electrophysiol* 2007;18:1086–1094

31. Fast VG, Rohr S, Gillis AM, Kléber AG. Activation of cardiac tissue by extracellular electrical shocks: formation of "secondary sources" at intercellular clefts in monolayers of cultured myocytes. *Circ Res* 1998;82:375–385

32. Spach MS, Dolber PC. Relating extracellular potentials and their derivatives to anisotropic propagation at a microscopic level in human cardiac muscle. Evidence for electrical uncoupling of side-to-side fiber connections with increasing age. *Circ Res* 1986;58:356–371

33. Le Grice IJ, Smaill BH, Chai LZ, Edgar SG, Gavin JB, Hunter PJ. Laminar structure of the heart: ventricular myocyte arrangement and connective tissue architecture in the dog. *Am J Physiol* 1995;38:H571–H582

34. Fast VG, Rohr S, Ideker RE. Non-linear changes of transmembrane potential caused by defibrillation shocks in strands of cultured myocytes. *Am J Physiol* 2000;278:H688–H697

35. Cheek ER, Ideker RE, Fast VG. Nonlinear changes of transmembrane potential during defibrillation shocks: role of Ca^{2+} current. *Circ Res* 2000;87:453–459

36. Fast VG, Cheek ER. Optical mapping of arrhythmias induced by strong electrical shocks in myocyte cultures. *Circ Res* 2002;90:664–670

37. Zhou XH, Rollins DL, Smith WM, Ideker RE. Responses of the transmembrane potential of myocardial cells during a shock. *J Cardiovasc Electrophysiol* 1995;6:252–263

38. Zhou XH, Smith WM, Rollins DL, Ideker RE. Transmembrane potential changes caused by shocks in guinea pig papillary muscle. *Am J Physiol* 1996;271:H2536–H2546

39. Fast VG, Sharifov OF, Cheek ER, Newton J, Ideker RE. Intramural virtual electrodes during defibrillation shocks in left ventricular wall assessed by optical mapping of membrane potential. *Circulation* 2002;106:1007–1014

40. Sharifov OF, Fast VG. Optical mapping of transmural activation induced by electrical shocks in isolated left ventricular wall wedge preparations. *J Cardiovasc Electrophysiol* 2003;14:1215–1222

41. Efimov IR, Cheng Y, Van Wagoner DR, Mazgalev T, Tchou PJ. Virtual electrode-induced phase singularity. A basic mechanism of defibrillation failure. *Circ Res* 1998;82:918–925

42. Efimov IR, Gray RA, Roth BJ. Virtual electrodes and deexcitation: new insights into fibrillation induction and defibrillation. *J Cardiovasc Electrophysiol* 2000;11:339–353

43. Cheek ER, Fast VG. Nonlinear changes of transmembrane potential during electrical shocks: role of membrane electroporation. *Circ Res* 2004;94:208–214

44. Fast VG, Cheek ER, Pollard AE, Ideker RE. Effects of electrical shocks on Ca_i^{2+} and V_m in myocyte cultures. *Circ Res* 2004;94:1589–1597

45. Raman V, Pollard AE, Fast VG. Shock-induced changes of Ca_i^{2+} and V_m in myocyte cultures and computer model: dependence on the timing of shock application. *Cardiovasc Res* 2006;73:101–110

46. Sharma V, Tung L. Ionic currents involved in shock-induced nonlinear changes in transmembrane potential responses of single cardiac cells. *Pflugers Arch* 2004;449:248–256

47. Yuan W, Ginsburg KS, Bers DM. Comparison of sarcolemmal calcium channel current in rabbit and rat ventricular myocytes. *J Physiol* 1996;493:733–746

48. Gomez JP, Potreau D, Branka JE, Raymond G. Developmental changes in Ca^{2+} currents from newborn rat cardiomyocytes in primary culture. *Pflugers Arch* 1994;428:241–249

49. Nikolski VP, Sambelashvili AT, Krinsky VI, Efimov IR. Effects of electroporation on optically recorded transmembrane potential responses to high-intensity electrical shocks. *Am J Physiol* 2004;286:H412–H418

50. Jones JL, Jones RE. Postshock arrhythmias—a possible cause of unsuccessful defibrillation. *Crit Care Med* 1980;8:167–171

51. Wharton JM, Wolf PD, Smith WM, Chen PS, Frazier DW, Yabe S, Danieley N, Ideker RE. Cardiac potential and potential gradient fields generated by single, combined, and sequential shocks during ventricular defibrillation. *Circulation* 1992;85:1510–1523

52. Cates AW, Wolf PD, Hillsley RE, Souza JJ, Smith WM, Ideker RE. The probability of defibrillation success and the incidence of postshock arrhythmia as a function of shock strength. *PACE* 1994;17:1208–1217

53. Kodama I, Sakuma I, Shibata N, Knisley SB, Niwa R, Honjo H. Regional differences in arrhythmogenic aftereffects of high intensity DC stimulation in the ventricles. *PACE* 2000;23:807–817

54. Gold JH, Schuder JC, Stoeckle H, Granberg TA, Hamdani SZ, Rychlewski JM. Transthoracic ventricular defibrillation in the 100 kg calf with unidirectional rectangular pulses. *Circulation* 1977;56:745–750

55. Ding L, Splinter R, Knisley SB. Quantifying spatial localization of optical mapping using Monte Carlo simulations. *IEEE Trans Biomed Eng* 2001;48:1098–1107
56. Hyatt CJ, Mironov SF, Vetter FJ, Zemlin CW, Pertsov AM. Optical action potential upstroke morphology reveals near-surface transmural propagation direction. *Circ Res* 2005;97:277–284
57. Sharifov OF, Fast VG. Intramural virtual electrodes in ventricular wall: effects on epicardial polarizations. *Circulation* 2004;109:2349–2356
58. Sharifov OF, Fast VG. Role of intramural virtual electrodes in shock-induced activation of left ventricle: optical measurements from the intact epicardial surface. *Heart Rhythm* 2006;3:1063–1073
59. Sharifov OF, Ideker RE, Fast VG. High-resolution optical mapping of intramural virtual electrodes in porcine left ventricular wall. *Cardiovasc Res* 2004;64:448–456
60. Cheek ER, Sharifov OF, Fast VG. Role of microscopic tissue structure in shock-induced activation assessed by optical mapping in myocyte cultures. *J Cardiovasc Electrophysiol* 2005;16:991–1000

Chapter 4.3

Virtual Electrode Theory of Pacing

John P. Wikswo and Bradley J. Roth

Introduction

One of the most important contributions of biomedical engineering to medicine is the development of pacemakers, external defibrillators, and implantable cardioverters/defibrillators.[1] Engineers have been quite successful in designing these devices empirically, without a fundamental understanding of the underlying biophysical mechanisms. Over the past 15 years, two areas of research – optical mapping of electrical activity in the heart[2] and mathematical modeling of the heart using the bidomain model[3] – have provided insight into the basic mechanisms by which cardiac electric fields are produced and how externally applied electric fields interact with cardiac tissue. The goal of this chapter is to describe this research and to summarize what has been learned from it. We survey the contributions of many researchers, but the emphasis is on our own work, which, of course, we know best. We focus on basic mechanisms; clinical applications are better described by other authors.[4] The fundamental knowledge gained from basic research in cardiac shock response is enabling the development of detailed mathematical models[5,6] that can guide the further optimization of implantable cardiac stimulators.

The electrical properties of the heart have been reviewed elsewhere. In 1993 Henriquez[3] summarized the bidomain model in a seminal paper that serves as an excellent foundation for the discussions in our chapter. Neu and Krassowska[7] examined the limitations of the bidomain as a continuum model. Roth[8] described mechanisms of electrical stimulation of excitable tissue, including cardiac tissue. In the past 10 years much work has been published in this field, particularly on comparing numerical simulations to experimental data. The agreement between theory and experiment is an important topic[9] and is the focus of this review.

John P. Wikswo Jr
Departments of Biomedical Engineering, Molecular Physiology & Biophysics, and Physics & Astronomy, The Vanderbilt Institute for Integrative Biosystems Research and Education, Vanderbilt University, Nashville, TN 37235, USA, john.wikswo@vanderbilt.edu

I. R. Efimov et al. (eds.), *Cardiac Bioelectric Therapy: Mechanisms and Practical Implications*.
© Springer Science+Business Media, LLC 2009

The bidomain model of cardiac tissue was first suggested by Otto Schmitt[10] and was developed by several researchers in the late 1970s.[11–13] It is a two- or three-dimensional cable model that accounts for the anisotropy of both the intracellular and extracellular spaces. Geselowitz and Miller[14] and Plonsey and Barr[15,16] made important contributions to our understanding of the model. By the late 1980s, many papers were appearing that described the importance of the bidomain model during action potential propagation.[17–20] The bidomain model is remarkable in cardiac electrophysiology in the extent to which it has supported quantitative predictions, the vast majority of which have been confirmed (Table 1). This review emphasizes the impact of the bidomain model during electrical stimulation, a field that began in earnest with our study of unipolar stimulation.[21]

Optical mapping was first used to study the response of cardiac tissue to an electric shock by Dillon[22] and Knisley and Hill[23] in the early 1990s. The membrane absorbs a fluorescent dye, and the amount of fluoresced light depends on the voltage across it. This technique allows the use of optical methods to make electrical recordings of transmembrane potential. Researchers can measure the transmembrane potential during the shock without electrical artifact, and they can study the repolarization phase of the action potential as well as the depolarization phase. The method has become the primary tool for recording the electrical behavior of the heart.[2]

Virtual Electrodes during Unipolar Stimulation of Cardiac Tissue

Sepulveda et al.[21,24–26] calculated the transmembrane potential, V_m, induced in a two-dimensional sheet of cardiac tissue during stimulation through a small, unipolar, extracellular electrode (Fig. 1). They found that the tissue was depolarized (yellow) under the electrode, and in contrast to the expected elliptical shape with the major axis aligned with the fiber direction (Fig. 2a), the region of direct electrotonic depolarization had a "dogbone" shape whose long axis was transverse to the fibers (Figs. 1 and 2c).

Concurrent with these numerical studies, Wikswo and his colleagues[27–33] used a circular electrode array with radial bipolar electrodes to measure not only the directional dependence of the propagation velocity of the action potential, but also the locus of points where propagation started at the end of the stimulus pulse. Their 1991 paper[33] provided a quantitative comparison of theory and experiment and confirmed not only the existence of the dog-bone–shaped region but also the need to utilize differing intracellular and extracellular anisotropies to explain the results (Fig. 2). This paper also provides the historical basis for the use of the term "virtual electrodes" in the context of extracellular stimulation. Wiederholt[34] reported in 1970 that for a sufficiently strong stimulus, 1–2 cm of nerve can be directly depolarized by the stimulus pulse, such that propagation begins not at the stimulus electrode, but at some distance from the electrode. Cummins et al.[35] showed how the measurements of two compound action potentials in nerves could be used to compute not only the conduction velocity but also the size of the region beyond which propagation excites, what they termed the "virtual cathode." Subsequently, Rattay[36–38]

Table 1: Bidomain predictions and experimental confirmation

Phenomena	Prediction	Confirmation
Magnetic field of closed wavefront	Sepulveda and Wikswo (1987)[19]	Staton et al. (1993),[197] Staton (1994),[199] Baudenbacher et al. (2002)[198]
Magnetic field at the apex of the heart	Wikswo and Barach (1982),[192] Roth et al. (1988)[210]	—[a]
Effect of perfusing bath on the interstitial potential	Roth and Wikswo (1986),[17] Roth (1988)[211]	Knisley et al. (1991)[212]
Effect of bath on rate of rise of action potential	Plonsey et al. (1988),[213] Wu et al. (1996, 1997),[214,215] Roth (1996, 2000)[216,217]	—[b]
Dog-bone shape of virtual cathode	Sepulveda et al. (1989)[21]	Wikswo et al. (1991)[33]
Virtual anode near unipolar cathode	Sepulveda et al. (1989)[21]	Knisley (1995),[47] Neunlist and Tung (1995),[48] Wikswo et al. (1995)[49]
Quatrefoil reentry	Roth and Saypol (1991),[218] Saypol and Roth (1992),[81] Roth (1997)[54]	Lin et al. (1999)[82]
Fiber curvature causes polarization during far-field stimulation	Trayanova et al. (1993),[120] Entcheva et al. (1998, 1999)[119,121]	Entcheva et al. (1998),[119] Knisley et al. (1999),[122c] Tung and Kleber (2000)[154c]
Make/break excitation	Roth (1995)[53]	Wikswo et al. (1995)[49d]
Shape of the strength–interval curve	Roth (1996)[66]	Sidorov et al. (2005)[56]
The no-response phenomenon	Roth (1997)[54,138]	Cranefield et al. (1957)[65]
Effect of bath on virtual electrodes	Latimer and Roth (1998)[182]	Knisley et al. (2000)[183]
Spiral wave meandering	Roth (1998, 2001)[219,220]	—[a]
Effect of interface on surface polarization	Latimer and Roth (1999),[123] Entcheva et al. (1998)[119]	Entcheva et al. (1998)[119]
Time dependence of the refractory period	Bennett and Roth (1999)[70]	Mehra et al. (1980)[69]
Magnetic field of planar wavefront	Roth and Woods (1999),[204] Murdick and Roth (2004)[207]	Holzer et al. (2004)[202]

(Cont.)

Table 1: (*Continued*)

Phenomena	Prediction	Confirmation
Fiber angle and polarization at a sealed boundary	Roth (1999)[185]	—[a]
S_1 refractory gradient is not essential for S_2 reentry	Roth (2000),[98] Winfree (2000, 2001)[96,97]	Cheng et al. (2000)[99]
Virtual electrodes and the pinwheel experiment	Lindblom et al. (2000, 2001)[101,102]	Sidorov et al. (2007)[100]
Effect of plunge electrodes	Langrill Beaudoin and Roth (2001, 2004)[144,145]	Woods et al. (2006)[146]
Effect of epicardial electrodes	Patel and Roth (2001)[148]	Knisley and Pollard (2005)[149]
High $[K]_o$ favors break excitation	Roth and Patel (2003)[58]	Sidorov et al. (2003)[55]
Prompt excitation of diastolic tissue with field stimulation	Fishler and Vepa (1998),[125,162] Hooks et al. (2002)[126]	Fast et al. (2002),[127] Sharifov and Fast (2003),[128] Woods et al. (2006, 2007)[134,135,164]
Quatrefoil reentry from burst pacing	Janks and Roth (2006)[221]	—[a]

[a] Not yet verified
[b] Not yet verified, but provides an alternative explanation of earlier data[222]
[c] These experiments were not a direct confirmation of the simulation, but nevertheless verified the main prediction: fiber curvature leads to membrane polarization
[d] Also consistent with previously unexplained data[42,50-52]

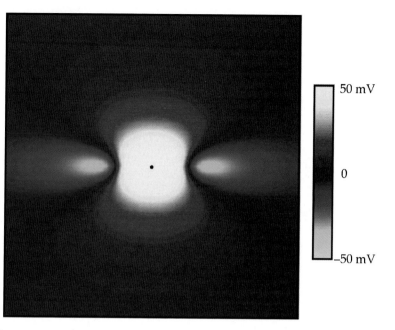

Figure 1: The transmembrane potential calculated during unipolar cathodal stimulation of an anisotropic, two-dimensional sheet of cardiac tissue with unequal intra- and extracellular electrical anisotropies. An 8 mm by 8 mm region is shown, with the electrode position at the center and fibers oriented horizontally (Computed according to Sepulveda et al.)[21]

provided a theoretical model for the activation function in nerves, and Sobie et al.[39] extended this concept to cardiac tissue.

The first reference we have been able to identify regarding the use of the term virtual cathode is in the 1955 book by Terman et al.[40] that discusses space charge effects in the vicinity of cathodes in vacuum tubes. There are a number of historical references in the cardiac literature regarding the use of the terms virtual cathode or virtual electrode, although it does not appear that all of these were made in the context of the site of initiation of propagation from strong, extracellular stimuli. Although Furman et al.[41] do use the term "virtual electrodes," it is in the context of the "ratio between chronic and acute thresholds, [that] depends upon the size and shape of the electrode and upon the thickness of the non-excitable fibrous tissue which forms about the electrode and separates it from the excitable myocardium." However, the work of Furman et al. has nothing to do with cable phenomena. Goto and Brooks[42] and Hoshi and Matsuda[43] examine membrane excitability during intracellular current injection into cardiac Purkinje fibers; the latter is particularly "modern" in the description of virtual electrodes, and it presents a diagram of hypothetical current flow through a fiber membrane resulting from cathodal or anodal surface electrodes and the resulting cathodal and anodal regions, which were determined by the sign of the transmembrane current. Hoshi and Matsuda also refer to Hoffman and Cranefield's[44] use of the term "virtual cathode."

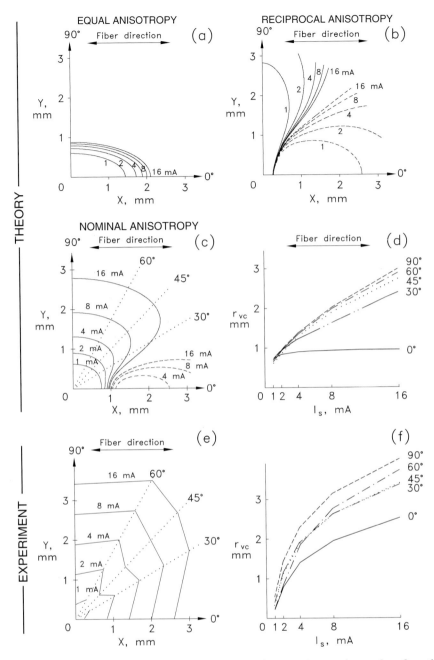

Figure 2: The first comparison of theoretical and experimental results for the two-dimensional virtual cathodes that result from injection of extracellular current into cardiac tissue. (**a–c**) The shape of the virtual cathode for five different stimulus currents for (**a**) equal tissue anisotropies (5.7:1), (**b**) reciprocal anisotropy (10:1), and (**c**) nominal anisotropy (10:1 intracellular space and 4:1 extracellular). (**d**) The dependence of virtual cathode size (r_{vc}) on stimulus current (I_s) for the model for five different angles, as determined from (**c**). (**e**) The experimentally inferred shape of the virtual cathode. (**f**) The dependence of r_{vc} on I_s, from the average data for five different angles, as determined from (**e**) (Adapted from Wikswo et al.)[33]

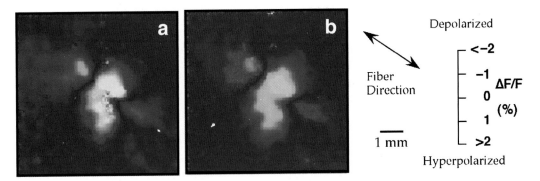

Figure 3: The transmembrane potential measured during unipolar stimulation of rabbit epicardium. (a) A cathodal and (b) an anodal 10 mA, 2 ms stimulus, applied when the tissue is refractory. $\Delta F/F$ is the fractional change of fluorescence caused by the dye di-4-ANEPPS and is proportional to the transmembrane potential (Wikswo et al., by permission of the authors and the Biophysical Society)[49]

In this historical context, the 1989 paper by Sepulveda et al.[21] and the 1991 paper by Wikswo et al.[33] and their preceding conference publications[24-36] clearly built upon existing knowledge of spatial, electronic effects in one-dimensional fibers, but these studies do represent the first predictions and observations of anisotropy related, multidimensional virtual cathode effects in cardiac tissue.

Returning to the modern effort, the Sepulveda et al.[21] two-dimensional model also predicted hyperpolarized (blue) "wings" in two regions adjacent to the electrode parallel to the fiber direction (Figs. 1 and 2b, c). These hyperpolarized regions are called *virtual anodes* because hyperpolarization occurs far from any anodal electrode. The virtual anodes arise because the tissue has "unequal anisotropy ratios": the ratio of conductivity parallel to the fibers to the conductivity perpendicular to the fibers is different in the intracellular and extracellular space.[45,46] Because of their small size, their then-unrecognized effect on conduction velocity, and their weak contribution to the extracellular potential, the predicted lateral virtual anodes in the transmembrane potential distribution during cathodal stimulation remained undetected until 1995, when three groups simultaneously used optical imaging of V_m to verify the calculation experimentally.[47-49] Figure 3 shows the V_m data from Wikswo's group during unipolar stimulation of rabbit epicardium. Figure 3a should be compared to Fig. 1, noting that the fiber direction is different in the two cases. Figure 3b was obtained by reversing the polarity of the stimulus current; the tissue is hyperpolarized under the anode, and virtual cathodes form along the fiber direction.

The single most important cardiac property underlying the virtual electrodes is the differences in the electrical anisotropy of the intracellular and extracellular resistivities. These differences ensure that current applied extracellularly will seek a spatially complex pathway into the intracellular space and may cross the membrane in opposite directions in adjacent regions (i.e., create adjacent virtual cathodes and anodes). Much of this review focuses on the role of these unequal anisotropies in the response of cardiac tissue to electrical stimulation.

Anode and Cathode Make and Break Excitation

The importance of the virtual electrodes surrounding the stimulating electrode became clear when analyzing the four mechanisms of electrical stimulation: cathode make, anode make, cathode break, and anode break. Dekker[50] identified these four distinct modes of stimulation, and Lindemans et al.[51] and others[42,52] studied them further. However, the mechanisms were not fully understood until the simulations by Roth[53] and experiments of Wikswo et al.[49] Because each of these four modes can play a role in defibrillation, it is particularly important to look at them in detail.

Cathode make stimulation is the easiest to understand. The depolarization under the cathode reaches threshold, triggering a wavefront that propagates outward. The excitation occurs soon after the start, or "make," of the stimulus pulse (Figs. 4a and 5a). For weak stimuli, the wavefront originates from a point directly under the electrode, but for stronger stimuli it begins from a point farther from the electrode that depends on both the direction of propagation and the stimulus strength.[33]

Anode make stimulation is analogous to cathode make, except that excitation begins at the edges of the virtual cathodes located on each side of the central dog-bone–shaped

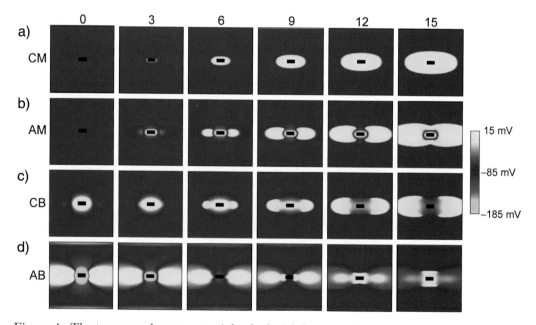

Figure 4: The transmembrane potential calculated during or following unipolar stimulation of cardiac tissue. The four rows correspond to cathode make (CM), anode make (AM), cathode break (CB), and anode break (AB) excitation. Each column corresponds to the time in milliseconds; in CM and AM the stimulus turns on at $t = 0$, and in CB and AB the stimulus turns off at $t = 0$ (Computed according to Roth)[53]

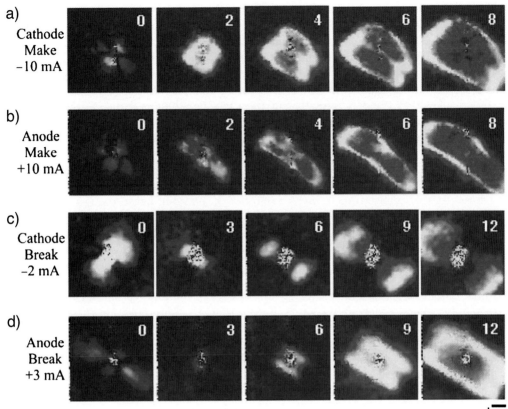

Figure 5: The transmembrane potential measured during unipolar stimulation of rabbit epicardium. The number in each frame is the time in milliseconds. The electrode is at the center, and the fibers are oriented from lower right to upper left (Wikswo et al., by permission of the authors and the Biophysical Society)[49]

anode (Figs. 4b and 5b). Because the depolarization under the electrode during cathodal stimulation is stronger than the depolarization at the virtual cathode during anodal stimulation, the threshold stimulus current is larger for anode make than cathode make stimulation.

Cathode break stimulation occurs following the end, or "break," of the stimulus pulse (Figs. 4c and 5c). The tissue under the cathode is depolarized and the sodium channels become unexcitable. However, the tissue at the virtual anode is hyperpolarized, so there the sodium channels are fully excitable. Following the end of the stimulus pulse, the depolarization under the cathode diffuses into the excitable tissue at the virtual anode, exciting it. The resulting wavefront propagates initially through the excitable path carved out by the virtual anode, which in this case is parallel to the fiber direction. The two crucial features of break excitation are the creation of an excitable path at the virtual anode (deexcitation) followed by electrotonic interaction (diffusion) of adjacent depolarization into the excitable tissue. Because the virtual anode must be strong enough to create an excitable path, the threshold stimulus current is higher for break excitation than for make excitation. In general, cathode make excitation will occur preferentially over cathode break excitation unless the tissue is refractory at the time the stimulus turns on, in which case make excitation is suppressed but break excitation can still occur.

The mechanism for anode break excitation is analogous to that for cathode break excitation, except that the excitable path, under the anode, is now in the direction perpendicular to the fibers, and the virtual cathodes are in the direction parallel to the fibers (Figs. 4d and 5d). The initial direction of propagation is therefore perpendicular to the fibers. At first glance, anode break excitation is puzzling because one might expect that the strong hyperpolarization under the anode would diffuse into the weaker virtual cathode and not result in excitation, rather than the weak depolarization diffusing into the strong hyperpolarization and triggering excitation. Anode break excitation works because the nonlinear behavior of the membrane causes the hyperpolarization to decay more rapidly than the depolarization, so that the remnant depolarization can then diffuse into the excitable tissue. Because nonlinear behavior is essential for this mechanism to work, the threshold for anode break excitation is higher than the threshold for the other three mechanisms.

One aspect of break excitation that is often underappreciated is that it is predicted to occur for pulses as short as 2 ms, albeit with very strong stimuli (15 mA).[54] Were it not for optical imaging of the distributed virtual electrode pattern, it would be difficult from timing alone to determine whether the excitation was make or break; high-speed, high-resolution optical imaging enables the identification of which region served as the site of activation, and hence can help identify break activation for short, 10 ms stimuli.[55] Measurements of strength–interval curves for an S_2 duration of 2–20 ms showed that for a 2 ms anodal stimulus, the curve still has a dip, which suggests break stimulation.[56]

Elevated extracellular potassium ion concentration, $[K]_o$, influences the mechanism of stimulation.[55,57] For normal $[K]_o$ (4 mM), diastolic stimulation occurs by the make mechanism. However, for elevated $[K]_o$ (10 mM), the mechanism switches to break (Fig. 6). Roth and Patel[58] found similar results using numerical simulations: high $[K]_o$ predisposes cardiac tissue to break excitation. Because ischemia raises $[K]_o$, break excitation may play a more important role in defibrillation than is suggested by simulations and experiments using normal $[K]_o$ levels.

Nikolski et al.[59] observed break excitation during diastole in tissue with normal $[K]_o$, but this may be caused by the output impedance of the quiescent current source used for stimulation.[60] Ranjan et al.[61,62] suggest that break excitation may arise because of a hyperpolarized activated membrane current. Although such a mechanism is possible,[63] the fact that break excitation typically originates from a hyperpolarized region adjacent to a depolarized region, rather than from the location where hyperpolarization is greatest, makes this explanation unlikely.

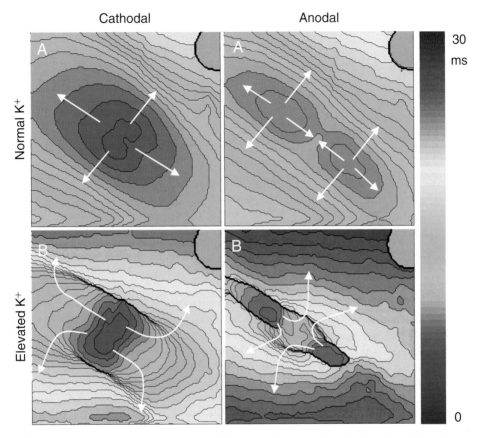

Figure 6: Activation isochrones for cathodal and anodal pacing during diastole with normal (4 mM) and elevated (10 mM) extracellular potassium ion concentration. Make excitation occurs with normal $[K]_o$ and break with elevated $[K]_o$ (Sidorov et al., by permission of the authors, ©2002 IEEE)[57]

Strength–Interval Curves

The four mechanisms of excitation have important implications for the strength–interval curve. This curve is generated by exciting the tissue with a weak electrical stimulus (S_1), triggering an outwardly propagating wavefront. After a delay, or "interval," the tissue is stimulated through the same electrode with a second stimulus (S_2). The strength–interval curve is a plot of the threshold S_2 strength versus the S_1–S_2 interval. For long intervals the tissue is completely recovered from the first action potential, so the S_2 threshold is low. However, as the interval is shortened to values less than the duration of an action potential, the S_2 threshold increases because the tissue is still refractory from the S_1 action potential.

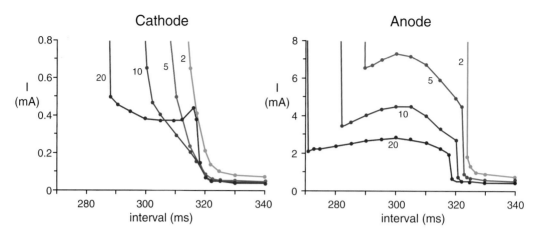

Figure 7: The calculated cathodal and anodal strength–interval curves for S_2 pulse durations of 2, 5, 10, and 20 ms (Adapted from Roth and Roth et al.)[66,223]

One interesting feature of the strength–interval curve is the presence of a "dip," or a region having a positive slope. A positive slope is counterintuitive because increasing the interval should decrease the refractoriness of the tissue and therefore decrease the stimulus threshold. Nevertheless, researchers observed a dip in the anodal strength–interval curve 50 years ago.[64,65] Dekker[50] used an epicardial surface stimulating electrode and an intramural bipolar recording electrode to show that the dip is associated with anode break excitation. At long intervals, the tissue is excitable when the S_2 stimulus turns on and anode make excitation occurs. At shorter intervals, the tissue is refractory when S_2 turns on so anode make excitation is suppressed, but anode break excitation still happens. A more detailed explanation for the dip arose from simulations based on the bidomain model.[66] The dip exists during the early part of the anode break section of the anodal strength–interval curve (Fig. 7). It appears because break excitation requires adjacent regions of depolarized and hyperpolarized tissue. Adequate hyperpolarization exists directly under the anode, so the limiting factor for break stimulation is the presence of sufficient depolarization at the virtual cathode to cause excitation by diffusion after the end of the stimulus pulse. However, another source of depolarization exists besides that caused directly by the S_2 stimulus. As the interval gets shorter, the surrounding tissue has higher levels of depolarization arising from the repolarization tail of the S_1 action potential. Thus, the S_2 stimulus current itself does not have to create as much depolarization as it would otherwise, lowering the S_2 stimulus threshold.

This mechanism was elegantly illustrated by Roth and Patel,[58] who computed strength–interval curves under conditions of high extracellular potassium ion concentration. High $[K]_o$ shortens the action potential and, more importantly, causes a significant refractoriness after the transmembrane potential recovers to its resting value.[67] In this case, shortening the interval does not cause an increase of the surrounding depolarization, and the resulting dip in the strength–interval curve disappears. Bray and Roth[68] performed a simulation

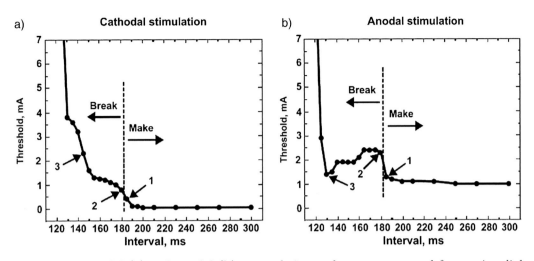

Figure 8: Cathodal (**a**) and anodal (**b**) strength–interval curves measured from epicardial unipolar stimulation of a rabbit heart. Note the "dip" in the anodal curve at about 130 ms, and the region of positive slope from 130 to 180 ms (Redrawn from Sidorov et al., with permission of *Am J Physiol Heart*)[56]

that came to a similar conclusion. When they added electroporation to their simulation, they found that break excitation was triggered not by the adjacent depolarization, but by electroporation under the anode that caused the tissue to recover to zero potential rather than the resting potential. Because the surrounding depolarization at short intervals no longer had a significant effect on the stimulus threshold, the break section of the strength–interval curve lost its dip.

The dip is not as prominent during cathodal stimulation because sufficient depolarization is supplied directly under the cathode, and the limiting factor determining if cathode break excitation occurs is if the hyperpolarization at the virtual anode is strong enough to create an excitable pathway for the S_2 wavefront to travel through. Shortening the interval does not assist in creating the excitable pathway (in fact, the surrounding depolarization makes it more difficult to "deexcite" the tissue), so the dip is usually not present. (Sometimes a small dip is present for very long S_2 pulse durations, as in Fig. 7.)

Sidorov et al.[56] recently tested these predictions about the strength–interval curve. Figure 8 shows the measured cathodal and anodal strength–interval curves and indicates their separation into make and break sections, as verified by optical mapping of the excitation wavefronts. The anodal curve shows that the section with positive slope is associated with break excitation. The dip is absent during cathodal stimulation, although the strength–interval curve is still divided into make and break sections.

As discussed by Janks and Roth (this volume), virtual electrodes are also useful in understanding the behavior of pacemaker electrode stimulus thresholds following implantation.[69,70]

Quatrefoil Reentry

Spiral-wave and figure-8 reentry (Fig. 9a–d) have been observed in cardiac tissue for over 15 years and play dominant roles in cardiac tachycardias and fibrillation.[71–76] One widely accepted mechanism for the induction of reentry by a shock is the critical point hypothesis.[76] Winfree[77] illustrated this hypothesis by considering the "pinwheel experiment." An S_1 planar wavefront propagates across a sheet of cardiac tissue. During the refractory tail of the S_1 action potential, a strong S_2 stimulus is applied through a point electrode (Fig. 9c). The S_1 refractory gradient interacts with the S_2 stimulus to produce two "critical points" about which a pair of oppositely rotating spiral waves form, resulting in figure-8 reentry. Shibata et al.[78] tested this prediction experimentally using epicardial mapping and found results consistent with Winfree's predictions.

As shown in Fig. 9e–f, the doubly anisotropic bidomain can support an additional topology, that of quatrefoil reentry. Matta et al.[79] performed S_1–S_2 stimulation through a single electrode and showed that a properly timed S_2 stimulus could induce fibrillation, a stimulation protocol that is not consistent with the formation of either spiral wave or figure-8 reentry. A mechanism for this type of reentry induction was first suggested by Winfree[80] and was simulated by Saypol and Roth.[81] Figure 10 shows a schematic of how quatrefoil reentry could be created experimentally and numerically for cathodal and anodal break stimulation and the resulting pattern of wavefronts. Figure 11 maps the predicted transmembrane potential at various times before, during, and after a cathodal S_2 stimulus.[54] Before the S_2 stimulus (280 ms), the tissue is refractory, so make excitation does not occur. However, at the end of the stimulus (300 ms), the tissue at the virtual anode has completely recovered excitability, and break excitation following the stimulus causes a wavefront that propagates parallel to the fibers (320 and 340 ms). As the surrounding tissue slowly recovers, this wavefront starts to propagate in the direction perpendicular to the fibers, and then back toward the stimulus (360 and 380 ms). By the time it reaches the tissue around the stimulus electrode, that tissue has recovered excitability and can support reentry (400 and 420 ms). The resulting reentrant loop is known as *quatrefoil reentry*. Quatrefoil reentry can occur following either cathodal or anodal S_2 stimuli, but for an anodal stimulus the wavefront propagates around the reentrant loop in the opposite direction, as shown in Fig. 10.

Lin et al.[82] observed quatrefoil reentry in a rabbit heart. Figure 12a shows an isochronal map of the wavefront location measured following a strong cathodal S_2 stimulus. Clearly the reentrant wavefront begins at the virtual anode, propagates initially parallel to the fibers, then arcs around and reenters the region near the electrode from the direction perpendicular to the fibers. Figure 12b shows the data for an anodal S_2 stimulus. The wavefront initially propagates perpendicular to the fibers, then reenters parallel to the fibers, exactly the opposite of cathodal stimulation.

Careful inspection of Fig. 11 reveals that during part of the reentrant circuit the wavefront has a low amplitude and propagates slowly (340 and 360 ms). Once the surrounding tissue recovers its excitability, propagation resumes its normal amplitude and speed (380 ms). This can be thought of as an example of "damped propagation," in which the wavefront propagates decrementally. A damped wavefront will either eventually die or,

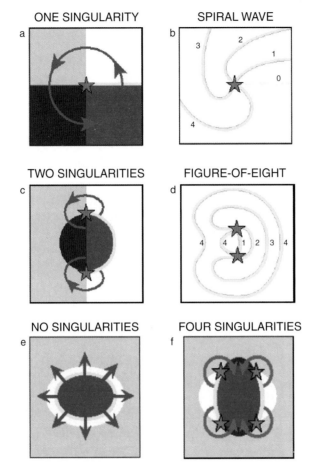

Figure 9: The creation of spiral wave and figure-8 reentries according to the critical point hypothesis. (a) Crossed-field stimulation begins with S_1 stimulation creating a plane wave moving from right to left (the refractory tail is *blue*), followed by strong S_2 stimulation from the bottom that creates a strong shock field (*red*). *Bright red* is excitable tissue that is stimulated by S_2, *dark red* is refractory (*red + light blue*). *White* is excitable tissue; S_2 is too weak to excite, but the wavefront (*yellow*) can move upward into this region. By the time the wavefront spirals into the upper left refractory region, that tissue will be excitable, producing the wavefront sequence in (b). In the middle row, S_1 line stimulation from the right followed by central stimulation produces figure-8 reentry (c, d). Equal anisotropies (e) will create elliptical S_1 and S_2 responses, with blocked or delayed propagation possible but no reentry. Unequal anisotropies are required for the creation of quatrefoil reentry (F), wherein the intersection of the transverse virtual cathode created by a strong S_2 stimulus intersects the tail of the elliptically expanding wavefront from weak S_1 stimulation

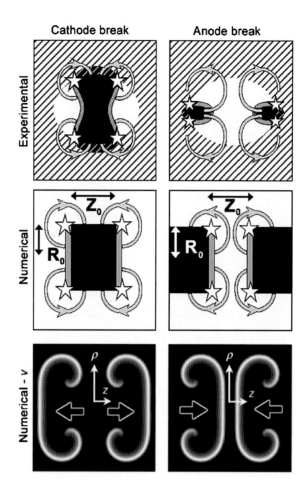

Figure 10: Cartoons showing quatrefoil reentry produced by cathodal break (*left column*) and anodal break (*right column*) for tissue with a horizontal fiber direction. *Top row* depicts the experimental configuration. *Black regions* are tissue stimulated by cathodal excitation, *gray border* is initial wavefront at the edge of excited tissue, *hatched regions* are refractory tissue, *white regions* are unexcited/hyperpolarized tissue, and *stars* show location of phase singularities. *Middle row* illustrates initial numerical approximation of the experimental configuration. *Black* is refractory, the *gray border* is excited, and *white* is unexcited. *Bottom row* depicts the spatial distribution of the fast variable a short time later. The *arrows* show the direction of the motion of the wavefront as it passes through the plane of the ring that is defined by the singular filament that encircles the z axis and the *black arrows* (Bray and Wikswo, reprinted with permission ©2003 by the American Physical Society [http://www.vanderbilt.edu/lsp/abstracts/9906-Bray-PRL-2003.htm])[88]

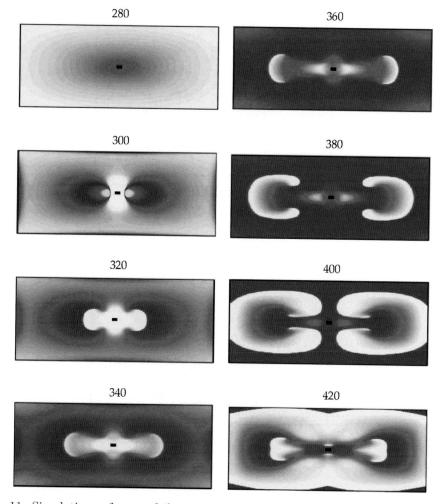

Figure 11: Simulations of quatrefoil reentry following a strong cathodal S_2 stimulus. An S_1 stimulus at time zero triggered an outwardly propagating wavefront. By 280 ms, the region around the electrode (*center black rectangle*) is in the refractory tail of the S_1 action potential. The S_2 stimulus lasts from 280 to 300 ms, followed by break excitation and quatrefoil reentry. The color scale for the transmembrane potential is the same as in Fig. 4 (Calculated according to Roth)[54]

as in Fig. 11, recover to become a steadily propagating wavefront. Sidorov et al.[83] and others[84,85] have examined the spatiotemporal dynamics of damped propagation in detail and concluded that the transition from a damped to a steadily propagating wavefront, illustrated in Fig. 13, is a key link in understanding defibrillation.

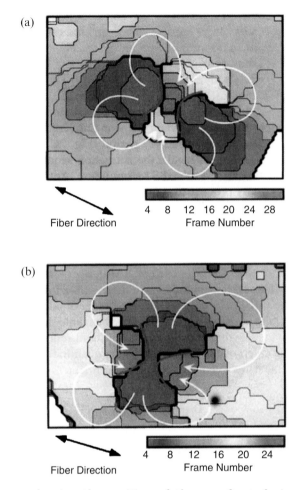

Figure 12: Isochrones showing the position of the wavefront during quatrefoil reentry, following a (**a**) cathodal and (**b**) anodal S_2 stimulus. Data were obtained from a rabbit heart (Lin et al.)[82]

Tracing the trajectories of phase singularities during quatrefoil reentry (Fig. 14) offers an excellent model system for studying the way phase singularities interact.[86–88] Gray et al.[89] have used measurements of the transmembrane potential together with calcium imaging to monitor reentry. Figure 15 shows that measuring both these variables simultaneously provides additional information about the dynamics of phase singularities. An interesting application of simultaneous imaging includes determining whether a particular arrhythmic focus is driven by calcium or voltage, which affects locally the direction of rotation in the phase plane.[90]

A third S_3 stimulus can terminate reentry induced by S_1–S_2 stimulation. The timing of S_3 is crucial, with certain times resulting in termination ("protective zones") and other times not.[91,92] These protective zones recur periodically.[93] Simulations by Hildebrandt and Roth[94] showed that quatrefoil reentry displays periodic protective zones that recur with the period of the quatrefoil reentrant circuit, and that the protective zones are wider for anodal than cathodal stimulation.

Traditionally, researchers have focused on the interaction of the S_1 refractory gradient and the S_2 stimulus gradient during the induction of reentry.[76,77] In fact Winfree's original prediction of quatrefoil reentry took just this point of view.[80,95] However, an S_1 gradient of refractoriness is not essential for reentry induction by an S_2 stimulus.[96–98] Figure 16 shows the induction of quatrefoil reentry when the S_1 action potential is uniform in space, so there is no refractory gradient. The S_2 shock (80 ms) has two roles: it creates a gradient of refractoriness during the shock by hyperpolarizing and deexciting the tissue at the virtual anode, and then initiates the wavefront by break excitation after the shock ends. This effect was experimentally verified by Cheng et al.[99] who observed that the direction of S_2 excitation and reentry did not depend on the direction of the S_1 refractory gradient.

Our discussion of reentry began with critical point theory and the pinwheel experiment (Fig. 9c) and culminated in our claim that the S_1 gradient of refractoriness is sometimes not even necessary because virtual electrodes alone are sufficient to trigger quatrefoil reentry (Fig. 16). Returning now to the pinwheel experiment, it is worthwhile to determine how it is influenced by the formation of virtual electrodes. Sidorov et al.[100] recently used optical mapping to study the pinwheel experiment and found that immediately after a cathodal S_2 shock delivered in the refractory period, virtual anodes formed along the fiber direction, as shown in Fig. 1. Depending on the timing of S_2, they observed make excitation, transitional make-break, break excitation, or damped waves. The fate of these excitation fronts depended on the direction of S_1 propagation relative to the fibers. Wavefronts initiated by virtual electrode mechanisms are shown in Fig. 13, but those wavefronts in more refractory tissue died, while wavefronts in more recovered tissue successfully propagated, consistent with the critical point hypothesis.

Sidorov et al.[100] used relatively weak shocks that did not induce reentry. Using numerical simulations, Lindblom et al.[101,102] performed a similar study with stronger S_2 shocks (to see these results explained with an extremely simple cellular automata model, see http://sprojects.mmi.mcgill.ca/heart/pages/rot/rothom.html). Depending on the S_2 timing and polarity and the direction of the S_1 wave relative to the fibers, they found figure-8 reentry (consistent with the pinwheel experiment) or quatrefoil reentry. Their simulations are consistent with the observations of Sidorov et al., and these studies demonstrate how to use the pinwheel experiment to reconcile two competing views of reentry induction: the critical point hypothesis and virtual electrodes.[101,103,104]

Defibrillation

The role of virtual electrodes during defibrillation has been examined experimentally by Efimov and his group[6,105–109] and in numerical simulations by Trayanova and her colleagues.[110–113] These authors have examined a variety of phenomena, such as defibrillation of ischemic tissue,[67,114,115] the isoelectric window,[116] biphasic shocks,[117] and differences

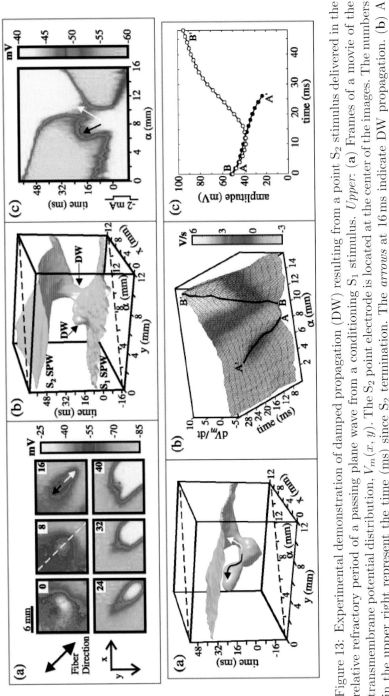

Figure 13: Experimental demonstration of damped propagation (DW) resulting from a point S_2 stimulus delivered in the relative refractory period of a passing plane wave from a conditioning S_1 stimulus. *Upper*: (a) Frames of a movie of the transmembrane potential distribution, $V_m(x, y)$. The S_2 point electrode is located at the center of the images. The numbers in the upper right represent the time (ms) since S_2 termination. The *arrows* at 16 ms indicate DW propagation. (b) A three-dimensional presentation of $V_m(x, y)$ following S_2 stimulation. The *dashed* α axis is parallel to the fiber direction and corresponds to the *white dashed line* in the 8 ms image in (a). (c) A time–space plot of the spatiotemporal dynamics of damped (*black arrow*) and steadily propagating (*white arrow*) waves. *Lower*: (a) Three-dimensional presentation of signal upstroke $[dV_m(x, y)/dt]$ following S_2 stimulation. The *arrows* indicate the DW propagation with decaying propagation (*black*) and the growing wave (*white*). (b) $dV_m(x, y)/dt$ as a function of time and space along the α axis. (c) The amplitude of waves A–A' (*filled circles*) and B–B' (*open circles*) from (b). In all panels, S_2 ended at time $= 0$ (Sidorov et al., reprinted with permission ©2003 by the American Physical Society [http://www.vanderbilt.edu/lsp/abstracts/1501-Sidorov-PRL-2003.htm])[83]

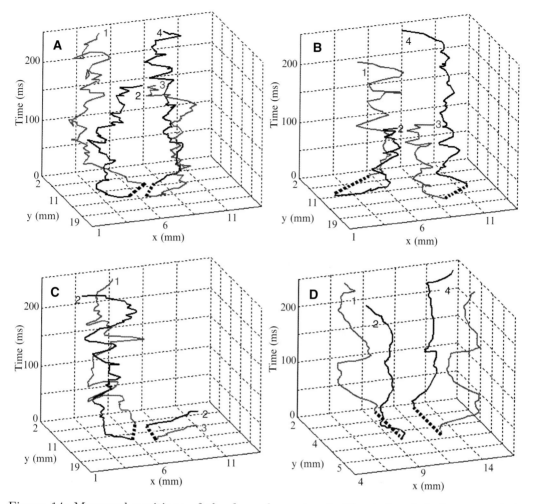

Figure 14: Measured positions of the four phase singularities induced during quatrefoil reentry as measured in a rabbit heart (Bray et al.)[86]

between the right and left chambers of the heart during defibrillation.[118] The agreement between these studies is impressive.[6,108,119] In addition to the now classic anisotropy-related membrane depolarization[120–122] and membrane depolarizations or hyperpolarizations at the locations where externally applied current enters or leaves the heart,[123,124] there are also predictions of heterogeneity related to intramural virtual electrodes,[125,126] which we discuss in additional detail later in this chapter. There are only a few experimental studies, primarily by the Fast,[127–130] Wikswo,[131–136] and Zemlin[137] groups, that address the predicted presence of these intramural virtual electrodes during defibrillation-strength shocks. Of particular interest is the transient nature of the virtual anodes during diastolic field shock and their being overrun by the virtual cathodes.[134–136]

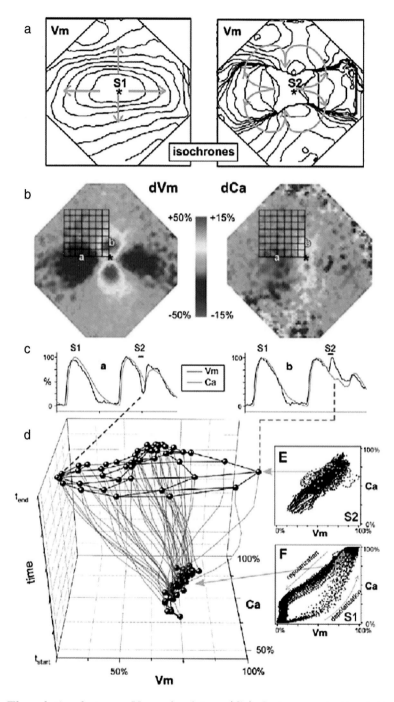

Figure 15: The relation between V_m and calcium (Ca) during point stimulation. (a) Isochrones following S_1 and S_2 stimulation. (b, c) Changes in transmembrane potential (dV_m) and intracellular calcium concentration (dCa) caused by the S_2 shock. (d) Dynamics in the V_m-Ca state space (Gray et al.)[89]

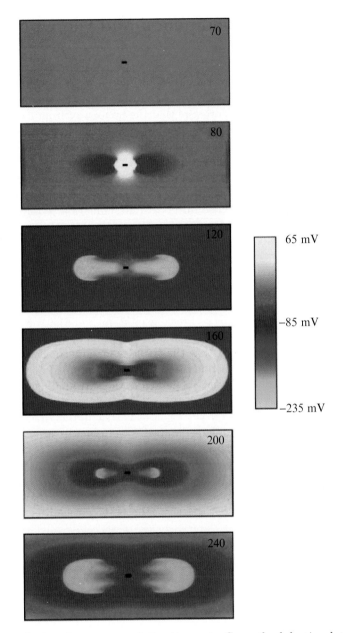

Figure 16: The calculated response of the tissue to S_2 cathodal stimulation following a uniform S_1 action potential. S_2 starts at 70 ms and lasts 5 ms (Roth, by permission of the author, © 2002 IEEE)[98]

The No-Response Phenomenon and the Upper Limit of Vulnerability

One question about the strength–interval curves in Figs. 7 and 8 is what causes the abrupt rise at very short intervals. The answer is that at this time the surrounding tissue is so refractory from the initial S_1 action potential that the break wavefront cannot propagate far from the stimulus electrode without encountering refractoriness, and the local electrotonic interaction cannot reach far enough for the electrode to overcome this situation. Break excitation initiates a wavefront at even very short intervals. Once this wavefront propagates away from the electrode, it reaches the edge of the virtual anode and then may be stopped by refractory tissue.[66] Whether the wavefront survives or dies is an all-or-none event, so the transition from successful stimulation to unsuccessful stimulation is abrupt.

An interesting feature of this short-interval section of the anodal strength–interval curve is the no-response phenomenon. Cranefield et al.[65] observed that at short intervals a weak anodal stimulus can fail to excite a wavefront, a somewhat stronger stimulus triggers excitation, and an even stronger stimulus causes the wavefront to fail. Roth[54,138] used simulations to determine the mechanism for the no-response phenomenon, as reviewed by Janks and Roth in their chapter in this book.[139] A weak stimulus cannot trigger break excitation. A stronger stimulus triggers break excitation and the wavefront successfully propagates away from the electrode. An even stronger stimulus triggers break excitation, but the hyperpolarization is so strong that the tissue is made ultraexcitable and the break wavefront propagates more quickly than normal. If the increase in speed is great enough, the wavefront reaches the edge of the virtual anode before the surrounding tissue has recovered from refractoriness and the wavefront dies. This behavior can be interpreted in terms of damped wavefronts.[83] When the wavefront reaches the edge of the virtual anode, it reaches refractory tissue and begins to decay. This damped wavefront will either die or recover and become a steadily propagating wavefront.

The no-response phenomenon would be a rather unimportant curiosity except for its relationship to the mechanism for the upper limit of vulnerability, or the strongest shock that can induce fibrillation.[140] Several investigators have suggested that the mechanism of the upper limit of vulnerability is essentially the same as the mechanism for the no-response phenomenon described above.[107,114,141–143] Because of the close relationship between the upper limit of vulnerability and the defibrillation threshold, this mechanism is central to understanding the mechanism of defibrillation.

Influence of Physical Electrodes During a Shock

Many studies of defibrillation use either epicardial or plunge electrodes to record the wavefront dynamics. These electrodes can perturb the state of cardiac tissue during the defibrillation shock. For instance, Langrill and Roth[144] predicted that an insulating plunge electrode in otherwise homogeneous tissue results in a complicated distribution of transmembrane potential, and this polarization influences how the tissue responds to the shock.[145]

This distribution arises because of the unequal anisotropy ratios of cardiac tissue. Woods et al.[146] observed this pattern of transmembrane potential surrounding a plunge electrode (Fig. 17). They conclude that insulated heterogeneities, such as plunge electrodes, could cause unintended experimental artifacts. Chattipakorn et al.[147] did not observe an effect of plunge electrodes on the shock response, but Langrill Beaudoin and Roth[145] showed that the electrodes only have an effect at specific timings of the shock.

An alternative to plunge electrodes is to use epicardial electrodes to record wavefront propagation. Patel and Roth[148] predicted that epicardial electrodes also induce a transmembrane potential during a defibrillation shock. The mechanism for this effect is quite different from plunge electrodes, and equal anisotropy ratios are not required. The electrode provides a low-resistance path for current, so as current approaches the electrode it leaves the intracellular space to take advantage of the low resistance path, thereby depolarizing the tissue (Fig. 18). On the other side of the electrode, current reenters the intracellular space, hyperpolarizing the tissue. This effect can be observed by optical mapping during a shock, but ordinarily the electrode blocks the view of the polarized region. Knisley and Pollard[149] have developed an indium tin oxide electrode that is transparent to light, so they can perform optical mapping of the area directly under the electrode. They used such an electrode to test Patel and Roth's prediction and observed the same effect experimentally. It is also useful that the reflectance of the indium tin oxide depends on the local current leaving the electrode surface, so that this approach can provide information about the spatial distribution of the current being delivered to the tissue under the electrode.

The Effect of Fiber Curvature on Stimulation of Cardiac Tissue

Trayanova et al.[120] were the first to realize that fiber curvature can induce polarization in cardiac tissue, and Trayanova's group has examined this effect in detail.[121,150,151] Roth and Langrill Beaudoin[152] found approximate analytical solutions to the bidomain equations for electrical stimulation of cardiac tissue with curving fibers and illustrated two mechanisms of polarization, both of which require unequal anisotropy ratios. In the first mechanism, the fiber orientation changes in the direction parallel to the electric field (Fig. 19a). On the left, the current is distributed evenly between the intracellular and extracellular spaces because they have similar conductivities in the direction parallel to the fibers.[153] On the right, most of the current is in the extracellular space because of the relatively small conductivity of the intracellular space in the direction perpendicular to the fibers. In the middle, the current must be moving from the intracellular to the extracellular space, thereby depolarizing the membrane. The key insight is that the current distributes according to the ratio of the conductivities (g) in the intracellular (i) and extracellular (e) spaces, and that this ratio is different in the longitudinal (L) and transverse (T) directions ($g_{iL}/g_{eL} \neq g_{iT}/g_{eT}$). This inequality is equivalent to the condition of unequal anisotropy ratios ($g_{iL}/g_{iT} \neq g_{eL}/g_{eT}$).

In the second mechanism, the fiber orientation changes in the direction perpendicular to the electric field (Fig. 19b). In this case, the current density J on the left and right

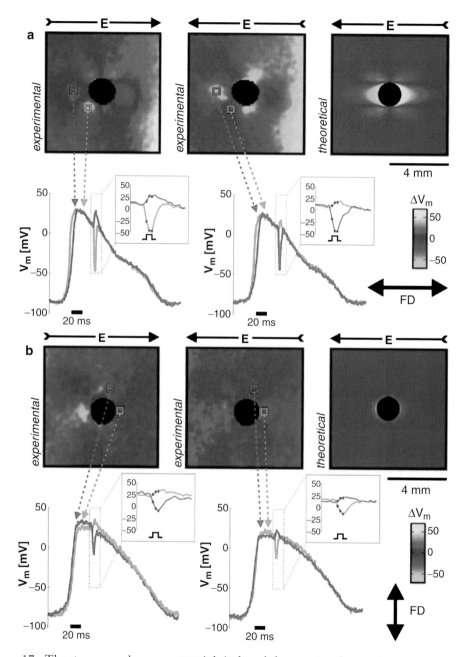

Figure 17: The transmembrane potential induced by an insulating heterogeneity in a uniform electric field (30 V/cm), with fibers (**a**) horizontal and (**b**) vertical. The *right panels* are numerical simulations. The *middle* and *left panels* are experimental data, for two polarities of the electric field. (Woods et al.)[146]

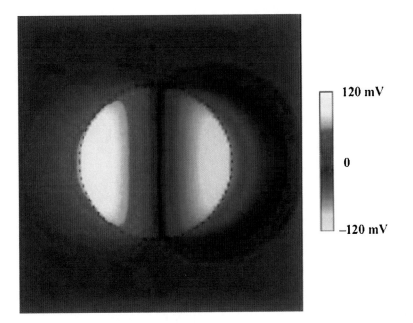

Figure 18: The calculated transmembrane potential under an epicardial electrode during an applied electric field (Patel and Roth, with kind permission of Springer Science and Business Media)[148]

sides is in the same direction as the electric field E. However, J in the middle is not aligned with E because of the anisotropy. The higher anisotropy in the intracellular space causes the intracellular current to rotate toward the fiber direction more than the extracellular current. This induces a horizontal component of the current density that is larger inside the cells than outside. The net result is current entering the cells on the left (thereby hyperpolarizing the tissue) and exiting the cells on the right (thereby depolarizing the tissue).

Figure 20 shows the transmembrane potential induced by a curving fiber geometry. The inset shows the individual contributions of the two mechanisms. Although the approximate analytical model used to calculate the results in Fig. 20 has significant limitations, it does provide useful insight into the mechanisms underlying polarization by fiber curvature.

The impact of fiber curvature during stimulation of the heart has been studied using a combination of whole-heart modeling and optical mapping. Efimov et al.[105] observed defibrillation shock-induced virtual electrodes that correlate well with simulations, albeit for epicardial polarizations.[119] Similarly, Knisley et al.,[122] using stimulation parallel to the surface of the heart, and Tung and Kleber,[154] using cultured, two-dimensional strands of cells, have found excellent agreement between theory and experiment. As discussed above, there remains a need for quantitative comparisons between model and experiment for intramyocardial fibers.

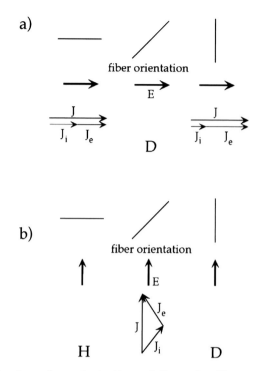

Figure 19: Two mechanisms for polarization of tissue by fiber curvature. (a) The fiber orientation changes in the direction of the electric field and (b) the fiber orientation changes in the direction perpendicular to the electric field (Roth and Langrill Beaudoin, reprinted with permission © 2003 by the American Physical Society [http://prola.aps.org/abstract/PRE/v67/i5/e051925])[152]

Heterogeneities

Another factor that influences the response of the heart to a shock is heterogeneities. Plonsey and Barr[155] and Krassowska et al.[156] concluded that periodic small-scale discontinuities in the intracellular conductivity associated with gap junctions cause small-scale regions of depolarization and hyperpolarization (the sawtooth effect). Keener[157] and Krinsky and Pumir[158] postulated that this behavior may underlie defibrillation. Experimentalists have not found these small-scale virtual electrodes,[159,160] but the averaging inherent in optical mapping could make them difficult to detect. Krassowska and Kumar[161] and Fishler and Vepa[125] and Fishler[162] suggested that heterogeneities in tissue properties distributed over several length scales could also cause excitation. Langrill Beaudoin and Roth[163] found that random changes in fiber direction would have the same effect and concluded that the high and low spatial frequency components of heterogeneities interact to cause reentry induction: low frequencies carve out excitable pathways, and high frequencies provide the large gradient of transmembrane potential required for break excitation.

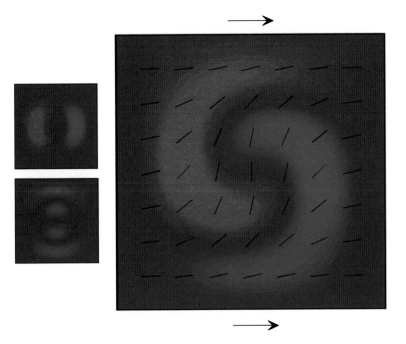

Figure 20: The transmembrane potential induced by curving fibers in the presence of an electric field. The fiber direction is indicated by the line segments, and the electric field by the *arrow*. The small panels on the *left* correspond to the two mechanisms of Fig. 19 individually (Roth and Langrill Beaudoin, reprinted with permission © 2003 by the American Physical Society [http://prola.aps.org/abstract/PRE/v67/i5/e051925])[152]

As we discussed in the section on defibrillation, recent evidence suggests that heterogeneities play an important role during whole-heart excitation. Woods et al.[134,135,164,165] observed widespread prompt excitation in a virtual anode, which may arise from heterogeneities that are at too small a spatial scale to observe in optical mapping. Sharifov and Fast[130] observed differences in the shock response between hearts stained with a voltage-sensitive dye only on the epicardium surface versus globally via coronary perfusion. Also, sophisticated modeling studies indicate the importance of heterogeneities.[166,167] Clearly this is a topic that requires additional study.

Averaging over Depth During Optical Mapping

Optical mapping does not measure V_m at the tissue surface, but instead averages over some depth below the surface.[168] Efimov et al.[169] observed double-humped action potentials during optical mapping, which they interpreted as being caused by three-dimensional scroll waves rotating below the tissue surface. Bray and Wikswo[170] simulated such scroll waves and found that shallow reentrant waves can indeed give rise to double-humped signals.

Averaging over depth also affects the measured V_m signal during electrical stimulation. Janks and Roth[171] found that if the electrical length constant is less than the optical decay constant, then the averaged signal severely underestimates the true surface transmembrane potential. Several researchers have observed evidence of electroporation after an electric shock,[172–174] but the optically measured transmembrane potential deviated from its resting value by less than 100 mV, which should not be sufficient to cause electroporation. Al-Khadra et al.[174] suggested that the optical signal might be collected over depth, with only the surface layer actually electroporated. Janks and Roth[175] examined this question using a numerical simulation and concluded that averaging over depth may indeed explain why a shock can cause electroporation while appearing to have a small transmembrane potential. However, they could not explain why the deviation of the resting potential, cited by the experimentalists as evidence for electroporation, was not also underestimated because of averaging over depth. Averaging over depth represents one of the pitfalls researchers face when comparing experimental data to numerical simulations,[9] but the development of good models of photon diffusion should remove major uncertainties in the comparison of theory and experiment.[176–179]

Boundary Conditions and the Bidomain Model

The boundary conditions[180,181] at the interface between cardiac tissue and an adjacent conductor can significantly influence the electrical behavior of the tissue, as is shown in Fig. 21a for field stimulation of a heart with a variable orientation in a bath.[124] Latimer and Roth[182] used the bidomain model to simulate unipolar stimulation of tissue when the electrode was in an adjacent conductive bath. They found results similar to those predicted by Sepulveda et al.,[21] that is, hyperpolarization at virtual anodes located along the fiber direction, near a cathode. Knisley et al.[183] observed similar results using optical mapping. Interestingly, in some cases the virtual anode could be "buried" below the tissue surface by boundary effects.[182,184]

Another interesting effect of the tissue boundary arises when the heart is stimulated using electrodes inside the heart, but is observed using optical mapping of the epicardial surface.[119,123] In this case not only the magnitude of the epicardial signal but even its sign depend on the boundary. Results obtained when the heart is placed against an insulating glass plate may be very different from those when the heart is superfused by a conducting solution (Fig. 21b).[124]

Yet another boundary effect arises when the myocardial fibers intersect an insulating surface at an angle. Typically, the sealed nature of an insulating surface prevents any transmembrane potential from being induced there. However, when the tissue has unequal anisotropy ratios and the fibers approach the boundary at an angle, the boundary condition causes the tissue to be polarized.[185] In most cases, myocardial fibers lie in a plane parallel to the tissue surface, so this effect is not important. Yet, when the tissue is cut to create a "wedge preparation" and then this cut surface is mapped optically, this boundary effect can play an important, and even dominant, role.[186]

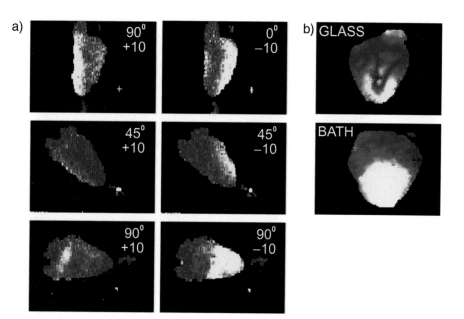

Figure 21: Examples of how boundary conditions can affect cardiac shock response. (a) The prompt response of an isolated rabbit heart to field stimulation by a horizontal electrical field at three different angles and shock polarities (± 10 V cm^{-1}). *Red/yellow* is depolarization. For $90°$, $+10$ V cm^{-1}, the valve ring may block the field. Otherwise, the pattern is clearly determined by the orientation and sign of the field and not the orientation of the heart, consistent with the monodomain/bidomain boundary between the surrounding bath and the heart. (b) The dye fluorescence image of the epicardial surface of an isolated rabbit heart during an intracardiac defibrillation-strength anodal shock. *Upper*: The heart is pressed against a glass plate to produce a horseshoe-shaped depolarized region (*yellow*) surrounding a hyperpolarized one (*blue*). *Lower*: The heart is suspended freely in the bath, and only depolarization is evident on the epicardium (Adapted from Lin and Wikswo)[124]

The Magnetic Field Produced by Cardiac Tissue

The original inquiries into the role of unequal anisotropies in the heart represented a convergence between Corbin and Scher's pioneering observations of phenomena that could not be explained by the uniform double-layer model of cardiac excitation,[187–189] the early bidomain model studies of Plonsey and Barr,[15,16] and the search by Wikswo et al.[190–194] for new information in the magnetocardiogram. Sepulveda and Wikswo[19] predicted a fourfold symmetric magnetic field pattern associated with an outwardly propagating wavefront in a two-dimensional sheet of cardiac tissue (Fig. 22). This magnetic field was only present when the tissue had unequal anisotropy ratios; if the anisotropy ratios were equal, the intracellular and extracellular currents exactly canceled each other and no magnetic field was produced.[19,195,196] Staton et al.[197] and Baudenbacher et al.[198] observed this behavior

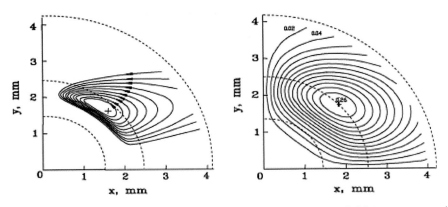

Figure 22: The calculated current lines (left) and the magnetic field isocontours (right) associated with an outwardly propagating circular wavefront (*dashed curves*). Only one quadrant of the x–y plane is shown (Adapted from Sepulveda and Wikswo by permission of the authors and the Biophysical Society)[19]

(Fig. 23) by measuring the magnetic field using a high-spatial-resolution superconducting quantum interference device (SQUID) magnetometer. Biomagnetic fields are important in cardiac electrophysiology because they provide a sensitive test of the bidomain model. Staton[199] considered the case when the anisotropy in the intracellular and extracellular space is described in terms of common-mode and differential-mode terms,[13] with the former corresponding to the average bulk anisotropy and the latter and more interesting representing the difference between the intracellular and extracellular anisotropies. He concluded that the observation of the effects of the differential mode required recording at spatial frequencies at least as high as $1\,\text{mm}^{-1}$, which represents a technical challenge only recently met with ultrahigh resolution scanning SQUID microscopes.[198,200–203]

Roth and Woods[204] theoretically examined the magnetic field produced by a plane wavefront. Their study elucidated the role of unequal anisotropy ratios in biomagnetism (Fig. 24). If the direction of propagation is different from the fiber direction, then the anisotropy rotates both the intracellular and extracellular current densities away from the direction of the potential gradient. However, the higher anisotropy of the intracellular space rotates the intracellular current more than the extracellular current. The result is a net current that is directed parallel to the wavefront.[204–206] This contribution to the biomagnetic field is as important as the one establishing the traditional view of a dipole directed perpendicular to the wavefront as the magnetic field source.[207]

Holzer et al.[202] measured the magnetic field produced by a planar wavefront, using both optical mapping of the electrical potential and magnetic mapping of the current (Fig. 25). They found that indeed the magnetic field pattern was consistent with a line of current directed parallel to the wavefront, and concluded that bidomain effects may play an important role in the production of the magnetocardiogram. The sensitivity and spatial resolution of magnetometers continues to improve,[200,201,208] providing a novel tool for measuring current in cardiac tissue.

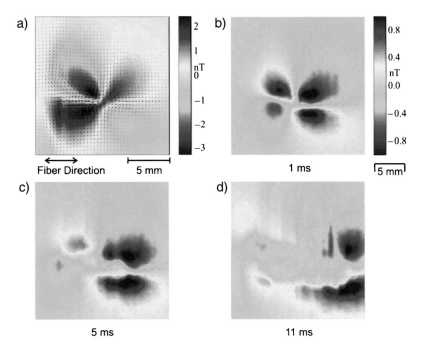

Figure 23: An experimental measurement of the magnetic fields associated with current injection and an expanding wavefront in cardiac tissue. (a) The magnetic field resulting from a cathodal stimulus current of 1.5 mA. The *overlaid arrows* schematically represent the current distribution under the assumption of two-dimensional sheet currents. (b–d) The magnetic fields generated by the subsequent propagation of action currents resulting from a cathodal point stimulus. Note the color bar, which reflects weaker fields in (b–d) than in (a). The octopolar patterns with four current loops can be explained in the framework of a bidomain model with unequal anisotropy ratios in the intra- and extracellular space; the phase reversal between (a) and (b) is consistent with the model predictions (Adapted from Baudenbacher et al.)[198]

Conclusion

From our discussions and the summary in Table 1, it should be clear that the bidomain model has been very successful in making qualitative predictions about the electrical behavior of the heart, possibly to a greater extent than any other tissue-level model. Quantitative predictions are still a challenge,[9] but progress is being made, particularly as both measurement techniques and models of the measurement process advance. Although much of the early research into the doubly anisotropic bidomain was focused on the information content of biomagnetic measurements,[19] the predicted response of the curved-fiber bidomain model to strong shocks[120] and the demonstrated presence of virtual electrodes[49]

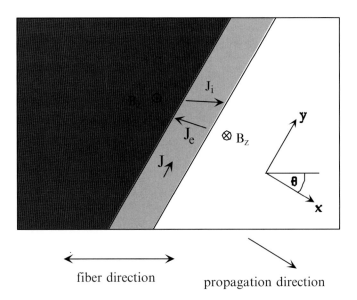

Figure 24: The current and magnetic field associated with a planar wavefront. The fiber direction is horizontal, and the direction of propagation is down and to the right. The intracellular and extracellular current densities, J_i and J_e, are both rotated away from the propagation direction, resulting in a net current J directed parallel to the wavefront (*light shading*) (Roth and Woods, by permission of the authors, © 1999 IEEE)[204]

provided the convincing evidence that the doubly anisotropic cardiac bidomain is central to the defibrillation process.[209] Today it is apparent that virtual electrodes, deexcitation, and break excitation play an important role in such vital events as defibrillation. The forthcoming challenges are to ascertain the role of heterogeneities in defibrillation (i.e., to probe the limits of the bidomain and to identify the spatial scale for which the bidomain in fact demonstrates behavior consistent with small-scale heterogeneities).[125,161,162]

Acknowledgments

We are indebted to Allison Price and Don Berry for their painstaking bibliographic, editorial, and graphical assistance in preparing this manuscript. We thank Veniamin Sidorov, Richard Gray, and Franz Baudenbacher for answering innumerable questions. We gratefully acknowledge the many contributions that our students and collaborators have made to the research that we describe in this chapter. This work was supported by the National Institutes of Health grants R01 HL57207 and HL58241.

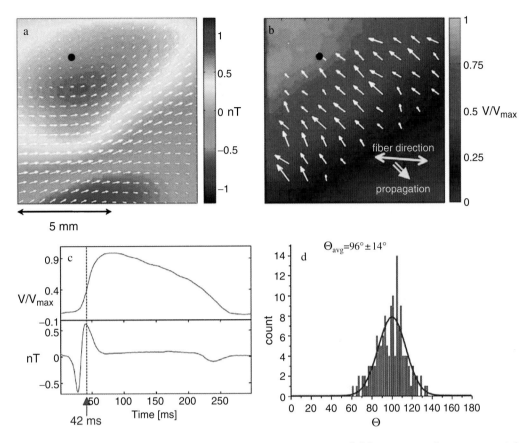

Figure 25: The relationships between the current, magnetic field, transmembrane potential, and the transmembrane potential gradient. (a) The current and magnetic field associated with a planar wavefront, (b) the transmembrane potential associated with the wavefront and *arrows* showing the direction of the potential gradient, (c) the action potential and magnetic field showing the time corresponding to panels (a) and (b), and (d) the average angle between the current and potential gradient (Holzer et al., by permission of the authors and the Biophysical Society)[202]

References

1. Jeffrey K. *Machines in Our Hearts: The Cardiac Pacemaker, the Implantable Defibrillator, and American Health Care.* Baltimore, MD: Johns Hopkins University Press; 2001
2. Rosenbaum DS, Jalife J. *Optical Mapping of Cardiac Excitation and Arrhythmias.* Armonk, NY: Futura; 2001

3. Henriquez CS. Simulating the electrical behavior of cardiac tissue using the bidomain model. *Crit Rev Biomed Eng* 1993;21:1–77

4. Zipes DP, Jalife J. *Cardiac Electrophysiology: From Cell to Bedside*, Ed. 4. Philadelphia, PA: Saunders; 2004

5. Burton RAB, Plank G, Schneider JE, Grau V, Ahammer H, Keeling SL, Lee J, Smith NP, Gavaghan D, Trayanova N, Kohl P. Three-dimensional models of individual cardiac histoanatomy: tools and challenges. *Ann N Y Acad Sci* 2006;1080:301–319

6. Efimov IR, Aguel F, Cheng Y, Wollenzier B, Trayanova N. Virtual electrode polarization in the far field: implications for external defibrillation. *Am J Physiol Heart* 2000;279:H1055–H1070

7. Neu JC, Krassowska W. Homogenization of syncytial tissues. *Crit Rev Biomed Eng* 1993;21:137–199

8. Roth BJ. Mechanisms for electrical stimulation of excitable tissue. *Crit Rev Biomed Eng* 1994;22:253–305

9. Roth BJ. Artifacts, assumptions, and ambiguity: pitfalls in comparing experimental results to numerical simulations when studying electrical stimulation. *Chaos* 2002;12:973–981

10. Schmitt OH. Biological information processing using the concept of interpenetrating domains. In: Leibovic KN, ed. *Information Processing in the Nervous System.* New York: Springer; 1969:325–331

11. Muler AL, Markin VS. Electrical properties of anisotropic nerve-muscle syncytia – I. Distribution of the electrotonic potential. *Biofizika* 1977;22:307–312

12. Miller WT III, Geselowitz DB. Simulation studies of the electrocardiogram I. The normal heart. *Circ Res* 1978;43:301–315

13. Tung L. A bi-domain model for describing ischemic myocardial D-C potentials. Ph.D. dissertation, Cambridge, MA: MIT; 1978

14. Geselowitz DB, Miller WT III. A bidomain model for anisotropic cardiac muscle. *Ann Biomed Eng* 1983;11:191–206

15. Plonsey R, Barr RC. Current flow patterns in two-dimensional anisotropic bisyncytia with normal and extreme conductivities. *Biophys J* 1984;45:557–571

16. Barr RC, Plonsey R. Propagation of excitation in idealized anisotropic two-dimensional tissue. *Biophys J* 1984;45:1191–1202

17. Roth BJ, Wikswo JP Jr. A bidomain model for the extracellular potential and magnetic field of cardiac tissue. *IEEE Trans Biomed Eng* 1986;33:467–469

18. Plonsey R, Barr RC. Interstitial potentials and their change with depth into cardiac tissue. *Biophys J* 1987;51:547–555

19. Sepulveda NG, Wikswo JP Jr. Electric and magnetic fields from two-dimensional anisotropic bisyncytia. *Biophys J* 1987;51:557–568

20. Henriquez CS, Trayanova NA, Plonsey R. Potential and current distributions in a cylindrical bundle of cardiac tissue. *Biophys J* 1988;53:907–918

21. Sepulveda NG, Roth BJ, Wikswo JP Jr. Current injection into a two-dimensional anisotropic bidomain. *Biophys J* 1989;55:987–999

22. Dillon SM. Optical recordings in the rabbit heart show that defibrillation strength shocks prolong the duration of depolarization and the refractory period. *Circ Res* 1991;69:842–856

23. Knisley SB, Hill BC. Optical recordings of the effect of electrical stimulation on action potential repolarization and the induction of reentry in two-dimensional perfused rabbit epicardium. *Circulation* 1993;88(Pt I):2402–2414

24. Sepulveda NG, Wikswo JP Jr. Electrical behavior of a cardiac bisyncytium during current injection. *Bull APS* 1987;32:2131

25. Sepulveda NG, Roth BJ, Wikswo JP Jr. Finite element bidomain calculations. In: Harris GF, Walker C, eds. *Proceedings of the Annual International Conference of the IEEE Engineering in Medicine and Biology Society.* Piscataway, NJ: IEEE; 1988:950–951

26. Wikswo JP Jr, Roth BJ, Sepulveda NG. Current distributions in bisyncytial tissue. *Phys Med Biol* 1988;33(Suppl 1):165

27. Wikswo JP Jr, Kopelman HA, Roden DM. Cardiac excitability and space constants measured in vivo using the virtual cathode effect. *Circulation* 1985;72:III-3

28. Kopelman HA, Bajaj AK, Wikswo JP Jr, Hondeghem LM, Woosley RL, Roden DM. Frequency- and direction-dependent effects of single and combinations of antiarrhythmic drugs on conduction velocity in vivo. *J Am Coll Cardiol* 1986;7:82a

29. Bajaj AK, Kopelman HA, Wikswo JP Jr, Cassidy F, Woosley RL, Roden DM. Frequency- and orientation-dependent effects of mexiletine and quinidine on conduction in the intact dog heart. *Circulation* 1987;75:1065–1073

30. Altemeier WA, Turgeon J, Wisialowski TA, Wikswo JP Jr, Roden DM. Contrasting effects of class I and class III antiarrhythmics on virtual cathode dimension. *Circulation* 1988;78(Suppl II): II-414

31. Wikswo JP Jr, Barach JP, Altemeier WA, Roden DM. Measurement and modeling of virtual cathode effects in cardiac muscle. *Phys Med Biol* 1988;33(Suppl 1):232

32. Wisialowski TA, Wikswo JP Jr, Roden DM. Lidocaine (LID) contracts the virtual cathode in a frequency-dependent fashion. *Circulation* 1990;82:SIII-99

33. Wikswo JP Jr, Wisialowski TA, Altemeier WA, Balser JR, Kopelman HA, Roden DM. Virtual cathode effects during stimulation of cardiac muscle: two-dimensional in vivo measurements. *Circ Res* 1991;68:513–530

34. Wiederholt WC. Threshold and conduction velocity in isolated mixed mammalian nerves. *Neurology* 1970;20:347–352

35. Cummins KL, Dorfman LJ, Perkel DH. Nerve-fiber conduction-velocity distributions. 2. Estimation based on 2 compound action potentials. *Electroencephalogr Clin Neurophysiol* 1979;46:647–658

36. Rattay F. Analysis of models for external stimulation of axons. *IEEE Trans Biomed Eng* 1986;33:974–977

37. Rattay F. Analysis of models for extracellular fiber stimulation. *IEEE Trans Biomed Eng* 1989;36:676–682

38. Rattay F. Modeling the excitation of fibers under surface electrodes. *IEEE Trans Biomed Eng* 1988;35:199–202

39. Sobie EA, Susil RC, Tung L. A generalized activating function for predicting virtual electrodes in cardiac tissue. *Biophys J* 1997;73:1410–1423

40. Terman FE, Helliwell RA, Pettit JM, Watkins DA, Rambo WR. *Electronic and Radio Engineering*, 4th edn. New York: McGraw Hill; 1955

41. Furman S, Hurzeler P, Parker B. Clinical thresholds of endocardial cardiac stimulation: a long-term study. *J Surg Res* 1975;19:149–155

42. Goto M, Brooks CM. Membrane excitability of the frog ventricle examined by long pulses. *Am J Physiol* 1969;217:1236–1245

43. Hoshi T, Matsuda K. Excitability cycle of cardiac muscle examined by intracellular stimulation. *Jpn J Physiol* 1962;12:433–446

44. Hoffman BF, Cranefield PF. Excitability. *Electrophysiology of the Heart*. New York: McGraw-Hill; 1960:211–256

45. Roth BJ. How the anisotropy of intracellular and extracellular conductivities influences stimulation of cardiac muscle. *J Math Biol* 1992;30:633–646

46. Roth BJ. Approximate analytical solutions to the bidomain equations with unequal anisotropy ratios. *Phys Rev E* 1997;55:1819–1826

47. Knisley SB. Transmembrane voltage changes during unipolar stimulation of rabbit ventricle. *Circ Res* 1995;77:1229–1239

48. Neunlist M, Tung L. Spatial distribution of cardiac transmembrane potentials around an extracellular electrode: dependence on fiber orientation. *Biophys J* 1995;68:2310–2322

49. Wikswo JP Jr, Lin S-F, Abbas RA. Virtual electrodes in cardiac tissue: a common mechanism for anodal and cathodal stimulation. *Biophys J* 1995;69:2195–2210

50. Dekker E. Direct current make and break thresholds for pacemaker electrodes on the canine ventricle. *Circ Res* 1970;27:811–823

51. Lindemans FW, Heetharr RM, Denier Van der Gon JJ, Zimmerman ANE. Site of initial excitation and current threshold as a function of electrode radius in heart muscle. *Cardiovasc Res* 1975;9:95–104

52. Ehara T. Rectifier properties of canine papillary muscle. *Jpn J Physiol.* 1971;21:49–69

53. Roth BJ. A mathematical model of make and break electrical stimulation of cardiac tissue by a unipolar anode or cathode. *IEEE Trans Biomed Eng* 1995;42:1174–1184

54. Roth BJ. Nonsustained reentry following successive stimulation of cardiac tissue through a unipolar electrode. *J Cardiovasc Electrophysiol* 1997;8:768–778

55. Sidorov VY, Woods MC, Wikswo JP. Effects of elevated extracellular potassium on the stimulation mechanism of diastolic cardiac tissue. *Biophys J.* 2003;84:3470–3479

56. Sidorov VY, Woods MC, Baudenbacher P, Baudenbacher F. Examination of stimulation mechanism and strength–interval curve in cardiac tissue. *Am J Physiol Heart* 2005;289:H2602–H2615

57. Sidorov VY, Woods MC, Wikswo JP Jr. Elevated potassium concentration converts excitation mechanism from make to break. In: *EMBS-BMES 2002, Proceedings of the Second Joint EMBS-BMES Conference, Oct. 23–26, Houston, TX*. Piscataway, NJ: IEEE, 2002:1377–1378

58. Roth BJ, Patel SG. Effects of elevated extracellular potassium ion concentration on anodal excitation of cardiac tissue. *J Cardiovasc Electrophysiol* 2003;14:1351–1355

59. Nikolski VP, Sambelashvili AT, Efimov IR. Mechanisms of make and break excitation revisited: paradoxical break excitation during diastolic stimulation. *Am J Physiol Heart* 2002;282:H565–H575

60. Nikolski V, Sambelashvili A, Efimov IR. Anode-break excitation during end-diastolic stimulation is explained by half-cell double layer discharge. *IEEE Trans Biomed Eng* 2002;49:1217–1220

61. Ranjan R, Chiamvimonvat N, Thakor NV, Tomaselli GF, Marban E. Mechanism of anode break stimulation in the heart. *Biophys J* 1998;74:1850–1863

62. Ranjan R, Tomaselli GF, Marban E. A novel mechanism of anode-break stimulation predicted by bidomain modeling. *Circ Res* 1999;84:153–156

63. Roth BJ, Chen J. Mechanism of anode break excitation in the heart: the relative influence of membrane and electrotonic factors. *J Biol Syst* 1999;7:541–552

64. van Dam RTh, Durrer D, Strackee J, van der Twell LH. The excitability cycle of the dog's left ventricle determined by anodal, cathodal and bipolar stimulation. *Circ Res* 1956;4:196–204

65. Cranefield PF, Hoffman BF, Siebens AA. Anodal excitation of cardiac muscle. *Am J Physiol* 1957;190:383–390

66. Roth BJ. Strength–interval curves for cardiac tissue predicted using the bidomain model. *J Cardiovasc Electrophysiol* 1996;7:722–737

67. Rodriguez B, Tice BM, Eason JC, Aguel F, Trayanova N. Cardiac vulnerability to electric shocks during phase 1A of acute global ischemia. *Heart Rhythm* 2004;1:695–703

68. Bray M-A, Roth BJ, The effect of electroporation on the strength–interval curve during unipolar stimulation of cardiac tissue. *19th Annual International Conference of the IEEE Engineering in Medicine and Biology Society, Oct. 30–Nov. 2.* Chicago: IEEE; 1997:15–18

69. Mehra R, McMullen M, Furman S. Time-dependence of unipolar cathodal and anodal strength–interval curves. *PACE* 1980;3:526–530

70. Bennett JA, Roth BJ. Time dependence of anodal and cathodal refractory periods in cardiac tissue. *PACE* 1999;22:1031–1038

71. El-Sherif N, Mehra R, Gough WB, Zeiler RH. Reentrant ventricular arrhythmias in the late myocardial infarction period. *Circulation* 1983;68:644–656

72. Davidenko JM, Pertsov AM, Salomonsz R, Baxter W, Jalife J. Stationary and drifting spiral waves of excitation in isolated cardiac muscle. *Nature* 1992;355:349–351

73. Pertsov AM, Davidenko JM, Salomonsz R, Baxter W, Jalife J. Spiral waves of excitation underlie reentrant activity in isolated cardiac muscle. *Circ Res* 1993;72:631–650

74. Gray RA, Jalife J, Panfilov AV, Baxter WT, Cabo C, Davidenko JM, Pertsov AM. Nonstationary vortexlike reentrant activity as a mechanism of polymorphic ventricular tachycardia in the isolated rabbit heart. *Circulation* 1995;91:2454–2469

75. Gray RA, Jalife J, Panfilov AV, Baxter WT, Cabo C, Davidenko JM, Pertsov AM. Mechanisms of cardiac fibrillation. *Science* 1995;270:1222–1225

76. Frazier DW, Wolf PD, Wharton JM, Tang ASL, Smith WM, Ideker RE. Stimulus-induced critical point: mechanism for electrical initiation of reentry in normal canine myocardium. *J Clin Invest* 1989;83:1039–1052

77. Winfree AT. *When Time Breaks Down: The Three-Dimensional Dynamics of Electro-chemical Waves and Cardiac Arrhythmias.* Princeton, NJ: Princeton University Press; 1987

78. Shibata N, Chen P-S, Dixon EG, Wolf PD, Danieley ND, Smith WM, Ideker RE. Influence of shock strength and timing on induction of ventricular arrhythmias in dogs. *Am J Physiol Heart* 1988;255:H891–H901

79. Matta RJ, Verrier RL, Lown B. Repetitive extrasystole as an index of vulnerability to ventricular fibrillation. *Am J Physiol* 1976;230:1469–1473

80. Winfree AT. Ventricular reentry in three dimensions. In: Zipes DP, Jalife J, eds. *Cardiac Electrophysiology: From Cell to Bedside.* Philadelphia: W.B. Saunders; 1990:224–234

81. Saypol JM, Roth BJ. A mechanism for anisotropic reentry in electrically active tissue. *J Cardiovasc Electrophysiol* 1992;3:558–566

82. Lin S-F, Roth BJ, Wikswo JP Jr. Quatrefoil reentry in myocardium: an optical imaging study of the induction mechanism. *J Cardiovasc Electrophysiol* 1999;10:574–586

83. Sidorov VY, Aliev RR, Woods MC, Baudenbacher F, Baudenbacher P, Wikswo JP. Spatiotemporal dynamics of damped propagation in excitable cardiac tissue. *Phys Rev Lett* 2003;91:208104

84. Gotoh M, Uchida T, Mandel WJ, Fishbein MC, Chen P-S, Karagueuzian HS. Cellular graded responses and ventricular vulnerability to reentry by a premature stimulus in isolated canine ventricle. *Circulation* 1997;95:2141–2154

85. Trayanova NA, Gray RA, Bourn DW, Eason JC. Virtual electrode-induced positive and negative graded responses: new insights into fibrillation induction and defibrillation. *J Cardiovasc Electrophysiol* 2003;14:756–763

86. Bray M-A, Lin S-F, Aliev RR, Roth BJ, Wikswo JP Jr. Experimental and theoretical analysis of phase singularity dynamics in cardiac tissue. *J Cardiovasc Electrophysiol* 2001;12:716–722

87. Bray M-A, Wikswo JP Jr. Considerations in phase plane analysis for non-stationary reentrant cardiac behavior. *Phys Rev E* 2002;65:051902

88. Bray M-A, Wikswo JP. Interaction dynamics of a pair of vortex filament rings. *Phys Rev Lett* 2003;90:238303

89. Gray RA, Iyer A, Bray M-A, Wikswo JP. Voltage-calcium state-space dynamics during initiation of reentry. *Heart Rhythm* 2006;3:247–248

90. Choi BR, Burton F, Salama G. Cytosolic Ca^{2+} triggers early after depolarizations and torsade de pointes in rabbit hearts with type 2 long QT syndrome. *J Physiol* 2002;543(2):615–631

91. Verrier RL, Brooks WW, Lown B. Protective zone and determination of vulnerability to ventricular-fibrillation. *Am J Physiol* 1978;234:H592–H596

92. Bonometti C, Hwang C, Hough D, Lee JJ, Fishbein MC, Karagueuzian HS, Chen P-S. Interaction between strong electrical stimulation and reentrant wavefronts in canine ventricular fibrillation. *Circ Res* 1995;77:407–416

93. Hwang C, Fan W, Chen PS. Recurrent appearance of protective zones after an unsuccessful defibrillation shock. *Am J Physiol Heart* 1996;40:H1491–H1497

94. Hildebrandt MC, Roth BJ. Simulation of protective zones during quatrefoil reentry in cardiac tissue. *J Cardiovasc Electrophysiol* 2001;12:1062–1067

95. Roth BJ. Art Winfree and the bidomain model of cardiac tissue. *J Theor Biol* 2004;230:445–449

96. Winfree AT. Various ways to make phase singularities by electric shock. *J Cardiovasc Electrophysiol* 2000;11:286–289

97. Winfree AT. *The Geometry of Biological Time.* New York: Springer; 2001

98. Roth BJ. An S_1 gradient of refractoriness is not essential for reentry induction by an S_2 stimulus. *IEEE Trans Biomed Eng* 2000;47:820–821

99. Cheng YN, Nikolski V, Efimov IR. Reversal of repolarization gradient does not reverse the chirality of shock-induced reentry in the rabbit heart. *J Cardiovasc Electrophysiol* 2000;11:998–1007

100. Sidorov VY, Woods MC, Baudenbacher F. Cathodal stimulation in the recovery phase of a propagating planar wave in the rabbit heart reveals four stimulation mechanisms. *J Physiol* 2007;583:237–250

101. Lindblom AE, Roth BJ, Trayanova NA. Role of virtual electrodes in arrhythmogenesis: pinwheel experiment revisited. *J Cardiovasc Electrophysiol* 2000;11:274–285

102. Lindblom AE, Aguel F, Trayanova NA. Virtual electrode polarization leads to reentry in the far field. *J Cardiovasc Electrophysiol* 2001;12:946–956

103. Roth BJ. The pinwheel experiment revisited. *J Theor Biol* 1998;190:389–393

104. Sambelashvili A, Efimov IR. The pinwheel experiment re-revisited. *J Theor Biol* 2002;214:147–153

105. Efimov IR, Cheng YN, Biermann M, VanWagoner DR, Mazgalev TN, Tchou PJ. Transmembrane voltage changes produced by real and virtual electrodes during monophasic defibrillation shock delivered by an implantable electrode. *J Cardiovasc Electrophysiol* 1997;8:1031–1045

106. Efimov IR, Cheng Y, Van Wagoner DR, Mazgalev TN, Tchou PJ. Virtual electrode-induced phase singularity: a basic mechanism of defibrillation failure. *Circ Res* 1998;82:918–925

107. Cheng Y, Mowrey KA, Van Wagoner DR, Tchou PJ, Efimov IR. Virtual electrode-induced reexcitation: a mechanism of defibrillation. *Circ Res* 1999;85:1056–1066

108. Efimov IR, Cheng Y, Yamanouchi Y, Tchou PJ. Direct evidence of the role of virtual electrode-induced phase singularity in success and failure of defibrillation. *J Cardiovasc Electrophysiol* 2000;11:861–868

109. Efimov IR, Gray RA, Roth BJ. Virtual electrodes and deexcitation: new insights into fibrillation induction and defibrillation. *J Cardiovasc Electrophysiol* 2000;11:339–353

110. Trayanova NA, Skouibine KB, Moore PB. Virtual electrode effects in defibrillation. *Prog Biophys Mol Biol* 1998;69:387–403

111. Skouibine KB, Trayanova NA. Anode/cathode make and break phenomena in a model of defibrillation. *IEEE Trans Biomed Eng* 1999;46:769–777

112. Skouibine K, Trayanova N, Moore P. Success and failure of the defibrillation shock: insights from a simulation study. *J Cardiovasc Electrophysiol* 2000;11:785–796

113. Trayanova N. Induction of reentry and defibrillation: the role of virtual electrodes. In: Virag N, Blanc O, Kappenberger L, eds. *Computer Simulation and Experimental Assessment of Cardiac Electrophysiology.* Armonk, NY: Futura; 2001:165–172

114. Cheng Y, Mowrey KA, Nikolski V, Tchou PJ, Efimov IR. Mechanisms of shock-induced arrhythmogenesis during acute global ischemia. *Am J Physiol Heart* 2002;282:H2141–H2151

115. Rodriguez B, Tice BM, Eason JC, Aguel F, Ferrero JM, Trayanova N. Effect of acute global ischemia on the upper limit of vulnerability: a simulation study. *Am J Physiol Heart* 2004;286:H2078–H2088

116. Hillebrenner MG, Eason JC, Trayanova NA. Mechanistic inquiry into decrease in probability of defibrillation success with increase in complexity of preshock reentrant activity. *Am J Physiol Heart* 2004;286:H909–H917

117. Anderson C, Trayanova N, Skouibine K. Termination of spiral waves with biphasic shocks: role of virtual electrode polarization. *J Cardiovasc Electrophysiol* 2000;11:1386–1396

118. Rodriguez B, Li L, Eason JC, Efimov IR, Trayanova NA. Differences between left and right ventricular chamber geometry affect cardiac vulnerability to electric shocks. *Circ Res* 2005;97:168–175

119. Entcheva E, Eason J, Efimov IR, Cheng Y, Malkin RA, Claydon F. Virtual electrode effects in transvenous defibrillation-modulation by structure and interface: evidence from bidomain simulations and optical mapping. *J Cardiovasc Electrophysiol* 1998;9:949–961

120. Trayanova NA, Roth BJ, Malden LJ. The response of a spherical heart to a uniform electric field: a bidomain analysis of cardiac stimulation. *IEEE Trans Biomed Eng* 1993;40:899–908

121. Entcheva E, Trayanova NA, Claydon FJ. Patterns of and mechanisms for shock-induced polarization in the heart: a bidomain analysis. *IEEE Trans Biomed Eng* 1999;46:260–270

122. Knisley SB, Trayanova NA, Aguel F. Roles of electric field and fiber structure in cardiac electric stimulation. *Biophys J* 1999;77:1404–1417

123. Latimer DC, Roth BJ. Effect of a bath on the epicardial transmembrane potential during internal defibrillation shocks. *IEEE Trans Biomed Eng* 1999;46:612–614

124. Lin S-F, Wikswo JP Jr. New perspectives in electrophysiology from the cardiac bidomain. In: Rosenbaum DS, Jalife J, eds. *Optical Mapping of Cardiac Excitation and Arrhythmias.* Armonk, NY: Futura Publishing; 2001:335–359

125. Fishler MG, Vepa K. Spatiotemporal effects of syncytial heterogeneities on cardiac far-field excitations during monophasic and biphasic shocks. *J Cardiovasc Electrophysiol* 1998;9:1310–1324

126. Hooks DA, Tomlinson KA, Marsden SG, LeGrice IJ, Smaill BH, Pullan AJ, Hunter PJ. Cardiac microstructure: implications for electrical propagation and defibrillation in the heart. *Circ Res* 2002;91:331–338

127. Fast VG, Sharifov OF, Cheek ER, Newton JC, Ideker RE. Intramural virtual electrodes during defibrillation shocks in left ventricular wall assessed by optical mapping of membrane potential. *Circulation* 2002;106:1007–1014

128. Sharifov OF, Fast VG. Optical mapping of transmural activation induced by electrical shocks in isolated left ventricular wall wedge preparations. *J Cardiovasc Electrophysiol* 2003;14:1215–1222

129. Sharifov OF, Ideker RE, Fast VG. High-resolution optical mapping of intramural virtual electrodes in porcine left ventricular wall. *Cardiovasc Res* 2004;64:448–456

130. Sharifov OF, Fast VG. Role of intramural virtual electrodes in shock-induced activation of left ventricle: optical measurements from the intact epicardial surface. *Heart Rhythm* 2006;3:1063–1073

131. Pitruzello AM, Woods MC, Wikswo JP Jr, Lin S-F. Differences in cardiac activation times for endocardium and epicardium in response to external electric shock. In: Blanchard SM, ed. *Proceedings of the First Joint BMES/EMBS Conference: Serving Humanity Advancing Technology, Atlanta*: Piscataway, NJ: IEEE; 1999:286

132. Woods MC, Pitruzello AM, Wikswo JP. Analysis of the shock-response of rabbit cardiac tissue. Presented at BMES Annual Fall Meeting, Philadelphia, PA, 2004

133. Woods MC. Field stimulation of the diastolic rabbit heart: the role of shock strength and duration on epicardial activation and propagation. In: *The Response of the Cardiac Bidomain to Electrical Stimulation*. Ph.D. Dissertation, Biomedical Engineering, Vanderbilt University; 2005:109–138

134. Woods MC, Maleckar MM, Sidorov VY, Holcomb MR, Mashburn DN, Trayanova NA, Wikswo JP. Negative virtual electrode polarization in the rabbit left ventricle delays activation during diastolic field stimulation. *Heart Rhythm* 2006;3(Suppl 1):S181–S182

135. Maleckar MM, Woods MC, Sidorov VY, Holcomb MR, Mashburn DN, Wikswo JP, Trayanova NA. Polarity reversal lowers activation time during diastolic field stimulation of the rabbit ventricles: insights into mechanisms. *Am J Physiol Heart Circ Physiol* 2008;295;doi:10.1152/ajpheart.00706.2008

136. Holcomb MR. *Measurement and Analysis of Cardiac Tissue during Electrical Stimulation*. Ph.D. Dissertation, Physics, Vanderbilt University; 2007

137. Zemlin CW, Mironov S, Pertsov AM. Near-threshold field stimulation: intramural versus surface activation. *Cardiovasc Res* 2006;69:98–106

138. Roth BJ. A mechanism for the "no-response" phenomenon during anodal stimulation of cardiac tissue. In: Jaeger RJ, Robert J, eds. *Proceedings of the 19th Annual International Conference of the IEEE Engineering in Medicine and Biology Society, Oct. 30–Nov. 2, Chicago, IL*. Piscataway, NJ: IEEE, 1997:176–179

139. Janks DL, Roth BJ. The bidomain theory of pacing. In: Efimov I, Kroll M, Tchou P, eds. *Cardiac Bioelectric Therapy: Mechanisms and Practical Implications*; New York: Springer; 2008:63–83

140. Chen P-S, Shibata N, Dixon EG, Martin RO, Ideker RE. Comparison of the defibrillation threshold and the upper limit of ventricular vulnerability. *Circulation* 1986;73:1022–1028

141. Banville I, Gray RA, Ideker RE, Smith WM. Shock-induced figure-of-eight reentry in the isolated rabbit heart. *Circ Res* 1999;85:742–752

142. Rodriguez B, Trayanova N. Upper limit of vulnerability in a defibrillation model of the rabbit ventricles. *J Electrocardiol* 2003;36:51–56

143. Langrill Beaudoin D, Roth BJ. The effect of the fiber curvature gradient on break excitation in cardiac tissue. *PACE* 2006;29:496–501

144. Langrill DM, Roth BJ. The effect of plunge electrodes during electrical stimulation of cardiac tissue. *IEEE Trans Biomed Eng* 2001;48:1207–1211

145. Langrill Beaudoin D, Roth BJ. Effect of plunge electrodes in active cardiac tissue with curving fibers. *Heart Rhythm* 2004;1:476–481

146. Woods MC, Sidorov VY, Holcomb MR, Langrill Beaudoin D, Roth BJ, Wikswo JP. Virtual electrode effects around an artificial heterogeneity during field stimulation of cardiac tissue. *Heart Rhythm* 2006;3:751–752

147. Chattipakorn N, Fotuhi PC, Chattipakorn SC, Ideker RE. Three-dimensional mapping of earliest activation after near-threshold ventricular defibrillation shocks. *J Cardiovasc Electrophysiol* 2003;14:65–69

148. Patel SG, Roth BJ. How epicardial electrodes influence the transmembrane potential during a strong shock. *Ann Biomed Eng* 2001;29:1028–1031

149. Knisley SB, Pollard AE. Use of translucent indium tin oxide to measure stimulatory effects of a passive conductor during field stimulation of rabbit hearts. *Am J Physiol Heart* 2005;289:H1137–H1146

150. Trayanova N, Skouibine K, Aguel F. The role of cardiac tissue structure in defibrillation. *Chaos* 1998;8:221–233

151. Trayanova NA, Skouibine KB. Modeling defibrillation: effects of fiber curvature. *J Electrocardiol* 1998;31(Suppl):23–29

152. Roth BJ, Langrill Beaudoin D. Approximate analytical solutions of the bidomain equations for electrical stimulation of cardiac tissue with curving fibers. *Phys Rev E* 2003;67:051925

153. Roth BJ. Electrical conductivity values used with the bidomain model of cardiac tissue. *IEEE Trans Biomed Eng* 1997;44:326–328

154. Tung L, Kleber AG. Virtual sources associated with linear and curved strands of cardiac cells. *Am J Physiol Heart* 2000;279:H1579–H1590

155. Plonsey R, Barr RC. Effect of microscopic and macroscopic discontinuities on the response of cardiac tissue to defibrillation (stimulating) currents. *Med Biol Eng Comput* 1986;24:130–136

156. Krassowska W, Pilkington TC, Ideker RE. Periodic conductivity as a mechanism for cardiac stimulation and defibrillation. *IEEE Trans Biomed Eng* 1987;34:555–560

157. Keener JP. Direct activation and defibrillation of cardiac tissue. *J Theor Biol* 1996;178:313–324

158. Krinsky VI, Pumir A. Models of defibrillation of cardiac tissue. *Chaos* 1998;8:188–203

159. Gillis AM, Fast VG, Rohr S, Kleber AG. Spatial changes in transmembrane potential during extracellular electrical shocks in cultured monolayers of neonatal rat ventricular myocytes. *Circ Res* 1996;79:676–690

160. Zhou XH, Knisley SB, Smith WM, Rollins D, Pollard AE, Ideker RE. Spatial changes in the transmembrane potential during extracellular electric stimulation. *Circ Res* 1998;83:1003–1014

161. Krassowska W, Kumar MS. The role of spatial interactions in creating the dispersion of transmembrane potential by premature electric shocks. *Ann Biomed Eng* 1997;25:949–963

162. Fishler MG. Syncytial heterogeneity as a mechanism underlying cardiac far-field stimulation during defibrillation-level shocks. *J Cardiovasc Electrophysiol* 1998;9:384–394

163. Langrill Beaudoin D, Roth BJ. How the spatial frequency of polarization influences the induction of reentry in cardiac tissue. *J Cardiovasc Electrophysiol* 2005;16:748–752

164. Woods MC, Holcomb MR, Sidorov VY, Gray RA, Wikswo JP. Transient virtual anodes during strong field shock of rabbit hearts. Presented at BMES Annual Fall Meeting, Los Angeles, CA, 2007

165. Woods MC. *The Response of the Cardiac Bidomain to Electrical Stimulation*. Ph.D. Dissertation, Biomedical Engineering, Vanderbilt University; 2005

166. Trew M, Sands GB. Shock-induced transmembrane potential fields in a model of cardiac microstructure. *J Cardiovasc Electrophysiol* 2005;16:1024

167. Plank G, Prassl AJ, Vigmond EJ, Burton RAB, Schneider J, Trayanova NA, Kohl P. Development of a microanatomically accurate rabbit ventricular wedge model. *Heart Rhythm* 2006;3(Suppl 1):S111–S112

168. Gray RA. What exactly are optically recorded "action potentials"? *J Cardiovasc Electrophysiol* 1999;10:1463–1466

169. Efimov IR, Sidorov V, Cheng Y, Wollenzier B. Evidence of three-dimensional scroll waves with ribbon-shaped filament as a mechanism of ventricular tachycardia in the isolated rabbit heart. *J Cardiovasc Electrophysiol* 1999;10:1452–1462

170. Bray MA, Wikswo JP. Examination of optical depth effects on fluorescence imaging of cardiac propagation. *Biophys J* 2003;85:4134–4145

171. Janks DL, Roth BJ. Averaging over depth during optical mapping of unipolar stimulation. *IEEE Trans Biomed Eng* 2002;49:1051–1054

172. Neunlist M, Tung L. Dose-dependent reduction of cardiac transmembrane potential by high-intensity electrical shocks. *Am J Physiol Heart* 1997;42:H2817–H2825

173. Kodama I, Sakuma I, Shibata N, Honjo H, Toyama J. Arrhythmogenic changes in action potential configuration in the ventricle induced by DC shocks. *J Electrocardiol* 1999;32(Suppl 1):92–99

174. Al Khadra A, Nikolski V, Efimov IR. The role of electroporation in defibrillation. *Circ Res* 2000;87:797–804

175. Janks DL, Roth BJ. Simulations of optical mapping during electroporation. *EMBC 2004, 26th Annual International Conference of the Engineering in Medicine and Biology Society, San Francisco, CA*. Piscataway, NJ: IEEE; 2004:3581–3584

176. Hyatt CJ, Mironov SF, Wellner M, Berenfeld O, Popp AK, Weitz DA, Jalife J, Pertsov AM. Synthesis of voltage-sensitive fluorescence signals from three-dimensional myocardial activation patterns. *Biophys J* 2003;85:2673–2683

177. Bernus O, Wellner M, Mironov SF, Pertsov AM. Simulation of voltage-sensitive optical signals in three-dimensional slabs of cardiac tissue: application to transillumination and coaxial imaging methods. *Phys Med Biol* 2005;50:215–229

178. Bishop MJ, Rodriguez B, Eason J, Whiteley JP, Trayanova N, Gavaghan DJ. Synthesis of voltage-sensitive optical signals: application to panoramic optical mapping. *Biophys J* 2006;90:2938–2945

179. Mironov SF, Vetter FJ, Pertsov AM. Fluorescence imaging of cardiac propagation: spectral properties and filtering of optical action potentials. *Am J Physiol Heart Circ Physiol* 2006;291:H327–H335

180. Krassowska W, Neu JC. Effective boundary conditions for syncytial tissues. *IEEE Trans Biomed Eng* 1994;41:143–150

181. Roth BJ. A comparison of two boundary-conditions used with the bidomain model of cardiac tissue. *Ann Biomed Eng* 1991;19:669–678

182. Latimer DC, Roth BJ. Electrical stimulation of cardiac tissue by a bipolar electrode in a conductive bath. *IEEE Trans Biomed Eng* 1998;45:1449–1458

183. Knisley SB, Pollard AE, Fast VG. Effects of electrode-myocardial separation on cardiac stimulation in conductive solution. *J Cardiovasc Electrophysiol* 2000;11:1132–1143

184. Trayanova NA. Effects of the tissue-bath interface on the induced transmembrane potential: a modeling study in cardiac stimulation. *Ann Biomed Eng* 1997;25:783–792

185. Roth BJ. Mechanism for polarisation of cardiac tissue at a sealed boundary. *Med Biol Eng Comput* 1999;37:523–525

186. Roth BJ, Patel SG, Murdick RA. The effect of the cut surface during electrical stimulation of a cardiac wedge preparation. *IEEE Trans Biomed Eng* 2006;53:1187–1190

187. Corbin LV II, Scher AM. The canine heart as an electrocardiographic generator. Dependence on cardiac cell orientation. *Circ Res* 1977;41:58–67

188. Roberts DE, Hersh LT, Scher AM. Influence of cardiac fiber orientation on wavefront voltage, conduction velocity, and tissue resistivity in the dog. *Circ Res* 1979;44:701–712

189. Roberts DE, Scher AM. Effect of tissue anisotropy on extracellular potential fields in canine myocardium in situ. *Circ Res* 1982;50:342–351

190. Barry WH, Fairbank WM, Harrison DC, Lehrman KL, Malmivuo JAV, Wikswo JP Jr. Measurement of the human magnetic heart vector. *Science* 1977;198:1159–1162

191. Wikswo JP Jr. A theoretical analysis of the relation between cardiac electric and magnetic fields. *Biophys J* 1978;21:91a

192. Wikswo JP Jr, Barach JP. Possible sources of new information in the magnetocardiogram. *J Theor Biol* 1982;95:721–729

193. Wikswo JP Jr, Barach JP, Gundersen SC, McLean MJ, Freeman JA. First magnetic measurements of action currents in isolated cardiac Purkinje fibers. *IL Nuovo Cimento* 1983;2D:368–378

194. Roth BJ, Wikswo JP Jr. Electrically silent magnetic fields. *Biophys J* 1986;50:739–745

195. Barach JP. A simulation of cardiac action currents having curl. *IEEE Trans Biomed Eng* 1993;40:49–58

196. Barach JP, Wikswo JP Jr. Magnetic fields from simulated cardiac action currents. *IEEE Trans Biomed Eng* 1994;41:969–974

197. Staton DJ, Friedman RN, Wikswo JP Jr. High-resolution SQUID imaging of octupolar currents in anisotropic cardiac tissue. *IEEE Trans Appl Supercond* 1993;3:1934–1936

198. Baudenbacher F, Peters NT, Baudenbacher P, Wikswo JP. High resolution imaging of biomagnetic fields generated by action currents in cardiac tissue using a LTS-SQUID microscope. *Physica C* 2002;368:24–31

199. Staton DJ. Magnetic imaging of applied and propagating action current in cardiac tissue slices: determination of anisotropic electrical conductivities in a two dimensional bidomain. Ph.D. dissertation, Physics, Vanderbilt University; 1994

200. Fong LE, Holzer JR, McBride KK, Lima EA, Baudenbacher F, Radparvar M. High-resolution room-temperature sample scanning superconducting quantum interference device microscope configurable for geological and biomagnetic applications. *Rev Sci Instrum* 2005;76:053703

201. Fong LE, Holzer JR, McBride K, Lima EA, Baudenbacher F, Radparvar M. High-resolution imaging of cardiac biomagnetic fields using a low-transition-temperature superconducting quantum interference device microscope. *Appl Phys Lett* 2004;84:3190–3192

202. Holzer JR, Fong LE, Sidorov VY, Wikswo JP Jr, Baudenbacher F. High resolution magnetic images of planar wave fronts reveal bidomain properties of cardiac tissue. *Biophys J* 2004;87:4326–4332

203. Baudenbacher F, Peters NT, Wikswo JP Jr. High resolution low-temperature super-conductivity superconducting quantum interference device microscope for imaging magnetic fields of samples at room temperatures. *Rev Sci Instrum* 2002;73:1247–1254

204. Roth BJ, Woods MC. The magnetic field associated with a plane wave front propagating through cardiac tissue. *IEEE Trans Biomed Eng* 1999;46:1288–1292

205. Barbosa CRH. Simulation of a plane wavefront propagating in cardiac tissue using a cellular automata model. *Phys Med Biol* 2003;48:4151–4164

206. dos Santos RW, Koch H. Interpreting biomagnetic fields of planar wave fronts in cardiac muscle. *Biophys J* 2005;88:3731–3733

207. Murdick RA, Roth BJ. A comparative model of two mechanisms from which a magnetic field arises in the heart. *J Appl Phys* 2004;95:5116–5122

208. Baudenbacher F, Fong LE, Holzer JR, Radparvar M. Monolithic low-transition-temperature superconducting magnetometers for high resolution imaging magnetic fields of room temperature samples. *Appl Phys Lett* 2003;82:3487–3489

209. Ideker RE, Chattipakorn N, Gray RA. Defibrillation mechanisms: the parable of the blind men and the elephant. *J Cardiovasc Electrophysiol* 2000;11:1008–1013

210. Roth BJ, Guo W-Q, Wikswo JP Jr. The effects of spiral anisotropy on the electric potential and the magnetic field at the apex of the heart. *Math Biosci* 1988;88:191–221

211. Roth BJ. The electrical potential produced by a strand of cardiac muscle: a bidomain analysis. *Ann Biomed Eng* 1988;16:609–637

212. Knisley SB, Maruyama T, Buchanan JW. Interstitial potential during propagation in bathed ventricular muscle. *Biophys J* 1991;59:509–515

213. Plonsey R, Henriquez CS, Trayanova NA. Extracellular (volume conductor) effect on adjoining cardiac muscle electrophysiology. *Med Biol Eng Comput* 1988;26:126–129

214. Wu J, Johnson EA, Kootsey JM. A quasi-one-dimensional theory for anisotropic propagation of excitation in cardiac muscle. *Biophys J* 1996;71:2427–2439

215. Wu J, Wikswo JP Jr. Effects of bath resistance on action potentials in the squid giant axon: myocardial implications. *Biophys J* 1997;73:2347–2358

216. Roth BJ. Effect of a perfusing bath on the rate of rise of an action potential propagating through a slab of cardiac tissue. *Ann Biomed Eng* 1996;24:639–646

217. Roth BJ. Influence of a perfusing bath on the foot of the cardiac action potential. *Circ Res* 2000;86:E19–E22

218. Roth BJ, Saypol JM. The formation of a re-entrant action potential wave front in tissue with unequal anisotropy ratios. *Int J Bifurcat Chaos* 1991;1:927–928

219. Roth BJ. Frequency locking of meandering spiral waves in cardiac tissue. *Phys Rev E* 1998;57:R3735–R3738

220. Roth BJ. Meandering of spiral waves in anisotropic cardiac tissue. *Phys D: Nonlinear Phenomena* 2001;150:127–136

221. Janks DL, Roth BJ. Quatrefoil reentry caused by burst pacing. *J Cardiovasc Electrophysiol* 2006;17:1362–1368

222. Spach MS, Miller WT III, Geselowitz DB, Barr RC, Kootsey JM, Johnson EA. The discontinuous nature of propagation in normal canine cardiac muscle. *Circ Res* 1981;48:39–54

223. Roth BJ, Lin S-F, Wikswo JP Jr. Unipolar stimulation of cardiac tissue. *J Electrocardiol* 1998;31(Suppl):6–12

Chapter 4.4

The Virtual Electrode Hypothesis of Defibrillation

Crystal M. Ripplinger and Igor R. Efimov

Introduction

Despite significant research efforts of investigators in academia, medicine, and the pharmaceutical industry, no effective pharmacological alternative to defibrillation by electric shock has been developed. Thus, defibrillation has evolved to become the only effective therapy against sudden cardiac death. Highly detailed knowledge of ion channel biophysics and cell signaling cascades has allowed for the development of numerous specific agonists and antagonists, but as of yet, has failed to deliver safe and effective antiarrhythmic therapy. In contrast to this approach, electrotherapy is steadily improving its efficacy and safety.

Despite major improvements over the past several decades, defibrillation is not free from side effects, which may include both contractile and electrical dysfunction.[1–3] In addition to physical damage to the heart, defibrillation is also associated with psychological side effects.[4,5] Therefore, reduction of defibrillation energy is highly desirable. However, the basic mechanisms of defibrillation still remain debatable a century after its inception, which has slowed further improvement of the therapy. This chapter explores one of the leading hypotheses of defibrillation, the virtual electrode hypothesis, which has emerged over the past decade through the successes of novel research methodologies, including optical mapping and bidomain modeling.

Historical Overview of Defibrillation Therapy

The motivation to explore the relationship between electrical activity of the heart and that of external electric stimuli began in the late nineteenth century, presumably due to the increasing electrification of urban areas.[6] In 1899, while studying induction of ventricular fibrillation in the dog heart, physiologists Prevost and Batelli working at the University

Igor R. Efimov
Department of Biomedical Engineering, Washington University, St. Louis, MO, USA, igor@wustl.edu

I. R. Efimov et al. (eds.), *Cardiac Bioelectric Therapy: Mechanisms and Practical Implications.*
© Springer Science+Business Media, LLC 2009

of Geneva discovered that they could defibrillate a dog heart by applying an appropriate high current shock directly to the surface of the myocardium: "We have shown that the fibrillatory tremulations produced in the dog, in which they are definitely established can under certain circumstances be arrested, the heart re-established its beats, if one submits the animal to passages of a high current of high voltage (of 4800 volts, for example)."[7]

In 1946 Russian physiologists Gurvich and Yuniev[8] reported defibrillation of the mammalian heart, with a capacitor discharge applied externally across the closed chest. The next year Beck et al.[9] reported the first successful human defibrillation in which they used two 110-V, 1.5-A alternating current (AC) current shocks to resuscitate a 14-year-old boy who suffered cardiac arrest during elective chest surgery. In 1956 Zoll et al.[10] performed the first successful human external defibrillation using a 15-A AC current that produced 710 V applied across the chest for 0.15 s. However, the superiority and safety of direct current (DC) over AC for defibrillation were demonstrated by several investigators such as Kouwenhouven and Milnor,[11] Lown et al.,[12] and Gurvich.[13] In 1969 Mirowski et al.[14,15] began research on the implantable cardioverter-defibrillator (ICD). In 1980 the first ICD was implanted in a human patient at Johns Hopkins Hospital. Since the advent of ICD technology, survival for those at high risk for ventricular tachycardia/fibrillation (VT/VF) has greatly improved.

Despite profound advancements in defibrillation therapy over the past century, little was known about the basic mechanisms of defibrillation until the past two decades due to the advent of fluorescent optical mapping with voltage-sensitive dyes. In parallel, advancements in numerical simulations using the bidomain model of cardiac tissue provided the theoretical means to interpret these complex experimental findings.

Bidomain Model

The bidomain model is now widely accepted for numerical and theoretical studies of cardiac electrophysiology. The tissue is represented by two interpenetrating intra- and extracellular domains with each of them having different conductivities along and across the direction of the fibers.[16,17] The state variables describing the system are intracellular (ϕ_i) and extracellular (ϕ_e) potentials defined everywhere in the domain of interest Ω. The transmembrane potential is defined as $V_m = \phi_i - \phi_e$. The following coupled reaction-diffusion equations constitute the bidomain model:

$$\nabla \cdot (\hat{\sigma}_i \nabla \phi_i) = I_m, \tag{1}$$

$$\nabla \cdot (\hat{\sigma}_e \nabla \phi_e) = -I_m - I_o, \quad \text{in } \Omega, \tag{2}$$

where $\hat{\sigma}_i$ and $\hat{\sigma}_e$ are intra- and extracellular conductivity tensors, respectively, I_m is the volume density of transmembrane current, and I_o is the volume density of the stimulation or shock current.

The transmembrane current is described as a sum of capacitive, ionic, and electroporation currents[18]:

$$I_m = \beta \left(C_m \frac{\partial V_m}{\partial t} + I_{\text{ion}}(V_m, t) + G(V_m, t) \cdot V_m \right), \tag{3}$$

where β is the surface-to-volume ratio (total membrane area divided by total tissue volume), C_{m} is the membrane capacitance, and $G(V_{\mathrm{m}}, t)$ is the electroporation conductance, which can be described by empirical equations.[19]

The ionic current, $I_{\mathrm{ion}}(V_{\mathrm{m}}, t)$, depends on the model of the cardiac myocyte used and can range from relatively simple and therefore less accurate (Beeler-Reuter,[20] BRDR[21]) to more complex (Luo-Rudy phase I[22] or II,[23] Hund-Rudy dynamic model[24]). These models describe individual ion channels kinetics and are based on Hodgkin-Huxley formalism.[25]

Fluorescent Optical Mapping

The development of optical recordings of membrane potential was driven by the need to overcome many obstacles in electrophysiology and the promise of a technology "for measuring membrane potential in systems where, for reasons of scale, topology, or complexity, the use of electrodes is inconvenient or impossible."[26] Based on our current experience in cardiac electrophysiology, this list needs to be extended to recordings of action potentials in the presence of external electric fields during stimulation and defibrillation; an impossible task with both extra- and intracellular electrodes due to the large electrical artifacts caused by external fields. Optical mapping techniques and potentiometric probes have now made major contributions to our understanding of cardiac electrophysiology in ways that could not have been accomplished with other approaches.

Over 30 years ago, investigators discovered molecular probes that bind to the plasma membrane of neuronal[27] and cardiac cells[28] and exhibit changes in fluorescence and/or absorption that mimic changes in transmembrane potential. Thus, the transmembrane potential can be measured by illuminating tissue stained with the fluorophore and detecting changes in the intensity or wavelength of the emitted light. Several useful classes of fluorophores have emerged over the past 30 years, including merocyanine, oxonol, and styryl dyes. However, styryl dyes represent the most popular family of dyes for cardiac electrophysiology applications, with RH-421 and di-4-ANEPPS being the most prominent members of this family. The spectroscopic properties of these dyes have been shown to have a linear response to transmembrane potential changes in the normal physiological range.[29–31]

The typical optical mapping experimental setup consists of an isolated tissue preparation or Langendorff-perfused heart that is perfused and/or superfused with an oxygenated physiologic crystalloid solution. The heart is stained with the voltage-sensitive fluorophore and illuminated with light at the correct excitation wavelength. The excitation light can be produced with lasers,[32] tungsten-halogen lamps,[28] or more recently with light emitting diodes (LEDs).[33–35] The emission light is filtered and can be collected by a charge-coupled device (CCD) camera, complementary metal-oxide semiconductor (CMOS) camera, or a photodiode array (PDA). The optical signals are typically digitized at 1–5 kHz and normalized, and two-dimensional maps of propagation can then be constructed. Many groups are now using one[36–38] or two[39] optical detectors in combination with a panoramic mirror arrangement, or three[40] optical detectors to record electrical activity on the entire surface of the heart and reconstruct propagation in three dimensions.

Virtual Electrodes and the Activating Function

The term *virtual electrode* was coined by Seymour Furman to explain the clinical observation of stimulation far from a chronically implanted pacemaker lead.[41] Later, this term was adopted by investigators studying both pacing and defibrillation in parallel with a synonymous but more rigorously defined term *activating function* to designate the "driving force," which drives transmembrane potential in either a depolarizing (positive) or hyperpolarizing (negative) direction following an externally applied electric field. The bidomain equations (1)–(2) can be rewritten in terms of the transmembrane ($V_m = \phi_i - \phi_e$) and extracellular (ϕ_e) potentials:

$$\nabla \cdot ((\hat{\sigma}_i + \hat{\sigma}_e)\nabla\phi_e) = -I_o - \nabla \cdot (\hat{\sigma}_i \nabla V_m), \tag{4}$$

$$I_m - \nabla \cdot (\hat{\sigma}_i \nabla V_m) = \nabla \cdot (\hat{\sigma}_i \nabla\phi_e). \tag{5}$$

During diastole, one can neglect the gradient of transmembrane potential in the left-hand side of (5) as well as the total transmembrane current. Therefore, the only source of transmembrane potential changes is the term in the right-hand side of (5), which is known as the generalized activating function:[42,43]

$$S = \nabla \cdot (\hat{\sigma}_i \nabla\phi_e) = \hat{\sigma}_i \Delta\phi_e + \nabla\hat{\sigma}_i \cdot \nabla\phi_e. \tag{6}$$

Quantitative investigation of virtual electrodes and the activating function started with the theoretical predictions of Sepulveda et al.,[44] who demonstrated that a unipolar stimulus produces both positive and negative polarization in a two-dimensional syncytium. These positive and negative polarizations are induced by virtual cathodes and virtual anodes, respectively.[45] The magnitude and location of positive and negative virtual electrodes depend on both the field configuration (ϕ_e) and tissue structure (σ_i and σ_e).[43]

These findings explained the phenomenon of anodal stimulation, which had eluded investigators for many years. According to classical cable theory, anodal stimulation hyperpolarizes tissue and thus cannot bring about an action potential. However, experimentalists had long observed excitation as a result of anodal stimulation. The virtual electrode theory predicts that virtual anodes are accompanied by virtual cathodes; therefore, action potentials can arise from these regions.

Early theories of predicted efficacy of defibrillation shocks were entirely based on the minimum external voltage gradient ($\nabla\phi_e$). As evident from the definition of the activating function (6), voltage gradient ($\nabla\phi_e$), while important, is not the only source of membrane polarization. Tissue structure (σ_i and σ_e) may be just as important. Microscopic and macroscopic tissue heterogeneities play an important role by providing the substrate for virtual electrodes during defibrillation shocks. What remains to be determined is the relative contribution of different scales of heterogeneities to defibrillation. Some groups argue that microscopic cell-size heterogeneities play the major role,[46] while other groups are convinced that large-scale heterogeneities are more important, because of the averaging effect of small-scale virtual electrodes by electrotonic interaction.[47]

Mechanisms of Defibrillation

In order to terminate an arrhythmia by electric shock, the shock must (1) terminate all or most wavefronts that sustain VT/VF; (2) not reinduce VT/VF; (3) suppress sources of VT/VF if they are focal in nature; and (4) not suppress postshock recovery of the normal sinus rhythm.

Theories of Defibrillation

In 1899 when Prevost and Battelli[7] discovered that large electric shocks could defibrillate the fibrillating myocardium, they posed the first theory of defibrillation, which was based on the "incapacitation" effects on the myocardium of strong electric shocks. It was not until 1939 that Gurvich and Yuniev proposed the first stimulatory theory of defibrillation.[48] They postulated directly stimulating and exciting the myocardium achieved defibrillation.

The stimulatory theory of defibrillation was later refined into the critical mass hypothesis in which experimentalists as well as theorists proposed that a critical mass of the myocardium (75–90%) needs to be directly defibrillated in order to fully terminate fibrillation.[49–51] This theory stated that the remaining fibrillating areas not affected by the shock would self-terminate.

In 1967 Fabiato and colleagues[52] demonstrated the first correlation between shock-induced fibrillation and defibrillation in a mechanism they called the "threshold of synchronous response." This idea was later extended by Chen and co-workers[53] into the now well-known "upper limit of vulnerability" hypothesis. This hypothesis states that the shock must terminate all wavefronts of fibrillation and that, in order to be successful, the shock must produce a sufficient voltage gradient (above the upper limit of vulnerability [ULV]) everywhere in the myocardium as not to reinduce fibrillation. This correlation was subsequently demonstrated in several experimental studies[54,55] and in humans.[56,57]

Although the concept of stimulus-induced reentry had been laid down decades earlier by Wiener and Rosenblueth,[58] Frazier and colleagues[59] were the first to obtain experimental evidence of this mechanism in 1989 in what they called the "stimulus-induced critical point" mechanism. Frazier et al. demonstrated that the chirality of reentry could be predicted based on the direction of the preshock repolarization gradient and the voltage gradient of the applied shock. After its discovery, the critical point mechanism was held responsible for reinduction of fibrillation after a failed defibrillation shock.[60,61]

In 1998 Dillon and Kwaku[62] proposed the "progressive depolarization" hypothesis of defibrillation and shock-induced fibrillation. This theory expanded on the critical mass, threshold of synchronous response, and ULV hypotheses but with a different interpretation of the supporting experimental evidence. The progressive depolarization hypothesis states that: "(1) Progressively stronger shocks depolarize, (2) Progressively more refractory myocardium, to (3) Progressively prevent postshock wavefronts, and (4) Prolong and synchronize post-shock repolarization, in a (5) Progressively larger volume of ventricle, to (6) Progressively decrease the probability of fibrillation after the shock." Thus, this theory is based on the prolongation of repolarization and refractory periods to effectively eliminate the excitable gap and terminate fibrillation.

However, contrary to this hypothesis, theoretical and experimental evidence supports the creation of virtual electrodes of opposite polarity in response to an applied stimulus.[44,45,63–66] Although the shock may prolong repolarization in some regions of the myocardium, it may be shortened in others. Thus, the virtual electrode mechanism casts doubt on all of the previously outlined theories of defibrillation, as these theories only account for the "stimulatory" response of defibrillation shocks. An alternative theory that accounts for both shock-induced excitation and deexcitation is the virtual electrode hypothesis of defibrillation.[66–68]

Virtual Electrode Hypothesis of Defibrillation: The Role of Deexcitation and Reexcitation

The virtual electrode hypothesis was the first to account for shock-induced deexcitation in both the mechanisms of defibrillation and shock-induced reentrant arrhythmias. When cardiac tissue is exposed to external field stimulation, areas of the tissue can be depolarized or hyperpolarized. Depolarization can result in prolongation of the action potential if the tissue is refractory (Fig. 1, middle trace) or activation if the tissue is excitable. Hyperpolarization can shorten the action potential and completely repolarize the tissue (Fig. 1, top trace) to restore excitability. This phenomenon is often referred to as "deexcitation" and is an all-or-none response. In addition, deexcitation may be followed by reexcitation caused by a postshock propagating wave (Fig. 1, bottom trace).

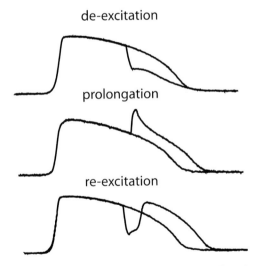

Figure 1: Tissue responses to virtual electrode polarization. The virtual anode deexcites the tissue and shortens the action potential and refractory period. The virtual cathode extends the action potential duration and refractory period. If deexcitation fully or partially restores excitability in the area of the virtual anode, and if the virtual cathode is within one space constant, reexcitation will take place

Further illustration of simultaneous shock-induced prolongation and shortening of the action potential is shown in Fig. 2.[69] The top panels of Fig. 2a show maps of postshock (+200 V) transmembrane potential (left), and action potential duration during a control beat (middle) and postshock (right). The action potentials were shortened in areas of negative polarization and prolonged in areas of positive polarization, resulting in dispersion of repolarization. In contrast, Fig. 2b shows a response that appears as action potential prolongation in all areas when the shock voltage was increased to +300 V. There is little difference in the areas of positive polarization (red traces), but dramatic differences in the areas of negative polarization (blue traces). In these areas, action potentials were shorted with a +200 V shock and lengthened due to reexcitation in response to a +300 V shock.

Virtual Electrode-Induced Phase Singularity Mechanism

Shock-induced arrhythmias were discovered over 150 years ago by Hoffa and Ludwig.[70] Since that time, experimentalists and theorists alike have investigated the relationship between defibrillation and shock-induced arrhythmogenesis. We can assume that shocks initiate arrhythmias via reentry, and that defibrillation shocks fail because they either leave fibrillating myocardium unaffected by the shock or because they produce a new reentrant arrhythmia. Therefore, it is relevant to discuss shock-induced arrhythmias in the settings of the virtual electrode hypothesis of defibrillation.

It is known that shocks delivered to refractory myocardium can induce reentry via break excitation.[67,71,72] Figure 3 shows how the postshock virtual electrode pattern can lead to reentry.[67] Figure 3a shows the postshock virtual electrode polarization (VEP). Deexcitation occurred only in the most negatively polarized region near the bottom right corner of the field of view. After the shock, the positively polarized region interacted electronically with the deexcited region (break excitation) to create a new wavefront that propagated from left to right (Fig. 3b). This new wavefront of activation then propagated slowly upward into the recovering myocardium to create a reentrant circuit (Fig. 3c). The circle in Fig. 3a indicates the point of shock-induced phase singularity[73] responsible for the initiation of reentrant activity.

It was subsequently demonstrated by Cheng et al.[69] that creation of reentrant arrhythmias via the virtual electrode-induced phase singularity mechanism is critically dependent on the magnitude of the applied electric field. Figure 4 shows examples of postshock VEP and resulting patterns of activation in response to an −80 (Fig. 4a), −160 (Fig. 4b), and −220 V (Fig. 4c) shocks. In Fig. 4a, complete deexcitation occurred only in the most negatively polarized region in the bottom right corner (darkest blue). As illustrated in the corresponding activation map, this region was excited first, followed by slower excitation spreading upward as these areas recovered. Excitation then spread to the left of the field of view producing a reentrant wavefront. At larger shocks strengths (Fig. 4b, c), larger regions were completely deexcited by the shock (darkest blue). Thus, a wavefront of reexcitation was produced in a larger area, promptly exciting the entire deexcited region. Such fast excitation does not allow for recovery of the incompletely deexcited regions; therefore, reentry is not produced in these cases. Thus, conduction velocity of the postshock wavefront depends on the magnitude of VEP (degree of shock-induced deexcitation).

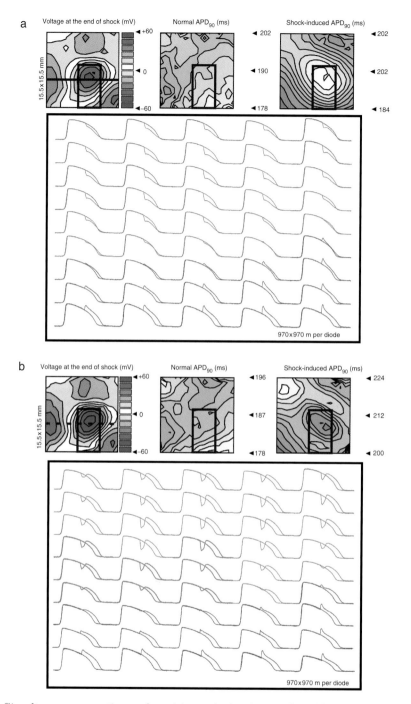

Figure 2: Simultaneous negative and positive polarizations induced by a monophasic anodal shock. (a) Response to a +200 V shock, which produced a high degree of dispersion of repolarization. (b) Response to a +300 V shock, which prolonged action potential duration everywhere in the region of interest. See text for details (Cheng et al. 1999)[69]

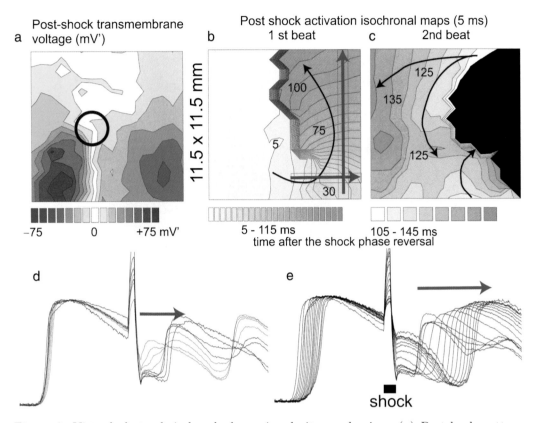

Figure 3: Virtual electrode-induced phase singularity mechanism. (a) Postshock pattern of virtual electrode polarization (VEP). (b) Immediately postshock, activation spreads to the deexcited region in the lower right corner and proceeds upward into the recovering myocardium to create a reentrant circuit (c). (d) Optical recordings from eight sites marked with the red arrow in (b). (e) Optical recordings from 16 sites marked with the blue arrow in (b) (Efimov et al. 1998)[67]

Presumably, the stronger negative polarization results in more complete recovery of sodium channels from inactivation and, therefore, faster conduction of postshock reexcitation. This relationship between conduction velocity and negative polarization is now thought to underlie the mechanisms of the upper and lower limits of vulnerability.[74] Low-intensity shocks producing inadequate negative polarization will result in failure of postshock conduction and, thus, failure to produce phase singularities. High-intensity shocks will produce a strong gradient of polarization, resulting in supernormal conduction, immediately extinguishing the excitable gap. Only shocks of "moderate" magnitude will produce conduction velocities appropriate for the creation of phase singularities and reentrant arrhythmias as in Fig. 4a.

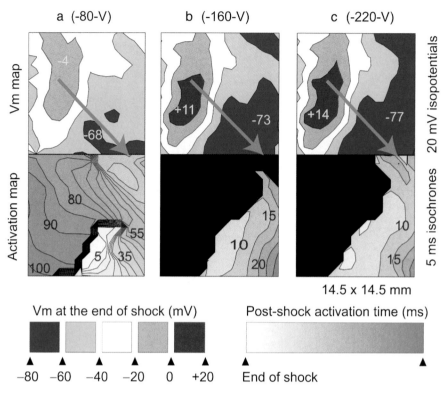

Figure 4: Modulation of virtual electrode polarization (VEP) magnitude and resulting conduction velocity by shock intensity. *Top*: Transmembrane potential at shock end. *Bottom*: Isochronal maps of postshock activation. (**a**–**c**) correspond to shock intensities of −80, −160, and −220 V, respectively (Cheng et al. 1999)[69]

Chirality of Shock-Induced Reentry Predicted by VEP Not the Repolarization Gradient

Frazier and colleagues[59] were the first to experimentally demonstrate the cross-field induced critical point (CFICP) mechanism of reentry induction by point stimulation. This mechanism predicts chirality (direction of rotation) of the induced reentrant circuit based on the directions of the preshock repolarization gradient as well as the applied voltage gradient. Reversal of either direction would result in reversal of chirality. The virtual electrode-induced phase singularity (VEIPS) mechanism,[67] on the other hand, suggests that chirality is predicted by postshock VEP alone and not by the direction of repolarization.

A series of experiments by Cheng et al.[75] successfully demonstrated this hypothesis. An example is shown in Fig. 5. The first two columns show isochronal maps of activation and repolarization, respectively, as a result of pacing from three different locations. The third and fourth columns show pre- and postshock transmembrane potential. As evident from the maps of postshock potential, shock-induced VEP dominates regardless of the

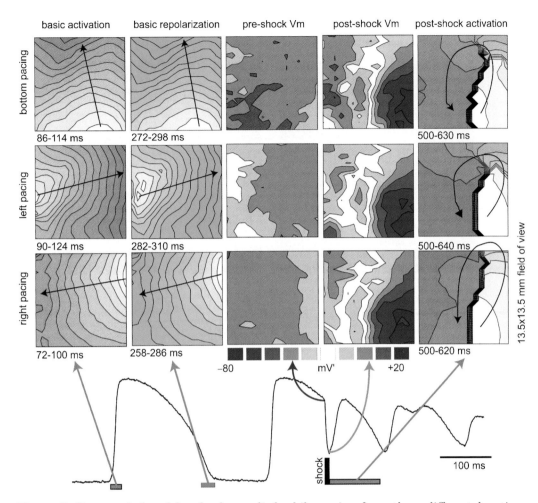

Figure 5: Reentry induced by shocks applied while pacing from three different locations (right ventricle [RV], left ventricle [LV], and apex). Columns from left to right are: activation, repolarization, preshock transmembrane potential, postshock transmembrane potential, and postshock activation. Rows from top to bottom are: apical pacing, RV pacing, and LV pacing. Chirality of shock-induced reentry is preserved regardless of the gradient of repolarization (Cheng et al. 2000)[75]

pattern of repolarization. The last column shows postshock activation with reentry rotating counterclockwise in all cases, thus the data support the VEIPS mechanism and contradict the CFICP hypothesis.

A more detailed analysis of the two mechanisms is shown in Fig. 6. In both panels, a planar wavefront propagates from top to bottom with the transmembrane potential indicated by differing shades of gray. The left panel depicts the CFICP hypothesis and assumes

Cross-field induced
critical points

Virtual electrode induced
phase singularity

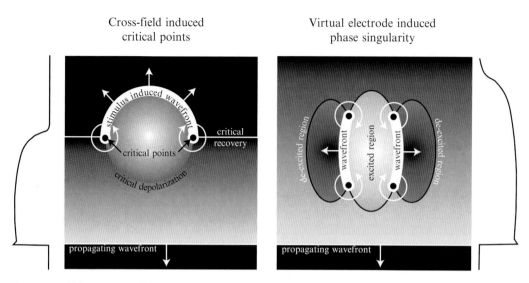

Figure 6: Schematics of the cross-field induced critical point (CFICP) and virtual electrode-induced phase singularity (VEIPS) mechanisms. See text for details (Cheng et al. 2000)[75]

that cathodal point stimulation produces positive polarization near the stimulation site. Two critical values are important in this mechanism: critical recovery, indicated by the line dividing refractory and excitable myocardium at the tail of the action potential, and critical depolarization, indicated with the circle dividing subthreshold from suprathreshold depolarization. The top of the circle of critical depolarization occurs in excitable myocardium, generating a new wavefront. The two points of intersection of critical depolarization and critical recovery represent the sites of wavebreak and are called critical points[59] or points of phase singularity.[73] In this mechanism, reversal of the direction of repolarization will result in wavefront generation along the bottom of the circle of critical depolarization and reversal of chirality.

The VEIPS hypothesis is shown in the right panel of Fig. 6 and predicts that point stimulation will produce regions of adjacent positive and negative polarization. For the case of cathodal stimulation, the stimulation site will be positively polarized (excited) with two negatively polarized (deexcited) regions on either side. The VEIPS mechanism does not rely on existence of an excitable region at the tail of the action potential, as the negatively polarized regions deexcite the tissue, creating an excitable region regardless of repolarization. Two wavefronts will be generated at the areas of adjacent positive and negative polarization, and a total of four wavebreaks or points of phase singularity will be induced. In Fig. 5, only one of the four phase singularities was observed. Reversal of the repolarization gradient can change the location of the two wavefronts of reexcitation, but it will not change their direction. Therefore, chirality will be preserved.

Shock-Induced VEP as a Mechanism for Defibrillation Failure

Thus far, the examples presented have all dealt with shock-induced arrhythmogenesis. However, shock-induced VEP is also present during ventricular arrhythmias and can be responsible for failed defibrillation shocks. Figure 7 illustrates an example of a failed monophasic −100 V defibrillation shock applied from an implantable right ventricle (RV) lead during ventricular tachycardia.[76] By panels 5 and 6, shock-induced VEP completely erases the existing tachycardia. However, due to the strong gradient of VEP, a new reentrant arrhythmia is immediately produced via the VEIPS mechanism.[67] The reentry core of

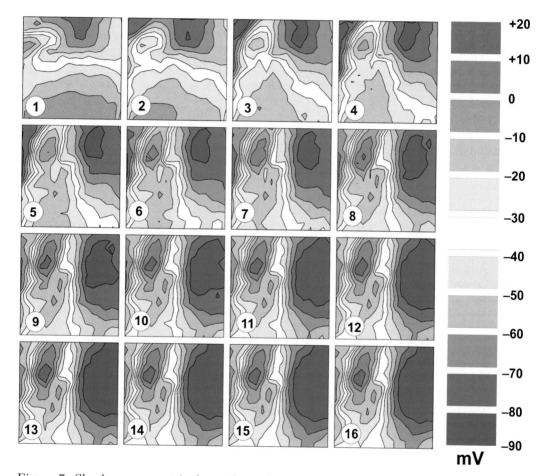

Figure 7: Shock erases ventricular tachycardia via virtual electrode effect. Maps of transmembrane potential during a failed 8 ms monophasic shock. *Panel 1* shows reentrant excitation just before shock application. By *panels 5–6*, reentrant activation is completely erased by typical virtual electrode polarization with simultaneous areas of positive (*red*) and negative (*blue*) polarization (Efimov et al. 2000)[76]

this arrhythmia is distinctly different from the preshock arrhythmia, indicating that the shock terminated the existing arrhythmia and reinitiated a new one, resulting in failed defibrillation.

The Role of Electroporation

Transmembrane polarization produced by virtual electrodes present during a defibrillation shock may reach significant amplitudes, which results in breakdown of the cell membrane.[77,78] This effect is known as *electroporation*. On one hand, electroporation imposes a limit on virtual electrode polarization, due to the formation of low resistance pores, which shunt the transmembrane potential and make it impossible to maintain even the resting potential until the pores are resealed.[78] On the other hand, electroporation may have important electrophysiological implications for arrhythmia maintenance. Experimental evidence suggests that electroporation occurring after a defibrillation shock may result in the creation of new centers of focal activity.[2] However, the pro- and antiarrhythmic effect of electroporation in the clinical setting remains a subject of debate.[1] However, data from implantable defibrillators clearly indicate that spontaneous sinus rhythm does not recover immediately postshock and requires pacing for several seconds. This period of time is consistent with the time course of resealing of electroporated membranes.

Clinical Implications of the Virtual Electrode Hypothesis of Defibrillation

The virtual electrode hypothesis of defibrillation, along with optical mapping techniques, has made great strides toward explaining many experimentally and clinically observed phenomena, which had remained a mystery to scientists and clinicians alike. Many of these discoveries have clinical implications for safe and efficient defibrillation.

The Role of Virtual Electrodes and Shock Polarity

Optical mapping experiments revealed the mechanism of superiority of anodal versus cathodal shocks when applied from transvenous defibrillation leads.[66,79] Figure 8 illustrates the general concept. During anodal shocks (Fig. 8a), the virtual cathodes created adjacent to the real anode produce wavefronts that propagate inward, toward the area of deexcitation. These wavefronts frequently collide and annihilate each other, whereas the positive polarization under the real cathode during cathodal shocks (Fig. 8b) creates wavefronts that propagate outward, having more "elbow room" (in Art Winfree's terms) for turning around and creating sustained reentry. These experimental findings were recently confirmed in a meta-analysis of clinical studies on ICD shock polarity, which revealed that anodal defibrillation shocks lower the defibrillation threshold (DFT) by 14.8% compared to cathodal shocks and result in a lower DFT in 83% of patients.[80] The lower DFT is presumably due to the decreased probability of reinitiating a reentrant arrhythmia postshock.

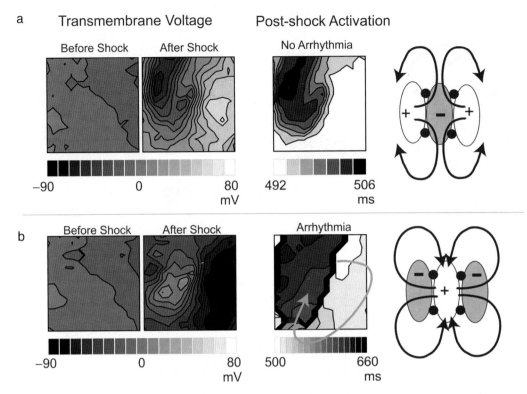

Figure 8: Anodal versus cathodal monophasic defibrillation shocks applied from an implantable lead. (a) *Left panels*: Transmembrane potential before and after an anodal shock (+100 V, 8 ms). *Middle*: Spread of postshock activation. The areas of first activation correspond to the virtual cathodes. Activation then spreads to the area of the real anode, collapsing on itself, and no arrhythmia is produced. *Right*: Diagram of postshock activation. (b) Similar panels as in (a) for a cathodal (−100 V, 8 ms) shock. In this case, activation spreads immediately outward from the real cathode to the virtual anodes where it has room to reenter, creating a sustained arrhythmia (Yamanouchi et al. 2001)[79]

Waveform Optimization

The efficacy of different defibrillation waveforms has also been determined with the virtual electrode hypothesis. It has been widely accepted that biphasic shocks have a lower defibrillation threshold than monophasic shocks,[81,82] but this phenomenon has its roots in the virtual electrode theory. Monophasic shocks must be greater than the ULV in order to avoid creation of a shock-induced phase singularity, which may reinduce reentry. However, the second phase of biphasic shocks acts to reverse the first phase polarization, thus eliminating the substrate for postshock reentry.[67] This phenomenon is illustrated in Fig. 9. The three maps in Fig. 9a show the postshock polarization in response to monophasic (+100 V), optimal biphasic (+100/−50 V), and nonoptimal biphasic

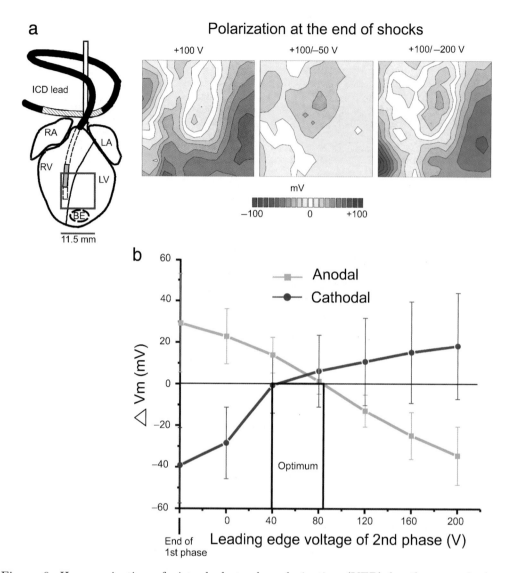

Figure 9: Homogenization of virtual electrode polarization (VEP) by the second phase of biphasic shocks. (a) Maps of polarization produced by monophasic (+100 V, 8 ms), optimal biphasic (+100/−50 V, 8/8 ms), and nonoptimal biphasic (+100/−200 V, 8/8 ms) defibrillation shocks. The area of recording is indicated by the *red box*. ICD, implantable cardioverter defibrillator; LA, left atrium; LV, left ventricle; RA, right atrium; RV, right ventricle (Efimov et al. 1998)[67] (b) Asymmetric reversal of first-phase polarization. Plot shows gradient of transmembrane potential after second phase of biphasic shocks in which the first phase voltage was held constant and the second phase voltage was varied. Positive polarization produced by anodal first phase was fully reversed by approximately 70 V or more, whereas negative polarization produced by cathodal first phase required only 40 V to reverse

$(+100/-200 \text{ V})$ defibrillation shocks. The optimal biphasic shock does not result in reentry due to the homogeneous pattern of VEP at shock end, whereas the large gradient of VEP produced by the monophasic and nonoptimal biphasic waveforms provides the substrate for reentry.

The "homogenization" of VEP by the second phase of a biphasic shock occurs in a nonlinear fashion. After the first phase, the deexcited hyperpolarized region is easily reexcited and completely depolarized, whereas the depolarized regions are only partially deexcited.[67] Therefore, not every biphasic shock will be able to produce this homogenization (Fig. 9a, right panel). If the energy of the second phase is below a certain threshold, it will not be able to reverse the hyperpolarization. If the energy of the second phase is above a certain level, it will reverse both the positive and negative polarization, creating a mirrored VEP pattern similar to a monophasic shock. Efimov et al.[67] found a ratio of between 0.2 and 0.7 of second- versus first-phase voltage for optimal biphasic shocks. This agrees with clinical observations of optimal biphasic waveforms.[82] Figure 9b illustrates these findings and suggests that optimal biphasic waveforms result in total positive polarization with no excitable hyperpolarized tissue remaining to provide the substrate for shock-induced arrhythmias.

Monophasic ascending defibrillation waveforms have also been shown to be superior to descending waveforms.[83] As shown in Fig. 10c, d, ascending waveforms produce maximum polarization at the end of the shock. Therefore, break excitation resulting from these shocks is likely to produce faster propagation into the deexcited regions and will not form reentry (Fig. 10f). However, descending waveforms tend to reach maximum polarization before the end of the shock (Fig. 10c) and typically have lower magnitude polarization at shock end (Fig. 10d), which contributes to slower conduction and provides the substrate for shock-induced reentry via the VEIPS mechanism (Fig. 10f).[67]

Toward Low-Energy Defibrillation

The virtual electrode hypothesis of defibrillation has not only allowed for explanation of the basic mechanisms of defibrillation, but it is also allowing us to entirely rethink our approach to conventional defibrillation. Reentrant VT is often pinned or anchored at a functionally or anatomically heterogeneous region that comprises the core of reentry. The theory of virtual electrode polarization and the activating function predict that areas near the reentry core will experience greater polarization in response to an applied electric field compared to the surrounding, more homogeneous tissue. Thus, the core of reentry can be preferentially excited with very small electric fields to destabilize and unpin reentrant VT from its stationary core. However, the external field must be applied at precisely the right moment for the virtual electrode-induced excitation to properly interact with and terminate VT. This idea has been recently validated both in theory[84] and in experiments.[85,86]

Takagi et al.[84] demonstrated this concept in a two-dimensional bidomain model with a nonconductive circular obstacle comprising the core of reentry. Figure 11 shows a successful and nonsuccessful shock application. At $t = 0 \text{ ms}$, a spiral wave (S) is shown anchored to the obstacle rotating counterclockwise. A 0.52 V/cm^{-1} uniform external field is applied at

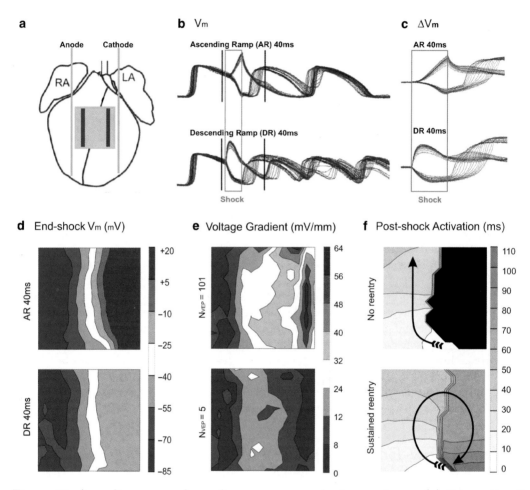

Figure 10: Ascending versus descending ramp monophasic waveforms. (a) Schematic of experimental setup showing shock electrode locations (*green lines*), field of view (*blue box*), and locations of individual optical traces shown in (b) and (c) (*blue and red lines*). RA, right atrium; LA, left atrium. (b) Optical action potentials during shock application for ascending and descending ramp defibrillation waveforms. (c) ΔV_m for the traces shown in (b). Ascending waveforms produce maximum polarization at shock end, whereas descending waveforms produce maximum polarization near the beginning of shock application. (d) Maps of polarization at shock end. (e) Voltage gradient at shock end. (f) Maps of postshock activation (Qu et al. 2005)[83]

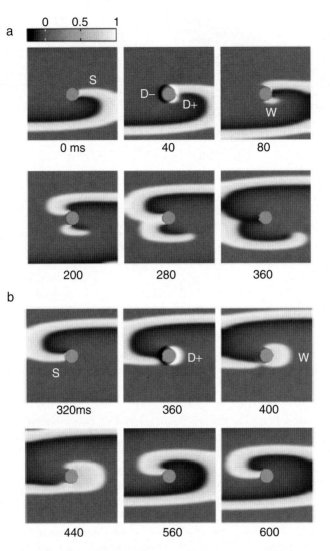

Figure 11: Bidomain simulations illustrating the low-energy "unpinning" concept. (a) Successful unpinning. $t = 0$ ms: spiral wave (S) is anchored to the obstacle rotating counterclockwise. $t = 40$ ms: a 0.52 V/cm^{-1} external field is applied. Positive and negative polarization (D+, D−) occur on opposite sides of the obstacle. $t = 80$ ms: the positive polarization results in a new wavefront (W), which rotates clockwise. $t = 280$ ms: the wavefronts collide resulting in detachment of both spiral waves. (b) An unsuccessful attempt due to improper timing of the applied field (Takagi et al. 2004)[84]

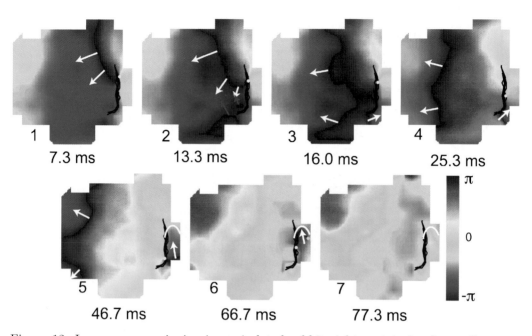

Figure 12: Low-energy unpinning in an isolated rabbit right ventricular free wall preparation. A $0.58\,\mathrm{V/cm^{-1}}$ shock is applied at $t = 13.3\,\mathrm{ms}$. Unpinning is similar to theoretical example presented in Fig. 11. See text for details (Ripplinger et al. 2006)[85]

$t = 40\,\mathrm{ms}$. Positive and negative polarization (D+, D-) can be seen on opposite sides of the obstacle. The positive polarization results in a new wavefront (W), which begins to rotate clockwise around the obstacle. Counterclockwise rotation of W is prevented due to refractory tissue in this direction. The wavefronts collide at $t = 280\,\mathrm{ms}$, which results in detachment of both spiral waves from the obstacle. The lower panels of Fig. 11 illustrate an unsuccessful attempt due to improper timing of the applied field. In this case, W can propagate in both directions and results in resetting of the spiral wave.

Our group recently validated this mechanism experimentally in a rabbit using isolated right ventricular preparation.[85] Figure 12 shows a spiral wave rotating counterclockwise around a line of block indicated with a black line (panel 1). At $t = 13.3\,\mathrm{ms}$, a $0.58\,\mathrm{V/cm^{-1}}$ external field is applied, creating a new wavefront that propagates in both directions around the line of block. The clockwise-propagating wavefront then collides with the existing spiral wave (panel 3) causing detachment from the core and termination at the tissue boundary (panels 4–5). The counterclockwise portion of the new wavefront eventually terminates upon hitting a refractory region (panel 6–7). Our experimental results in this model indicate that a 20-fold reduction in defibrillation energy may be obtained compared to conventional defibrillation. In a follow-up study, our group demonstrated a similar 20-fold reduction in defibrillation energy required to terminate sustained VT in a canine 4-day healed myocardial infarction model.[86] This new low energy approach may provide a promising alternative to conventional high-energy defibrillation and may alleviate many of the side effects currently associated with strong electric shocks.

Conclusion

The virtual electrode hypothesis of defibrillation has emerged as a result of the combined efforts of the theoretical and experimental research communities, which have developed bidomain modeling and optical mapping. These two research methodologies have allowed us to formulate novel hypotheses and to test them in various models of defibrillation. However, clinical advances are still to be gained from this theory. We believe that further improvement of the virtual electrode hypothesis of defibrillation will result in the development of low-energy electrotherapy of ventricular and atrial tachyarrhythmias.

References

1. Al Khadra A, Nikolski V, Efimov IR. The role of electroporation in defibrillation. *Circ Res* 2000;87(9):797–804
2. Kodama I, Shibata N, Sakuma I, Mitsui K, Iida M, Suzuki R, Fukui Y, Hosoda S, Toyama J. Aftereffects of high-intensity DC stimulation on the electromechanical performance of ventricular muscle. *Am J Physiol* 267(1 Pt 2):H248–H258
3. Neunlist M, Tung L. Dose-dependent reduction of cardiac transmembrane potential by high-intensity electrical shocks. *Am J Physiol* 273(6 Pt 2):H2817–H2825
4. Godemann F, Butter C, Lampe F, Linden M, Schlegl M, Schultheiss HP, Behrens S. Panic disorders and agoraphobia: side effects of treatment with an implantable cardioverter/defibrillator. *Clin Cardiol* 27(6):321–326
5. Kamphuis HC, de Leeuw JR, Derksen R, Hauer RN, Winnubst JA. Implantable cardioverter defibrillator recipients: quality of life in recipients with and without ICD shock delivery: a prospective study. *Europace* 5(4):381–389
6. Fye WB. Ventricular fibrillation and defibrillation: historical perspectives with emphasis on the contributions of John MacWilliam, Carl Wiggers, and William Kouwenhoven. *Circ* 1985;71(5):858–865
7. Prevost JL, Battelli F. Sur quel ques effets des dechanges electriques sur le coer mammifres. *C R Seances Acad Sci* 1899;129:1267
8. Gurvich NL, Yuniev GS. Restoration of regular rhythm in the mammalian fibrillating heart. *Am Rev Sov Med* 1946;3:236–239
9. Beck CS, Pritchard WH, Feil HS. Ventricular fibrillation of long duration abolished by electric shock. *JAMA* 1947;135:985
10. Zoll PM, Linethal AJ, Gibson W, et al. Termination of ventricular fibrillation in man by externally applied electric shock. *N Engl J Med* 1956;254:727
11. Kouwenhoven WB, Milnor WR. Treatment of ventricular fibrillation using a capacitor discharge. *J Appl Physiol* 1954;7(3):253–257

12. Lown B, Neuman J, Amarasingham R, Berkovits BV. Comparison of alternating current with direct electroshock across the closed chest. *Am J Cardiol* 1962;10:223–233

13. Gurvich NL. *The Main Principles of Cardiac Defibrillation.* Moscow: Medicine; 1975

14. Mirowski M, Mower MM, Reid PR. The automatic implantable defibrillator. *Am Heart J* 1980;100(6 Pt 2):1089–1092

15. Mirowski M, Reid PR, Mower MM, Watkins L, Gott VL, Schauble JF, Langer A, Heilman MS, Kolenik SA, Fischell RE, Weisfeldt ML. Termination of malignant ventricular arrhythmias with an implanted automatic defibrillator in human beings. *N Engl J Med* 1980;303(6):322–324

16. Tung L. *A Bidomain Model for Describing Ischemia Myocardial DC Potentials.* Cambridge, MA: Massachusetts Institute of Technology; 1978

17. Henriquez CS. Simulating the electrical behavior of cardiac tissue using the bidomain model. *Crit Rev Biomed Eng* 1993;21(1):1–77

18. Skouibine K, Trayanova N, Moore P. A numerically efficient model for simulation of defibrillation in an active bidomain sheet of myocardium. *Math Biosci* 2000;166(1):85–100

19. Krassowska W. Effects of electroporation on transmembrane potential induced by defibrillation shocks. *Pacing Clin Electrophysiol* 1995;18(9 Pt 1):1644–1660

20. Beeler GW, Reuter H. Reconstruction of the action potential of ventricular myocardial fibres. *J Physiol (Lond)* 1977;268(1):177–210

21. Drouhard JP, Roberge FA. A simulation study of the ventricular myocardial action potential. *IEEE Trans Biomed Eng* 1982;29(7):494–502

22. Luo CH, Rudy Y. A model of the ventricular cardiac action potential. Depolarization, repolarization, and their interaction. *Circ Res* 1991;68(6):1501–1526

23. Luo CH, Rudy Y. A dynamic model of the cardiac ventricular action potential. I. Simulations of ionic currents and concentration changes. *Circ Res* 1994;74(6):1071–1096

24. Hund TJ, Rudy Y. Rate dependence and regulation of action potential and calcium transient in a canine cardiac ventricular cell model. *Circulation* 2004;110(20):3168–3174

25. Hodgkin AL, Huxley AF. Propagation of electrical signals along giant nerve fibers. *Proc R Soc Lond B Biol Sci* 1952;140(899):177–183

26. Cohen LB, Lesher S, De Weer P, Salzberg BM. Optical monitoring of membrane potential: methods of multisite optical measurement. *Optical Methods in Cell Physiology.* New York: Wiley-Interscience; 1986:71–100

27. Davila HV, Salzberg BM, Cohen LB, Waggoner AS. A large change in axon fluorescence that provides a promising method for measuring membrane potential. *Nat New Biol* 1973;241(109):159–160

28. Salama G, Morad M. Merocyanine 540 as an optical probe of transmembrane electrical activity in the heart. *Science* 1976;191(4226):485–487

29. Morad M, Salama G. Optical probes of membrane potential in heart muscle. *J Physiol (Lond)* 1979;292:267–295

30. Ross WN, Salzberg BM, Cohen LB, Grinvald A, Davila HV, Waggoner AS, Wang CH. Changes in absorption, fluorescence, dichroism, and birefringence in stained giant axons: optical measurement of membrane potential. *J Membr Biol* 1977;33(1–2):141–183

31. Salama G, Loew LM. Optical measurements of transmembrane potential in heart. *Spectroscopic Membrane Probes*. Boca Raton, FL: CRC; 1988:137–199

32. Dillon S, Morad M. A new laser scanning system for measuring action potential propagation in the heart. *Science* 1981;214(4519):453–456

33. Kodama I, Sakuma I, Shibata N, Knisley SB, Niwa R, Honjo H. Regional differences in arrhythmogenic aftereffects of high intensity DC stimulation in the ventricles. *Pacing Clin Electrophysiol* 2000;23(5):807–817

34. Entcheva E, Kostov Y, Tchernev E, Tung L. Fluorescence imaging of electrical activity in cardiac cells using an all-solid-state system. *IEEE Trans Biomed Eng* 2004;51(2):333–341

35. Amino M, Yamazaki M, Nakagawa H, Honjo H, Okuno Y, Yoshioka K, Tanabe T, Yasui K, Lee JK, Horiba M, Kamiya K, Kodama I. Combined effects of nifekalant and lidocaine on the spiral-type re-entry in a perfused 2-dimensional layer of rabbit ventricular myocardium. *Circ J* 2005;69(5):576–584

36. Bray MA, Lin SF, Wikswo JP. Panoramic epifluorescent visualization of cardiac action potential activity. *Proc SPIE* 1999;3658:99–107

37. Lin SF, Wikswo JP. Panoramic optical imaging of electrical propagation in isolated heart. *J Biomed Opt* 1999;4(2):200–207

38. Bray MA, Lin SF, Wikswo J. Three-dimensional visualization of phase singularities on the isolated rabbit heart. *J Cardiovasc Electrophysiol* 2002;13(12):1311

39. Kay MW, Amison PM, Rogers JM. Three-dimensional surface reconstruction and panoramic optical mapping of large hearts. *IEEE Trans Biomed Eng* 2004;51(7):1219–1229

40. Qu F, Ripplinger CM, Nikolski VP, Grimm C, Efimov IR. Three dimensional panoramic imaging of cardiac arrhythmias in the rabbit heart. *J Biomed Opt* 2007;12(4):044019

41. Furman S, Hurzeler P, Parker B. Clinical thresholds of endocardial cardiac stimulation: a long-term study. *J Surg Res* 1975;19:149–155

42. Rattay F. Analysis of models for extracellular fiber stimulation. *IEEE Trans Biomed Eng* 1989;36(7):676–682

43. Sobie EA, Susil RC, Tung L. A generalized activating function for predicting virtual electrodes in cardiac tissue. *Biophysical J* 1997;73(3):1410–1423

44. Sepulveda NG, Roth BJ, Wikswo JP. Current injection into a two-dimensional anisotropic bidomain. *Biophysical J* 1989;55(5):987–999

45. Wikswo JP, Lin SF, Abbas RA. Virtual electrodes in cardiac tissue: a common mechanism for anodal and cathodal stimulation. *Biophysical J* 1995;69(6):2195–2210

46. Fast VG, Rohr S, Gillis AM, Kleber AG. Activation of cardiac tissue by extracellular electrical shocks: formation of 'secondary sources' at intercellular clefts in monolayers of cultured myocytes. *Circ Res* 1998;82(3):375–385

47. Trayanova N, Skouibine K, Aguel F. The role of cardiac tissue structure in defibrillation. *Chaos* 1998;8(1):221–233

48. Gurvich NL, Yuniev GS. Restoration of regular rhythm in the mammalian fibrillating heart. *Byull Eksper Biol Med* 1939;8(1):55–58

49. Zipes DP, Fischer J, King RM, Nicoll Ad, Jolly WW. Termination of ventricular fibrillation in dogs by depolarizing a critical amount of myocardium. *Am J Cardiol* 1975;36(1):37–44

50. Witkowski FX, Penkoske PA, Plonsey R. Mechanism of cardiac defibrillation in open-chest dogs with unipolar DC-coupled simultaneous activation and shock potential recordings. *Circulation* 1990;82(1):244–260

51. Krinskii VI, Fomin SV, Kholopov AV. [Critical mass during fibrillation]. *Biofizika* 1967;12(5):908–914

52. Fabiato A, Coumel P, Gourgon R, Saumont R. The threshold of synchronous response of the myocardial fibers. Application to the experimental comparison of the efficacy of different forms of electroshock defibrillation. *Arch Mal Coeur Vaiss* 1967;60(4):527–544

53. Chen PS, Shibata N, Dixon EG, Martin RO, Ideker RE. Comparison of the defibrillation threshold and the upper limit of ventricular vulnerability. *Circulation* 1986;73(5):1022–1028

54. Shibata N, Chen PS, Dixon EG, Wolf PD, Danieley ND, Smith WM, Ideker RE. Influence of shock strength and timing on induction of ventricular arrhythmias in dogs. *Am J Physiol* 1988;255(4 Pt 2):H891–H901

55. Fabritz CL, Kirchhof PF, Behrens S, Zabel M, Franz MR. Myocardial vulnerability to T wave shocks: relation to shock strength, shock coupling interval, and dispersion of ventricular repolarization. *J Cardiovasc Electrophysiol* 1996;7(3):231–242

56. Chen PS, Feld GK, Kriett JM, Mower MM, Tarazi RY, Fleck RP, Swerdlow CD, Gang ES, Kass RM. Relation between upper limit of vulnerability and defibrillation threshold in humans. *Circulation* 1993;88(1):186–192

57. Hwang C, Swerdlow CD, Kass RM, Gang ES, Mandel WJ, Peter CT, Chen PS. Upper limit of vulnerability reliably predicts the defibrillation threshold in humans. *Circulation* 1994;90(5):2308–2314

58. Wiener N, Rosenblueth A. The mathematical formulation of the problem of conduction of impulses in a network of connected excitable elements, specifically in cardiac muscle. *Arch Inst Cardiol Mexico* 1946;16(3–4):205–265

59. Frazier DW, Wolf PD, Wharton JM, Tang AS, Smith WM, Ideker RE. Stimulus-induced critical point. Mechanism for electrical initiation of reentry in normal canine myocardium. *J Clin Invest* 1989;83(3):1039–1052

60. Walcott GP, Walcott KT, Knisley SB, Zhou X, Ideker RE. Mechanisms of defibrillation for monophasic and biphasic waveforms. *Pacing Clin Electrophysiol* 1994;17(3 Pt 2):478–498

61. Walcott GP, Walcott KT, Ideker RE. Mechanisms of defibrillation. Critical points and the upper limit of vulnerability. *J Electrocardiol* 1995;28(Suppl):1–6

62. Dillon SM, Kwaku KF. Progressive depolarization: a unified hypothesis for defibrillation and fibrillation induction by shocks. *J Cardiovasc Electrophysiol* 1998;9(5):529–552

63. Roth BJ. A mathematical model of make and break electrical stimulation of cardiac tissue by a unipolar anode or cathode. *IEEE Trans Biomed Eng* 1995;42(12):1174–1184

64. Knisley SB, Hill BC, Ideker RE. Virtual electrode effects in myocardial fibers. *Biophysical J* 1994;66(3 Pt 1):719–728

65. Neunlist M, Tung L. Spatial distribution of cardiac transmembrane potentials around an extracellular electrode: dependence on fiber orientation. *Biophysical J* 1995;68(6):2310–2322

66. Efimov IR, Cheng YN, Biermann M, Van Wagoner DR, Mazgalev T, Tchou PJ. Transmembrane voltage changes produced by real and virtual electrodes during monophasic defibrillation shock delivered by an implantable electrode. *J Cardiovasc Electrophysiol* 1997;8:1031–1045

67. Efimov IR, Cheng Y, Van Wagoner DR, Mazgalev T, Tchou PJ. Virtual electrode-induced phase singularity: a basic mechanism of defibrillation failure. *Circ Res* 1998;82(8):918–925

68. Efimov IR, Gray RA, Roth BJ. Virtual electrodes and de-excitation: new insights into fibrillation induction and defibrillation. *J Cardiovasc Electrophysiol* 2000;11(3):339–353

69. Cheng Y, Mowrey KA, Van Wagoner DR, Tchou PJ, Efimov IR. Virtual electrode induced re-excitation: a basic mechanism of defibrillation. *Circ Res* 1999;85(11):1056–1066

70. Hoffa M, Ludwig C. Einige neue Versuche uber Herzbewegung. *Zeitschrift Rationelle Medizin* 1850;9:107–144

71. Skouibine K, Trayanova NA, Moore P. Anode/cathode make and break phenomena in a model of defibrillation. *IEEE Trans Biomed Eng* 1999;46(7):769–777

72. Lin SF, Roth BJ, Wikswo JP. Quatrefoil reentry in myocardium: an optical imaging study of the induction mechanism. *J Cardiovasc Electrophysiol* 1999;10:574–586

73. Winfree AT. *When Time Breaks Down: The Three-Dimensional Dynamics of Electrochemical Waves and Cardiac Arrhythmias.* Princeton, NJ: Princeton University Press; 1987

74. Cheng Y, Van Wagoner D, Tchou PJ, Efimov IR. Defibrillation shock-induced waves of re-excitation: implications to upper and lower limits of vulnerability. *PACE* 1999;22(4(II)):809

75. Cheng Y, Nikolski V, Efimov IR. Reversal of repolarization gradient does not reverse the chirality of shock-induced reentry in the rabbit heart. *J Cardiovasc Electrophysiol* 2000;11(9):998–1007

76. Efimov IR, Cheng Y, Yamanouchi Y, Tchou PJ. Direct evidence of the role of virtual electrode induced phase singularity in success and failure of defibrillation. *J Cardiovasc Electrophysiol* 2000;11(8):861–868

77. Jones JL, Jones RE, Balasky G. Microlesion formation in myocardial cells by high-intensity electric field stimulation. *Am J Physiol* 1987;253(2 Pt 2):H480–H486

78. Nikolski VP, Sambelashvili AT, Krinsky VI, Efimov IR. Effects of electroporation on optically recorded transmembrane potential responses to high-intensity electrical shocks. *Am J Physiol Heart Circ Physiol* 2004;286(1):H412–H418

79. Yamanouchi Y, Cheng Y, Tchou PJ, Efimov IR. The mechanisms of vulnerable window: the role of virtual electrodes and shock polarity. *Can J Physiol Pharmacol* 2001;79(1):25–33

80. Kroll MW, Efimov IR, Tchou PJ. Present understanding of shock polarity for internal defibrillation: the obvious and non-obvious clinical implications. *Pacing Clin Electrophysiol* 2006;29(8):885–891

81. Chapman PD, Vetter JW, Souza JJ, Troup PJ, Wetherbee JN, Hoffmann RG. Comparative efficacy of monophasic and biphasic truncated exponential shocks for nonthoracotomy internal defibrillation in dogs. *J Am Coll Cardiol* 1988;12(3):739–745

82. Feeser SA, Tang AS, Kavanagh KM, Rollins DL, Smith WM, Wolf PD, Ideker RE. Strength-duration and probability of success curves for defibrillation with biphasic waveforms. *Circulation* 1990;82(6):2128–2141

83. Qu F, Li L, Nikolski VP, Sharma V, Efimov IR. Mechanisms of superiority of ascending ramp waveforms: new insights into mechanisms of shock-induced vulnerability and defibrillation. *Am J Physiol Heart Circ Physiol* 2005;289(2):H569–H577

84. Takagi S, Pumir A, Pazo D, Efimov I, Nikolski V, Krinsky V. Unpinning and removal of a rotating wave in cardiac muscle. *Phys Rev Lett* 2004;93(5):058101

85. Ripplinger CM, Krinsky VI, Nikolski VP, Efimov IR. Mechanisms of unpinning and termination of ventricular tachycardia. *Am J Physiol Heart Circ Physiol* 2006;291(1):H184–H192

86. Fedorov VV, Schuessler RB, Lall S, Ripplinger CM, Sakamoto S, Efimov IR. Low voltage defibrillation of sustained ventricular tachycardia in infarcted canine hearts. *Heart Rhythm* 2007;4 (5S):S171

Chapter 4.5

Simultaneous Optical and Electrical Recordings

Stephen B. Knisley, Herman D. Himel IV, and John H. Dumas III

Introduction to Electrooptical Measurements

Development of antiarrhythmic electrical therapies requires knowledge of the characteristics of cardiac arrhythmias and effects of electrical stimulation on the heart. Much of the available knowledge is obtained from measurements of extracellular potentials or transmembrane potentials in the heart using electrical or optical methods. With an extracellular electrode in contact with the heart, activation of the cells is detected by observing the intrinsic negative deflection of the extracellular potential. (In this chapter, the occurrence of a rapid increase in inwardly directed membrane current during the phase zero depolarization is termed *activation*, whereas the transition of a dye molecule to the excited state by light absorption is termed *excitation*.) Maps constructed from the times of these deflections at several locations in the heart indicate the spatiotemporal distributions of activation. Also maps of the distribution of extracellular potentials in the heart during a shock reveal characteristics of the electric field, which can be correlated with effects of shocks on the activation. Extracellular potential measurements can also indicate repolarization using t-wave analysis, and action potential contour using the monophasic action potential produced by pressure or suction near the electrode. Most electrical measurements do not detect activation during a shock pulse because of interference by the shock's electric field.

Another way to examine arrhythmic activation and effects of shocks is by optical action potential measurements. An isolated heart or heart tissue specimen is stained with a transmembrane voltage-dependent fluorescent dye and illuminated with excitation light. Absorption of light by dye molecules induces an excited molecular state. The molecules emit fluorescence photons as part of the process of decay to the ground state. The

Stephen B. Knisley
Department of Biomedical Engineering, The University of North Carolina at Chapel Hill, Chapel Hill, NC, USA,
sknisley@email.unc.edu

I. R. Efimov et al. (eds.), *Cardiac Bioelectric Therapy: Mechanisms and Practical Implications.*
© Springer Science+Business Media, LLC 2009

spectrum of emitted fluorescence from di-4-ANEPPS shifts toward shorter wavelengths when the heart cells depolarize. This shift reverses when cells repolarize. Therefore, intensity of the long wavelength portion of the fluorescence spectrum (e.g., red light containing wavelengths >570 nm in rabbit heart containing di-4-ANEPPS excited with blue light at 488 nm) decreases when cells depolarize, and then increases during repolarization. The resulting signal contains an inverted optical action potential that is linearly related to the transmembrane potential. However, there is not an absolute calibration between the optical signal and membrane voltage.

The optical signal may be affected by undesired factors that alter intensity of the fluorescence spectrum, most notably fluctuations in excitation intensity, dye bleaching, or heart motion. To remove these effects in some applications, blue light (488 nm) is used for excitation, and a signal containing the short wavelength portion of the fluorescence spectrum (e.g., green light ranging from the excitation wavelength to 570 nm) is measured simultaneously with the long wavelength signal. The signal from the green fluorescence contains an upright action potential. The ratio of the two fluorescence signals is then computed.

The tissue activation is detected using the optical phase zero depolarization. Activation isochrone maps are produced with methods similar to those produced with electrical mapping. The action potential duration and repolarization time are also measured optically. A characteristic of optical signals that is important for study of electric shocks is that an extracellular electric field itself does not alter the fluorescence, whereas a change in transmembrane potential that may occur in the presence on an extracellular electric field does alter fluorescence. This allows optical measurements of transmembrane potentials during shocks.

The availability of a translucent electrode material, indium tin oxide (ITO), makes it possible to map both extracellular potentials and optical transmembrane potentials simultaneously. ITO is a combination of indium oxide and tin oxide that can be sputtered onto a substrate to form an electrically conductive and translucent thin film. Lithographic patterning of an ITO film on a glass substrate produces electrodes through which light passes for optical mapping in underlying tissue. This enables electrical stimulation or mapping while optically mapping at the same sites. Our laboratory has examined pertinent electrical and optical properties of ITO and employed ITO in studies of cardiac stimulation and activation. Some of the experiments are discussed below.

ITO Properties

For a 200 nm film of ITO on a 1.1 mm-thick borosilicate glass, transmittance is 0.85–0.9 in the range of light wavelengths from 488 to 818 nm.[1] The surface appears optically flat as evident from absence of visible distortion of images viewed through the plate. Examination of a transmitted laser beam failed to indicate measurable scatter.[1]

One consequence of ITO's high optical transmittance is that the presence or absence of ITO at a particular location on one side of a glass plate and identification of which side contains ITO are not visually obvious. Since ITO is electrically conductive, an ohmmeter provides a simple way to find which side of the glass contains the conductive ITO film. If the film is lithographically patterned, examination of the specular reflection image can reveal the pattern. A microscope containing a coaxial illuminator indicates ITO patterns on plates that are positioned normal to the illumination axis.

Resistivity and interfacial resistance between an electrode and biological material affect usability for stimulation or recording. The sheet resistivity of a thin film indicates the ability to carry current along runs or from one part of a thin film electrode to another part of the electrode.[2] Sheet resistivity is ~15 Ω per square for ITO films having a thickness of 200 nm. A thicker film has lower sheet resistivity and light transmittance. For example, a film having thickness 850 nm exhibits ~1–2 Ω per square and transmittance of 0.75 for 550 nm light.

Interfacial conductance of ITO film with Tyrode's solution is reported to be $880 \, S/m^{-2}$ when the ITO is an anode and $1{,}500 \, S/m^{-2}$ when the ITO is a cathode.[3] These values are much higher than the interfacial conductance for gold or stainless steel electrodes and are more comparable to values for Ag/AgCl electrodes.[4]

The ITO film can be etched by immersion in a solution containing HCl and HNO_3 concentrates to produce patterned arrays of ITO electrodes for electrical mapping in hearts.[1] A pattern is produced by application of acid-resistant material to the ITO by photographic techniques or other methods, followed by immersion of the plate in the acid.[1,5,6] The plate often remains immersed for a sufficient time to remove all ITO in those areas not covered by acid-resistant material. The plate may also be immersed for a limited time to thin the ITO film, which increases sheet resistivity of the remaining ITO in that area.[7]

The optical transmittance of ITO changes when current crosses the interface between ITO and the heart.[3] This is produced by oxidation or reduction reactions that transfer current carried by electrons and ions. The specific reactions have been studied for certain metals used for stimulation.[8] There are several possible oxidation or reduction reactions for ITO.[9] Reactions can darken metallic shock electrodes, indicating the distribution of interfacial current.[10–12] A map of the changes in ITO transmittance indicates the distribution of the ITO–heart interfacial current.

Ratiometric Optical Mapping

A laser scanner system is the simplest approach for multiwavelength band fluorescence mapping. The scanner controls localization by directing a single excitation light beam to one spot at a time. All bands of fluorescence measured at an instant in time originate from the same spot. The number of bands that can be practically measured is limited by the space available to position photomultiplier tubes near the heart and by the number of photons in each band.[5] The ratiometric methods require light detectors that register signals proportional to the intensities of fluorescence. For measurements described here, it is not necessary that the light detectors for different wavelength bands have identical sensitivity.

The nonratiometric signals that contain motion artifacts and ratiometric signals have been used to distinguish the heart motion–induced components from the transmembrane potential component.[13] Measurements in three bands have been used for ratiometry with simultaneous coloaded calcium and transmembrane potential–sensitive fluorescent dyes to reduce motion artifacts and drift.[14] Ratiometric methods were used to cancel effects of ITO transmittance changes when mapping under ITO electrodes.[3]

Role of the Second Spatial Derivative of the Extracellular Potential in Field Stimulation

Initial tests were performed with nonsimultaneous electrical and optical mapping.[15] Cable theory predicts transmembrane current is proportional to the second spatial derivative of the extracellular potential (i.e., Laplacian component).[16,17] A Laplacian component differs from the extracellular potential gradient (first spatial derivative of extracellular potential), which has been used to quantify stimulatory strength and thresholds of the shock-induced electric field in tissue.[18,19]

To produce Laplacian components in two dimensions on the heart surface, electrical stimulation was applied with metallic wire or mesh electrodes to produce either nonuniform or approximately uniform electric fields on the epicardium. Optical mapping in a region between the electrodes indicated the changes in transmembrane potential produced by the electric fields. In separate measurements, extracellular potentials were mapped with a roving linear electrode array while the stimuli were repeated for each position of the array. Results were compared with bidomain models that incorporated the heart's epicardial fiber structure.

Results showed that the location of the detectable Laplacian components of the extracellular potentials qualitatively match locations of changes in transmembrane potential. As illustrated in Fig. 1, regions undergoing positive changes in transmembrane potential exhibit a mostly negative Laplacian, while regions undergoing negative changes in transmembrane potential exhibit a positive Laplacian. The changes in transmembrane potential correspond to the Laplacian components more than they correspond to the potential gradient. Also the results demonstrated that fiber structure of the tissue distorts the extracellular electric field.

In a study to test the activating function theory,[20,21] ITO was used to create an extracellular electric field containing an activating function.[7] Half of the ITO film was etched in stirred acid solution for a brief time to thin the ITO and increase its sheet resistivity. Then leads were attached to the etched and nonetched ends of the ITO film as shown in Fig. 2. Current applied to the ITO produced a large potential gradient in the etched ITO region, while it produced a smaller potential gradient in the nonetched ITO. An activating function occurred at the boundary between the two regions where the potential gradient changed.

In experiments with rabbit hearts stained with di-4-ANEPPS, the ITO was placed on the heart so that the ventricular epicardial surface was exposed to the activating function. Optical mapping was performed in the underlying tissue. The excitation light and fluorescence passed through the ITO and glass plate. Results are illustrated in Fig. 3.

a

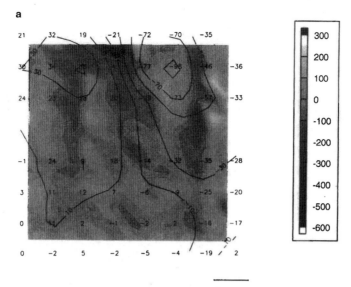

1 mm

b

$\nabla^2 \Phi_e$ (V/cm^2); NUS2

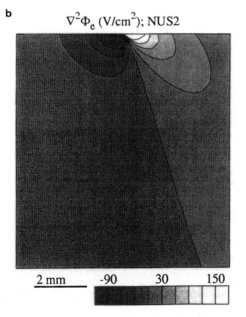

2 mm   -90   30   150

Figure 1: Maps of the Laplacian of extracellular potential during electric field stimulation performed with a small electrode above the center of the map and a large electrode below the map to produce a nonuniform electric field. (**a**) Epicardial measurements (V/cm^2) from a rabbit heart. Transmembrane potential changes (numbers and contour lines) are overlaid on a gray-scale Laplacian from the same heart. (**b**) Bidomain model results. The current strength was 56 mA in the heart and 44 mA in the model. (From Knisley et al., Biophysical Journal 77, 1404–1417, 1999, figure 12 © 1999 Biophysical Society, Reproduced with permission.)

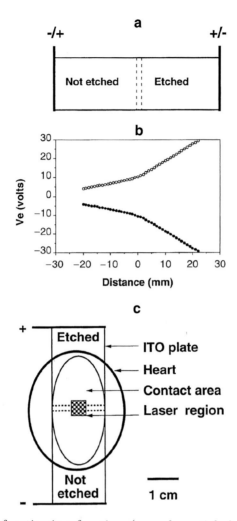

Figure 2: Production of activating function (second spatial derivative of extracellular potential) with indium tin oxide (ITO). (a) Right half of conductive ITO on glass plate was etched in acid to decrease thickness of the ITO film and increase film resistance. Shock current was delivered at plate ends. (b) Current produced potential gradients along the plate measured with roving electrode. Potential gradient in etched half was 2.5 times that in nonetched half. Second spatial derivative of extracellular potential occurred in central region. (c) Plate was positioned on ventricles of hearts stained with di-4-ANEPPS. Laser scanner measured transmembrane potential changes in central region. (From Knisley, IEEE Transactions on Biomedical Engineering 47, 1114–1119, 2000, figure 1, © 2000, IEEE, Reproduced with permission.)

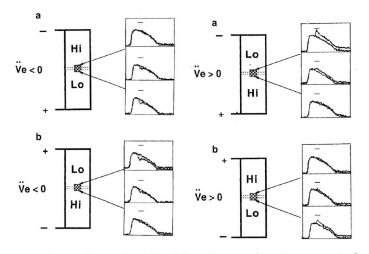

Figure 3: Outcome of experimental trials with activating function in central region (*dotted lines*) produced by nonuniformly etched indium tin oxide (ITO) plate. Action potentials with and without the shock are overlaid. The d^2V_e/dt^2 was negative (*left column*, $V_e'' < 0$) or positive (*right column*, $V_e'' > 0$). When the positive lead was attached to the low-gradient end of the ITO (*left column*), negative transmembrane potential changes occurred during the shock both before and after the plate was rotated. When the positive lead was attached to the high-gradient end of the ITO (*right*), positive transmembrane potential changes occurred before and after rotation. (From Knisley, IEEE Transactions on Biomedical Engineering 47, 1114–1119, 2000, figures 3 and 4, © 2000, IEEE, Reproduced with permission.)

Results show that contact with the ITO containing an activating function introduces a change in transmembrane potential that has the corresponding sign. Other tests with only a potential gradient showed that transmembrane potential changes are due to a variation in heart conductance between the base and apex, corresponding to increased heart width near the base. These results are consistent with the generalized activating function that contains a term for the extracellular potential gradient scaled by the change in tissue conductance, and a term for the change in the potential gradient.[21]

The sign of the second derivative of the extracellular potential matches the sign of the transmembrane potential change in the experiments shown in Figs. 2 and 3, whereas it is the opposite of the sign of the transmembrane potential change in Fig. 1. This is due to differences in experimental conditions in the two studies. The experiments in which the ITO produced an activating function are more applicable to the Rattay formulation.[20] The ITO resistance is sufficiently low that the electric field produced by ITO is not greatly affected by the tissue. That differs from the conditions used for the study in Fig. 1, in which the extracellular electric field was affected by the tissue.[15,20]

Stimulatory Effects of a Spatial Variation of Extracellular Conductance in an Electric Field

According to theory, spatial variations in extracellular resistance introduce transmembrane currents at borders between regions of high and low extracellular resistance due to redistribution of current between intracellular and extracellular spaces.[22] For example, a decrease in extracellular resistance at a certain location along the direction of intracellular and extracellular current flow will produce a larger current extracellularly by redistribution of some of the intracellular current to the extracellular space. This redistribution produces outward transmembrane current and a positive change in transmembrane potential. Effects of some heart interfaces and alterations in extracellular conductance on the transmembrane potential have been demonstrated.[7,23] Redistribution due to extracellular structures of the heart, such as a region of connective tissue or a blood vessel, might produce far-field stimulatory effects. However, that hypothesis has not been experimentally validated.

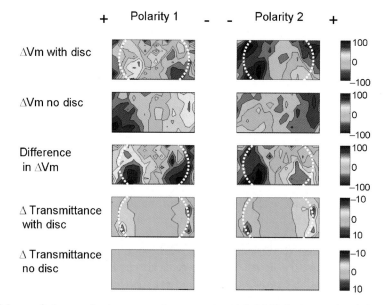

Figure 4: Maps of change in transmembrane potential (ΔV_{m}) determined from the ratio, and transmittance of the indium tin oxide (ITO) (Δ transmittance) determined with red fluorescence in a rabbit heart during field stimulation pulse given in action potential plateau. *Top row* shows ΔV_{m} for each S_2 polarity with ITO disc on the heart. *Second row* shows ΔV_{m} for identical S_2 after disc was removed. The *third row* shows the difference in ΔV_{m} between the above plots, an estimate of the effect produced by the disc. The ΔV_{m} and difference in ΔV_{m} are expressed as a percentage of the action potential amplitude. *Rows 4 and 5* show the Δ transmittance with and without the disc as percentages. (From Knisley and Pollard, Am J Physiol Heart Circ Physiol 289, H1137–H1146, 2005, figure 4. Reproduced with permission.)

Tests with an inactive extracellular conductor were performed to see whether such changes in transmembrane potentials occur in tissue under the conductor and correspond to the current redistribution hypothesis. These experiments used ITO as the conductor, while the shock was applied to the heart from mesh electrodes to produce an electric field in the region containing the ITO. Optical mapping was performed in the tissue under and on either side of the ITO. Figure 4 illustrates an example of results.

The maps illustrate fluorescence measurements both with an inactive ITO disc on the heart and without the disc, which serves as a control. A control is useful because there are transmembrane potential changes in the far field in hearts even when no artificial change in extracellular resistance is introduced. The difference between the map with the disc and the control represents the effect of the disc. ITO-heart interfacial current estimated from the red fluorescence signal indicates opposite interfacial currents at the left and right edges of the disc, consistent with redistribution of current between the heart and ITO. The results essentially show a cathodal stimulatory effect near the edge of the inactive disc facing the real shock anode, and an anodal stimulatory effect near the edge of the disc facing the real shock cathode.

Effect of Unipolar Stimulation in the Tissue under the Electrode

Unipolar stimulation of ventricles produces anisotropic effects in which a cathodal stimulus depolarizes cells in tissue away from the electrode near the transverse axis (axis perpendicular to the cardiac fibers) while it hyperpolarizes near the fiber axis.[12,24-29] The anisotropy of these polarizations, or "virtual electrodes," during the pulse is qualitatively accounted for by just the linear tissue properties. The polarizations produce a number of important nonlinear responses. These include a difference in the magnitudes of the positive and negative polarizations at the same site during an anodal pulse versus that during a cathodal pulse, a "no-switch" region oblique to fibers at which the direction of polarization is the same for both stimulation polarities, quatrefoil reentry, phase singularities, and direction-dependent action potential prolongation.[30-32]

A theoretical prediction that was not measured in the experiments described is that tissue under a unipolar electrode is depolarized during the pulse when the electrode is a cathode, whereas the tissue is hyperpolarized when the electrode is an anode. Optical measurement in tissue under the electrode is difficult due to the blockage of the light by a metal electrode. Thus experiments used point electrodes that minimized blockage or used optrode-based methods.[33]

ITO has been used to map multiple sites under a unipolar stimulation electrode. The ITO pattern contained a 1-cm disc electrode and an insulated run from the electrode to the edge of the plate.[3] Optical mapping was performed with a ratiometric method and correction algorithm that enabled transmembrane potential measurements with minimal effects of changes in ITO transmittance.

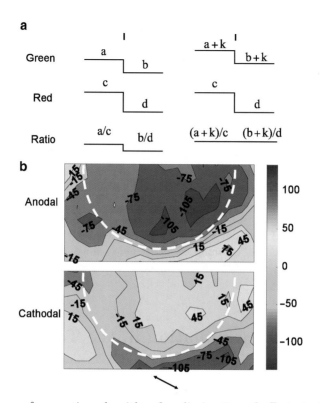

Figure 5: Cartoon of correction algorithm for elimination of effects in the ratio produced by a difference between the fractional changes of green and red fluorescence signals due to alteration in indium tin oxide (ITO) transmittance, and contour maps from anterior heart showing changes in transmembrane potential under anodal and cathodal stimulation electrodes. (a) *Left part* represents a case in which the changes in green and red signals measured during cardiac cycles before and after the pulse are not identical, which produces a change in ratio. Baselines are illustrated without action potentials for clarity. The value, k, satisfying $(a + k)/c = (b + k)/d$ is added to the green signal (*right*) to eliminate change in ratio. (b) Changes in transmembrane potential measured during action potential plateau are given as a percentage of action potential height. The *double-headed arrow* at the *bottom* indicates mean fiber direction assessed from minute epicardial grooves in the region of the optical grid. (From Lian et al., Annals of Biomedical Engineering 32, 1202–1210, 2004, figure 2, © Biomedical Engineering Society with kind permission of Springer Science and Business Media.)

The changes in transmembrane potential during shocks given in the action potential plateau were nonuniform under the electrode, as shown in Fig. 5. Changes produced by anodal stimulation were negative at all locations under the electrode, and their magnitudes varied by a factor of ~2 at different sites under the electrode. For cathodal stimulation, the changes were positive at most locations under the electrode. Negative transmembrane

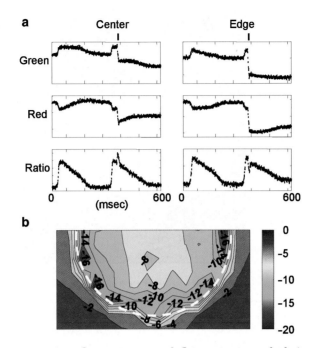

Figure 6: Simultaneous green fluorescence, red fluorescence and their ratio, and contour map of the change in red fluorescence during a cathodal stimulus applied from indium tin oxide (ITO) disc electrode on rabbit heart. (a) Optical recordings from spots under the center and edge of the disc during two heartbeats. A single stimulation pulse from disc was delivered during the plateau of the second action potential (*vertical bar* above recordings). Green and red fluorescence signals decreased during the pulse (downward deflection). The ITO transmittance decreased during the shock. Ratio indicates change in transmembrane potential during the pulse. (b) Map shows percentage decrease in red fluorescence during the pulse. Edge of disc electrode is indicated (*white dotted line*). (From Lian et al., Annals of Biomedical Engineering 32, 1202–1210, 2004, figure 3, © Biomedical Engineering Society with kind permission of Springer Science and Business Media.)

potential changes occurred at some locations under the electrode during the cathodal stimulation.

The changes in fluorescence intensity caused by changes in ITO transmittance indicated interfacial current between the ITO electrode and the heart flowed in the same direction at all locations under the electrode. The interfacial current had its greatest magnitude near the edge of the disc, as shown in Fig. 6. The transmembrane potential changes were qualitatively accounted for by superposition of the reported effects of unipolar point stimulation[28] scaled by the interfacial current distribution, as is evident by comparing Fig. 7 with Fig. 5b.

A bidomain model produced qualitatively similar variations in magnitudes of the transmembrane potentials under the electrode. However, the model and experiments disagreed

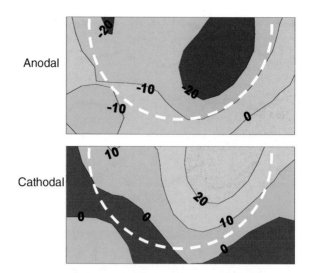

Figure 7: The transmembrane potential changes predicted by superposition of the changes produced by currents from points on the disc electrode surface. Currents at locations on the disc were estimated using the square root of changes in red fluorescence. The transmembrane potential changes produced by individual currents from the locations were based on experiments using point stimulation in hearts. These were scaled in proportion to current and located relative to their respective point before summation. (From Lian et al., Annals of Biomedical Engineering 32, 1202–1210, 2004, figure 6, © Biomedical Engineering Society with kind permission of Springer Science and Business Media.)

at the edge of the electrode, where the model predicted larger transmembrane potential changes compared with those found in hearts.

When the stimuli were applied during electrical diastole in the experiments, early sites of excitation sometimes corresponded to the sites at which the positive changes in transmembrane potential were found during the plateau-phase shocks. For weaker stimuli in diastole, anomalous sites of excitation were found at which no positive change in transmembrane potential were measured during the plateau-phase shocks.

Electrooptical Mapping of Cardiac Excitation

An important assumption in cardiac electrophysiology is that the rapid negative deflection in the extracellular potential is simultaneous with the phase-zero depolarization of cardiac cells near the electrode. This has been considered for some time, since Sir Thomas Lewis described the graphic registration of the heartbeat.[34] Currently the negative deflection is used in many clinical and experimental studies of arrhythmias as a standard index of the depolarization. The accepted relationship between the extracellular potential and the transmembrane potential has been verified by numerous computational models of heart tissue and in vitro tissue experiments in which the transmembrane action potential is examined together with the extracellular potential.[35,36] Interestingly, few or none of the experimental validations were performed in intact heart tissue or during arrhythmias. It is conceivable abnormal conduction in arrhythmias changes the relationship. A method that provides both optical and electrical maps simultaneously may provide insights into the relationship between these measurements during arrhythmias.

Electrode arrays produced with photolithographically patterned ITO allow electrical mapping and simultaneous optical mapping of a region of the heart by passing the excitation and fluorescence light through the ITO electrodes. Two studies have been performed that employed this approach with isolated rabbit hearts. One examined epicardially paced beats and sinus beats, and the other examined ventricular fibrillation.

Method of Electrooptical Mapping

The process for array fabrication begins with a glass plate containing an ITO thin film. A positive photoresist is spun onto the ITO, dehydrated, and exposed with ultraviolet light using a mask that contains the electrode pattern. Examples of masks are illustrated in Fig. 8. Photoresist is developed, dehydrated, and then etched in an acid solution to remove ITO in all regions except electrodes, runs, or wire attachment areas. A wash with acetone and dehydration removes the remaining photoresist. Insulation is then added on the ITO runs so that they do not contact the heart during experiments. Insulation consists of a layer of either photoresist or polyimide that is patterned with another mask to cover the runs from the electrodes to the wire attachment areas located at edges of the plate.

Wires are attached with conductive cement. Attachment areas are then covered with epoxy to eliminate the possibility of contact of the leads with saline during experiments. The leads are connected to isolation amplifiers having gain of 10 and passband of direct current to 16 KHz. The isolation prevents damage to the recording system in case a shock produces large common-mode voltage at the electrodes. Low-pass filtering is employed when necessary. The reference electrode for all ITO recording channels is an Ag–AgCl electrode attached to the aortic root. Amplified signals are passed to a computer and digitized using a ± 10 V range synchronously with optical signals. Digitization rates are 4–8 KHz.

The laser spots are aligned with the electrodes by adjusting the size of the scanned laser grid to match the size of the electrode array, and then positioning the grid so that laser light for the spots passes to the centers of the corresponding electrodes. This is verified before recordings by examination with a magnifying loupe, using the specular reflected light at low power. Under these conditions, laser beam locations and perimeters of electrodes are visible. Fine alignment is performed with a micrometer mechanism attached to the mirror that directs laser light to the electrode array. The apparatus is mounted on a rigid optical table so that alignment remains stable.

The heart is placed in contact with the ITO array. Slight pressure is applied from the opposite side of the heart using a flexible arm to produce a 1–2 cm contact region of epicardium with the array.

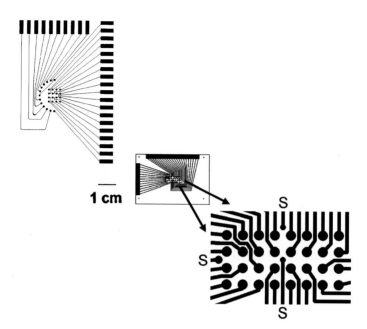

Figure 8: Indium tin oxide (ITO) patterns used for electrode arrays. *Upper left*: Pattern used in study of paced beats and sinus beats. ITO was sputtered onto a glass plate. Photolithographically produced ITO electrode pattern contained a $7 \times 7\,mm$ array of 16 circular recording electrodes having 1-mm diameter with center-to-center interelectrode distance of 2 mm in directions parallel to principal array axes, and a semicircular array of 13 stimulation electrodes evenly spaced 8 mm from the center of the recording array. ITO runs having width of 0.1 mm passed from each electrode to rectangular wire attachment area at an edge of plate. Wires (not shown) were attached with conductive cement. *Lower*: Pattern used in study of ventricular fibrillation. *Lower right* shows enlargement of central region containing 32 translucent circular 1-mm diameter recording electrodes arranged in a $6 \times 14\,mm^2$ array, and three circular stimulation electrodes (S). (Adapted from Knisley and Neuman, Annals of Biomedical Engineering 31, 32–41, 2003, figure 1, and Himel and Knisley, Physiological Measurement 28, 707–719, 2007, figure 1, with permission from IOP Publishing Limited.)

Electrooptical Mapping of Epicardially Paced Beats and Sinus Beats

The initial electrooptical mapping of cardiac activations employed a square array containing 16 ITO electrodes used for recording and a semicircular array containing 13 electrodes used for stimulation.[1]

Recordings of a stimulation-induced beat are shown in Fig. 9. The maximum magnitudes of the first time derivatives of the optical transmembrane potential recordings and

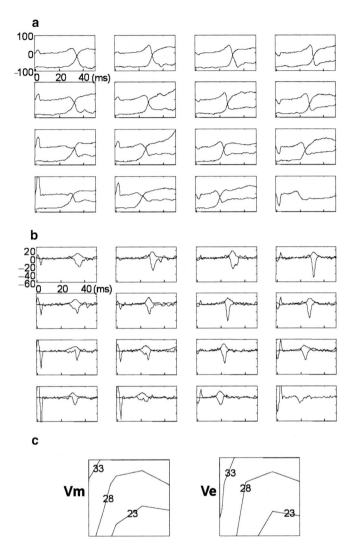

Figure 9: Recordings (**a**), time derivatives (**b**), and activation isochrone maps (**c**) for optical V_m and V_e on posterior epicardium. Activation was produced by stimulation below the array. (**a**) Optical V_m and V_e. Vertical units are millivolts for optical V_m and 10^{-4} V for V_e. Optical V_m was calibrated assuming 100 mV action potential amplitude and -80 mV resting membrane potential. Each V_e contained a stimulation artifact, delay due to propagation, and downward deflection. (**b**) Time derivatives of optical V_m and V_e. Vertical units are V/s for optical V_m and V/dekasecond for V_e. (**c**) Contour maps of times of maximum optical dV_m/dt and minimum dV_e/dt in milliseconds indicate upward propagation. (From Knisley and Neuman, Annals of Biomedical Engineering 31, 32–41, 2003, figure 2, © 2003 Biomedical Engineering Society. Reproduced with permission.)

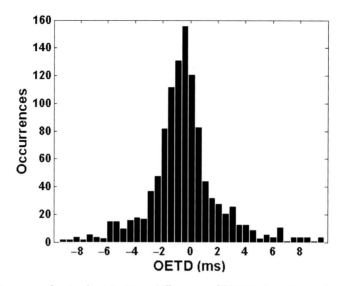

Figure 10: Histogram of optoelectric time differences (OETD, i.e., time of maximum optical dV_m/dt minus time of minimum dV_e/dt at each spot) for pacing-induced heartbeats. Action potentials in anterior or posterior ventricular regions of two hearts were produced by biphasic stimuli at individual sites within semicircular electrode array to produce propagation in various directions relative to the epicardial fibers. The OETD was -0.46 ± 2.6 ms (mean $\pm$ SD, $p <.000001$ for value vs. zero, $n = 1{,}112$). (From Knisley and Neuman, Annals of Biomedical Engineering 31, 32–41, 2003, figure 4, © 2003 Biomedical Engineering Society. Reproduced with permission.)

extracellular potential recordings corresponded temporally to within a few milliseconds. Isochrone contours constructed from the two types of recordings were similar. The optoelectric time difference (OETD) was defined as the time between the maximum optical dV_m/dt and the minimum dV_e/dt measured at a laser spot and its corresponding electrode. Beats produced by bipolar pacing from all adjacent pairs of stimulation electrodes in the semicircular array produced a distribution of OETD shown in Fig. 10. The mean OETD is -1/2 ms (negative value indicates earlier mean activation time for the optical measurements).

Results indicate there is a greater depth of interrogation for the optical method compared with the electrical method. The theoretical depth to width ratio of the interrogated volume for optical V_m is greater than the ratio for V_e.[1,37] Figure 11 shows dimensions of interrogated volumes determined with computer models. Also, electrooptical mapping of sinus beats indicates the maximum optical dV_m/dt is earlier than the minimum dV_e/dt, as shown in Fig. 12. For beats that propagate from deeper tissue to the surface, a measurement that interrogates deeper will detect the activation earlier. In addition, when stimulation was applied at electrodes that produced propagation along epicardial fibers, activation time measured from optical V_m was later than the time measured from V_e. However, when pacing produced propagation across epicardial fibers, the activation measured from optical V_m was

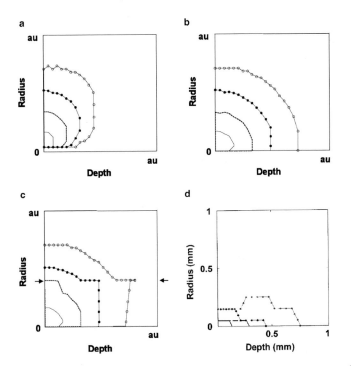

Figure 11: Computer-generated relative dimensions of regions interrogated by V_e under various conditions (**a–c**) and by optical V_m (**d**). (**a–c**) Borders of subsets of nodes in dipole models that contribute fractions of total potential at origin (*solid line* 20%, *dashed line* 40%, *filled circles* 60%, *open circles* 80%). Radius and depth scales are identical. (**a**) Dipoles were oriented randomly and within planes parallel to the surface. (**b**) Dipoles were oriented randomly. (**c**) Dipoles were oriented randomly and strength of all dipoles at a given radius (*arrows*) was increased 1.5-fold. (**d**) Borders of subsets of nodes in a Monte Carlo light transport model that contribute fractions of the total fluorescence emitted from the tissue surface when laser excitation beam with a radius of 0.1 mm is directed toward origin from the left (*solid line* 20%, *dashed line* 40%, *filled circles* 60%, *open circles* 80%). (From Knisley and Neuman, Annals of Biomedical Engineering 31, 32–41, 2003, figure 7, © 2003 Biomedical Engineering Society. Reproduced with permission.)

earlier than that measured from V_e. The dependence of the time difference on orientation is illustrated in Fig. 13. For propagation along epicardial fibers, the fiber rotation with depth in myocardium produces the observed lag of activation in deeper fibers because the deeper fibers are not aligned with the propagation direction. For propagation across epicardial fibers, the deeper fibers interrogated optically lead activation because they are more aligned with the propagation direction, again consistent with optical interrogation deeper than the electrical interrogation.

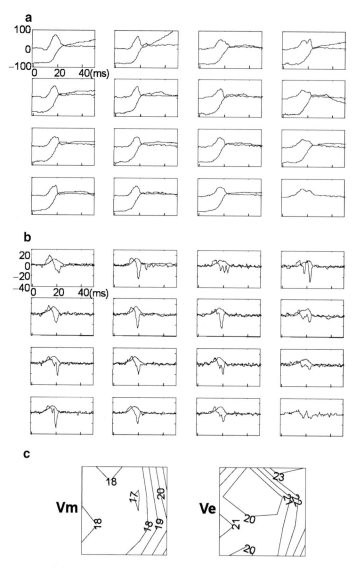

Figure 12: Recordings (**a**), computed time derivatives (**b**), and activation isochrone maps (**c**) for optical V_m and V_e during a sinus beat. Results indicated activation in the recording region approximately 3 ms earlier for optical V_m compared with V_e. Units are same as in Figure 9. (From Knisley and Neuman, Annals of Biomedical Engineering 31, 32–41, 2003, figure 5, © 2003 Biomedical Engineering Society. Reproduced with permission.)

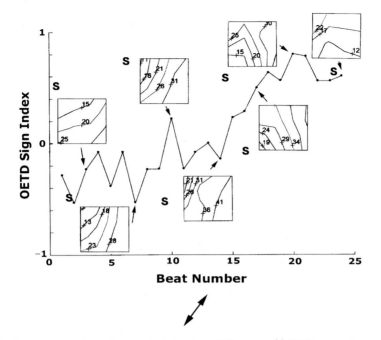

Figure 13: Indices of the sign of optoelectric time difference (OETD, i.e., time of maximum optical dV_m/dt minus time of minimum dV_e/dt at each spot) for various directions of propagation in the recording region in a single heart. The index for each beat is defined as the number of spots with positive OETD minus the number with negative OETD, divided by their total. Indices are plotted versus beat number for a train of 24 beats produced by bipolar pacing at individual sites (S) within semicircular electrode array. Stimulation sites scanned counterclockwise beginning above the mapped region with two stimuli given at each site. Activation isochrone maps (*insets*) illustrate changes in propagation produced by switching to a different stimulation site. Average epicardial fiber direction is indicated (*double-headed arrow*). (From Knisley and Neuman, Annals of Biomedical Engineering 31, 32–41, 2003, figure 6, © 2003 Biomedical Engineering Society. Reproduced with permission.)

Electrooptical Mapping of Fibrillation

Simultaneous electrical and optical mapping was performed with rabbit hearts in which fibrillation was induced electrically.[6] The deflections in the optical V_m and V_e occur at shorter and less regular intervals compared with the deflections during sinus rhythm or pacing. Magnitudes of the fibrillatory deflections vary among beats.

Results from representative spots are illustrated in Fig. 14. The times of downward deflections in V_e are qualitatively similar to the times of the upward deflections of optical V_m. Expansion of the time axis shows there were quantitative differences between times of the maxima and minima of the slopes of these deflections. The majority of deflections

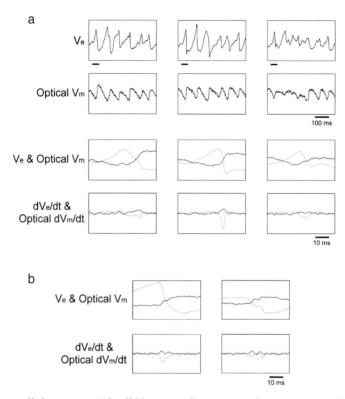

Figure 14: Extracellular potentials (V_e), optical transmembrane potentials (optical V_m), and their first time derivatives during ventricular fibrillation. (**a**) *Top row* shows V_e at three adjacent spots during a single 500-ms segment of VF. The simultaneous optical V_m at each spot is shown below each V_e. *Horizontal bar* below each V_e indicates 50-ms segment that is shown in third and fourth rows with expanded time scale. *Third row* shows overlaid V_e (*dotted trace*) and optical V_m (*solid trace*). *Fourth row* shows their first time derivatives (*dotted and solid*, respectively). For row 1, the y-axis range is from -10 to 10 mV. For row 2, the y-axis range is from -5 to $+5\%$ of the mean ratiometric signal. Row 3 has these y-axis ranges. Row 4 has a y-axis range from -1.5 to $+1.5$ mV/ms for the *dotted curve*, and from -1.5 to $+1.5\%$/ms for the *solid curve*. (**b**) The V_e (*dotted*), optical V_m (*solid*), and their first time derivatives at two laser spots that exhibit complex morphology. Time segment is different from that in (**a**). The y-axis ranges are same as in rows 3 and 4 of (**a**). (From Himel and Knisley, Physiological Measurement 28, 707–719, 2007, figure 3, with permission from IOP Publishing Limited.)

were consistent with a single local maximum or minimum, although morphologies of the deflections varied. A small fraction of recordings had more complex morphologies and exhibited two distinct local maxima of optical dV_m/dt or local minima of dV_e/dt.

The magnitudes of OETD during fibrillation were typically less than a few milliseconds for the deflections in which the magnitudes of the slopes exceeded 75% of the largest slopes

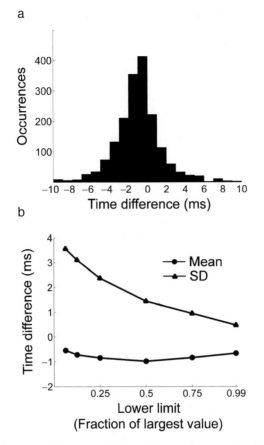

Figure 15: Optoelectric time differences (time of maximum optical dV_m/dt minus time of minimum dV_e/dt at each spot) during ventricular fibrillation. (a) Histogram of optoelectric time differences from all spots in a single heart. Minima of dV_e/dt and maxima of optical dV_m/dt having magnitudes that exceeded 0.25 of the greatest magnitude at each spot were included. (b) Dependence of mean and standard deviation of optoelectric time difference on lower limit in three hearts. Lower limit is expressed as fraction of the largest magnitude of dV_e/dt or optical dV_m/dt at each spot. (From Himel and Knisley, Physiological Measurement 28, 707–719, 2007, figure 5, with permission from IOP Publishing Limited.)

at each spot. When the analysis included deflections in which the magnitudes of slopes were smaller, including those as small as 6% of the largest slopes, time differences become increasingly variable. This is seen in the standard deviations shown in Fig. 15. Variability in the measurements is partly accounted for by effects of noise, which was demonstrated with a computer model in which noise was added to simulated derivatives.

In the combined results for fibrillation, the steepest part of the optical deflection is earlier than the steepest part of the electrical deflection by an average of 0.84 ms. This result, taken together with the deeper optical interrogation, indicates most fibrillatory beats have a propagation component oriented toward the surface, producing an earlier optical deflection. Origination of beats below the surface may be expected due to the greater amount of tissue within the ventricular wall.

Conclusion

It is important to recognize that neither of the measurement methods described here interrogates just from a single cell. One can interpret each recording obtained from hearts optically or with an extracellular electrode as a weighted summation of contributions from many cells within an interrogated volume. In hearts, the optically interrogated volume is relatively large (approximate millimeter scale) because significant scatter of light allows some photons that originate from regions surrounding the center of the recording site to get into the light detector. Enhanced volume of interrogation due to scattering is not specific to laser scanner methods. Monte Carlo models also indicate that the interrogated width exceeds the imaged surface area due to scattering when the broad-field illumination and photodiode array-based or camera-based optical mapping methods are used.[37]

Due to optical summation in the heart studies, it would not have been possible to observe shock-induced changes in transmembrane potentials on a cellular size scale. If microscopic membrane polarization does exist in hearts, this might be a mechanism for electric field stimulation. The anomalous activation observed in experiments might be produced by microscopic membrane polarizations. From a theoretical perspective, small structures including capillaries, connective tissues, and individual cells or cell bundles, are capable of producing membrane polarization by the local redistribution of current.

The conclusion that the interrogated volume for the optical method extends deeper than that for the electrical methods opens possibilities for more detailed study of surface and subsurface activation in the heart. These two mapping methods used together provide limited information on three-dimensional distributions of activation near the surface.

Future research may achieve subcellular optical mapping in hearts. Multiphoton excitation, which is capable of microscopic resolution, has been used to excite transmembrane potential dependent fluorescence in hearts.[38,39] This suggests possibilities to examine subcellular membrane polarizations during shocks. Also optical measurements with cellular resolution in hearts may enable a more complete understanding of the activations during arrhythmias.

References

1. Knisley SB, Neuman MR. Simultaneous electrical and optical mapping in rabbit hearts. *Ann Biomed Eng* 2003;31:32–41
2. Blech IA. Properties of materials. In: Christiansen D, ed. *Electronics Engineers' Handbook*, 4th edn. New York: McGraw-Hill; 1997:9.4
3. Liau J, Dumas J, Janks D, Roth BJ, Knisley SB. Cardiac optical mapping under a translucent stimulation electrode. *Ann Biomed Eng* 2004;32:1202–1210

4. Das DP, Webster JG. Defibrillation recovery curves for different electrode materials. *IEEE Trans Biomed Eng* 1980;27:230–233

5. Liau J, Knisley SB. Microprocessor-controlled laser scanner system for multiwavelength cardiac optical mapping. *IEEE Comput Cardiol* 2002;29:549–552

6. Himel IV HD, Knisley SB. Comparison of optical and electrical mapping of fibrillation. *Physiol Meas* 2007;28:707–719

7. Knisley SB. Evidence for roles of the activating function in electric stimulation. *IEEE Trans Biomed Eng* 2000;47:1114–1119

8. Geddes LA, Baker LE, Moore AG. Optimum electrolytic chloriding of silver electrodes. *Med Biol Eng* 1969;7:49–56

9. Kotz JC, Paul Treichel J. *Chemistry and Chemical Reactivity*, 4th ed. Fort Worth: Saunders College Publishing; 1999

10. Baynham TC, Knisley SB. Development of a current sensing electrode to determine current distribution in cardiac tissue. *Ann Biomed Eng* 1996;24:S60 (abstract)

11. Knisley SB, Johnson PL. Evaluating current distribution of the surface of a stimulation electrode. *Proceedings of the 18th Annual International Conference IEEE, Engineering in Medicine and Biology Society* (CD ROM); 1996:18

12. Knisley SB, Baynham TC. Line stimulation parallel to myofibers enhances regional uniformity of transmembrane voltage changes in rabbit hearts. *Circ Res* 1997;81:229–241

13. Himel IV HD, Knisley SB. Imaging of cardiac movement using ratiometric and nonratiometric optical mapping: effects of ischemia and 2, 3-butanedione monoxime. *IEEE Trans Med Imaging* 2006;25:122–127

14. Kong W, Walcott GP, Smith WM, Johnson PL, Knisley SB. Emission ratiometry for simultaneous calcium and action potential measurements with coloaded dyes in rabbit hearts: reduction of motion and drift. *J Cardiovasc Electrophysiol* 2003;14:76–82

15. Knisley SB, Trayanova N, Aguel F. Roles of electric field and fiber structure in cardiac electric stimulation. *Biophys J* 1999;77:1404–1417

16. Weidmann S. Electrical constants of trabecular muscle from mammalian heart. *J Physiol* 1970;210:1041–1054

17. Hodgkin AL, Rushton WAH. The electrical constants of a crustacean nerve fibre. *Proc Roy Soc Lond B* 1946;133:444–479

18. Lepeschkin E, Jones JL, Rush S, Jones RE. Local potential gradients as a unifying measure for thresholds of stimulation, standstill, tachyarrhythmia and fibrillation appearing after strong capacitor discharges. *Adv Cardiol* 1978;21:268–278

19. Tang ASL, Reiser SL, Wolf PD, Daubert JP, Ideker RE. Gradient shock fields from intracardiac catheter and cutaneous patch. *Circulation* 1988;78:II-45

20. Rattay F. Analysis of models for extracellular fiber stimulation. *IEEE Trans Biomed Eng* 1989;36:676–682

21. Sobie EA, Susil RC, Tung L. A generalized activating function for predicting virtual electrodes in cardiac tissue. *Biophys J* 1997;73:1410–1423

22. Fishler MG, Vepa K. Spatiotemporal effects of syncytial heterogeneities on cardiac far-field excitations during monophasic and biphasic shocks. *J Cardiovasc Electrophysiol* 1998;9:1310–1324

23. Entcheva E, Eason J, Efimov IR, Cheng Y, Malkin R, Claydon F. Virtual electrode effects in transvenous defibrillation-modulation by structure and interface: evidence from bidomain simulations and optical mapping. *J Cardiovasc Electrophysiol* 1998;9:949–961

24. Neunlist M, Tung L. Optical recordings of ventricular excitability of frog heart by an extracellular stimulating point electrode. *PACE* 1994;17:1641–1654

25. Neunlist M, Tung L. Spatial distribution of cardiac transmembrane potentials around an extracellular electrode: dependence on fiber orientation. *Biophys J* 1995;68:2310–2322

26. Wikswo JP Jr, Lin SF, Abbas RA. Virtual electrodes in cardiac tissue: a common mechanism for anodal and cathodal stimulation. *Biophys J* 1995;69:2195–2210

27. Knisley SB, Hill BC, Ideker RE. Virtual electrode effects in myocardial fibers. *Biophys J* 1994;66:719–728

28. Knisley SB. Transmembrane voltage changes during unipolar stimulation of rabbit ventricle. *Circ Res* 1995;77:1229–1239

29. Knisley SB. Left ventricular transmembrane voltage changes produced by suprapericardial point and line stimulation. *Circulation* 2001;104:II-772 (abstract)

30. Lin S-F, Roth BJ, Wikswo JP. Quatrefoil reentry in myocardium: an optical imaging study of the induction mechanism. *J Cardiovasc Electrophysiol* 1999;10:574–586

31. Baynham TC, Knisley SB. Roles of line stimulation-induced virtual electrodes and action potential prolongation in arrhythmic propagation. *J Cardiovasc Electrophysiol* 2001;12:256–263

32. Knisley SB, Pollard AE, Ideker RE. Changing shock polarity causes a "no-switch" region where transmembrane voltage hyperpolarizes with either polarity. *PACE* 1998;21:847 (abstract)

33. Neunlist M, Zou S-Z, Tung L. Design and use of an "optrode" for optical recordings of cardiac action potentials. *Pflugers Arch* 1992;420:611–617

34. Lewis ST. *The Mechanism and Graphic Registration of the Heart Beat.* London: Shaw and Sons; 1925

35. Spach MS, Kootsey JM. Relating the sodium current and conductance to the shape of transmembrane and extracellular potentials by simulation: effects of propagation boundaries. *IEEE Trans Biomed Eng* 1985;32:743–755

36. Spach MS, Miller WT III, Miller-Jones E, Warren RB, Barr RC. Extracellular potentials related to intracellular action potentials during impulse conduction in anisotropic canine cardiac muscle. *Circ Res* 1979;45:188–204

37. Ding L, Splinter R, Knisley SB. Quantifying spatial localization of optical mapping using Monte Carlo simulations. *IEEE Trans Biomed Eng* 2001;48:1098–1107

38. Krishnan RV, Knisley SB. Spatial localization of cardiac optical mapping with multiphoton excitation. *J Biomed Opt* 2003;8:253–263

39. Dumas III JH, Knisley SB. Two-photon excitation of di-4-ANEPPS for optical recording of action potentials in rabbit heart. *Ann Biomed Eng* 2005;33:1802–1807

Chapter 4.6

Optical Mapping of Multisite Ventricular Fibrillation Synchronization

Liang Tang and Shien-Fong Lin

Defibrillation with strong shocks of several hundred volts is still the most effective way to terminate life-threatening cardiac rhythm abnormalities such as ventricular fibrillation (VF). The standing puzzle that has lasted for several decades is why defibrillate with such a high voltage when the activation threshold of cardiac myocytes is much less than $100\,\mathrm{mV}$. Such a conceptual conflict has prompted many theoretical and experimental studies to understand the action of strong shocks.[1–7]

An important goal in defibrillation study is to reduce the shock energy requirement. Because the quality of life in patients carrying implantable cardioverter-defibrillators (ICDs) is significantly affected by the occurrence of shocks, efforts have been made to decrease the shock energy for less pain and battery drain.[8–10] Major progress came in the 1980s when it was realized that biphasic shocks were far superior to monophasic shocks for defibrillation.[11,12] Since then, empirical studies of defibrillation waveforms have identified only marginal improvements, suggesting that empirical variation of defibrillation waveform is unlikely to result in conceptual breakthroughs or significant improvements in defibrillation efficacy.

Alternatively, defibrillation theories may be used to guide the defibrillation optimization efforts. Although no comprehensive theory of defibrillation presently relates mechanisms, shock timing, and waveform optimization, recent advances in the understanding of electrical stimulation and the initiation and maintenance of VF may serve as a signpost. The bidomain model[13–16] of both intra- and extracellular spaces has provided insights into the mechanism of tissue activation with direct implication for the defibrillation mechanism. Cardiac conduction and activation have been modeled mathematically using complex representations of cardiac cells with detailed ionic currents connected in networks. Predictions of these

Shien-Fong Lin

Krannert Institute of Cardiology, Indiana University School of Medicine, Indianapolis, IN 46202, USA, linsf@iupui.edu

I. R. Efimov et al. (eds.), *Cardiac Bioelectric Therapy: Mechanisms and Practical Implications.*
© Springer Science+Business Media, LLC 2009

models have been bootstrapped with experimental results based on computerized high-resolution multielectrode[17,18] and optical mapping[19] studies to develop testable hypotheses, such as "chaos control,"[20] "electrical restitution,"[21] and "mother rotor."[22] It is expected that research methods based on information regarding the mechanistic action of electrical pulses on cardiac tissue may be more likely to provide a "silver bullet" for arrhythmia treatment than empirical methods.

Pacing to Terminate Ventricular Fibrillation

During VF, as fibrillatory wavefronts propagate across the surface of a tissue, there are regions of tissue that can still be excited by external stimulation; these regions are known as excitable gaps.[23,24] The concept of pacing during VF is premised on the use of low-energy pulses to capture the fibrillatory tissue, preferably during the excitable gaps,[24–26] and enlargement of the captured region may eventually lead to VF termination. Defibrillation studies have led to many attempts to design low-energy defibrillation or pacing strategies.[23,27–29] These strategies may be categorized as either passive or interactive. The passive paradigm, such as overdrive pacing and antitachycardia pacing, delivers a constant frequency pulse train seeking to capture the rhythm and gain control. Overdrive pacing has been shown to be effective in capturing a small region of the heart;[23,28] however, the limited success of this approach to VF termination may be attributable to the instability of VF frequency. Antitachycardia pacing is effective in terminating slow ventricular tachycardia (VT), but it is not effective in terminating faster VT or VF. On the other hand, the interactive paradigm, such as chaos control,[20,30,31] seeks to deliver energy based on real-time feedback control. The stimuli are delivered irregularly based on the nonlinear dynamics of the heart. Application of nonlinear control has allowed termination of pacing-induced alternans[32] and conversion of VF to a different "state" of arrhythmia,[20] but spontaneous termination of VF has not been demonstrated.

New Opportunities in Improving Ventricular Defibrillation

A new opportunity exists in taking advantage of the VF organization concept to reduce defibrillation requirements. Technical breakthroughs and high-resolution mapping studies of VF over the past few years have opened up new prospects of improving ventricular defibrillation. These breakthroughs include the development of high-resolution optical mapping techniques to study membrane responses to defibrillation without prolonged saturation of amplifiers. Advanced analytical tools have been developed to study the organization and progression of VF. High-resolution mapping studies have identified spatiotemporal organization in VF of functional or structural origins.[33–36] Such an organization was suggested to correlate with defibrillation energy requirement.[37,38] Tools have been designed to analyze the complexity and organization of VF especially from high-resolution electrical and optical mapping data.

A second new opportunity comes from the feasibility of using multiple electrical leads for defibrillation. Parallel to the improvements in defibrillation study in the animal laboratory, clinical studies have recently entered a new era by the development of biventricular pacing and defibrillation. Previous efforts in defibrillation study focused on shock-timing control or waveform optimization to reduce the energy requirement based on the assumption that the energy is delivered between two electrodes at fixed locations. On the other hand, biventricular defibrillation is accomplished by placing an additional defibrillation electrode through the coronary sinus in the cardiac veins in the left ventricle. With biventricular pacing gaining acceptance and biventricular defibrillation resulting in improved defibrillation efficacy,[39,40] the idea of extra leads in the left ventricle may soon be adopted for general clinical application. While biventricular defibrillation is possible, it carries a risk of venous rupture or vascular damage if too much current is given to a small cardiac vein in the left ventricle. The study by Butter et al.[39] limited the shock strength to 10 J to avoid complications. Consequently, although biventricular defibrillation offers new opportunities in defibrillation, it also carries a higher risk and has presented a new challenge to both clinicians and investigators. It is therefore even more important to develop novel approaches to deliver the defibrillation shocks that maximize benefits and minimize risk.

Optical Mapping of Multisite Synchronization of Ventricular Fibrillation

The high-resolution optical mapping technique has led to the development of an optical recording guided real-time feedback system. Pacing with feedback control attempts to deal with the variability of VF frequencies and has shown more promise in tissue capture.[41–43] During feedback pacing, tissue polarization is continuously monitored in real time, thus allowing pacing pulses to be delivered in the excitable gaps. More important, the pacing current is only delivered upon activation of a "reference site," which provides a timing reference for wavefront synchronization.

The core technology of this project is a real-time imaging and control system that is capable of measuring action potential characteristics and controlling the delivery of pacing/defibrillation pulses. The software was designed using a LabVIEW platform (National Instruments, Austin, TX). Currently, the acquisition program allows real-time monitoring and threshold detection of optical potentials of up to five pixels. Within the same program, the delivery of electrical stimuli is controlled based on real-time measurement of these action potential signals. Different modes of electrical stimulation have been tested using this software. The stimulation protocols that we have used include (1) excitable gap pacing, (2) protective zone pacing, (3) synchronization of activation, (4) subthreshold pulse train, and (5) overdrive pacing. Due to the flexibility of the software, new pacing protocols are constantly added to this program.

To allow fast visualization of experimental results, a data viewer has been designed to accompany the acquisition program. The interactive front-panel control of the viewer is shown in Fig. 1. Main areas on the front panel include (1) a movie player to dynamically play

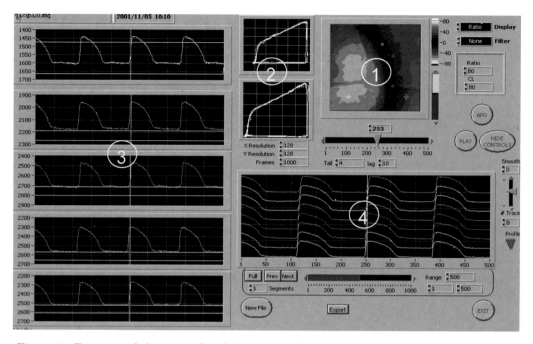

Figure 1: Front-panel diagram of real-time optical imaging acquisition/analysis program

back large sequences of data, so the user can select the display mode from raw data, optical potential, wavefront, isochrones, phase, and phase singularities; (2) two animated trajectory plots of $V(t)$ versus $V(t - \tau)$ from selected pixels in the image; (3) transmembrane potential displays of five control pixels (one reference site and four pacing site), where timing of pacing pulses is superimposed under these traces to validate detection of threshold crossing; and (4) a spatial profile of optical potential along a user-selected straight line on the image.

Pak et al.[41] evaluated the defibrillation efficacy of the novel multisite pacing algorithm using the optical recording guided, synchronized pacing (SyncP) in excitable gaps. The effects of feedback pacing (FBP, $n = 106$, n is the number of episodes), overdrive pacing (ODP, $n = 48$, 90% VF cycle length [VFCL]), and high-frequency pacing (HFP, $n = 129$, 43–215 Hz) on isolated rabbit hearts in VF were compared. Four pacing electrodes (denoted with "e" in Fig. 2a) were placed on the optical mapping field of the left ventricular anterior wall. The electrodes were made with Teflon-coated stainless steel, and the interelectrode spacing was about 10 mm.

For FBP, the optical action potentials were monitored from four different pacing electrode sites and one reference site in real time (430 frames per second; Fig. 2a). The reference site was selected arbitrarily after observing the common direction of VF wave propagation along the fiber orientation. Figure 2b shows the algorithm of FBP. When (1) the reference mapping site was depolarized during VF to above 40% of optical action potential amplitude and (2) the optical action potential of a pacing site was below threshold, electrical current was delivered at electrode sites and one reference site in real time (430 frames per second;

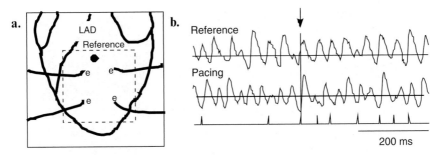

Figure 2: (a) Configuration of pacing electrodes and reference site for synchronized feedback pacing. (b) Illustration of the algorithm for feedback pacing

Fig. 2a). Each electrode was independently controlled following the same algorithm. An important feature of SyncP was the use of depolarization of a local reference site to guide the pacing pulse delivery. Pacing current was delivered only when the reference site was depolarized. This reference site served as an endogenous timing reference whose frequency varied with the overall progression of VF but could be distinctive from neighboring sites. The experimental results support the concept that adaptive pacing is superior to the fixed frequency pacing in synchronizing and terminating irregular wavefronts.

The results (Fig. 3) show that (1) the defibrillation efficacy of independent FBP was 14.8%, and those of ODP and HFP were 2.1% ($p < .01$) and 1.6% ($p < .0001$), respectively. Energy consumption for FBP (4 mJ) was significantly lower than that of ODP ($p < .0001$). (2) FBP, but not ODP or HFP, decreased spatial dispersion of fibrillation cycle length during pacing ($p < .01$) and postpacing ($p < .05$) periods compared to the prepacing period in paced area. (3) FBP with 2 or 5 mA current was more effective in decreasing SDCL than FBP with 10 mA ($p < .001$).

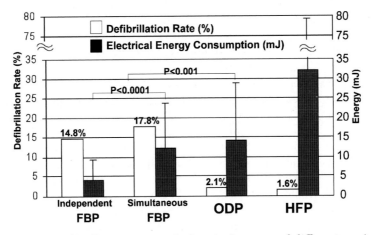

Figure 3: Defibrillation rate and electrical energy of different pacing

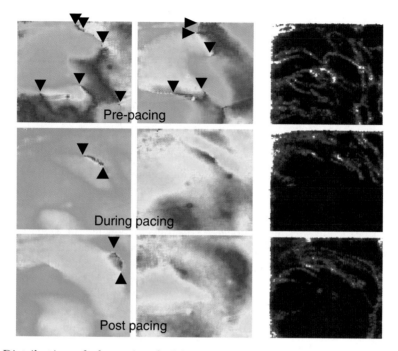

Figure 4: Distribution of phase singularities in prepacing, during pacing, and postpacing periods. Propagation in the controlled area is synchronized during pacing, as no phase singularities exit in this area. The wave synchronization persists even after pacing

The synchronized FBP algorithm was intended to synchronize depolarization of tissue under the pacing electrode with that of the reference site. The degree of wave synchronization was determined using phase maps and the distribution of phase singularities. As shown in Fig. 4, the phase singularities in the phase maps are indicated with arrows. During the prepacing period, various phases coexisted, and three to six phase singularity points were always present. During the pacing period, however, color phase maps became homogeneous, and the number of phase singularities decreased. This kind of synchronization sustained for a while in the postpacing period. One hundred–frame (230 ms) cumulative phase singularity point maps, the right-most column of Fig. 4, with light color representing more phase singularities, also showed a decrease in phase singularities during pacing and immediate postpacing periods in the area surrounded by the pacing electrodes.

One possible explanation of the defibrillation mechanism of SyncP is the electrical reduction of available tissue mass to sustain VF. Kim et al.[17] demonstrated that as tissue mass was decreased, the number of wavefronts decreased, and the life span of reentrant wavefronts increased, resulting in a parallel decrease of the dynamic complexity of VF. Although SyncP did not mechanically reduce tissue mass, pacing could have induced a "virtual reduction" of tissue mass that enlarged the synchronized area and decreased the dynamic complexity of VF, leading to the termination of fibrillation. It was estimated that the approximate tissue mass surrounded by the pacing electrodes was 9–11% of ventricular mass. A second possible mechanism is that SyncP eliminated the excitable gap in a small heart and led to conduction block, halting the reentrant circuit. This is likely the case when pacing in the excitable gaps without a reference site. Another potential mechanism is that the pacing was performed in a dominant domain where it halted the mother rotor.[36]

Optical Recording-Guided Pacing to Create Functional Block during VF

VF propagation can be effectively blocked by creating tissue damage through ablation procedures.[44,45] These procedures create irreversible tissue damage with unknown long-term consequences. However, functional blocks created without permanently damaging the tissue are more desirable. Recently, Ravi et al.[64] tested the idea of creating a functional block in the ventricle during VF via multiple-electrode configurations. In other words, the study was to apply a SyncP protocol[41,46] along a linearly distributed array of electrodes to create a linear functional block. If the defibrillation mechanism of SyncP for the electrical reduction of available tissue mass to sustain VF is correct, a significant functional block for VF is an important factor to improve multisite pacing efficacy to terminate VF.

SyncP was performed in isolated rabbit hearts during VF using optical recording to control the delivery of pacing pulses in real time. The electrodes were arranged in a line configuration in along-fiber and cross-fiber directions (Fig. 5). SyncP caused synchronized activation along the line of pacing electrodes. Figure 6 shows examples of independent and simultaneous SyncP in the fiber direction (Fig. 6a, b) and cross-fiber direction (Fig. 6c, d). In Fig. 6a, when the reference site was activated (frame 581), sites e3 and e4 were in the excitable gap. Therefore, stimulation current was delivered to e3 and e4, but not to e1 or e2. The stimulation resulted in synchronized activation (frame 587) and repolarization (frame 599). In Fig. 6b, when the reference site was activated, all electrodes fired at the same

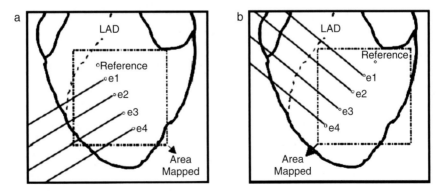

Figure 5: Orientation of multisite pacing along or cross-fiber direction

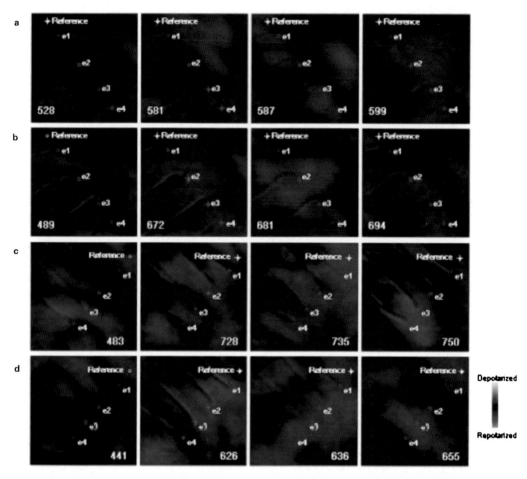

Figure 6: Voltage maps indicating linear functional block created by synchronized pacing (SyncP). The *red* represents depolarization, and *blue* represents repolarization. *Small circles* in the maps show locations of the pacing electrodes (e1–e4). A *plus sign* in the *circle* represents the delivery of pacing current. The *frame numbers* are indicated in the corners of each map. (**a**) Independent SyncP, fiber direction; (**b**) Simultaneous SyncP, fiber direction; (**c**) Independent SyncP, cross-fiber direction; (**d**) Simultaneous SyncP, cross-fiber direction

time, causing synchronized activation (frame 681) and repolarization (frame 694). The same electrode firing protocols were used in the cross-fiber configuration as shown in Fig. 6c, d.

The increased synchronicity was not restricted solely to the pacing sites, but also occurred along the line connecting the electrodes. The effect of wavefront synchronization by multisite pacing may decrease at the myocardium away from the pacing electrodes. Ravi et al.[64] quantified the variable degree of synchronization (the effect of pacing) away from the electrode line. The drop in variance between prepacing and pacing periods was calculated along lines parallel to, but shifted outward from, the original electrode line. Values were normalized by dividing variance drops at increasing distances from the electrode line by the variance change (between prepacing and pacing) at the electrode line. In the independent SyncP mode, pacing was 70% as effective at 1.2 mm and 50% as effective at 2.2 mm. In the simultaneous SyncP mode, the amount of synchronization dropped to 70% at 1.5 mm and to 50% at 2.4 mm.

The configuration of a linear electrode array is preferable in clinical situations because it can be placed on a catheter. The recent advancement of catheter design and pacing technology has allowed pacing with multiple, spatially distributed electrodes. Byrd et al.[47] showed that biventricular antitachycardia pacing is superior to conventional antitachycardia pacing in situations where the additional ventricular lead advanced the orthodromic wavefront. This advancement may increase the likelihood of orthodromic termination on refractory tissue and termination of reentry. Since many ICDs have an additional lead available for pacing, this concept of biventricular pacing might also prove beneficial to VF termination via increased capture area and increased conduction blocks.

It should be noted that only one line of functional block has been tested. It is feasible to create multiple lines of functional block with this approach. Note that the successful defibrillation rate with synchronized multipacing was only 16%.[41] This rate may be significantly increased through a combination of area and linear synchronized pacing methods.

Improvement of Defibrillation Efficacy with Synchronized Multisite Pacing

According to the upper limit of vulnerability (ULV) hypothesis,[48–50] the timing of electrical shocks in the low-voltage gradient area[51,52] is an important determinant of the defibrillation outcome. If the shock is delivered on the effectively refractory myocardium, the same shock cannot reinitiate VF in the low-voltage gradient area and results in successful defibrillation.[53] This concept might be supported by observations of the protective zone.[54–56] Protective zone is defined as a period of time during which a critically timed second stimulus (S_3) can terminate local reentry induced by an earlier stimulus (S_2), and thereby prevent VF.[57] However, the concept of the protective zone has been limited to the temporal dimension and newly initiated Wiggers's stage I VF or VF with only a limited number of reentrant wavefronts.[57–59] The spatiotemporal protective zone or VF termination by timed stimulation in persistent disorganized VF has not been explored. This is because when the wavefront in the low-voltage gradient area is not completely synchronized, shock could be delivered to refractoriness in only part of the low-voltage gradient area. This leads to heterogeneous repolarization and local-reentry–induced defibrillation failure. To overcome these limitations of classical temporal protective zone, Pak et al.[41] tried defibrillation shock at the spatiotemporal protective zone, which was implemented by two strategies and demonstrated better defibrillation efficacy: (1) multisite SyncP for wavefront synchronization and

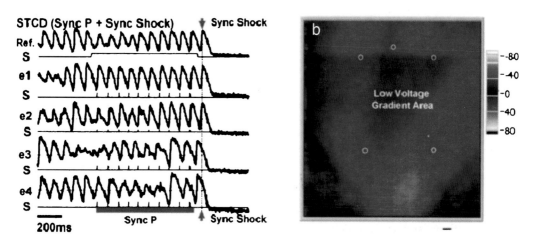

Figure 7: Low-voltage gradient area in isolated rabbit heart. Four unipolar electrodes and a reference point were positioned around the area. (b) Preshock synchronized pacing (SyncP) protocol. *Thick red horizontal bar* represents the SyncP period, and *vertical dotted line* represents the timing of the shock

(2) Sync shock (timed shock) to induce a higher proportion of unexcitable shock in the low-voltage gradient area under the synchronized state.

Wavefront synchronization and synchronization of repolarization are known to be important for VF termination.[60,61] Optical recording guided real-time detection and stimulation of spatiotemporal excitable gaps – SyncP – via multisite pacing was demonstrated to cause pace termination of VF with millijoule energy.[41] Therefore, wavefront synchronization and a subsequent timed shock on the unexcitable low-voltage gradient area may improve defibrillation efficacy. In the study by Pak et al.,[41] spatiotemporally controlled defibrillation (STCD), which is composed of SyncP and following Sync shock, was explored (Fig. 7a).

In order to measure the low-voltage gradient area in isolated rabbit heart, a diastolic shock (100 V) was delivered during optical recording. The area not directly depolarized by the shock (Fig. 7b) was defined as the low-voltage gradient area,[4] which was usually located on the left ventricular anterior wall. The methods of multisite Sync pacing have been reported previously.[10] To perform STCD, left ventricular anterior wall is paced with SyncP protocol for 0.92 s and followed by timed Sync defibrillating shock [STCD=SyncP (0.92 s)+Sync shock]. The optical mapping data of STCD consisted of 0.46 s of prepacing VF, 0.92 s of SyncP, and then Sync shock, followed by 0.46 s of postpacing period.

Preshock SyncP was shown to reduce the reinitiation of VF wavefronts in the low-voltage gradient area. As a result, the DFT_{50} (defibrillation threshold) of the timed shock with pre-multisite pacing method was decreased as compared to control random shocks in the rabbit model. Table 1 shows that the DFT_{50} of the STCD (154.0 ± 61.4 V) was 10.3% lower than that of the random shocks (174.3 ± 75.7 V, $p < .05$, $Z = -2.3664$). The STCD effects were more prominent when prepacing VF was disorganized and had a short VFCL. When tissues with a greater than 10% reduction of DFT_{50} by STCD (Table 1, tissues 1, 3,

Table 1: STCD decreases DFT_{50} compared to random shock

$DFT_{50}(V)$

Tissue	Random shock	STCD	% Decrease
1 $(n = 5)$	274.0 ± 32.1	240.0 ± 21.2	12.41
2 $(n = 5)$	86.6 ± 15.1	82.4 ± 14.0	5.07
3 $(n = 5)$	118.0 ± 11.2	97.6 ± 5.4	17.29
4 $(n = 5)$	128.8 ± 11.5	127.0 ± 6.0	1.40
5 $(n = 5)$	146.4 ± 10.9	142.4 ± 12.0	2.73
6 $(n = 5)$	189.0 ± 11.5	157.2 ± 16.1	16.83
7 $(n = 5)$	277.2 ± 29.5	231.6 ± 38.6	16.45
Total $(n = 35)$	174.3 ± 75.7	$154.0 \pm 61.4^*$	10.31

$^*p < .018, Z = -2.3664$. STCD, spatiotemporally controlled defibrillation; DFT, defibrillation threshold

6, and 7) were compared to those with a less than 10% decrease (Table 1, tissues 2, 5, and 6), the former had a significantly shorter VFCL (83.0 ± 9.6 ms vs. 111.3 ± 28.3 ms, $p < .001$) and higher spatial dispersion of VFCL (9.5 ± 5.0 ms vs. 5.0 ± 2.6 ms, $p < .01$), suggesting more disorganized preshock VF than the latter. This is also indirect evidence showing the importance of VF synchronization in lowering defibrillation energy requirement.

More recently, Tang et al.[62] explored a timely synchronized pacing to terminate VF following failed defibrillating shock (postshock SyncP) to improve defibrillation efficacy. Instead of randomly continuous triggering of pacing after shock, an optical recording guided real-time detection feedback mechanism was used to apply synchronized (i.e., properly timed) pacing (i.e., electrical stimulus) to cardiac tissues to intervene the postshock organized activation. Figure 8 shows a series of optical frames in a successful VF termination episode by the postshock SyncP strategy. The heart tissue was completely depolarized by a defibrillating shock at 200 V (frame 496), followed by a quiescent period of 76 ms (frame 526), during which no electrical activity was observed. The shock was not successful, and there were four repetitive responses after the defibrillating shock, as shown in the optical signal. Panels 1–4 show the propagation of the four beats and the corresponding stimulation of the postshock pacing electrode, respectively. The first activation started from the upper right corner of the mapped region (frame 534). When the tissue around the reference site was depolarized by the early activation, the pacing electrode was activated to deliver a 5-mA electric stimulus to the myocardium around the pacing sites (frame 538). The interaction between the stimulus-initiated wavefronts and the reinitiated VF fronts resulted in wavefront synchronization (frame 548). The following three beats showed the similar interaction between reinitiated VF wavefronts and stimulus-induced fronts (panels 2–4). As shown in the optical recording data, sinus rhythm resumed after four repetitive responses with postshock pacing stimuli. This result showed that the novel strategy can improve the current defibrillation efficacy by converting unsuccessful shocks to successful ones without additional shock delivery.

It was demonstrated that maximizing the extent of myocardium captured by electrical-induced stimulation was important for successful VF defibrillation. Nanthakumar et al.[63]

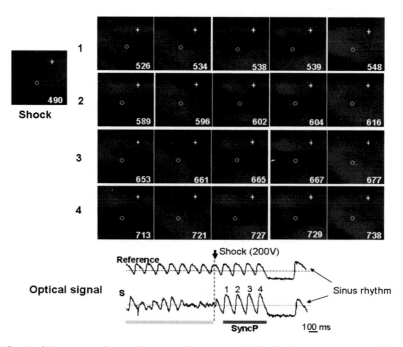

Figure 8: Optical imaging data showing the novel defibrillation strategy with postshock synchronized pacing (SyncP). *Asterisk* designates the reference site, and the *circle* shows the postshock pacing site. *Numbers* indicate the frame numbers

reported that pacing in the posterior swine left ventricle resulted in a greater incidence and extent of myocardial capture than in the anterior left ventricle. In isolated rabbit hearts, with the same shock strength, successful and failed defibrillation episodes were associated with 50 and 15% of the myocardium, respectively, captured by the SyncP $(p < .001)$. To maximize the myocardial capture by optimizing the SyncP site, we compared the postshock SyncP in both anterior and posterior left ventricle. The isoelectric window (IEW) duration was found to be similar for both cases, which was approximately 60–65 ms $(n = 0.05;$ Fig. 9). However, the myocardium capture rate and the defibrillation rate were significantly different. The pacing in the anterior and posterior left ventricle resulted in approximately 55 and 75% myocardium capture, respectively $(p < .01)$. Correspondingly, the defibrillation rate for anterior pacing (14%) was more than four times higher than posterior pacing (3.7%).

In the postshock SyncP strategy, only one pacing site was explored, and the misplaced pacing electrode in myocardium accounted for approximately 20% of failed pace termination of VF after failed shock. A combination of multipacing strategy and global reference site is expected to provide insights into further improvements of the efficacy of this novel defibrillation strategy.

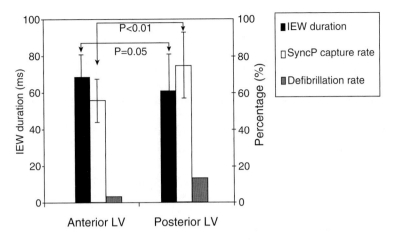

Figure 9: Comparison of postshock synchronized pacing (SyncP) in anterior and posterior left ventricle

Conclusion

Spatiotemporal organization of VF and distributed pacing/defibrillation leads offer unprecedented opportunities to renew our concepts of defibrillation and promote new possibilities in delivering defibrillation energy. Theoretically it is possible to calculate VF organization in real time and shock or pace the tissue when fibrillation is most organized. Results from a pacing study also found that organized VF was easier to capture with pulse train than unorganized VF.[29] However, using previously proposed algorithms to calculate VF organization is still computationally costly and not suitable for real-time control. The synchronized feedback multipacing approach is a means to achieve "enforced" organization that can produce large synchronized areas. Most important, such a pacing method has been demonstrated to result in defibrillation with extremely low energy requirement. The ability to pace directly in the excitable gaps lowers the electrical energy, and a large area of induced synchronized activation might be equivalent to a reduction of critical mass, thus terminating VF. Further development along this line of interactive pacing could bring about new adaptive, antifibrillatory-pacing strategies using millijoule pulses on a cycle-to-cycle basis in a spatially distributed manner.

References

1. Zhou X, Knisley SB, Smith WM, Rollins D, Pollard AE, Ideker RE. Spatial changes in the transmembrane potential during extracellular electric stimulation. *Circ Res* 1998;83(10):1003–1014

2. Sharma V, Tung L. Theoretical and experimental study of sawtooth effect in isolated cardiac cell-pairs. *J Cardiovasc Electrophysiol* 2001;12(10):1164–1173

3. Newton JC, Knisley SB, Zhou X, Pollard AE, Ideker RE. Review of mechanisms by which electrical stimulation alters the transmembrane potential. *J Cardiovasc Electrophysiol* 1999;10(2):234–243

4. Pumir A, Krinsky VI. Two biophysical mechanisms of defibrillation of cardiac tissue. *J Theor Biol* 1997;185(2):189–199

5. Swerdlow CD, Fan W, Brewer JE. Charge-burping theory correctly predicts optimal ratios of phase duration for biphasic defibrillation waveforms. *Circulation* 1996;94(9):2278–2284

6. Fishler MG. Syncytial heterogeneity as a mechanism underlying cardiac far-field stimulation during defibrillation-level shocks. *J Cardiovasc Electrophysiol* 1998;9(4): 384–394

7. Anderson C, Trayanova NA. Success and failure of biphasic shocks: results of bidomain simulations. *Math Biosci* 2001;174(2):91–109

8. Wathen MS, Sweeney MO, DeGroot PJ, Stark AJ, Koehler JL, Chisner MB, Machado C, Adkisson WO. Shock reduction using antitachycardia pacing for spontaneous rapid ventricular tachycardia in patients with coronary artery disease. *Circulation* 2001;104(7):796–801

9. Israel CW, Hugl B, Unterberg C, Lawo T, Kennis I, Hettrick D, Hohnloser SH. Pace-termination and pacing for prevention of atrial tachyarrhythmias: results from a multi-center study with an implantable device for atrial therapy. *J Cardiovasc Electrophysiol* 2001;12(10):1121–1128

10. Huang J, Rogers JM, Killingsworth CR, Walcott GP, KenKnight BH, Smith WM, Ideker RE. Improvement of defibrillation efficacy and quantification of activation patterns during ventricular fibrillation in a canine heart failure model. *Circulation* 2001;103(10):1473–1478

11. Jones JL, Jones RE. Improved defibrillator waveform safety factor with biphasic waveforms. *Am J Physiol* 1983;245(1):H60–H65

12. Dixon EG, Tang AS, Wolf PD, Meador JT, Fine MJ, Calfee RV, Ideker RE. Improved defibrillation thresholds with large contoured epicardial electrodes and biphasic waveforms. *Circulation* 1987;76(5):1176–1184

13. Knisley SB. Transmembrane voltage changes during unipolar stimulation of rabbit ventricle. *Circ Res* 1995;77:1229–1239

14. Roth BJ. A mathematical model of make and break electrical stimulation of cardiac tissue by a unipolar anode or cathode. *IEEE Trans Biomed Eng* 1995;42(12):1174–1184

15. Wikswo JP Jr, Lin S-F, Abbas RA. Virtual electrodes in cardiac tissue: a common mechanism for anodal and cathodal stimulation. *Biophys J* 1995;69:2195–2210

16. Efimov IR, Cheng YN, Biermann M, Van Wagoner D, Mazgalev TN, Tchou PJ. Transmembrane voltage changes produced by real and virtual electrodes during monophasic defibrillation shock delivered by an implantable electrode. *J Cardiovasc Electrophysiol* 1997;8:1031–1045

17. Kim YH, Garfinkel A, Ikeda T, Wu TJ, Athill CA, Weiss JN, Karagueuzian HS, Chen PS. Spatiotemporal complexity of ventricular fibrillation revealed by tissue mass

reduction in isolated swine right ventricle. Further evidence for the quasiperiodic route to chaos hypothesis. *J Clin Invest* 1997;100(10):2486–2500

18. Walcott GP, Knisley SB, Zhou X, Newton JC, Ideker RE. On the mechanism of ventricular defibrillation. *Pacing Clin Electrophysiol* 1997;20(2 Pt 2):422–431

19. Efimov IR, Cheng Y, Van Wagoner DR, Mazgalev T, Tchou PJ. Virtual electrode-induced phase singularity: a basic mechanism of defibrillation failure. *Circ Res* 1998;82(8):918–925

20. Garfinkel A, Spano ML, Ditto WL, Weiss JN. Controlling cardiac chaos. *Science* 1992;257(5074):1230–1235

21. Weiss JN, Chen PS, Qu Z, Karagueuzian HS, Garfinkel A. Ventricular fibrillation: how do we stop the waves from breaking? *Circ Res* 2000;87(12):1103–1107

22. Jalife J. Ventricular fibrillation: mechanisms of initiation and maintenance. *Annu Rev Physiol* 2000;62:25–50

23. KenKnight BH, Bayly PV, Gerstle RJ, Rollins DL, Wolf PD, Smith WM, Ideker RE. Regional capture of fibrillating ventricular myocardium: evidence of an excitable gap. *Circ Res* 1995;77:849–855

24. Taneja T, Horvath G, Racker DK, Goldberger J, Kadish A. Excitable gap in canine fibrillating ventricular myocardium: effect of subacute and chronic myocardial infarction. *J Cardiovasc Electrophysiol* 2001;12(6):708–715

25. Kamjoo K, Uchida T, Ikeda T, Fishbein MC, Garfinkel A, Weiss JN, Karagueuzian HS, Chen PS. Importance of location and timing of electrical stimuli in terminating sustained functional reentry in isolated swine ventricular tissues: evidence in support of a small reentrant circuit. *Circulation* 1997;96(6):2048–2060

26. Gu Y, Patwardhan A. Multiple spatially distributed stimulators and timing programs for entrainment of activation during ventricular fibrillation. *Biomed Sci Instrum* 2002;38:295–299

27. Allessie M, Kirchhof C, Scheffer GJ, Chorro F, Brugada J. Regional control of atrial fibrillation by rapid pacing in conscious dogs. *Circulation* 1991;84(4):1689–1697

28. Province R, Qian Y-W, Lin S-F, Sung RJ. Effects of pulse train amplitude and waveform on ability to entrain fibrillating rabbit ventricle with epicardial pacing. *PACE* 1999;22:A66

29. Newton JC, Huang J, Rogers JM, Rollins DL, Walcott GP, Smith WS, Ideker RE. Pacing during ventricular fibrillation: factors influencing the ability to capture. *J Cardiovasc Electrophysiol* 2001;12(1):76–84

30. Watanabe M, Gilmour RF, Jr. Strategy for control of complex low-dimensional dynamics in cardiac tissue. *J Math Biol* 1996;35(1):73–87

31. Christini DJ, Stein KM, Markowitz SM, Mittal S, Slotwiner DJ, Lerman BB. The role of nonlinear dynamics in cardiac arrhythmia control. *Heart Dis* 1999;1(4):190–200

32. Christini DJ, Stein KM, Markowitz SM, Mittal S, Slotwiner DJ, Scheiner MA, Iwai S, Lerman BB. Nonlinear-dynamical arrhythmia control in humans. *Proc Natl Acad Sci USA* 2001;98(10):5827–5832

33. Berenfeld O, Pertsov AM, Jalife J. What is the organization of waves in ventricular fibrillation? *Circ Res* 2001;89(3):E22

34. Walcott GP, Kay GN, Plumb VJ, Smith WM, Rogers JM, Epstein AE, Ideker RE. Endocardial wave front organization during ventricular fibrillation in humans. *J Am Coll Cardiol* 2002;39(1):109–115

35. Damle RS, Kanaan NM, Robinson NS, Ge YZ, Goldberger JJ, Kadish AH. Spatial and temporal linking of epicardial activation directions during ventricular fibrillation in dogs. Evidence for underlying organization. *Circulation* 1992;86(5):1547–1558

36. Zaitsev AV, Berenfeld O, Mironov SF, Jalife J, Pertsov AM. Distribution of excitation frequencies on the epicardial and endocardial surfaces of fibrillating ventricular wall of the sheep heart. *Circ Res* 2000;86(4):408–417

37. Hsia PW, Fendelander L, Harrington G, Damiano RJ. Defibrillation success is associated with myocardial organization. Spatial coherence as a new method of quantifying the electrical organization of the heart. *J Electrocardiol* 1996;29(Suppl):189–197

38. Patwardhan A, Moghe S, Wang K, Wright H, Leonelli F. Correlation between defibrillation shock outcome and coherence in electrocardiograms. *Pacing Clin Electrophysiol* 2001;24(9 Pt 1):1354–1362

39. Butter C, Meisel E, Tebbenjohanns J, Engelmann L, Fleck E, Schubert B, Hahn S, Pfeiffer D. Transvenous biventricular defibrillation halves energy requirements in patients. *Circulation* 2001;104(21):2533–2538

40. Walker RG, Kenknight BH, Ideker RE. Critically timed auxiliary shock to weak field area lowers defibrillation threshold. *J Cardiovasc Electrophysiol* 2001;12(5):556–562

41. Pak HN, Liu YB, Hayashi H, Okuyama Y, Chen PS, Lin SF. Synchronization of ventricular fibrillation with real-time feedback pacing: implication to low-energy defibrillation. *Am J Physiol Heart Circ Physiol* 2003;285(6):H2704–H2711

42. Wu R, Patwardhan A. Restitution of action potential duration during sequential changes in diastolic intervals shows multimodal behavior. *Circ Res* 2004;94(5):634–641

43. Jordan PN, Christini DJ. Adaptive diastolic interval control of cardiac action potential duration alternans. *J Cardiovasc Electrophysiol* 2004;15(10):1177–1185

44. Keane D. New catheter ablation techniques for the treatment of cardiac arrhythmias. *Card Electrophysiol Rev* 2002;6(4):341–348

45. Pak HN, Oh YS, Liu YB, Wu TJ, Karagueuzian HS, Lin SF, Chen PS. Catheter ablation of ventricular fibrillation in rabbit ventricles treated with beta-blockers. *Circulation* 2003;108(25):3149–3156

46. Pak H-N, Okuyama Y, Oh Y-S, Hayashi H, Liu Y-B, Chen P-S, Lin S-F. Improvement of defibrillation efficacy with preshock synchronized pacing. *J Cardiovasc Electrophysiol* 2004;15(5):581–587

47. Byrd IA, Rogers JM, Smith WM, Pollard AE. Comparison of conventional and biventricular antitachycardia pacing in a geometrically realistic model of the rabbit ventricle. *J Cardiovasc Electrophysiol* 2004;15(9):1066–1077

48. Wang NC, Lee MH, Ohara T, Okuyama Y, Fishbein GA, Lin SF, Karagueuzian HS, Chen PS. Optical mapping of ventricular defibrillation in isolated swine right ventricles: demonstration of a postshock isoelectric window after near-threshold defibrillation shocks. *Circulation* 2001;104(2):227–233

49. Chen PS, Shibata N, Dixon EG, Wolf PD, Danieley ND, Sweeney MB, Smith WM, Ideker RE. Activation during ventricular defibrillation in open-chest dogs. Evidence of

complete cessation and regeneration of ventricular fibrillation after unsuccessful shocks. *J Clin Invest* 1986;77(3):810–823

50. Chen P-S, Wolf PD, Ideker RE. Mechanism of cardiac defibrillation: a different point of view. *Circulation* 1991;84:913–919

51. Chen PS, Wolf PD, Claydon FJ, Dixon EG, Vidaillet HJ Jr, Danieley ND, Pilkington TC, Ideker RE. The potential gradient field created by epicardial defibrillation electrodes in dogs. *Circulation* 1986;74(3):626–636

52. Chen PS, Swerdlow CD, Hwang C, Karagueuzian HS. Current concepts of ventricular defibrillation. *J Cardiovasc Electrophysiol* 1998;9(5):553–562

53. Kwaku KF, Dillon SM. Shock-induced depolarization of refractory myocardium prevents wave-front propagation in defibrillation. *Circ Res* 1996;79(5):957–973

54. Tamargo J, Moe B, Moe GK. Interaction of sequential stimuli applied during the relative refractory period in relation to determination of fibrillation threshold in the canine ventricle. *Circ Res* 1975;37(5):534–541

55. Euler DE, Moore EN. Continuous fractionated electrical activity after stimulation of the ventricles during the vulnerable period: evidence for local reentry. *Am J Cardiol* 1980;46(5):783–791

56. Hwang C, Fan W, Chen PS. Recurrent appearance of protective zones after an unsuccessful defibrillation shock. *Am J Physiol* 1996;271(4 Pt 2):H1491–H1497

57. Wiggers CJ. The mechanism and nature of ventricular defibrillation. *Am Heart J* 1940;20:399–412

58. Verrier RL, Brooks WW, Lown B. Protective zone and the determination of vulnerability to ventricular fibrillation. *Am J Physiol* 1978;234:H592–H596

59. Bonometti C, Hwang C, Hough D, Lee JJ, Fishbein MC, Karagueuzian HS, Chen PS. Interaction between strong electrical stimulation and reentrant wavefronts in canine ventricular fibrillation. *Circ Res* 1995;77(2):407–416

60. Kirchhof PF, Larissa Fabritz C, Franz MR. Phase angle convergence of multiple monophasic action potential recordings precedes spontaneous termination of ventricular fibrillation. *Basic Res Cardiol* 1998;93(5):412–421

61. Dillon SM. Synchronized repolarization after defibrillation shocks. a possible component of the defibrillation process demonstrated by optical recordings in rabbit heart. *Circulation* 1992;85(5):1865–1878

62. Tang L, Hwang GS, Song J, Chen PS, Lin SF. Post-shock synchronized pacing in isolated rabbit left ventricle: evaluation of a novel defibrillation strategy. *J Cardiovasc Electrophysiol* 2007;18:740–749

63. Nanthakumar K, Johnson PL, Huang J, Killingsworth CR, Rollins DL, McElderry HT, Smith WM, Ideker RE. Regional variation in capture of fibrillating swine left ventricle during electrical stimulation. *J Cardiovasc Electrophysiol* 2005;16(4):425–432

64. Ravi K, Nihei M, Willmer A, Hayashi H, Lin S-F. Optical recording-guided pacing to create functional line of block during ventricular fibrillation. *J Biomed Opt* 2006;11:021013-1-8 (PMID 16674188)

Part V

Methodology

Chapter 5.1

The Bidomain Model of Cardiac Tissue: From Microscale to Macroscale

Craig S. Henriquez and Wenjun Ying

Introduction

Cardiac tissue can be viewed as connected cells (myocytes), organized and tethered through an extracellular matrix to produce a contraction of the heart that is triggered by a highly coordinated spread of electrical activity. The currents underlying the propagation of impulses from cell to cell flow across the cell membrane and through both the intracellular and extracellular spaces in the heart. Over the past 30 years there has been considerable interest in the structures that couple the intracellular spaces of myocytes to one another and their role in arrhythmia.[1,2] In cardiac tissue, this coupling takes place though the intercalated discs. The *intercalated disc* is an interwoven membrane separating adjacent cells and contains both adherens junctions, which anchor the contractile proteins and maintain mechanical strength during contraction, and gap junctions that permit small molecules and ions to pass freely between the cells.[3] A gap junction is composed of two hemichannels (connexons), one in each cell, that come together and form a pore, which essentially establishes electrical connectivity.[4,5] Under normal conditions, the propagation of action potentials involves both the flux of ions across voltage and ligand gated ion channels and from cell to cell. For the most part, the majority of the gap junctions are found at the ends of the irregularly shaped cardiac cells, although some appear at the lateral faces. The number of gap junctions between cells, in part, determines the strength of connection. It is widely believed that the more gap junctions present, the lower the electrical coupling resistance. These pores act like resistors in parallel in an electrical circuit. The type of proteins (connexins) that form the connexon also helps determine its electrical properties or conductance. Different connexin proteins are found in different regions of the heart.[4]

Craig S. Henriquez
Department of Biomedical Engineering, Duke University, Durham, NC 27708, USA, ch@duke.edu

I. R. Efimov et al. (eds.), *Cardiac Bioelectric Therapy: Mechanisms and Practical Implications.*
© Springer Science+Business Media, LLC 2009

The other component of the intracellular resistance is determined by the micro- and nanostructures inside the cell itself. Like most muscle cells, most cardiac cells contain contractile proteins actin and myosin that are anchored by Z-lines. Ventricular mycotyes also possess a highly organized transverse-tubule (T-tubule) system. A T-tubule is a deep invagination of the plasma membrane that allows depolarization of the membrane to quickly penetrate to the interior of the cell. It effectively acts to bring the extracellular environment in proximity to the intracellular space of the cell.[6] The presence of the T-tubules, proteins, and other structures will affect or limit ion mobility and flux and hence increase the intracellular resistance of the cell. In some heart cells (atrial cells, conduction system), however, the T-tubule system is less organized or effectively absent, and hence the electrical properties of these cells are expectedly different.[6]

Like the intracellular space, the extracellular space of cardiac tissue is similarly complex. But unlike the intracellular space, the role of the interstitial space on the spread of electrical activity is less well understood or appreciated. The extracellular space or interstitium occupies from 20 to 25% of the total heart volume.[7] It includes the extracellular matrix (ECM), which includes the interstitial matrix and the basement membrane that acts to protect cells from compression and provide a site of anchorage. Gels of polysaccharides and fibrous proteins like collagen fill the spaces between cells. The interstitial space also includes fibroblasts, which act to synthesize an array of proteins that maintain the ECM.[8] The fibroblasts also secrete noncollagenous components of ECM known as the *ground substance*. Ground substance is distributed in a homogeneous mat throughout the space and within the T-tubules and includes proteoglycans, which are involved in binding cations (such as sodium, potassium, and calcium), and water, which regulates the movement of molecules through the ECM.[7] It is often surprising to learn that fibroblasts are about twice as numerous as myocytes in the heart. Finally, the largest fraction of the interstitial space consists of blood vessels. In one of the more comprehensive studies of the interstitium of cardiac muscle, Frank and Langer[7] found that about one third of the circumference of each myocyte in the heart is within 2,000 Å of a capillary. Through their quantitative stereological methods, Frank and Langer found that the extracellular space is occupied by ground substance (23%), blood vessels (60%), connective tissue cells (e.g., fibroblasts) (7%), collagen (4%), and 6% "empty" space.

Because current must flow in a closed circuit, the transmembrane ion flux must flow through both the intracellular and interstitial spaces. For a given membrane potential gradient, the total current in each space and, ultimately, the speed of propagation of the action potential impulse depends on the resistance of the space, which in turn depends on the geometry at the micro- and macroscales and material composition. Factors that modulate the resistance of the intracellular space, such as cell geometry and size, changes in the number and kind of gap junctions, have all been implicated in conduction disturbances.[9] Surprisingly, factors that modulate the resistance of the interstitial space, such as changes in the number of fibroblasts, changes in the proportion of collagen, changes in the permeability of the ground substance, changes in the vessel size, and so forth, have been generally ignored or considered to be negligible in changing impulse conduction. Although the studies are less numerous, there is growing evidence that the properties of the interstitial space must be considered in propagation disturbances.[10,11]

Microscopic Modeling Cardiac Tissue

Computer models have been used to study cardiac conduction since the late 1970s.[12,13] At that time, computational power limited investigations to very simple geometries corresponding to single fibers or monolayer sheets of cells. With the evolution of computer technologies, computational models of the heart have become three dimensional and increasingly more realistic, providing a broader range of investigations to study how changes in the tissue structure and ionic properties affect propagation, arrhythmogenesis, and the response to externally applied stimuli.

When building models of cardiac tissue, it is necessary to make judicious choices about the amount of structural detail that should be included. A reasonable starting point is to assume each cell has a uniform, resistive cytoplasmic resistive space Ω_i that is bounded by a membrane Γ and is surrounded uniformly by a conductive extracellular space, Ω_e (Fig. 1a.) For simplicity, we can assume that the junction between cells is represented by a local change in geometry (e.g., the formation of narrow tubule) so the potential and currents are continuous from cell to cell.

In the absence of an external stimulus, the intracellular and extracellular spaces are source-free and thus the intracellular and extracellular potentials Φ_i and Φ_e are solutions to the Laplace equations:

$$\Delta\Phi_i = 0 \quad \text{in } \Omega_i, \tag{1}$$

$$\Delta\Phi_e = 0 \quad \text{in } \Omega_e. \tag{2}$$

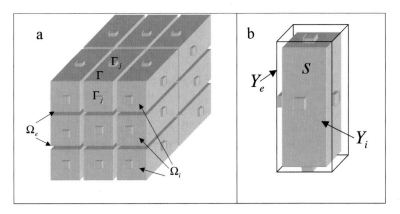

Figure 1: (a) Idealized lattice of cardiac cells connected through gap junctions. The intracellular space, Ω_i, is separated from the extracellular space, Ω_e, by the membrane, Γ. The portion of the membrane associated with gap junction (local change in geometry connecting adjacent cells) is denoted by Γ_j. (b) Portion of the intracellular space, Y_i, extracellular space, Y_e, and membrane, S, associated with a unit cell

In the case that a stimulation current is applied to the intra- and extracellular spaces, the potentials are instead governed by the Poisson equations:

$$\Delta\Phi_i = I_i^s \quad \text{in } \Omega_i, \tag{3}$$

$$\Delta\Phi_e = I_e^s \quad \text{in } \Omega_e, \tag{4}$$

where I_i^s and I_e^s denote the stimulation currents applied. For the sake of simplicity, the remainder of the presentation assumes no current stimulation is applied.

The current that crosses the membrane is continuous with the intracellular and extracellular currents that are normal to the surface Γ. This defines the boundary conditions to (1) and (2) and are given by

$$-\sigma_i \partial_n \Phi_i = C_m \frac{\partial}{\partial t} V_m + I_{ion}(V_m, q), \tag{5}$$

$$-\sigma_e \partial_n \Phi_e = C_m \frac{\partial}{\partial t} V_m + I_{ion}(V_m, q), \tag{6}$$

$$\frac{\partial q}{\partial t} = M(V_m, q), \tag{7}$$

where the normal derivative, ∂_n, is taken with the normal pointing outside of the cell, the transmembrane potential is the difference between Φ_i and Φ_e at the membrane and given by

$$V_m = \Phi_i - \Phi_e \quad \text{on } \Gamma. \tag{8}$$

The left-hand sides of (5) and (6) represent the intra- and extracellular currents evaluated on the membrane, Γ. The right-hand sides of (5) and (6) describe the current across the membrane as having two components: a capacitive component that depends on the membrane capacitance C_m and the time derivative of the transmembrane potential V_m, and the nonlinear current–voltage relationship $I_{ion}(V_{ion}, q)$ and $M(V_m, q)$ that corresponds to the chosen excitability model of the membrane dynamics.

The model described by (5)–(7) gives the microscopic representation of the electric potentials in the tissue. Although it is possible to model propagation from cell to cell using this model, such an approach requires that the geometry of the intracellular and extracellular space be represented separately. Although this is possible for a small number of cells, the practical implementation is both technically challenging and computationally expensive.

Macroscopic Modeling Cardiac Tissue

An alternative approach to modeling at the microscale is to assume the properties of cardiac tissue can be averaged in some sense. Neu and Krassowska[14] first showed that it is possible to derive such a macroscopic model of tissue from an idealized version of the microscopic model. This approach has been expanded and adopted by others.[15,16]

We begin by assuming that the tissue is spatially periodic in which all the cells are identical in shape, arranged in a regular fashion, and have the same pattern of connections with neighbors. The smallest repeatable pattern of this structure is called the *unit cell* (Fig. 1b). In this idealized structure, a few fundamental material constants can be defined:

d_{cell} : A typical measure of the cell dimension (units: L) (e.g., the cell diameter of a unit cell).

σ_i : Conductivity of the cytoplasm filling the inside of cell (units: $R^{-1}L^{-1}$). The conductivity of the fluid filling the extracellular space σ_e has the same order of magnitude as σ_i and, hence, does not need to be considered a fundamental material constant.

R_m : Surface specific resistivity of the membrane that separates the inside and the outside of cell (RL^2).

C_m : Capacitance of the membrane ($R^{-1}L^{-2}T$).

Here R denotes an arbitrary unit of resistance, L is a unit of length, and T a unit of time.

We can define a dimensionless combination of the first three fundamental parameters described above:

$$\varepsilon = \left(\frac{d_{cell}}{R_m \sigma_i} \right)^{1/2}. \tag{9}$$

For a typical cardiac cell, $d_{cell} = 25\,\mu m$, $l_{cell} = 100\,\mu m$ (cell length), $\sigma_i = 5\,mS\,cm^{-1}$ and $R_m = 10,000\,\Omega\,cm^2$, leading to $\varepsilon = 7.1 \times 10^{-3}$. This dimensionless parameter ε is closely associated with the characteristic scale of the microscopic model.

Using all four fundamental material constants, several additional time and length constants can be formulated. For convenience, the macroscopic units of length is defined as $L = d_{cell}/\varepsilon$, and the time constant associated with charging the membrane by the transmembrane current is given by $\tau = R_m C_m$. After that, we can convert the cellular problem into a nondimensional form by scaling space and time with the constants, such as,

$$\hat{x} = x/L, \quad \hat{t} = t/\tau, \tag{10}$$

and scaling the potentials Φ_i, Φ_e, and V_m by a convenient unit ΔV of measure for them, such as,

$$\hat{\Phi}_i = \Phi_i/\Delta V \quad \hat{\Phi}_e = \Phi_e/\Delta V, \quad \hat{V}_m = V_m/\Delta V. \tag{11}$$

Assuming that the typical state variables q can be scaled by $q = Q^{-1}q$, with Q a convenient unit (matrix) of measure for the state variables to make dimensionless, the nondimensional current–voltage relationship $I_{ion}(V_m, q)$ has the following form:

$$\hat{I}_{ion}(\hat{V}_m, q) = \frac{R_m}{\Delta V} I_{ion}(V_m, q), \tag{12}$$

and the dimensionless nonlinear reactions for state variables are:

$$\hat{M}(\hat{V}_m, q) = \frac{\tau}{Q} M(V_m, q). \tag{13}$$

After substitition, we obtain the following dimensionless boundary conditions:

$$-\partial_n \Phi_i = \varepsilon \left\{ C_m \frac{\partial}{\partial t} V_m + I_{ion}(V_m, q) \right\}, \tag{14}$$

$$-\mu \partial_n \Phi_e = \varepsilon \left\{ C_m \frac{\partial}{\partial t} V_m + I_{ion}(V_m, q) \right\}, \tag{15}$$

$$\frac{\partial q}{\partial t} = M(V_m, q), \tag{16}$$

where μ is the ratio of extracellular and intracellular conductivities, i.e.,

$$\mu = \frac{\sigma_e}{\sigma_i}, \tag{17}$$

and ε is the dimensionless small parameter defined by (9). For convenience, the superscripts $\hat{}$ of the dimensionless variables are omitted. Note that the Laplace equations in (1) and (2) are invariant with respect to the scaling above.

Homogenization

If the period of a structure is assumed to be very small compared to the size of the domain of interest, then a formal mathematical process, known as *homogenization*, can be applied.[17] For boundary value problems with periodic structure, perturbation analysis can be used to obtain an asymptotic expansion of the solution in terms of a small parameter, which is the ratio of the period of the structure to a typical length in the region. Homogenization theory can be used to study the limit of Φ_i and Φ_e as $\varepsilon \to 0$. In particular, it is desirable to identify the equations that are satisfied in this limit. Physically, the limit $\varepsilon \to 0$ corresponds to the case where the heterogeneities become vanishingly small. Thus as Hornung[17] notes, through homogenization, the original, highly *heterogeneous* material, characterized by the rapidly oscillating coefficients, can be replaced by an effective, *homogeneous* material that is characterized by constant coefficients.

Assuming the network of cardiac cells is a periodic structure, similar to a regular lattice of interconnected cylinders, then we can define portions of intra- and extracellular spaces Ω_i and Ω_e that belong to a unit cell as Y_i and Y_e, respectively. Similarly, the unit cell portion of the membrane Γ is denoted by S (Fig. 1b).

Introducing a microscopic variable $\xi = x/\varepsilon$, associated with the dimension of a unit cell, we assume the electric potentials, Φ_i, Φ_e, V_m, and the state variables q are functions of both the slow (macroscopic) variable x and the fast (microscopic) variable ξ. The potentials and state variables have the following asymptotic expansion in powers of the dimensionless parameter ε:

$$\begin{aligned}
\Phi_i(x, \xi) &= \Phi_i^{(0)}(x, \xi) + \varepsilon \Phi_i^{(1)}(x, \xi) + \varepsilon^2 \Phi_i^{(2)}(x, \xi) + \cdots, \\
\Phi_e(x, \xi) &= \Phi_e^{(0)}(x, \xi) + \varepsilon \Phi_e^{(1)}(x, \xi) + \varepsilon^2 \Phi_e^{(2)}(x, \xi) + \cdots, \\
V_m(x, \xi) &= V_m^{(0)}(x, \xi) + \varepsilon V_m^{(1)}(x, \xi) + \varepsilon^2 V_m^{(2)}(x, \xi) + \cdots, \\
q(x, \xi) &= q^{(0)}(x, \xi) + \varepsilon q^{(1)}(x, \xi) + \varepsilon^2 q^{(2)}(x, \xi) + \cdots.
\end{aligned} \tag{18}$$

The slow and fast variables correspond respectively to the global and local structure of the field.

Using this approach, the gradients with respect to x and ξ are ∇_x and ∇_ξ, respectively, and the full gradient operator is given by:

$$\nabla = \frac{1}{\varepsilon}\nabla_\xi + \nabla_x. \tag{19}$$

The full Laplacian operator Δ is represented as

$$\Delta = \frac{1}{\varepsilon^2}\Delta_{\xi\xi} + \frac{1}{\varepsilon}(\nabla_\xi \cdot \nabla_x + \nabla_x \cdot \nabla_\xi) + \Delta_{xx}. \tag{20}$$

Substituting the asymptotic expansions (18) and into the Laplace equation (1) and (2) and equating the coefficients of the powers -2, -1, 0 of the dimensionless parameter ε to zero, we obtain the following equations:

$$\frac{1}{\varepsilon^2} : \Delta_{\xi\xi}\Phi_i^{(0)} = 0 \quad \text{in } Y_i,$$

$$\frac{1}{\varepsilon} : \Delta_{\xi\xi}\Phi_i^{(1)} + (\nabla_\xi \cdot \nabla_x + \nabla_x \cdot \nabla_\xi)\Phi_i^{(0)} = 0 \quad \text{in } Y_i, \tag{21}$$

$$1 : \Delta_{\xi\xi}\Phi_i^{(2)} + (\nabla_\xi \cdot \nabla_x + \nabla_x \cdot \nabla_\xi)\Phi_i^{(1)} + \Delta_{xx}\Phi_i^{(0)} = 0 \quad \text{in } Y_i.$$

Similarly, substituting the asymptotic expansions into the boundary condition equation (5) and (6), we obtain the following equations:

$$\frac{1}{\varepsilon} : n \cdot \nabla_\xi\Phi_i^{(0)} = 0 \quad \text{on } S,$$

$$1 : n \cdot \left(\nabla_\xi\Phi_i^{(1)} + \nabla_x\Phi_i^{(0)}\right) = 0 \quad \text{on } S, \tag{22}$$

$$\varepsilon : n \cdot \left(\nabla_\xi\Phi_i^{(2)} + \nabla_x\Phi_i^{(1)}\right) = -\left\{\frac{\partial}{\partial t}V_m^{(0)} + I_{\text{ion}}\left(V_m^{(0)}, q^{(0)}\right)\right\} \quad \text{on } S.$$

The following three boundary value problems can be formulated.

For the coefficient $\Phi_i^{(0)}$ of 1 in the asymptotic expansion for the intracellular potential Φ_i, the first boundary value problem is given by:

$$\Delta_{\xi\xi}\Phi_i^{(0)} = 0 \quad \text{in } Y_i,$$

$$n \cdot \nabla_\xi\Phi_i^{(0)} = 0 \quad \text{on } S. \tag{23}$$

For the coefficient $\Phi_i^{(1)}$ of ε in the asymptotic expansion for the intracellular potential Φ_i, the second boundary value problem is given by:

$$\Delta_{\xi\xi}\Phi_i^{(1)} + (\nabla_\xi \cdot \nabla_x + \nabla_x \cdot \nabla_\xi)\Phi_i^{(0)} = 0 \quad \text{in } Y_i,$$

$$n \cdot \nabla_\xi\Phi_i^{(1)} + n \cdot \nabla_x\Phi_i^{(0)} = 0 \quad \text{on } S. \tag{24}$$

For the coefficient $\Phi_i^{(2)}$ of ε^2 in the asymptotic expansion for the intracellular potential Φ_i, the third boundary value problem is given by:

$$\Delta_{\xi\xi}\Phi_i^{(1)} + (\nabla_\xi \cdot \nabla_x + \nabla_x \cdot \nabla_\xi)\Phi_i^{(1)} + \Delta_{xx}\Phi_i^{(0)} = 0 \quad \text{in } Y_i,$$

$$n \cdot \nabla_\xi \Phi_i^{(2)} + n \cdot \nabla_x \Phi_i^{(1)} + \left\{ \frac{\partial}{\partial t} V_m^{(0)} + I_{\text{ion}}\left(V_m^{(0)}, q^{(0)}\right) \right\} = 0 \quad \text{on } S. \tag{25}$$

Then, the coefficients $\Phi_i^{(0)}$, $\Phi_i^{(0)}$ and $\Phi_i^{(2)}$ $\Phi_i^{(2)}$ in the expansion for the intracellular potential Φ_i can be computed as functions of ξ by solving one by one the Neumann boundary value problems (BVP) in the local portion Y_i of a unit cell. Under reasonable assumptions on the domain Y_i, its boundary S and the data on the right-hand side of problems, the Neumann BVP has a unique solution up to a constant.

From the first BVP, which only has a constant solution with respect to ξ, we find that the solution $\Phi_i^{(0)}$ depends only on the macroscopic variable x. Actually, it represents a potential average over Y_i by letting ε go to zero.

With the ξ independence of $\Phi_i^{(0)}$, the second BVP becomes:

$$\Delta_{\xi\xi}\Phi_i^{(1)} = 0 \quad \text{in } Y_i,$$

$$n \cdot \nabla_\xi \Phi_i^{(1)} + n \cdot \nabla_x \Phi_i^{(0)} = 0 \quad \text{on } S. \tag{26}$$

It is not difficult to show that the unique zero mean solution of the BVP can be represented as:[15]

$$\Phi_i^{(1)} = -w_i(\xi) \cdot \nabla_x \Phi_i^{(0)} + \tilde{\Phi}_i^{(1)}(x,t), \tag{27}$$

where $w_i = (w_i^1(\xi), w_i^2(\xi), w_i^3(\xi))^{\mathrm{T}}$ and its components $w_i^k(\xi)$ $(k = 1,2,3)$, satisfy

$$\Delta_{\xi\xi}w_i^k(\xi) = 0, \quad \text{in } Y_i,$$

$$\nabla_\xi w_i^k(\xi) \cdot n_i = n_{i,\xi_k} \quad \text{on } S, \tag{28}$$

where $n_i = (n_{i,\xi_1}, n_{i,\xi_1}, n_{i,\xi_1})^{\mathrm{T}}$ is the unit outward normal to the membrane portion with respect to the intracellular portion Y_i. The problems for $w_i^k(\xi)$ $(k = 1,2,3)$ are solvable up to a constant, and the solutions can be fixed (e.g., by the condition $\int_S w_i^k(\xi)d\xi = 0$). Note that the macroscopic component $\tilde{\Phi}_i^{(1)}(x,t)$ and $\Phi_i^{(0)}$ in the representation of the coefficient $\Phi_i^{(1)}$ (27) are independent of the microscopic variable.

Rewriting the third BVP as

$$\nabla_\xi \cdot \left(\nabla_\xi \Phi_i^{(2)} + \nabla_x \Phi_i^{(1)}\right) = -\Delta_{xx}\Phi_i^{(0)} - \nabla_x \cdot \nabla_\xi \Phi_i^{(1)} \quad \text{in } Y_i,$$

$$n \cdot \left(\nabla_\xi \Phi_i^{(2)} + \nabla_x \Phi_i^{(1)}\right) = -\left\{ \frac{\partial}{\partial t} V_m^{(0)} + I_{\text{ion}}\left(V_m^{(0)}, q^{(0)}\right) \right\} \quad \text{on } S, \tag{29}$$

and integrating the equation over the unit cell portion Y_i of the intracellular space Ω_i and applying the divergence theorem and the boundary conditions, we obtain the following identity:

$$\int_{Y_i} (\Delta_{xx}\Phi_i^{(0)} + \nabla_x \cdot \nabla_\xi \Phi_i^{(1)})d\xi = \int_S \left\{ \frac{\partial}{\partial t} V_m^{(0)} + I_{ion}(V_m^{(0)}, q^{(0)}) \right\} ds. \tag{30}$$

Substituting (27) into (30), we obtain

$$\nabla_x \cdot \left\{ |Y_i|I - \int_{Y_i} \nabla_\xi w_i d\xi \right\} \cdot \nabla_x \Phi_i^{(0)} = |S| \left\{ \frac{\partial}{\partial t} V_m^{(0)} + I_{ion}(V_m^{(0)}, q^{(0)}) \right\}, \tag{31}$$

where $\nabla_\xi w_i = [\nabla_\xi w_i^1, \nabla_\xi w_i^2, \nabla_\xi w_i^3]$ and $|Y_i|, |S|$ denote the volume and the area of the unit cell portions Y_i, S of the intracellular space Ω_i and the membrane Γ, respectively.

If we define $\hat{\beta}$ to be the dimensionless surface-to-volume ratio, such that $\hat{\beta} = \frac{|S|}{|Y|}$, where $|Y|$ is the volume of a unit cell, then we obtain the following expression from (31):

$$\nabla_x \cdot \left\{ \frac{1}{|Y|} \left(|Y_i|I - \int_{Y_i} \nabla_\xi w_i d\xi \right) \right\} \cdot \nabla_x \Phi_i^{(0)} = \hat{\beta} \left\{ \frac{\partial}{\partial t} V_m^{(0)} + I_{ion}(V_m^{(0)}, q^{(0)}) \right\}. \tag{32}$$

A tensor $\hat{D}_i$ can be defined as the integral

$$\hat{D}_i = \frac{1}{|Y|} \left\{ |Y_i|I - \int_{Y_i} \nabla_\xi w_i d\xi \right\}. \tag{33}$$

This dimensionless tensor is effectively related to the geometry of the unit cell.

Finally, we obtain the following equation for the intracellular potential directly from the identity:

$$\nabla_x \cdot (\hat{D}_i \nabla_x \Phi_i^{(0)}) = \hat{\beta} \left\{ \frac{\partial}{\partial t} V_m^{(0)} + I_{ion}(V_m^{(0)}, q^{(0)}) \right\}. \tag{34}$$

where the intracellular potential Φ_i is independent of the microscopic scale.

Similarly, we can obtain the dimensionless *averaged equation* for the extracellular potential:

$$\nabla_x \cdot (\hat{D}_e \nabla_x \Phi_e^{(0)}) = -\hat{\beta} \left\{ \frac{\partial}{\partial t} V_m^{(0)} + I_{ion}(V_m^{(0)}, q^{(0)}) \right\}, \tag{35}$$

where the dimensionless tensor $\hat{D}_e$ of extracellular conductivity is given by:

$$\hat{D}_e = \frac{\mu}{|Y|} \left\{ |Y_e|I - \int_{Y_e} \nabla_\xi w_e d\xi \right\}, \tag{36}$$

where μ is the ratio of extracellular and intracellular conductivities, defined in (17) and $w_e = (w_e^1(\xi), w_e^2(\xi), w_e^3(\xi))^T$ and its components $w_e^k(\xi)$ $(k = 1, 2, 3)$ satisfy

$$\begin{aligned} \Delta_{\xi\xi} w_e^k(\xi) &= 0 \quad \text{in } Y_e, \\ \nabla_\xi w_e^k(\xi) n_e &= n_{e,\xi_k} \quad \text{on } S, \end{aligned} \tag{37}$$

where $n_e = (n_{e,\xi_1}, n_{e,\xi_2}, n_{e,\xi_3})^T$ is the unit outward normal to the membrane portion S with respect to the extracellular portion of Y_e.

Bidomain Model of Cardiac Tissue

Using (10) and the definitions of macroscopic time and space units τ and L, we can rescale the dimensionless equations to the following dimensional averaged equations for the macroscopic intra- and extracellular potentials:

$$\nabla_x \cdot (D_i \nabla_x \Phi_i) = \beta \left\{ C_m \frac{\partial}{\partial t} V_m + I_{ion}(V_m, q) \right\}, \tag{38}$$

$$\nabla_x \cdot (D_e \nabla_x \Phi_e) = -\beta \left\{ C_m \frac{\partial}{\partial t} V_m + I_{ion}(V_m, q) \right\}, \tag{39}$$

where the dimensional surface-to-volume ratio is defined as $\beta = \hat{\beta}/d_c$ and the dimensional conductivity tensors D_i and D_e are given by

$$D_i = \sigma_i \hat{D}_i \quad \text{and} \quad D_e = \sigma_e \hat{D}_e. \tag{40}$$

Equations (38) and (39) describe the bidomain model of cardiac tissue.[18,19] As presented, the bidomain model can be viewed as a macroscopic model that represents the asymptotic behavior of the potentials and currents in a periodic, discrete cellular model.[14] In the bidomain, the intracellular space, the extracellular space, and the membrane that separates them exist at every point in the region of interest.[19] Each point effectively represents a unit cell, and thus it is assumed that the amount of extracellular space and the membrane properties around each unit cell do not vary (i.e., axially symmetric). In this continuous, micro- to macroscale derivation of the bidomain model, the conductivity tensor is assumed to be constant, and the properties come from the geometry of the cell and its associated extracellular space.

In the intracellular space, the magnitude of the tensor involves both the cytoplasmic properties and the gap properties. Equation (33) assumes the gap is a microtubule of very small length (i.e., on order of that of two cell membranes) and width such that the potentials are everywhere continuous. Because of the small dimensions of the gap, it is possible to represent it as an interface such that the potentials have a jump in discontinuity.

If we assume Ω_i be the intracellular space and Γ_j the portion of the cellular membrane associated with the gap junction, then for the intracellular potential Φ_i to be continuous across the junction interface between two cells (A and B), the following is satisfied:

$$\Phi_i^B - \Phi_i^A = 0 \quad \text{on } \Gamma_j$$

$$\sigma_i \frac{\partial \Phi_i^B}{\partial n} - \sigma_i \frac{\partial \Phi_i^A}{\partial n} = 0 \quad \text{on } \Gamma_j. \tag{41}$$

For the potential to be discontinuous or have a jump, then:

$$-\sigma \frac{\partial \Phi_i^A}{\partial n} = \frac{\Phi_i^B - \Phi_i^A}{R_j} \quad \text{on } \Gamma_j,$$

$$\sigma_i \frac{\partial \Phi_i^B}{\partial n} - \sigma_i \frac{\partial \Phi_i^A}{\partial n} = 0 \quad \text{on } \Gamma_j. \tag{42}$$

where R_j is the specific resistance of the portion of the membrane associated with gap junction (approximately $1.0\,\Omega\,\mathrm{cm}^2$).

In the "continuous" view, the geometry (shape and orientation) of the cellular membrane Γ, including the small tubules, determines the effective conductivities as indicated by (33).

In the "discontinuous" view, the portion of the membrane associated with the junction is simply a resistive interface. In general, the flux flowing out of the cell into the extracellular space across the cellular membrane is much smaller than the flux across the junction, as the membrane flux is normally on the order of ε, and the junctional flux is typically on the order of

$$\eta = \frac{d_c}{R_j \sigma_i} \approx 0.5. \tag{43}$$

Thus, to compute the effective conductivity, we can assume the cell membrane is a perfect insulator.

The continuous and discontinuous approaches to deriving the effective conductivity of the unit cell (cell plus gap junctions) are essentially equivalent. The *continuous* approach emphasizes the geometry of the cell membrane, while the *discontinuous* approach emphasizes more on the local effects of the presence of the gap junctions, and accounts for the gap through an effective gap junction resistance, R_j.

Bidomain Properties at the Tissue Level

Perhaps the most challenging aspect of setting up the bidomain model is determining the components of the conductivity tensors associated with the intra- and extracellular spaces that are consistent with the underlying structure. Often the cellular structure is either not precisely known or it cannot be determined a priori. In some cases, the properties are determined by making a series of measurements on the preparation and interpreting the data using the bidomain model. More often the properties are simply assumed using literature values from measurements from simpler preparations or from other modeling studies.[20]

Intuitively, the conductivity tensors, D_i and D_e, are related to the geometry, coupling, orientation, and degree of packing of cells in the tissue. The tensors are symmetric and positive definite matrices where the three eigenvalues of the tensor are associated with the average electrical properties in the directions given by the three orthogonal eigenvectors.

We can obtain a simple estimate for the magnitude of the components of the tensor by assuming cardiac tissue is a lattice of coupled, identical rectangular parallelepiped cells (Fig. 1a). We assume that each unit cell is isotropic with conductivity σ_i surrounded by a uniform layer of fluid with conductivity σ_e, and connected to six neighbors through small tubules on the end and lateral faces. Although clearly an idealization, this cell arrangement gives rise to reasonable estimates for tissue conductivities for reasonable cell dimensions and gap resistances.

As shown in Fig. 2, we can imagine each unit cell has a width, d_{cell}, height d_{cell}, and length l_{cell} such that the total cell volume is:

$$\mathrm{Vol}_{cell} = d_{cell} \times d_{cell} \times l_{cell}. \tag{44}$$

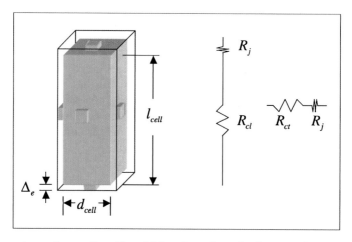

Figure 2: Dimension of a unit cell: width, d_{cell}; length, l_{cell}, and the thickness of the extracellular fluid, Δ_{e}. The unit cell has a total intracellular resistance (cytoplasmic and gap junction) along the cell, $R_{\text{il}} = R_{\text{cl}} + R_{\text{j}}$, and across the cell, $R_{\text{it}} = R_{\text{ct}} + R_{\text{j}}$

The fluid that surrounds each cell is relatively small and has a thickness of Δ_{e} such that the total volume occupied by the cell and extracellular fluid is

$$\text{Vol}_{\text{cell}} = d_{\text{tot}} \times d_{\text{tot}} \times l_{\text{tot}}, \tag{45}$$

where

$$d_{\text{tot}} = d_{\text{cell}} + 2\Delta_{\text{e}}, \tag{46}$$

$$l_{\text{tot}} = l_{\text{cell}} + 2\Delta_{\text{e}}. \tag{47}$$

The fraction of intracellular space is given by:

$$f_{\text{i}} = \frac{\text{Vol}_{\text{cell}}}{\text{Vol}_{\text{tot}}}. \tag{48}$$

Because $\Delta_{\text{e}}, d_{\text{cell,tot}} \ll l_{\text{cell,tot}}$, the intracellular fraction is usually defined as the ratio of the cross-sectional areas, namely

$$f_{\text{i}} \approx \frac{d_{\text{cell}}^2}{d_{\text{tot}}^2}. \tag{49}$$

The extracellular fraction is

$$f_{\text{e}} = 1 - f_{\text{i}}. \tag{50}$$

The total resistance of the cell is the sum of the resistance of the cytoplasm along the cell, R_{cl}, or across the cell, R_{ct}, namely

$$R_{\text{cl}} = \frac{l_{\text{cell}}}{\sigma_{\text{i}} d_{\text{cell}}^2} \quad \text{or} \quad R_{\text{ct}} = \frac{d_{\text{cell}}}{\sigma_{\text{i}} d_{\text{cell}} l_{\text{cell}}} = \frac{1}{\sigma_{\text{i}} l_{\text{cell}}}, \tag{51}$$

and the resistance of the gap junction, R_j. If we assume a typical connexon has a conductance g_j, then the total resistance of the gap junction is

$$R_j = \frac{1}{Ng_j}, \tag{52}$$

where N is the number of connexons in the gap junction. For simplicity, we assume that the number of connexons is the same on the end and lateral faces. Thus, the total resistance of the cell and junction along the cell is

$$R_{il} = R_{cl} + R_j = \frac{l_{cell}}{\sigma_i d_{cell}^2} + R_j \tag{53}$$

and across the cell is

$$R_{it} = R_{ct} + R_j = \frac{1}{\sigma_i l_{cell}} + R_j \approx R_j. \tag{54}$$

The total interstitial resistance along the cell is

$$R_{el} = \frac{l_{tot}}{\sigma_e \left(d_{tot}^2 - d_{cell}^2 \right)} \tag{55}$$

and across the cell is

$$R_{et} = \frac{d_{tot}}{\sigma_e (d_{tot} l_{tot} - d_{cell} l_{cell})}. \tag{56}$$

If we assume the intracellular space and the extracellular space occupy the same total volume, V_{tot}, then we can compute an effective conductivity (i.e., the bidomain conductivity) that would yield the same total resistance as that computed for the actual intracellular and interstitial volumes. For example, if intrinsic intracellular or interstitial resistance along the cell is $R_{il,el}$, then the effective conductivity, $s_{il,el}$, that would yield the same resistance in V_{tot} is

$$s_{il,el} = \frac{1}{R_{il,el} d_{tot}^2 / l_{tot}} = \frac{l_{tot}}{R_{il,el} d_{tot}^2}. \tag{57}$$

Similarly, the effective conductivity across the cell is

$$s_{it,et} = \frac{1}{R_{it,et} \, d_{tot} l_{tot} / d_{tot}} = \frac{1}{R_{it,et} l_{tot}}. \tag{58}$$

Substituting (53) and (55) into (57), we obtain

$$s_{il} = \frac{l_{tot}}{\left(\frac{l_{cell}}{\sigma_i d_{cell}^2} + R_j \right) d_{tot}^2} = \frac{\left(d_{cell}^2 / d_{tot}^2 \right) \sigma_i}{\left(\frac{l_{cell}}{l_{tot}} + R_j \sigma_i \frac{d_{cell}^2}{l_{tot}} \right)} \tag{59}$$

and

$$s_{el} = \frac{l_{tot}}{\left(\frac{l_{tot}}{\sigma_e (d_{tot}^2 - d_{cell}^2)} \right) d_{tot}^2} = \sigma_e \left(1 - \frac{d_{cell}^2}{d_{tot}^2} \right). \tag{60}$$

Substituting (54) and (56) into (58), yields

$$s_{\text{it}} = \frac{1}{\left(\frac{1}{\sigma_i l_{\text{cell}}} + R_j\right) l_{\text{tot}}} = \frac{1}{\left(\frac{l_{\text{tot}}}{\sigma_i l_{\text{cell}}} + R_j l_{\text{tot}}\right)} \tag{61}$$

and

$$s_{\text{et}} = \frac{1}{\left(\frac{d_{\text{tot}}}{\sigma_e (d_{\text{tot}} l_{\text{tot}} - d_{\text{cell}} l_{\text{cell}})}\right) l_{\text{tot}}} = \left(1 - \frac{d_{\text{cell}} l_{\text{cell}}}{d_{\text{tot}} l_{\text{tot}}}\right) \sigma_e. \tag{62}$$

Although the above expressions for the effective bidomain conductivities assume a relatively simple geometry, they are consistent with other estimates that assume a more complicated cell geometry and connectivity. Neu and Krassowska[14] derived expressions for the effective conductivity, assuming parallelepiped cells with hexagonal cross-sections in which each cell was connected to six neighboring cells only at the ends of the cell through lateral gap junctions arranged on a jutting triangular face. For this unique cell arrangement, they obtained the following estimates:

$$s_{\text{il}} = \frac{f_i \sigma_i}{\left(1 + \frac{R_j}{3R_c}\right)}, \quad s_{\text{it}} = \frac{1}{\sqrt{3}} \frac{1}{R_j l_{\text{cell}}}, \quad s_{\text{el}} = f_e \sigma_e, \quad s_{\text{et}} = \frac{f_e}{2} \sigma_e. \tag{63}$$

Under certain reasonable assumptions such as $l_{\text{tot}} \approx l_{\text{cell}}$, the conductivity of the intracellular space is relatively high and the fraction of intracellular space f_i, given by (49), is close to 1, then (59)–(62) for a regular lattice or rectangular parallelepiped cells can be approximated as

$$s_{\text{il}} = \frac{f_i \sigma_i}{\left(1 + \frac{R_j}{R_{\text{cl}}}\right)}, \quad s_{\text{it}} = \frac{1}{R_j l_{\text{cell}}}, \quad s_{\text{el}} = f_e \sigma_e, \quad s_{\text{et}} = \left(1 - \sqrt{f_i}\right) \sigma_e. \tag{64}$$

The two sets of expressions are very similar, except for the geometric factors of 3 and $\sqrt{3}$ in the estimates of the intracellular properties.

We can obtain some estimates for the bidomain conductivities (g's) by considering some reasonable values for the cell dimensions, fraction of intracellular space, intracellular conductivity, and gap resistance. As noted earlier a typical myocyte has an average cell width of $d_{\text{cell}} = 25\,\mu\text{m}$, an average cell length of $l_{\text{cell}} = 100\,\mu\text{m}$, and an intracellular conductivity $\sigma_i = 5\,\text{mS cm}^{-1}$. These dimensions lead to $R_{\text{cl}} = 320\,\text{k}\Omega$, $R_{\text{ct}} = 20\,\text{k}\Omega$. Frank and Langer[7] estimated that the intracellular volume fraction is 75–80%. But since some of the extracellular space is nonconducting, we can assume a fraction of $f_e = 15\%$, with a conductivity of $\sigma_e = 20\,\text{mS cm}^{-1}$. For the given cell length and cell width, this corresponds to an extracellular gap of about $1\,\mu\text{m}$ around the entire cell, leading to $d_{\text{tot}} = 27\,\mu\text{m}$ and $l_{\text{tot}} = 102\,\mu\text{m}$. The unitary conductance of a single channel comprised of connexin-43 is $g_j = 75\,\text{pS}$.[21]

Perhaps the most uncertain parameter in the analysis is the number of open connexons in a gap junction connecting two cells. Some studies have suggested that the fraction of open channels may decrease with increasing gap junction area, such that the gap junction conductance per area is not constant.[21] In understanding their measurements on isolated rat

Table 1: Estimates for the bidomain conductivities for a lattice of parallelepiped cells (57–60) for different number of connexons (N) in the gap junction region.

$N = 3,000$ $(R_j = 4.44\,\mathrm{M\Omega})(\mathrm{mS\ cm^{-1}})$	$N = 30,000$ $(R_j = 444\,\mathrm{k\Omega})(\mathrm{mS\ cm^{-1}})$
$s_{il} = 0.29$	$s_{il} = 2.0$
$s_{it} = 0.0219$	$s_{it} = 0.213$
$s_{el} = 3.0$	$s_{el} = 3.0$
$s_{et} = 1.9$	$s_{et} = 1.9$

myocyte cell pairs, Weingart and Maurer[22] argued that 90–95% of the available connexons in the cell may be closed at any given time. They estimated that 2,500–5,000 of the 50,000 connexons were open to be consistent with the measured gap resistance of 2.0–5.0 MΩ, with an assumed $g_j = 100\,\mathrm{pS}$. Somewhat surprisingly, simulation studies on propagation suggest that a much smaller gap resistance of 83–500 kΩ is required to obtain reasonable propagation velocities.[21,23] This range is consistent with a very large number of open channels.

It is interesting to compare the estimated conductivities over the range of open connexons. Using the parameters for dimensions of the intra- and extracellular space, intra- and extracellular conductivities, and the unitary connexon conductance of $g_j = 75\,\mathrm{pS}$, the conductivities and anisotropy ratios can be computed from (57) to (60). Table 1 shows the values for $N = 3,000$ and $N = 30,000$.

For $N = 30,000$ the anisotropy ratio ($AR = s_{il}/s_{it}$) is approximately 9.5:1, and for $N = 3,000$, $AR = 13.5:1$. Although the two AR's are roughly consistent with experimental measurements of a 3:1 ratio of conduction velocity along and across fibers, the values of conductivities for $N = 30,000$ are more consistent with those used in simulation studies to obtain conduction velocities in the range of 50–80 cm s^{-1}.[20] This suggests that the number of open channels in the gap may on the high end of the estimate.

The fact that the AR is relatively insensitive to the magnitude of the gap resistance suggests that it depends more on the assumed geometry of the cell. Using the approximate expressions (64), we can see that for large R_j ($R_j \gg R_c$), the anisotropy ratio is roughly proportional to the square of the ratio of the length of the cell to the width of the cell, namely

$$AR \approx \frac{f_i l_{\mathrm{cell}}^2}{d_{\mathrm{cell}}^2}. \tag{65}$$

For the assumed dimensions, this yields an $AR = 13.6:1$.

Interestingly enough, for the arrangement assumed by Neu and Krassowska (63), the limiting ratio for large R_j is

$$AR \approx 3\sqrt{3}\frac{f_i l_{\mathrm{cell}}^2}{d_{\mathrm{cell}}^2}, \tag{66}$$

or roughly five times bigger than that for the regular lattice of rectangular parallelepipeds. In their analysis, they assumed a much narrower cell of width $d_{\mathrm{cell}} = 15\,\mu\mathrm{m}$ for the length $l_{\mathrm{cell}} = 100\,\mu\mathrm{m}$. This leads to a limiting value of $AR = 196:1$, which they admit is significantly outside the experimentally measured ratios.[14] Even for the rectangular parallelepipid cells, $AR = 37.8$ for the narrower cell, which is very extreme.

This simple analysis shows that the properties of cardiac tissue are very much dependent on cell shape and connectivity, and significant variations in the magnitudes of the components of the conductivity tensor may arise under conditions where the cell size and gap junction distributions change, such as hypertrophy and ischemia.

Bidomain Properties at the Heart Level

In general, the orientations of the cells in the heart are not uniform. As a result, the conductivity tensors will vary spatially. The direction of the cells can be obtained through careful histology,[24,25] or through the use of imaging methods such as diffusion tensor magnetic resonance imaging (MRI),[26,27] optical coherence tomography,[28] or confocal and two-photon microscopy.[29]

Using histological methods, Legrice et al.[24] found that the ventricular myocardium was comprised of sheets of cells running radially from epicardium to endocardium, and the three eigenvectors of the intra- or extracellular conductivity tensor at any position correspond to the three principal directions of the cardiac microstructure one along the myocardial fiber $(e_l(x))$, a second orthogonal to the fiber direction and lying in the myocardial sheet plane $(e_t(x))$, and a third orthogonal to the first two in the cross-sheet direction $(e_n(x))$. In other words, $e_l(x)$ parallels to the local fiber direction; $e_t(x)$ and $e_n(x)$ are tangential and normal to the muscle sheet, respectively. The effective conductivities of intra- and extracellular spaces always have the same principal axes: $e_l(x)$, $e_t(x)$, and $e_n(x)$.

Based on the arguments above, the intra- and extracellular conductivity tensors D_i and D_e may be given by:

$$D_i = s_{il} e_l(x) e_l^T(x) + s_{it} e_t(x) e_t^T(x) + s_{in} e_n(x) e_n^T(x), \tag{67}$$

$$D_e = s_{el} e_l(x) e_l^T(x) + s_{et} e_t(x) e_t^T(x) + s_{en} e_n(x) e_n^T(x). \tag{68}$$

Sometimes the expression for the intra- and extracellular conductivity tensors can be simplified by assuming that the transverse coupling is the same in all angular directions orthogonal to the fiber axis ($s_{il,el} = s_{in,en}$). This is known as *transverse isotropy*. Note that the three principal directions, $e_l(x)$, $e_t(x)$, and $e_n(x)$, are orthogonal to one another. The x coordinate system can be locally oriented such that

$$e_l(x) e_l^T(x) + e_t(x) e_t^T(x) + e_n(x) e_n^T(x) = I, \tag{69}$$

where I is the 3×3 identity matrix. Substituting (69) into (67) and (68), we recover the conductivity tensors:

$$D_i = s_{in} I + (s_{il} - s_{in}) e_l(x) e_l^T(x), \tag{70}$$

$$D_e = s_{en} I + (s_{el} - s_{en}) e_l(x) e_l^T(x). \tag{71}$$

Generally, the principal conductivity in each direction is not equal (i.e., $s_{il,el} \neq s_{it,et} \neq s_{in,en}$). The heart is sometimes referred to as being transversely orthotropic.[13]

Macroscopically, the gobal orientation of the cells in the heart defines the so-called fiber orientation, although true fibers do not exist. In the free wall of the ventricle, the "fibers" can rotate up to $120°$. The rotational anisotropy creates quite different conditions for wave propagation in three dimensions when initiated from a point or focal source.[30,31] In many implementations of the bidomain, the conductivities in the three principal directions are assumed to be constant throughout the domain. In reality, the conductivities will vary slightly in space in normal tissue and perhaps vary significantly in diseased tissue.

Conclusion

Most clinical measurements and electrical interventions take place through the interstitial space. Analysis of the spread of electrical activity takes place by interpreting extracellular signals measured either at the surface of the heart via arrays of electrodes on a catheter or at the body surface through standard or nonstandard electrocardiogram (ECG) electrode placement. Pacemakers to initiate impulse propagation or defibrillators to extinguish fibrillation act by introducing currents first through the extracellular space. The bidomain model of cardiac tissue was developed and has evolved over the past 30 years to help elucidate the role of the interstitial space on the action potential shape and conduction velocity, the morphology of electrograms under normal and diseased conditions, and the patterns of transmembrane potential produced through point and field stimulation.[32–34] The model, which began as a mathematical curiosity, is now firmly established as a practical tool in the field of cardiac electrophysiology.[19]

The original implementations of the bidomain model made key assumptions regarding the material properties that facilitated the computation.[18,35] In fact, under the assumption that the anisotropies of the intracellular space and the interstitial space are equal ($D_i = kD_e$), (the equations (38) and (39)) defining the bidomain model reduce to a single equation, known as the monodomain model.[19] As such, we can view the monodomain model as a derivative of the bidomain model. As algorithms advanced, it became possible to consider general properties and bidomain theory, and simulations revealed behaviors that strongly depend on the nature of the conductivity tensors in both spaces. Perhaps the most striking was the prediction of a bidomain model with unequal anisotropy that a unipolar stimulus gives rise to unique pattern of transmembrane potential in which a central, nonelliptical region of depolarization is flanked by regions of hyperpolarization.[36] The so-called dog-bone prediction was later validated using optical measurements of the heart.[37] The effect of unequal anisotropy has also explained directional variations in the morphology of the electrograms measured on the heart.[31,38,39]

There has been a recent trend to consider the effects of the microstructure of the intracellular and interstitial spaces on conduction and the response to externally applied stimuli, particularly in modeling diseased tissue.[40–42] It is here where the application of the classical bidomain becomes more challenging. In heterogeneous tissue, the properties are clearly not uniform and can possibly vary on the length scale smaller than a cell width. Although it is possible to develop a "discrete" bidomain in which the effects of intracellular and interstitial inhomogeneities are explicitly included, the biggest uncertainty in the model is relating the microstructure to bidomain conductivities, particularly in three dimensions. The common belief is that the bidomain model requires that the magnitude of the effective conductivities be uniform and continuous and represent the spatial average over many cells. Such averaging is only necessary when the spatial discretization used to solve the bidomain equations is larger than the length or width of a single cell, and the assumption of uniformity is often one of convenience. If willing to use descretization smaller than the width of a single cell, it is possible to explicitly incorporate the gap junction resistance and account for variations in cell geometry by appropriately modifying the cytoplasmic and interstitial conductivities. The process to determine the properties for the general case, however, will involve some combination of parameter estimation from measurements and data and clever statistical analysis.

Computing a solution of the model at a subcellular scale over the whole heart is currently impractical and perhaps unnecessary. It is expected that the desire to incorporate such microheterogeneity will bring with it advanced computational techniques that retain the features of the small scale in larger computational elements. A promising approach is multiscale finite elements (MsFEM) that numerically construct coarse representations based on the model and parameters defined at the microscale.[43] Using this approach, the domain solved using MsFEM method usually has a much smaller number of elements, while the fine scale effects are incorporated and preserved.

Ultimately, the value of the bidomain model, like any physiological model, will be judged on its ability, as Beard et al.[44] argue, to simulate, predict, and optimize procedures, experiments, and therapies, and to disprove and define new hypotheses. Using advanced imaging methods and experimental measurements, it is now possible to develop models of the preparation of interest, with detailed representations of the tissue structure and corresponding properties.[39,45] The use of the preparation-specific models of the heart represents a paradigm shift in the ability to design new experiments and test hypotheses to help reveal important and previously unknown features of cardiac electrophysiology. By integrating information at multiple scales, the combined use of the bidomain model and experiments should provide greater insight into molecular mechanisms of arrhythmia initiation, maintenance, and termination than could be obtained from either approach alone.

References

1. Severs NJ, Coppen SR, Dupont E, Yeh HI, Ko YS, Matsushita T. Gap junction alterations in human cardiac disease. *Cardiovasc Res* 2004;62:368–377
2. Saffitz JE, Davis LM, Darrow BJ, Kanter HL, Laing JG, Beyer EC. The molecular-basis of anisotropy – role of gap-junctions. *J Cardiovasc Electrophysiol* 1995;6:498–510
3. Severs NJ. Microscopy of the gap junction – a historical-perspective. *Microsc Res Tech* 1995;31:338–346
4. Evans WH, Martin PE. Gap junctions: structure and function (review). *Mol Membr Biol* 2002;19:121–136

5. Saffitz JE, Hoyt RH, Luke RA, Kanter HL, Beyer EC. Cardiac myocyte interconnections at gap-junctions – role in normal and abnormal electrical-conduction. *Trends Cardiovasc Med* 1992;2:56–60

6. Brette F, Orchard C. T-tubule function in mammalian cardiac myocytes. *Circ Res* 2003;92:1182–1192

7. Frank JS, Langer GA. Myocardial interstitium – its Structure and its role in ionic exchange. *J Cell Biol* 1974;60:586–601

8. Baudino TA, Carver W, Giles W, Borg TK. Cardiac fibroblasts: friend or foe? *Am J Physiol Heart Circ Physiol* 2006;291:H1015–H1026

9. Kleber AG, Rudy Y. Basic mechanisms of cardiac impulse propagation and associated arrhythmias. *Physiol Rev* 2004;84:431–488

10. Kleber AG. Conduction of the impulse in the ischemic myocardium – implications for malignant ventricular arrhythmias. *Experientia* 1987;43:1056–1061

11. Fleischhauer J, Lehmann L, Kleber AG. Electrical resistances of interstitial and microvascular space as determinants of the extracellular electrical-field and velocity of propagation in ventricular myocardium. *Circulation* 1995;92:587–594

12. Henriquez CS, Papazoglou AA. Using computer models to understand the roles of tissue structure and membrane dynamics in arrhythmogenesis. *Proc IEEE* 1996;84:334–354

13. Pullan AJ, Cheng LK, Buist ML. *Mathematically Modelling the Electrical Activity of the Heart: From Cell to Body Surface and Back Again.* Hackensack, NJ: World Scientific; 2005

14. Neu JC, Krassowska W. Homogenization of syncytial tissues. *Crit Rev Biomed Eng* 1993;21:137–199

15. Pennacchio M, Savare G, Franzone PC. Multiscale modeling for the bioelectric activity of the heart. *Siam J Math Anal* 2006;37:1333–1370

16. Keener JP, Sneyd J. *Mathematical Physiology*, corrected 2nd edn. New York: Springer; 2001

17. Hornung U. *Homogenization and Porous Media.* New York: Springer; 1997

18. Miller WT, Geselowitz DB. Simulation studies of electrocardiogram. 1. Normal heart. *Circ Res* 1978;43:301–315

19. Henriquez CS. Simulating the electrical behavior of cardiac tissue using the bidomain model. *Crit Rev Biomed Eng* 1993;21:1–77

20. Plonsey R, Barr RC. A critique of impedance measurements in cardiac tissue. *Ann Biomed Eng* 1986;14:307–322

21. Jongsma HJ, Wilders R. Gap junctions in cardiovascular disease. *Circ Res* 2000;86:1193–1197

22. Weingart R, Maurer P. Action-potential transfer in cell pairs isolated from adult-rat and guinea-pig ventricles. *Circ Res* 1988;63:72–80

23. Shaw RM, Rudy Y. Ionic mechanisms of propagation in cardiac tissue – roles of the sodium and L-type calcium currents during reduced excitability and decreased gap junction coupling. *Circ Res* 1997;81:727–741

24. Legrice IJ, Smaill BH, Chai LZ, Edgar SG, Gavin JB, Hunter PJ. Laminar structure of the heart – ventricular myocyte arrangement and connective-tissue architecture in the dog. *Am J Physiol Heart Circ Physiol* 1995;38:H571–H582

25. Streeter DD Jr, Spotnitz HM, Patel DP, Ross J Jr, Sonnenblick EH. Fiber orientation in the canine left ventricle during diastole and systole. *Circ Res* 1969;24:339–347

26. Hsu EW, Henriquez CS. Myocardial fiber orientation mapping using reduced encoding diffusion tensor imaging. *J Cardiovasc Mag Reson* 2001;3:339–347

27. Scollan DF, Holmes A, Winslow R, Forder J. Histological validation of myocardial microstructure obtained from diffusion tensor magnetic resonance imaging. *Am J Physiol Heart Circ Physiol* 1998;44:H2308–H2318

28. Gupta M, Rollins AM, Izatt JA, Efimov IR. Imaging of the atrioventricular node using optical coherence tomography. *J Cardiovasc Electrophysiol* 2002;13:95

29. LeGrice I, Sands G, Hooks D, Gerneke D, Smaill B. Microscopic imaging of extended tissue volumes. *Clin Exp Pharmacol Physiol* 2004;31:902–905

30. Franzone PC, Guerri L, Pennacchio M, Taccardi B. Spread of excitation in 3-D models of the anisotropic cardiac tissue. III. Effects of ventricular geometry and fiber structure on the potential distribution. *Math Biosci* 1998;151:51–98

31. Taccardi B, Macchi E, Lux RL, Ershler PR, Spaggiari S, Baruffi S, Vyhmeister Y. Effect of myocardial fiber direction on epicardial potentials. *Circulation* 1994;90:3076–3090

32. Franzone PC, Guerri L, Pennacchio M, Taccardi B. Anisotropic mechanisms for multiphasic unipolar electrograms: simulation studies and experimental recordings. *Ann Biomed Eng* 2000;28:1326–1342

33. Roth BJ, Lin SF, Wikswo JP. Unipolar stimulation of cardiac tissue. *J Electrocardiol* 1998;31:6–12

34. Trayanova NA, Roth BJ, Malden LJ. The Response of a spherical heart to a uniform electric-field – a bidomain analysis of cardiac stimulation. *IEEE Trans Biomed Eng* 1993;40:899–908

35. Miller WT, Geselowitz DB. Simulation studies of electrocardiogram. 2. Ischemia and infarction. *Circ Res* 1978;43:315–323

36. Sepulveda NG, Roth BJ, Wikswo JP Jr. Current injection into a two-dimensional anisotropic bidomain. *Biophys J* 1989;55:987–999

37. Wikswo JP, Lin SF, Abbas RA. Virtual electrodes in cardiac tissue: a common mechanism for anodal and cathodal stimulation. *Biophys J* 1995;69:2195–2210

38. Colli Franzone P, Guerri L, Taccardi B. Potential distributions generated by point stimulation in a myocardial volume: simulation studies in a model of anisotropic ventricular muscle. *J Cardiovasc Electrophysiol* 1993;4:438–458

39. Muzikant AL, Hsu EW, Wolf PD, Henriquez CS. Region specific modeling of cardiac muscle: comparison of simulated and experimental potentials. *Ann Biomed Eng* 2002;30:867–883

40. Spach MS, Barr RC. Effects of cardiac microstructure on propagating electrical waveforms. *Circ Res* 2000;86:E23–E28

41. Spach MS, Heidlage JF, Dolber PC, Barr RC. Extracellular discontinuities in cardiac muscle: evidence for capillary effects on the action potential foot. *Circ Res* 1998;83:1144–1164

42. Hooks DA, Tomlinson KA, Marsden SG, LeGrice IJ, Smaill BH, Pullan AJ, Hunter PJ. Cardiac microstructure – implications for electrical, propagation and defibrillation in the heart. *Circ Res* 2002;91:331–338

43. Hou TY, Wu XH. A multiscale finite element method for elliptic problems in composite materials and porous media. *J Comput Phys* 1997;134:169–189

44. Beard DA, Bassingthwaighte JB, Greene AS. Computational modeling of physiological systems. *Physiol Genomics* 2005;23:1–3

45. Trew ML, Caldwell BJ, Sands GB, Hooks DA, Tai DCS, Austin TM, LeGrice IJ, Pullan AJ, Smaill BH. Cardiac electrophysiology and tissue structure: bridging the scale gap with a joint measurement and modelling paradigm. *Exp Physiol* 2006;91:355–370

Chapter 5.2

Multielectrode Mapping of the Heart

Edward J. Berbari and Haris Sih

Introduction

Multielectrode cardiac mapping has at least a 50-year history in cardiac research, and the development of this methodology has closely followed the technological advances in instrumentation and computing. The methodology has proven to be quite effective in characterizing potential distributions on both the body surface and the epicardial surface of the heart.[1–4] However, the more challenging problem for multielectrode systems is the identification and display of cardiac activation or isochronal maps. In the earlier era of cardiac mapping, hardware limitations, particularly the speed of computer processing and digital data acquisition, were the major challenges for obtaining continuous data from a high number of recording channels. For the current generation of digital electronics and computers this is no longer a significant challenge. The analysis and interpretation of the data still pose a number of challenges, since in many cases, such as diseased myocardium or during complex tachyarrhythmias, the biophysical basis of conduction is not fully developed. For example, the use of contour-generation software often does not consider the actual nature of the underlying pathophysiology. Many standard interpolation algorithms will indeed create contours overlying scar tissue within infarcted regions. This is an inherent error.

A number of newer mapping approaches rely on mathematical models to create images based on data at some distance from the actual sources. In some cases these systems are proprietary and may have indeed conquered some long-standing problems. In other cases, because the systems produce "good looking" images that fit a preconceived model of activation, their underlying models are not challenged. This chapter focuses on the issues surrounding direct contact, multielectrode mapping approaches and will concentrate on the problems associated with producing activation maps, especially from regions surrounding and within infarct regions.

Edward J. Berbari
Department of Biomedical Engineering, Indiana University Purdue University, Indianapolis, IN, USA,
eberbari@iupui.edu
Haris Sih
St Jude Medical, Inc, St Paul, MN, USA

I. R. Efimov et al. (eds.), *Cardiac Bioelectric Therapy: Mechanisms and Practical Implications.*
© Springer Science+Business Media, LLC 2009

Methods

To acquire enough data from direct contact electrodes to produce an activation map of the entire three-dimensional extent of the entire heart would indeed be impossible. (This of course is the driving force behind the model-based approach alluded to above.) A system that records from hundreds or even thousands of sites requires an integrated system of hardware and software. Because the computer technology has advanced so rapidly in recent years, the computational component of the mapping problem is not a major concern. Additionally, the ready availability of high-capacity disk drives no longer limits the storage issues of long periods of continuous data acquisition. The number of channels used by the system will still drive the major cost of the system with relatively expensive analog amplifiers and high-count analog-to-digital converters. The authors have published previous reviews that provide a background for this chapter.[5,6]

Typically, activation mapping of the heart uses bipolar recording electrodes, while unipolar electrodes are used for isopotential mapping. These electrodes are often used in evenly spaced arrays overlying the epicardial surface in experimental studies, while many clinical studies rely on catheter-based electrodes and sequential placement of the catheter. Since all recordings are done differentially (i.e., with a respect to a reference electrode), the term unipolar refers to the situation where the reference is at some distance from the source of interest (>1 cm). This reference point is not critical. A bipolar measurement is between two electrodes that are often closely ($\leq$1 cm) spaced with respect to the source of interest. Often the activation time of the cells beneath the electrode needs to be determined. Criteria used to derive activation times from the recorded signals are discussed in detail below. For normal tissue the maximum negative derivative is the most widely used criterion for defining activation time in a unipolar electrogram. The most widely used criterion for bipolar electrograms is the peak of the main deflection.[7] Within infarct regions these criteria have been challenged.

Using either unipolar or bipolar electrodes, one can map sequentially from a single roving electrode or simultaneously from multiple electrodes along the length of a catheter or embedded in a hand probe. Such approaches have been used in both open chest (epicardial mapping) and endocardially using catheters. Such approaches do not require sophisticated, high-speed, multichannel digital acquisition systems; however, the actual maps are usually hand created and often do not provide reliable information. The visualization of cardiac activation requires knowledge of the anatomy and a good imagination to mentally reconstruct the sequence of activation. The use of multielectrode catheters placed under fluoroscopic guidance and the use of multichannel electrophysiology recording systems facilitate sequential mapping, but the mental reconstruction of activation is still an integral part of this process. Although obviously a useful clinical tool, sequential mapping relies on reproducible activation sequences and low spatial variation (i.e., low spatial frequency content) of activation and thus can be insufficient for some research applications.

Multielectrode array mapping entails simultaneously recording the electrical activity of the heart from a large number of sites (typically more than 100). Endocardial mapping can be accomplished with basket catheters that have electrodes placed on thin wire-like splines. When the catheter is inserted into a vein or artery, the splines are contracted to fit into the diameter of the catheter. Once the catheter is positioned in the chamber of interest, the splines are expanded like the opening of an umbrella, and the electrodes are exposed and hopefully in contact with the tissue. Although basket catheters allow for closed-chest, endocardial recordings, they are limited by several factors, including the lack of control over which electrodes are in contact with the tissue, unevenly spaced electrodes between splines, and the difficulty in precise anatomic location of the splines.

An epicardial approach avoids these issues, at least to some degree, at the expense of requiring an open-chest procedure. Often, but not always, epicardial electrode arrays are arranged in a regular grid pattern and are of varying construction and dimension. Since epicardial mapping is seldom used in the clinical setting, and since each experiment may require unique arrays, most epicardial arrays are made "in-house" with the materials and methods convenient to each researcher. Regardless of the construction, investigators minimally need to be aware of the contact quality between the electrodes and the tissue, the necessary interelectrode spacing, whether bipolar or unipolar electrodes are prudent, and the stability and reproducibility of the array placement. Regardless of whether endocardial or epicardial arrays are used, the hardware requirements are identical, generally consisting of a bank of amplifiers, filters, multiplexers, and analog-to-digital converters, and then some means to store the data to digital media.

As digital hardware speeds have gone up and their prices have come down, the conceivable number of simultaneous channels that can be acquired has increased. However, data management issues, such as electrogram display/review, activation visualization, and so forth, are more problematic with ever-increasing numbers of channels. These issues are especially troublesome when studying activation in a complex substrate such as regions within or surrounding an infarct and for studying rapid and irregular rhythms.

Determining Activation Time

The voltages recorded from the electrodes represent the sum of all potentials that are present throughout the heart at each instant of the cardiac cycle. They represent both locally generated potentials (e.g., from those cells in direct contact with the electrode) and the potentials from cells throughout the rest of the myocardium. This potential field is continuous in nature, meaning that there are no abrupt changes within the heart or on its surface. This is true even for the tissues and cells that are not excitable (e.g., blood and its constituent cells, blood vessels, connective tissue, scar tissue, and so forth), since they all have resistive properties that allow for the spread of the potential filed. Hence voltages measured from these unexcitable tissues will only reflect those potentials from distant depolarizing cells. Regardless of the algorithm used to determine a unique depolarization time, electrodes over these unexcitable cells will not have an activation time.

Following are data obtained from a 4-day-old canine infarction model[8] that has been excised and placed in a chamber with superfused Tyrode's solution. This model has been well documented as having a surviving epicardial layer of cells. However, it is not homogeneous and exhibits many of the problems of inexact activation time determination alluded to above.

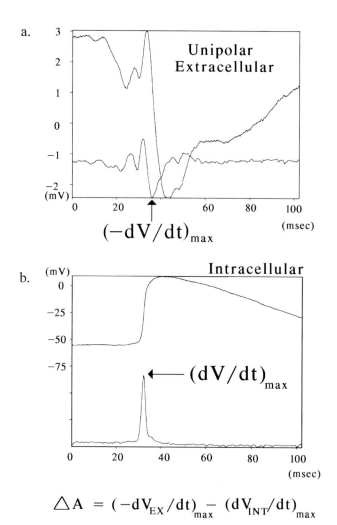

$$\triangle A \;=\; (-dV_{EX}/dt)_{max} - (dV_{INT}/dt)_{max}$$

Figure 1: The role of the derivative for determining activation time from a unipolar, extracellular recording as shown in the *top trace* of (**a**), and an intracellular microelectrode as shown in the *top trace* in (**b**). (**a**) The criterion for choosing the activation time is the maximum negative derivative. (**b**) The criterion is the maximum of the derivative

The most common criterion for determining activation time from a unipolar extracellular recording is to take the time derivative (dV/dt) and find its maximum negative value, as shown in Fig. 1a. The upper trace in this panel is an extracellular recording obtained from the canine infarction model. In this case it has a prominent intrinsic deflection. The lower trace is the derivative of this signal. The maximum negative value is shown at the arrow. In very close proximity to this extracellular recording a transmembrane potential, recorded with a microelectrode, was also obtained. Figure 1b shows such a transmembrane

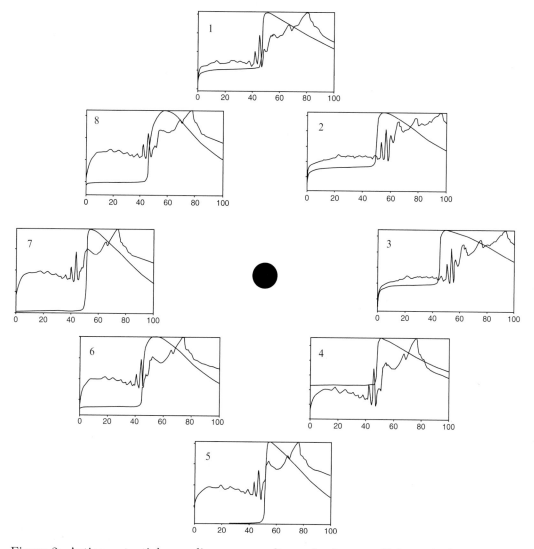

Figure 2: Action potential recordings surrounding a fixed extracellular unipolar recording (*black dot*) obtained from an in vitro preparation of canine infarct model. Each panel shows the multiphasic recording at the position of the *black dot*. All microelectrode recordings were obtained as close to this site as possible, and all cases were less than 1.0 mm. The maximum timing difference of the microelectrodes was measured at 18 ms between panels 2 and 7

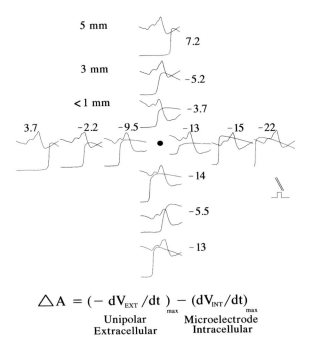

$$\triangle A = (- \, dV_{EXT}/dt \,)_{max} - (dV_{INT}/dt)_{max}$$

Unipolar   Microelectrode
Extracellular   Intracellular

Figure 3: Action potential recordings obtained from a similar infarct preparation as shown in Fig. 2. Each set of recordings shows the multiphasic extracellular recording obtained from a unipolar electrode at the *black dot*. This preparation was stimulated with bipolar electrodes at the approximate position in the lower right corner. The microelectrode recordings were obtained in a cross pattern at distances of less than 1, 3, and 5 mm. The number next to each panel represents the difference calculated by the formula at the *bottom* of the figure. The arc where the timing differences change sign is between the 3 and 5 mm recording sites in the upper-left set of recordings

potential in the top trace, and the bottom trace is the respective time derivative. The maximum time derivative is the most commonly used criterion for defining activation time from a microelectrode recording and is shown in this panel with an arrow. At the bottom of this figure is the formula for determining the difference between these separately obtained measures of activation. If indeed they represent the same population of cells, then this difference would be zero.

This concept was tested within the infarct region, and Figs. 2 and 3 are based on this approach. Figure 2 shows a series of eight panels each with the same unipolar extracellular recording obtained from the position in the center (black dot) and with a roving microelectrode recording obtained as close to this central electrode as possible (< 1 mm) and at the relative position around this electrode, as depicted by the position of each panel. Note the wide variation between the intrinsic deflections of the extracellular recording and the timing of the action potential upstroke. Within this 1-mm diameter there is a difference

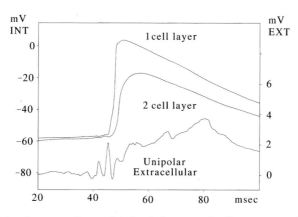

Figure 4: Microelectrode recordings obtained from a similar preparation as data in the previous figures. The *top trace* is the microelectrode recording from the first viable cell in the epicardial surface. The *second trace* is from the second cell layer, demonstrating an activation timing difference about 3 ms

of about 18 ms between the respective activation times. This demonstrates the difficulty in determining activation times within these infarct regions.

Figure 3 is from a similar preparation, but the roving microelectrode recording was obtained in a cross-like pattern. Again each panel has the extracellular recording and the transmembrane recording, and the panel position is the relative position of the microelectrode recording, less than 1, 3, and 5 mm. The central black dot is the site of the extracellular recording. The number next to each recording site represents the difference of the two activation times. Note that there are two places where the sign changes from negative to positive, and that it was assumed that between these sign changes is the position where the two activation times are equal to zero. From this one would conclude that using these traditional measures of activation time would result in an error of 3–5 mm. This is often times more than the spacing of electrodes in dense multielectrode systems.

To further complicate the issue of isochronal mapping in the infarct region Fig. 4 shows two microelectrode recordings in the upper two traces. In this case one was from the first layer of cells and the other was obtained during the same "stick" but advanced to the second layer of cells. Note that there is an approximate 3-ms difference in the timing of the upstrokes. This difference provides evidence that the activation wavefronts may not be perpendicular to the epicardial surface.

Most mapping studies of infarct regions will show electrograms that are highly ambiguous in nature. These electrograms are problematic since they often have a multiphasic or so-called fractionated appearance. Figure 5 demonstrates one such set of recordings. These were obtained from unipolar recordings spaced 2 mm apart and placed over an infarct region during an in vitro study. In the top left corner of the map, the unipolar recordings show fairly typical biphasic electrograms. Recordings in the bottom section of the map, however, are fractionated. Over a distance as small as 2 mm, the character of an electrogram changes dramatically, from unambiguous to highly fractionated. It would appear that

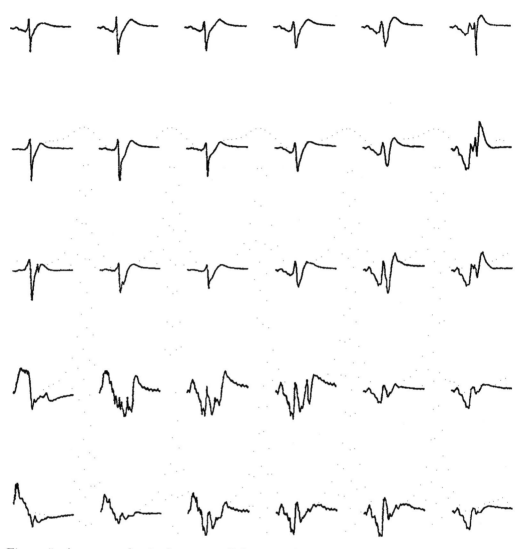

Figure 5: An array of unipolar extracellular recordings obtained from a plaque electrode placed over the epicardial infarct region obtained during an in vitro study. Each electrode was spaced 2 mm apart. Note the relatively normal, single intrinsicoid recordings in the *upper/left* portion of the recording set and the multiphasic (multiple intrinsic) deflections in the lower/right portion of the recording set

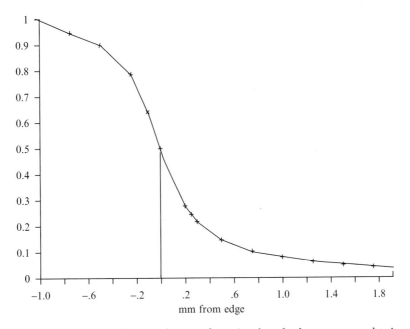

Figure 6: Plot of the normalized voltage of a simulated electrogram obtained from a 2-mm long activation wavefront over a thin layer model of the ventricle as function of the lateral distance away from the recoding site. At −1.0 mm the wavefront is centered under the recording site. At 0.0 mm the edge of the wavefront is at the recording site. Greater negative values further remove the wavefront from the recording site

no mathematical formula could identify the actual activation time for these multiphasic recordings. Other explanations, beyond the scope of this chapter, would point to a different biophysical basis for these recordings based on the role of passive cell coupling.

Biophysical models can help explain other common expressions heard in electrophysiologic recording jargon such as "How far does the electrode see?" A study by Geselowitz et al.[9] modeled activation wavefronts and used a 2-mm long wavefront to determine the relative voltage amplitude recorded as the wavefront moved progressively to the side of the recording electrode. Figure 6 is the plot of this normalized voltage versus distance to the side of the electrode. Note that when the horizontal scale is zero the edge of the 2-mm long wavefront is just at the electrode site. As this number becomes increasingly positive the wavefront is no longer under the electrode, and at a distance of 1 mm the amplitude is decreased by 90% of the original normalized voltage. Hence in answer to the above question a unipolar recording will not "see" much beyond a few millimeters for small sources. Applying this knowledge to the bottom two rows of recordings in Fig. 5 one would argue that these multiphasic waveforms are not likely from multiple sources at distances greater than 1 mm.

Generating Contours

Although several studies have been performed to correlate activation times to extracellular electrogram features, little has been studied about the mechanics of contour generation for activation maps. Some investigators use a visual approach and manually draw the maps. Others use "canned" contour programs available in scientific subroutine software libraries, and still others use custom written software. Only a few references exist on the mechanics of contour generation as applied to cardiac activation.[1–4] The field of cartography has evolved around and is usually applied to geophysical problems,[10,11] and it include methods employing minimum least square fitting. It is difficult to determine to what extent these methods have been used in either the published reports or from commercial vendors in cardiac applications.

It is our premise that many conclusions about activation sequences have been deduced from poorly constructed contour maps. Some general issues have been discussed by Ideker et al.[12] In essence, a fundamental assumption about the underlying structure of activation is implicitly or explicitly made without regard to problems concerning spatial sampling or the assumption of spatial continuity. However, there have been few formal attempts to define the spatial sampling necessary for cardiac activation maps.[13] Spatial continuity is the two-dimensional property similar to time domain continuity. Most linear mathematical approaches to signal processing require that there be no abrupt changes in the values of the measured quantity; that is, the time derivatives are not infinite. This is also true for the two-dimensional problem where the spatial derivatives are not infinite. Put into other terms, no point in the spatial representation can be multivalued. Unfortunately, mapping in infarct regions almost ensures discontinuous regions. The inhomogeneity in conduction properties is well known, and the presence of dead tissue (i.e., nonconducting regions) must be accounted for in the contour generation process. In geophysical terms, such discontinuities are called faults, and generating contours around a fault region should be considered in cardiac map generation.

Contour generation can be done by hand. It obviously interjects an element of bias, but more importantly it does not allow for a mathematical description of the data. Such descriptions allow the use of transformations such as directional derivatives, smoothing with two-dimensional filters, and the measurement of error in the contours when compared to the actual underlying data. At this stage, the values chosen from the individual raw data waveforms would be considered unambiguous. The next assumption in contour generation is that the spatial sampling is adequate. The previous discussion implied that at present there is no known way to ensure this since the minimum wavefront length is not known. The next assumption in contour generation is that the data fit some underlying mathematical structure. The simplest structure is the linear model assumed by simple triangulation methods. In essence this assumes that if a straight line connects the sample data points, the values under the line vary linearly between the two points. Triangulation has several drawbacks in that there is no physiologic basis for the linear assumption, and that depending on how the data points are linked, there is no unique solution. For unevenly spaced recording sites, there are many ways in which the data points can be linked. There are no a priori

Table 1: Example Data Points and Coordinates

	X	Y	D	V	V/D
Grid	2	3			
Data A	1.5	3.6	0.78	6	7.69
Data B	3.0	3.0	1.0	6	6.00
Data C	2.0	2.4	0.6	7	11.67
Data D	1.0	2.9	1.0	7	7.0

restrictions on the formation of triangles as the data in the entire region are linked together. Older software algorithms were even susceptible to the order of data entry. Hence, in the early 1970s, triangulation fell into disuse by cartographers as the method is not well defined. More recently, some efforts have been made to regularize the triangulation methods, but other more mathematically based methods are favored.

Gridding is a method whereby the data points (usually unevenly spaced) are converted to an underlying, evenly spaced set of points. The grid can be defined to have many more points than the sample points. The value assigned to each intersecting grid line can be a linear combination (e.g., an average) of nearest data points. The term "nearest" can be defined in a radial sense (e.g., all data points within 5 mm). Alternatively, using the radial search criterion, the grid value can be weighted with a distance measure. Thus, data points closer to the grid point will have a larger influence in calculating the grid value than data points farther away. Much of what has been said can be more succinctly stated in mathematical terms:

$$\overline{V}_G = \frac{\sum_{i=1}^{4} (V_i/D_{iG})}{\sum_{i=1}^{4} (1/D_{iG})}. \tag{1}$$

Here, $\overline{V}_G$ is the value computed at the gridded data point, V_i are the values at the four original data points, and D_{iG} are the distances from those original data points to the new grid point. For a more intuitive approach, however, these concepts can be described graphically with a set of simulated data points. Figure 7 has six panels. Figure 7a shows a set of irregularly spaced data points with values ranging from 5 to 8. Figure 7b is a regularly spaced grid, with the open circles at the line intersections representing the new underlying grid points. Figure 7c demonstrates the variable spacing between the data and grid points by overlapping Fig. 7a and 7b. Figure 7d is an example of one grid point and its four surrounding nearest neighbors. The simplest way to evaluate the value of the grid point is to average the surrounding data points. This value is 6.5. However, one can also use the weighting approach described by (1). Table 1 shows the actual coordinates and data points for this problem.

Substituting values into (1), $\overline{V}_G = (7.69 + 6.0 + 11.67 + 7.0)/4.95 = 6.54$. In this example, the calculation is very close to the simple average of 6.5. The rest of the grid points, to one decimal point, are shown in Fig. 7f. Now that the data have been converted to a

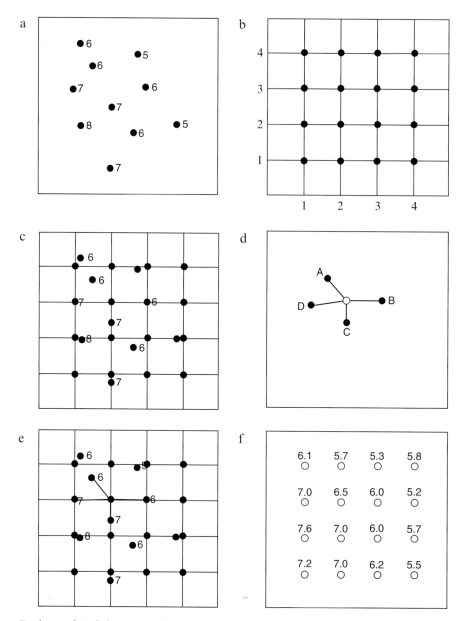

Figure 7: A graphical depiction of generating a grid of evenly spaced data points from a set of nonuniformly spaced data points (see the text for a full description)

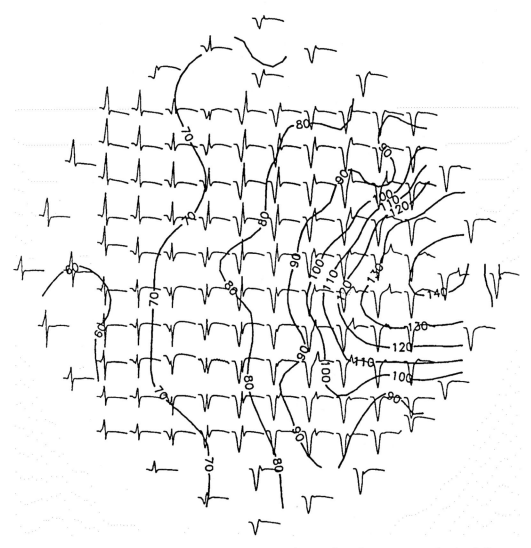

Figure 8: An activation map overlying the set of unipolar electrograms obtained from a grid (4 mm spacing in the central 10 × 10 grid, greater spacing distances along each edge) of electrodes obtained from a canine infarct model in vivo. This set of electrodes was analyzed with late potential activation times as the primary mapped isochrones

regularized grid, many types of operations can be performed. The method of deriving the contours can be based on one of many different schemes, such as cubic spline fitting or even linear interpolations. Many schemes can be used in forming the grid. For example, one could require that there be data points in all four quadrants surrounding the grid point, except in the case of boundary grid points. Krige[14] proposed a statistically based method that

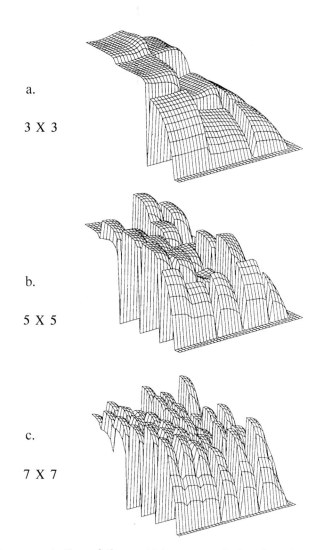

Figure 9: Visual representation of the spatial autocorrelation function with an increasing analysis grid size ($\mathbf{a} = 3 \times 3$ set of data points, $\mathbf{b} = 5 \times 5$, and $\mathbf{c} = 7 \times 7$). The relative amplitude of these data represents higher levels of correlation among the underlying data points

minimizes the variance of data points that coincide with or are very close to the grid points. This minimum variance method, often referred to as Kriging, now allows for estimates of error in the map. Detailed discussion of this is beyond the scope of this chapter, but in essence such a statistical approach would allow for the generation of an optimal map and clear delineation of regions with the highest uncertainty.

An example of gridding to generate an activation map over the infarct is shown in Fig. 8. The underling electrograms are shown at each recording site, spaced approximately 4 mm apart. The isochronal lines were derived from a uniform and Kriged grid where the data from each electrogram were assumed to be spatially continuous (no dead inactive regions), and where each electrogram has a unique activation time.[15,16] Each isochrone represents 10 ms, with early activation on the left and late activation on the right. The specifics of timing are not considered, and the emphasis is on the actual generation of the contour lines. It is a first-order polynomial approximation and assumes uniform, constant velocity, conduction. It was derived from the grid.

The creation of a contour map that takes into consideration a faulted region (e.g., dead nonconducting tissue) is another example of how a gridded structure can be used. It is not enough to just declare that an electrogram site generates no activation time. Without a clear definition of a fault zone, most algorithms will simply interpolate across the dead tissue. The drawing of an isochrone or the inclusion of a data point in the interpolation that is "across" the fault should be considered an invalid approach. It is not known how this has been dealt with in prior studies.

One solution to this sense of uncertainty is to understand the degree to which the data points to be contoured are related. Theoretically only data that are highly correlated can be interpolated with a high degree of confidence. If the data points are not correlated, then interpolating among them is not a valid exercise. The use of correlation functions is widely used in many applications when comparing data sets. A similar two-dimensional approach for studying spatial correlation of data points is also possible and in particular the spatial-autocorrelation function can be used to assess the degree to which the surrounding data are correlated. The details of this approach in cardiac mapping are beyond the scope of this chapter.[13] Figure 9 was obtained from the data that were contoured in Fig. 8. There are three panels in this figure, each obtained with different regional resolution. Figure 8a performed the spatial autocorrelation function around a 3×3 set of data points; Fig. 8b used a 5×5 set; Fig. 8c used a 7×7 set. The feature to recognize in these panels is the lower amplitudes to the right-center portion of the figure. This is the region of the late potentials and was the most uncertain point of defining the late activation times. Hence the spatial autocorrelation function can be used to highlight the regions of greatest uncertainty in a contour map. As one might attempt to interpret contour-generated data, the information from the autocorrelation function could bolster or temper the level of confidence of the interpretation, much as one does with the correlation coefficient of one-dimensional data.

Conclusion

The question may be asked, "Why are these details about map generation important?" Most of the theories regarding cardiac activation and arrhythmogenesis are derived from the visual examination of contour maps. However, there has been very little attention given to the creation of these maps. Even if the problems of selecting activation times from the electrograms are solved, the validity of the mapping assumptions has not been critically examined. It is quite possible to generate visually different maps, all correct according to their mathematical basis, from the same data sets. Hence, differences of interpretation concerning a particular activation sequence may in fact be due to different algorithms used in contour generation rather than the underlying pathophysiology.

The methods used to generate a contour map should be examined in greater detail as it applies to cardiac mapping. Investigators must become cognizant of various methods and the strengths and weaknesses of these approaches. Until that time, the conclusions drawn from contour maps should be tempered so that investigators can develop the technical skills to deal with the problems associated with the data presentation. Various mapping approaches will change the interpretation of the data, and greater care must be taken in presenting the methods used and the impact these methods have on interpretation.

The interpolation of activation times is perhaps the greatest possible source of error in creating activation maps from infarcted regions of the heart. Because there can be dead or nonactivating regions, one can never assign a valid activation time to such regions due to the discontinuity of activation that this implies. A more accurate method would be to consider interpolating the isopotential data, as there are no discontinuities. The role of the spatial autocorrelation function would provide a level of confidence when dealing with uncertain data.

References

1. Barr RC, Gallie TM, Spach MS. Automated production of contour maps for electrophysiology: I. Problem definition, solution strategy, and specification of geometric model. *Comput Biomed Res* 1980;13:142–153
2. Barr RC, Gallie TM, Spach MS. Automated production of contour maps for electrophysiology: III. Construction of contour maps. *Comput Biomed Res* 1980;13:171–191
3. Barr RC, Gallie TM, Spach MS. Automated production of contour maps for electrophysiology: II. Triangulation, verification, and organization of the geometric model. *Comput Biomed Res* 1980;13:154–170
4. Monro DM. Interpolation methods for surface mapping. *Comput Programs Biomed* 1980;11:145–157
5. Berbari EJ, Lander P, Geselowitz DB, Scherlag BJ, Lazzara R. The methodology of cardiac mapping. In: Breithardt G, Borgreffe M, Shenasa M, eds. *Cardiac Mapping*. Armonk, NY: Futura; 1993:63–79
6. Sih H, Berbari EJ. The methodology of cardiac mapping. In: Breithardt G, Borgreffe M, Shenasa M, eds. *Cardiac Mapping*, 2nd edn. Armonk, NY: Futura; 2003:41–58
7. Biermann M, Shenasa M, Borggrefe M, Hindricks G, Haverkamp W, Breithardt G. The interpretation of cardiac electrograms. In: Breithardt G, Borgreffe M, Shenasa M, eds. *Cardiac Mapping*. Armonk, NY: Futura; 1993:11–34
8. Scherlag BJ, El-Sherif N, Hope R, Lazzara R. Characterization and localization of ventricular arrhythmias resulting from myocardial ischemia and infarction. *Circ Res* 1974;35:372–383

9. Geselowitz DB, Smith S, Mowrey K, Berbari EJ. Model studies of extracellular electrograms arising from an excitation wave propagating in a thin layer. *IEEE Trans Biomed Eng* 1991;38:526–531

10. Robinson JE. *Computer Applications in Petroleum Geology*. New York: Van Nostrand Reinhold; 1982

11. Davis JC. *Statistics and Data Analysis*. New York: Wiley; 1986

12. Ideker RE, Smith WM, Blanchard SM, Reiser SL, Simpson EV, Wolf PD, Danieley ND. The assumptions of isochronal cardiac mapping. *Pacing Clin Electrophysiol* 1989;12:456–478

13. Ramachandran D, Berbari EJ, Lander P. Comparison of interpolation methods used in epicardial activation map. In: *Computers in Cardiology*. Los Alamitos, CA: IEEE Computer Society Press; 1993:129–136

14. Krige DG. Two dimensional weighted moving average trend surfaces for ore evaluation. *J S Afr Inst Min Metall* 1966;13:3815

15. Berbari EJ, Lander P, Geselowitz DB. A cardiac mapping system for identifying late potentials: correlation with signal averaged surface recordings. *Comput Cardiol* 1988:369–372

16. Berbari EJ, Lander P, Scherlag BJ, Lazzara R, Geselowitz DB. Ambiguities of epicardial mapping. *J Electrocardiol* 1992;24(Suppl):16–20

Chapter 5.3

The Role of Electroporation

Vladimir P. Nikolski and Igor R. Efimov

Abstract A therapeutical application of electrical current to cardiac tissue for reviving the normal function (defibrillation, pacing) or for ablating pathological conduction pathways inevitably has to take into account the phenomenon of electroporation, the electric field–induced rupture of sarcolemma that is usually evidenced by a drastic unselective increase in cell membrane permeability to small ions and large molecules. This chapter describes some aspects of this phenomenon in relation to cardiac therapy and research. Particularly, it provides evidences that (1) electroporation of the heart tissue can occur during clinically relevant intensities of the external electrical field and (2) electroporation can affect the outcome of defibrillation therapy, being both pro- and antiarrhythmic.

Role of Electroporation in Defibrillation

Defibrillation has become first-line therapy for cardiac tachyarrhythmias. However, despite a century of research, basic mechanisms of defibrillation remain debatable. An issue of major controversy is the role of electroporation in success or failure of defibrillation. In particular, it remains a subject of hot debate whether electroporation is pro- or antiarrhythmic in clinical settings.

Discovery of defibrillation by Prevost and Battelli[1] resulted from observation of transient incapacitation of myocardium caused by strong electric shock with intensities above a certain threshold. Incapacitation was evident as complete halt of electrical activity in the heart. Prevost and Battelli were successful in induction of fibrillation by small intensity shocks, following the protocols of Vulpian[2] and Hoffa and Ludwig,[3] as well as in arresting ventricular fibrillation by "faradization" or strong electrical discharge. Although electroporation was not known at the time of this seminal discovery, it is reasonable to assume that the observed incapacitation was associated with electroporation. Based on their experimental observations, Prevost and Battelli formulated a theory of defibrillation, according to which fibrillation

Vladimir P. Nikolski

CRDM Research, Medtronic, Inc., Minneapolis, MN, USA, vladimir.p.nikolski@medtronic.com

I. R. Efimov et al. (eds.), *Cardiac Bioelectric Therapy: Mechanisms and Practical Implications.*
© Springer Science+Business Media, LLC 2009

stops due to shock-induced transient incapacitation of myocardium. Many investigators of the first half of twentieth century have adhered to the theory that electrical therapy treats by temporarily suppressing cardiac electrical function, resulting in cessation of any activity including fibrillation for seconds until excitability is recovered.[4] Initial experience of defibrillation in animal models of sudden cardiac death and in clinical settings required application of direct heart massage due to depression of cardiac electrical and mechanical function, which followed the incapacitating shock.[5] Thus, incapacitation, which is likely to result from electroporation, was associated with antiarrhythmic effects and was successfully used in clinical practice.

On the other hand, experimental evidence from isolated papillary muscle,[6] cell,[7] and cell culture[8] suggests that electroporation can be proarrhythmic, resulting in short bursts of focal activity. Such bursts have also been observed clinically[9] and in vivo.[10] Yet their role in reinducing ventricular fibrillation remains to be determined. For example, Osswald et al.[10] observed that "such brief runs of accelerated junctional rhythm or ideoventricular rhythm . . . terminated spontaneously within a few seconds" and "none of them induced VF." Gurvich[9] characterized each defibrillation waveform not only by its defibrillation threshold (DFT), the main measure of efficacy, but also by the injury threshold (IT), which was measured as minimal intensity of shocks inducing brief runs of extrasystolic activity. He postulated that a clinically applicable waveform must have a large window between DFT and IT, or large ratio IT:DFT. However, some waveforms, applied in the early age of defibrillation had unacceptably low ratio IT:DFT. For example alternating current (AC) defibrillation waveform, which was used by Beck et al.[5] in the first clinically successful case of defibrillation, had a ratio below 1.[9] Thus, shock-induced injury was associated with successful defibrillation by such AC waveforms.

Subsequent improvement of safety and efficacy of defibrillation therapy resulted in drastic reduction of electromechanical dysfunction associated with electric shock, with an electroporation being considered as an undesirable adverse effect. This improvement of defibrillation therapy was primarily due to optimization of defibrillation waveforms and lead configurations resulting from hard work of several generations of basic and clinical electrophysiologists. Gurvich and Yuniev[11] introduced monophasic critically damped sine waveform to replace less efficient AC defibrillation[5] based on his estimates of DFT and IT. Subsequently he introduced an optimized biphasic waveform to replace the monophasic waveform, due to its lower DFT and higher IT.[9] Having observed a significant reduction of damaging effects of defibrillation, Gurvich and his colleages[11–13] formulated "stimulatory" theory of defibrillation, suggesting that "momentary electrical stimulation of the fibrillating heart" by a shock abolishes fibrillation by "synchronization of separate heart elements"[14] rather than incapacitation of myocardium. Gurvich acknowledged that defibrillation also had a suppressive effect on cardiac function, which may be injurious, and thus necessitated limiting the magnitude of shock current.

Since its original formulation,[9,11] the stimulatory theory of defibrillation was significantly advanced by several generations of investigators.[15–18] Present understanding of defibrillation has been extensively reviewed recently.[17–19] Despite some degree of disagreement on the theory of defibrillation, it appears to be generally accepted that the following effects of defibrillation shock are necessary in order to succeed: (1) shock must extinguish all or a critical number of fibrillation wavefronts;[20] (2) shock must not induce a new fibrillation by creating new reentrant circuits or ectopic foci.[21]

Extinguishing the wavefronts that support fibrillation is achieved through (1) depolarization of myocardium by either inducing active response in excitable areas of fibrillating myocardium or extending the refractory period of unexcitable myocardium;[9,22] (2) deexcitation[23] of myocardium with subsequent reexcitation[24] upon shock withdrawal via break excitation[25] or via application of the second phase of biphasic shock with a smaller amplitude.[23]

However, in addition to the ability to extinguish arrhythmia, shock is known to be able to induce fibrillation[3,26,27] via mechanisms not related to electroporation. Therefore, the same shock that succeeded in extinguishing ongoing fibrillation can induce new fibrillation. There are several theories of such induction. According to the virtual electrode-induced phase singularity theory,[18,23] defibrillation shock induces virtual electrode polarization, which is characterized by the presence of shock-induced transmembrane polarization of both positive and negative polarities. As a result, the proximity of the two oppositely polarized regions can produce wavefronts of break-excitation and phase singularities, also known as virtual electrode-induced phase singularity.[23] Degeneration of such phase singularities into sustained arrhythmia leads to defibrillation failure.[23,28]

Most likely these two theories of defibrillation, namely, the incapacitation theory and the stimulation theory, are extreme in their assessment of the role of electroporation. One places electroporation as the foundation of mechanisms of defibrillation, while the other ignores its role in defibrillation. The truth is likely to be in the middle. Indeed, despite significant improvement in defibrillation efficacy, which resulted in radical reduction of defibrillation thresholds and myocardial damage, there is still extensive clinical and basic electrophysiology data indicating that defibrillation shocks are accompanied with adverse effects, which are likely to be associated with electroporation. These adverse effects are (1) transient ectopy, tachycardia, or induction of ventricular fibrillation;[8,29,30] (2) depression of electrical and mechanical functions;[6,31–34] (3) bradycardia, complete heart block, and increased pacing thresholds;[30,35,36] (4) atrial and ventricular mechanical dysfunction (stunning), which is directly related to the strength of shocks;[37–40] (5) significant elevation of troponin I serum level in patients after spontaneous implantable cardioverter defibrillator shocks;[41] (6) decrease of the myocardial lactate extraction rate by mitochondria;[10] and (7) ST segment elevation.[35,42]

Profibrillatory effects of electroporation and tissue damage are supported by clinical observations of postshock ectopy and arrhythmia, reviewed above, as well as by basic studies, including classical studies of Gurvich[9] as well as several recent studies.[6,8,43] Antifibrillatory effects of electroporation were made known with the seminal work of Prevost and Battelli.[1] Animal experimental data also support antifibrillatory effects of electroporation.[33] Figures 1 and 2 show that strong electroporating shock reduces vulnerability to shock-induced arrhythmia applied during a period of electroporation. Figure 1 shows an example of preconditioning with strong electroporating shock in one heart. As seen in the upper trace, a single test shock applied during the vulnerable phase of an action potential induces a sustained arrhythmia (gray bar). Application of a preconditioning shock with the peak voltage equal to the defibrillation threshold voltage ($\times 1$ DFT) creates the conditions for

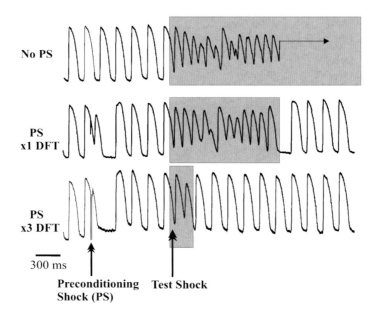

Figure 1: Preconditioning with electroporating shock reduces shock-induced vulnerability (see text for detail). PS, preconditioning shock; DFT, defibrillation threshold. Traces show optically recorded action potential from left ventricular epicardium

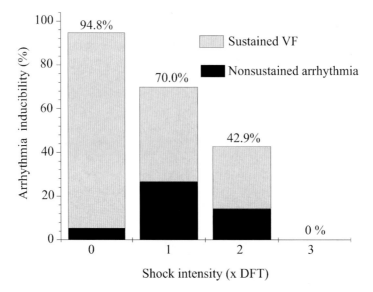

Figure 2: Inducibility of ventricular fibrillation by T-wave shock versus preconditioning shock applied 1,200 or 1,500 ms prior to that shock. Preconditioning shock peak intensity is expressed as 0×, 1×, 2×, and 3× defibrillation threshold voltages

the induction of a short nonsustained arrhythmia by a subsequent test shock. Finally, an application of a shock with a voltage three times larger then DFT ($3 \times$ DFT) prevented the induction of the arrhythmia, allowing only one extra-beat posttest shock.

A summary of the statistics for these experiments[33] is shown in Figure 2 test shock applied during the T wave induces arrhythmias in 94.8% cases without a preconditioning shock (left bar). Most of them are sustained (gray bar). Application of the preconditioning shock with the peak voltage equal to DFT reduces inducibility to 70%. Application of the electroporating preconditioning shock with the peak voltage equal to $3 \times$ DFT completely eliminates vulnerability.

Electroporation has a lesser effect on transthoracic defibrillation because of the relative uniformity of voltage gradients inside the heart as compared to the intracardiac shocks. There was no elevation in troponin T and only a slight increase in troponin I in a few patients after transthoracic cardioversions with shocks up to 360 J.[44] In other study troponin I did not show any significant changes at all.[45] Direct measurements of the electrical field inside the heart during the delivery of 120–360 J shocks from external defibrillators in swine animal model[46] showed that the maximum voltage gradients are around $20 \, \text{V/cm}^{-1}$. This is less than 60–$70 \, \text{V/cm}^{-1}$ that caused conduction block in previous studies[34] and consequently should not cause significant electroporation effects in the ventricles (the recent data suggest that the electroporation threshold for an atrial tissue can be two to five times smaller than in the ventricle[47]). At the same time during intracardiac defibrillation the potential gradient near the electrode had to be almost $200 \, \text{V/cm}^{-1}$ to guarantee the electrical field strength greater than 6–$7 \, \text{V/cm}^{-1}$ throughout the whole myocardium, which is necessary for successful defibrillation.[48] As a result an intracardiac defibrillation is likely to induce electroporation of the endocardial structures located in the vicinity of the shock electrode.

Experiments on isolated rabbit heart showed that the endocardium is significantly more susceptible to electroporation than the epicardium.[49] Electroporation can selectively affect small trabeculated structures and bundles of the conduction system of the heart while sparing the bulk of the ventricular wall.[33] This could result in transient suppression of excitability and conduction block.[34] Conduction in a small papillary muscle in the rabbit heart can be transiently inhibited by a strong electric shock, and such transient block can last from one beat to many seconds, depending on the shock strength.[33,50] Potentially, such transient inhibition of conduction in bundles of the heart can lead to initiation of a reentrant or focal arrhythmia, or on the other hand, can have an antiarrhythmic effect via isolation of ectopic foci and the reduction of tissue mass available for arrhythmia maintenance. Recent study has shown that endocardial bundles may create focal sites of abnormal automaticity or triggered activity during ventricular fibrillation.[51] If such bundles, being more prone to electroporation, are located close enough to the defibrillation electrode, then the shock-induced electroporation could suppress ectopic foci or small-sized reentrant cores that otherwise may lead to defibrillation failure.

In summary, both clinical and basic experimental evidence suggests that electroporation is induced[52] by defibrillation shocks and plays a role in defibrillation[53] as well as in postshock metabolism and electromechanical function of the heart. However, the antifibrillatory role of electroporation remains controversial, since conflicting data suggest both pro- and antiarrhythmic effects of electroporation.[17,19]

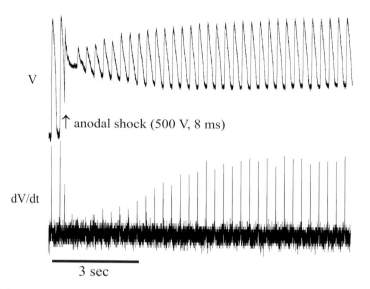

Figure 3: Evidence of shock-induced electroporation. Optical recording of transmembrane potential V (*upper trace*) shows time-dependent postshock reduction of resting potential and action potential amplitude. Maximal upstroke rate of rise (dV/dt) is also reduced and slowly recovers after shocks (*lower trace*)

Contribution of Electroporation to Optically Recorded Cellular Responses

Direct real-time recording or visualization of electroporation for in vivo or in vitro tissue or organ system remains to be developed. Presently, the information about electroporation can be indirectly inferred from (1) the staining of the tissue with fluorescent dyes that can penetrate the cells only through the pores and subsequent histological imaging of intracellular space and (2) from electroporation-induced depression of excitability, resulting in depolarization of cellular membrane during diastolic interval,[6,7,32,33] reduction of amplitude of action potentials and of the rate of rise of upstroke (dV/dt)max, and elevation of intracellular calcium concentration.[7] Understanding the effects of electroporation at the cardiac tissue or whole heart level during application of an external electric field is much less developed than for single cell experiments. One of the problems of such experiments is related to the strong spatial heterogeneity of electroporation effects, which complicate their interpretation.[6,32,33,54]

Optical mapping technique revealed evidence of diastolic depolarization in both ventricles and atria in response to strong electric shocks. Figure 3 shows an example of such reversible elevation of resting potential, reduction of dV/dt, and action potential amplitude in ventricles of rabbit heart after shock of high intensity. Electroporation, which is responsible for these effects in the rabbit model of defibrillation, manifests itself at shock intensities above the defibrillation threshold.[33]

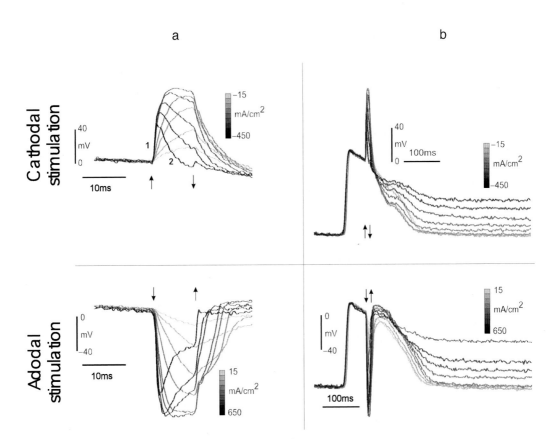

Figure 4: Optical recording of transmembrane potential transients under the electrode during stimulation with different current densities. (a, b) show the same data at small and large time scales. *Arrows* mark stimulus onset and withdrawal. Current strength is gray-scale coded. Electroporation is evident from saturation of ΔV_m and elevation of the postshock diastolic potential

Spatiotemporal patterns and voltage dependence of electroporation were studied in several types of preparations, such as the whole, intact Langendorff-perfused heart,[33,55] the isolated endocardium and septum preparations,[49] and 6-mm diameter areas of epicardium under the stimulating electrode.[56] In these studies it was found that electroporation is dependent on shock intensity, tissue structure, and electrode configuration. Optically recorded membrane potential transients were multiphasic, consisting of relatively slow (#2) and fast (#1) components (Fig 4a.)

Such kinetics were reported earlier by several groups of investigators who interpreted this morphology of shock response as evidence of existence of a hyperpolarization-activated ionic channel.[57,58] However, the shock-induced electroporation could be a more plausible explanation because it induces diastolic depolarization, regardless of the polarity of the shock and the shock-induced response. Figure 4 shows the responses to anodal and cathodal stimuli shown at different time scales, in order to illustrate shock response (Fig. 4a, at 10-ms scale) and postshock resting potential elevation (Fig. 4b, at 100-ms scale). Shocks of moderate intensity (light gray lines), which do not produce postshock elevation of resting potential (Fig. 4b), result in depolarizing or hyperpolarizing exponential responses during application of the shocks (Fig. 4a). Strong shocks resulting in reversal of depolarization or hyperpolarization during shock application (dark lines in Fig. 4a) also show clear postshock diastolic depolarization (dark lines in Fig. 4b).

Electroporation Assessment by Membrane Impermeable Dye Diffusion

Previously mentioned results used the changes in optical action potentials as a surrogate to estimate electroporation. However, a shock-induced facilitation of transport of macromolecules across the cell membrane is the most convincing indicator of electroporation. The poration of the rabbit heart was assessed more directly by recording *propidium iodide* (PI) uptake.[56] In this study shocks were applied at the rabbit epicardium from 6-mm diameter electrode. The upper panel of Fig. 5 shows PI fluorescence recorded inside the stimulated area (solid line) and 3 mm outside the stimulated area (dashed line). At the start of perfusion with $30 \mu M$ PI there was an initial rapid increase of PI fluorescence. In 10–15 min it reached the plateau. After strong shock application ($1,600 \, \text{mA/cm}^{-2}$, 20 ms, marked with an arrow) there was an accelerated accumulation of fluorophore in the tissue under the electrode but not outside the electrode. PI was allowed to accumulate for 10 min. After that PI was washed out from the heart for 30 min, the heart was frozen in embedding media and cryosectioned. The lower panel of Fig. 5 shows the low- and high-resolution images of a 20-μm slice sectioned throughout the stimulated area. The electroporated region is clearly demarcated by the PI stained nuclei.

To relate the changes in optical potentials to the PI uptake the heart was dual stained with PI and voltage sensitive dye RH237. RH237 and PI fluorescence was collected at the same spot beneath the electrode. Figure 6 shows that the $15 \, \text{V/cm}^{-1}$ ($300 \, \text{mA/cm}^{-2}$) shocks caused neither diastolic optical potential elevation (gray traces on an upper graph) nor PI fluorescence increase (nonrising trace on lower graph after $\pm 15 \, \text{V/cm}^{-1}$ mark). The $35 \, \text{V/cm}^{-1}$ ($700 \, \text{mA/cm}^{-2}$) shocks caused diastolic potential elevation (black traces on the upper graph) and onset of PI fluorescence increase (rising trace after $\pm 35 \, \text{V/cm}^{-1}$ mark on lower graph). No shock-induced PI fluorescence increase was observed 3 mm outside the electrode edge after $35 \, \text{V/cm}^{-1}$ shock. Histological evaluation of the same tissue slice cut through the center of stimulated area (right panels) showed that PI staining was localized at the cell nuclei near the epicardium in the area adjacent to the electrode, confirming occurrence of electroporation.

Despite the fact that cell electropermeabilization is already a routine technique, the complete understanding of its mechanisms remains to be formulated. The most fundamental questions remain unknown: What is the size and density of pores created by the shock, do pores grow after the shock, and what is the time of their resealing? In experiments

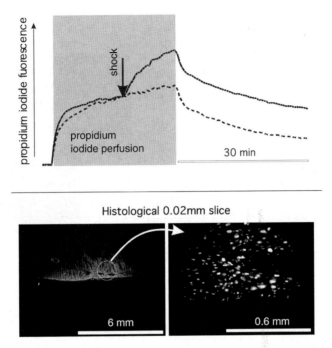

Figure 5: Uptake of membrane impermeable dye propidium iodide after a strong shock. *Upper panel* shows the initial increase of propidium iodide fluorescence after beginning of perfusion recorded inside the stimulating hole and 3 mm outside the hole. After shock application ($1,600\,\mathrm{mA/cm^{-2}}$, 20 ms) there was an accelerated accumulation of fluorophore in the tissue inside the hole. *Lower panel* shows the fluorescent images made with 4× and 40× lenses for a 20-μm slice sectioned throughout the stimulated area. Electroporated region is clearly demarcated by the propidium iodide–stained cell nuclei

with propidium iodide there was no immediate PI fluorescence increase during the shock.[56] It suggests that the amount of PI molecules that penetrated through the electroporation holes during the 20-ms stimulus was undetectable in this protocol. This also explains why there was no difference in PI uptake for shocks of different polarities despite the positive charge of the PI molecule. Slow diffusion of PI into the cells takes place when the external electrical field is already turned off, thus fluorescence is continuously rising after the shock during dye perfusion in whole heart experiments,[56] as it did in cell culture studies.[59] These data suggest that electroporated cells were repaired within minutes rather than seconds. Potentially, optically recorded diastolic potential (DP) elevation might be a more sensitive indicator of electroporation than PI uptake because DP elevation can be detected within 1 s after shock application. However, this method cannot be used in depth of three-dimensional tissues.

Although PI is used widely in electroporation research, these studies are usually conducted on cell suspensions. There were concerns that this molecule may not be well suited for studies in tissues with interconnected cells due to its relatively small molecular weight

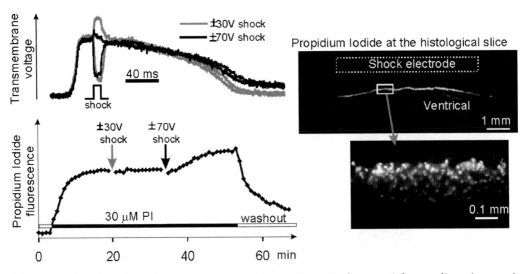

Figure 6: Manifestation of electroporation changes in optical potential recordings is associated with an increase of propidium iodide fluorescence under the stimulation electrode. No increase was observed at sites not under the electrode. Histological images showed typical pattern of nuclear stain at the thin layer of epicardium at the areas where optical potentials had signs of electroporation

(668 Da) with a radius about 0.6 nm, which is smaller than the pore of the gap junction channel (about 0.8 nm). Thus, it was suggested that PI may diffuse to neighboring cells, creating an appearance of electroporation in intact cells. Experimental data show that the area of electroporation, identified by PI staining, could be as narrow 0.1 mm, which means that perhaps the diffusion of PI molecules does not occur over large distances due to rapid binding of PI to the nuclei.

Modeling work has shown that electroporation occurs only in a very small region of the tissue, perhaps only a one-cell layer adjacent to the electrode.[60,61] In contrast the experiments with PI uptake show that the extent of electroporation is much farther than that spreading for many cell layers. However, PI accumulation during the strong shock could be related to other factors (barotrauma, hyperthermia), leading to cell death. If such factors are less dependant on proximity to the tissue boundaries then electroporation,[60,61] it can explain the much larger depth of affected tissue after the 1.6 A/cm^{-2} shock in comparison to the 0.7 A/cm^{-2} shock. A single cell study showed that during 2 kV/cm^{-1}, 20 μs shocks, the cells with irreversible membrane electroporation accumulate a five times larger amount of PI than cells that restored their membrane within 10 min after field exposure.[59] It was also shown that 1.8 A/cm^{-2} stimuli cause irreversible cell damage.[62] It is also possible that the different results obtained by modeling studies are due to limitations of the model, such as lack of realistic representation of three-dimensional myofiber/fibroblast architecture and behavior of ion channels at extreme transmembrane potentials.

Role of Electroporation in Pacing

Traditionally, electroporation is not a concern during cardiac pacing. However, the current density near the surface of the pacing electrode in implantable devices could be as high as 0.5 A/cm^{-2} (0.06 cm^2 electrode surface area, 6 V pacing amplitude, 200 Ω pacing impedance) that is sufficient to cause electroporation in the surrounding myocytes. This may be an additional factor that causes pacing electrode encapsulation and pacing threshold increase. In the short term the electroporation causes an increase of virtual electrode polarization in hyperpolarized regions near the electrode tip; however, the damage resulting from electroporation might be the direct cause of subsequent virtual electrode polarization elimination and pacing threshold increase.[63]

Irreversible Electroporation in Cardiac Surgery

Irreversible electroporation[64] is a novel ablation modality that utilizes the bursts of short 20–1,000 μs high-voltage pulses ~1–3 kV to induce nonthermal cell necrosis in a target tissue. Irreversible electroporation does not cause the denaturation of proteins typical to thermal ablation and spares the tissues scaffold. Thus it preserves the blood flow through the ablated areas while it blocks arrhythmic pathways during atrial ablation procedure.[65] Clinical devices that use this ablation technique have to generate fields above 800 V/cm^{-1} that requires the delivery of 50 A current pulses.[66] The procedure takes only 1–4 s with no local temperature change, and the shape of ablated tissue is not affected by the direction of the blood flow. This facilitates the creation of transmural lesions on a beating heart without the minute-long exposure and broadening of the lesion volumes, as occurs with the radio-frequency ablation technique.[67]

Conclusion

Electroporation is the inevitable complement of the electrical therapy and can be an undesirable drawback for cardiac pacing or a useful tool for ablation. In the case of defibrillation therapy, its role is more obscure, suggesting that a moderate reversible electroporation, especially in the case of intracardiac shocks, may help to suppress an arrhythmogenic substrate. Yet electroporation may cause proarrhythmic effects in the heart as well. Electroporation effects precede the immediate tissue damage that can be induced by extremely high-intensity fields generated inside the cardiac tissue. Electroporation can be monitored by changes in the morphology of the transmembrane polarization transients during anodal and cathodal shocks from monotonic to nonmonotonic response, elevation of the resting potential, and postshock action potential amplitude reduction. Electroporation changes in transmembrane potential traces are present for hyperpolarized as well as depolarized stimuli of a similar strength. Membrane impermeable dye (i.e., propidium iodide) uptake signifies that recovery of membrane integrity in cardiac cells can take minutes after shock termination. Partially this may be caused by a slow diffusion of the dye molecules to the nuclei. Further improvement of defibrillation therapy may be able to direct electroporation power precisely to the reentry substrate in order to minimize the adverse effects on contractile heart properties or for delivering gene therapy to the arrhythmogenic zones.

References

1. Prevost JL, Battelli F. Sur quel ques effets des dechanges electriques sur le coer mammifres. *C R Seances Acad Sci* 1899;129:1267
2. Vulpian A. Note sur les effets de la faradisation directe des ventricules du coeur le chien. *Arch de Physiol* 1874;i:975
3. Hoffa M, Ludwig C. Einige neue Versuche uber Herzbewegung. *Zeitschrift Rationelle Medizin* 1850;9:107–144
4. Hooker DR, Kouwenhoven WB, Langworthy OR. The effects of alternating electrical current on the heart. *Am J Physiol* 1933;103:444–454
5. Beck CS, Pritchard WH, Feil HS. Ventricular fibrillation of long duration abolished by electric shock. *JAMA* 1947;135:985–986
6. Kodama I, Shibata N, Sakuma I, Mitsui K, Iida M, Suzuki R, Fukui Y, Hosoda S, Toyama J. Aftereffects of high-intensity DC stimulation on the electromechanical performance of ventricular muscle. *Am J Physiol* 1994;267:H248–H258
7. Krauthamer V, Jones JL. Calcium dynamics in cultured heart cells exposed to defibrillator-type electric shocks. *Life Sci* 1997;60:1977–1985
8. Fast VG, Cheek ER. Optical mapping of arrhythmias induced by strong electrical shocks in myocyte cultures. *Circ Res* 2002;90:664–670
9. Gurvich NL. *The Main Principles of Cardiac Defibrillation.* Moscow: Medicine; 1975
10. Osswald S, Trouton TG, O'Nunain SS, Holden HB, Ruskin JN, Garan H. Relation between shock-related myocardial injury and defibrillation efficacy of monophasic and biphasic shocks in a canine model. *Circulation* 1994;90:2501–2509
11. Gurvich NL, Yuniev GS. Restoration of regular rhythm in the mammalian fibrillating heart. *Byull Eksper Biol Med* 1939;8:55–58
12. Gurvich NL, Yuniev GS. Restoration of regular rhythm in the mammalian fibrillating heart. *Am Rev Soviet Med* 1946;3:236–239
13. Gurvich NL, Tabak VY, Bogushevich MS, Vanin IV, Makarychev VA. Defibrillation of the heart with a diphasic impulse in experiment and in the clinic. *J Cardiol* 1971;10:104–107
14. Negovsky VA, Gurvich NL, Tabak VY, Bogushevich MS. The nature of electric defibrillation of the heart. *Resuscitation* 1973;2:255–259
15. Fabiato A, Coumel P, Gourgon R, Saumont R. The threshold of synchronous response of the myocardial fibers. Application to the experimental comparison of the efficacy of different forms of electroshock defibrillation. *Arch Mal Coeur Vaiss* 1967;60:527–544
16. Chen PS, Shibata N, Dixon EG, Martin RO, Ideker RE. Comparison of the defibrillation threshold and the upper limit of ventricular vulnerability. *Circulation* 1986;73:1022–1028
17. Dillon SM, Kwaku KF. Progressive depolarization: a unified hypothesis for defibrillation and fibrillation induction by shocks. *J Cardiovasc Electrophysiol* 1998;9:529–552

18. Efimov IR, Gray RA, Roth BJ. Virtual electrodes and re-excitation: new insights into fibrillation induction and defibrillation. *J Cardiovasc Electrophysiol* 2000;11:339–353

19. Chen PS, Swerdlow CD, Hwang C, Karagueuzian HS. Current concepts of ventricular defibrillation. *J Cardiovasc Electrophysiol* 1998;9:553–562

20. Zipes DP, Fischer J, King RM, Nicoll A deB, Jolly WW. Termination of ventricular fibrillation in dogs by depolarizing a critical amount of myocardium. *Am J Cardiol* 1975;36:37–44

21. Frazier DW, Wolf PD, Wharton JM, Tang AS, Smith WM, Ideker RE. Stimulus-induced critical point. Mechanism for electrical initiation of reentry in normal canine myocardium. *J Clin Invest* 1989;83:1039–1052

22. Dillon SM. Synchronized repolarization after defibrillation shocks. A possible component of the defibrillation process demonstrated by optical recordings in rabbit heart. *Circulation* 1992;85:1865–1878

23. Efimov IR, Cheng Y, Van Wagoner DR, Mazgalev T, Tchou PJ. Virtual electrode-induced phase singularity: a basic mechanism of failure to defibrillate. *Circ Res* 1998;82:918–925

24. Cheng Y, Mowrey KA, Van Wagoner DR, Tchou PJ, Efimov IR. Virtual electrode induced re-excitation: a basic mechanism of defibrillation. *Circ Res* 1999;85:1056–1066

25. Roth BJ. A mathematical model of make and break electrical stimulation of cardiac tissue by a unipolar anode or cathode. *IEEE Trans Biomed Eng* 1995;42:1174–1184

26. Ferris LP, King BG, Spence PW, Williams HB. Effect of electric shock on the heart. *Electrical Eng* 1936;55:498–515

27. Wiggers CJ, Wegria R. Ventricular fibrillation due to single localized induction in condenser shock supplied during the vulnerable phase of ventricular systole. *Am J Physiol* 1939;128:500

28. Banville I, Gray RA, Ideker RE, Smith WM. Shock-induced figure-of-eight reentry in the isolated rabbit heart. *Circ Res* 1999;85:742–752

29. Donoso E, Cohn LJFCK. Ventricular arrhythmias after precordial electric shock. *Am Heart J* 1967;73:595–601

30. Waldecker B, Brugada P, Zehender M, Stevenson W, Welens HJ. Ventricular arrhythmias after precordial electric shock. *Am J Cardiol* 1986;57:120–123

31. Tovar O, Tung L. Electroporation of cardiac cell membranes with monophasic or biphasic rectangular pulses. *Pacing Clin Electrophysiol* 1991;14(Pt 2):1887–1892

32. Neunlist M, Tung L. Dose-dependent reduction of cardiac transmembrane potential by high-intensity electrical shocks. *Am J Physiol* 1997;273:H2817–H2825

33. Al-Khadra AS, Nikolski V, Efimov IR. The role of electroporation in defibrillation. *Circ Res* 2000;87:797–804

34. Yabe S, Smith WM, Daubert JP, Wolf PD, Rollins DL, Ideker RE. Conduction disturbances caused by high current density electric fields. *Circ Res* 1990;66:1190–1203

35. Eysmann SB, Marchlinski FE, Buxton AE, Josephson ME. Electrocardiographic changes after cardioversion of ventricular arrhythmias. *Circulation* 1986;73:73–81

36. Stickney RE, Doherty A, Kudenchuk PJ, Morud SA, Walker C, Chapman FW, Cummins RO. Survival and postshock ECG rhythms for out-of-hospital defibrillation. *PACE* 1999;22(4-II):740

37. Sparks PB, Kulkarni R, Vohra JK, Mond HG, Jayaprakash S, Yapanis AG, Grigg LE, Kalman JM. Effect of direct current shocks on left atrial mechanical function in patients with structural heart disease. *J Am Coll Cardiol* 1998;31:1395–1399

38. Sparks PB, Jayaprakash S, Mond HG, Vohra JK, Grigg LE, Kalman JM. Left atrial mechanical function after brief duration atrial fibrillation. *J Am Coll Cardiol* 1999;33:342–349

39. Grimm RA, Stewart WJ, Arheart K, Thomas JD, Klein AL. Left atrial appendage "stunning" after electrical cardioversion of atrial flutter: an attenuated response compared with atrial fibrillation as the mechanism for lower susceptibility to thromboembolic events. *J Am Coll Cardiol* 1997;29:582–589

40. Kam RM, Garan H, McGovern BA, Ruskin JN, Harthorne JW. Transient right bundle branch block causing R wave attenuation postdefibrillation. *Pacing Clin Electrophysiol* 1997;20:130–131

41. Hasdemir C, Shah N, Rao AP, Acosta H, Matsudaira K, Neas BR, Reynolds DW, Po S, Lazzara R, Beckman KJ. Analysis of troponin I levels after spontaneous implantable cardioverter defibrillator shocks. *J Cardiovasc Electrophysiol* 2002;13:144–150

42. Ambler JJ, Deakin CD. A randomized controlled trial of efficacy and ST change following use of the Welch-Allyn MRL PIC biphasic waveform versus damped sine monophasic waveform for external DC cardioversion. *Resuscitation* 2006;71:146–151

43. Ohuchi K, Fukui Y, Sakuma I, Shibata N, Honjo H, Kodama I. A dynamic action potential model analysis of shock-induced aftereffects in ventricular muscle by reversible breakdown of cell membrane. *IEEE Trans Biomed Eng* 2002;49:18–30

44. Lund M, French JK, Johnson RN, Williams BF, White HD. Serum troponins T and I after elective cardioversion. *Eur Heart J* 2000;21:245–253

45. Ricard P, Levy S, Boccara G, Lakhal E, Bardy G. External cardioversion of atrial fibrillation: comparison of biphasic vs monophasic waveform shocks. *Europace* 2001;3:96–99

46. Niemann JT, Walker RG, Rosborough JP. Intracardiac voltage gradients during transthoracic defibrillation: implications for postshock myocardial injury. *Acad Emerg Med* 2005;12:99–105

47. Fedorov VV, Kostecki G, Hemphill M, Efimov IR. Atria are more susceptible to electroporation than ventricles: Implications for atrial stunning, shock-induced arrhythmia and defibrillation failure. *Circ Res* 2008;5(4):593–604

48. Walcott GP, Killingsworth CR, Ideker RE. Do clinically relevant transthoracic defibrillation energies cause myocardial damage and dysfunction? *Resuscitation* 2003;59:59–70

49. Al-Khadra AS, Cheng Y, Tchou PJ, Efimov IR. Electroporation in defibrillation: difference in susceptibility between endocardium and epicardium. *PACE* 1999;22(4-II):834

50. Al-Khadra AS, Nikolski V, Efimov IR. Electroporation and conduction failure in endocardial bundles in response to defibrillation shocks. *PACE* 2000;23(4-II):706

51. Tabereaux PB, Walcott GP, Rogers JM, Kim J, Dosdall DJ, Robertson PG, Killingsworth CR, Smith WM, Ideker RE. Activation patterns of Purkinje fibers during long-duration ventricular fibrillation in an isolated canine heart model. *Circulation* 2007;116:1113–1119

52. Jones JL, Jones RE, Balasky G. Microlesion formation in myocardial cells by high-intensity electric field stimulation. *Am J Physiol* 1987;253:H480–H486

53. Peleska B. [Problems of defibrillation and stimulation of the myocardium]. *Zentralbl Chir* 1965;90:1174–1188

54. Tung L, Tovar O, Neunlist M, Jain SK, O'Neill RJ. Effects of strong electrical shock on cardiac muscle tissue. *Ann N Y Acad Sci* 1994;720:160–175

55. Cheng Y, Tchou PJ, Efimov IR. Spatio-temporal characterization of electroporation during defibrillation. *Biophysical J* 1999;76(1):A85

56. Nikolski VP, Sambelashvili AT, Krinsky VI, Efimov IR. Effects of electroporation on optically recorded transmembrane potential responses to high-intensity electrical shocks. *Am J Physiol Heart Circ Physiol* 2004;286:H412–H418

57. Fast VG, Rohr S, Ideker RE. Nonlinear changes of transmembrane potential caused by defibrillation shocks in strands of cultured myocytes. *Am J Physiol Heart Circ Physiol* 2000;278:H688–H697

58. Cheng DK, Tung L, Sobie EA. Nonuniform responses of transmembrane potential during electric field stimulation of single cardiac cells. *Am J Physiol* 1999;277:H351–H362

59. Shirakashi R, Kostner CM, Muller KJ, Kurschner M, Zimmermann U, Sukhorukov VL. Intracellular delivery of trehalose into mammalian cells by electropermeabilization. *J Membr Biol* 2002;189:45–54

60. DeBruin KA, Krassowska W. Electroporation and shock-induced transmembrane potential in a cardiac fiber during defibrillation strength shocks. *Ann Biomed Eng* 1998;26:584–596

61. Aguel F, DeBruin KA, Krassowska W, Trayanova NA. Effects of electroporation on the transmembrane potential distribution in a two-dimensional bidomain model of cardiac tissue. *J Cardiovasc Electrophysiol* 1999;10:701–714

62. Koning G, Veefkind AH, Schneider H. Cardiac damage caused by direct application of defibrillator shocks to isolated Langendorff-perfused rabbit heart. *Am Heart J* 1980;100:473–482

63. Sambelashvili AT, Nikolski VP, Efimov IR. Virtual electrode theory explains pacing threshold increase caused by cardiac tissue damage. *Am J Physiol Heart Circ Physiol* 2004;286:H2183–H2194

64. Rubinsky B. Irreversible electroporation in medicine. *Technol Cancer Res Treat* 2007;6:255–260

65. Lavee J, Onik G, Mikus P, Rubinsky B. A novel nonthermal energy source for surgical epicardial atrial ablation: irreversible electroporation. *Heart Surg Forum* 2007;10:E162–E167

66. Bertacchini C, Margotti PM, Bergamini E, Lodi A, Ronchetti M, Cadossi R. Design of an irreversible electroporation system for clinical use. *Technol Cancer Res Treat* 2007;6:313–320

67. Thomas SP, Guy DJ, Boyd AC, Eipper VE, Ross DL, Chard RB. Comparison of epicardial and endocardial linear ablation using handheld probes. *Ann Thorac Surg* 2003;75:543–548

Part VI

Implications for Implantable Devices

Chapter 6.1

Lessons for the Clinical Implant*

Mark W. Kroll and Charles D. Swerdlow

Our goal in this chapter is to provide a practical review for clinicians of how our understanding of defibrillation scientific results can help with their clinical practice. Some of the typical implant practices are found to be driven by dogma and not by science.

Electrical Parameters of Defibrillation Waveforms

Parameters that Influence Defibrillation

Although no simple electrical descriptor provides a good measure of defibrillation efficacy, the waveform parameters that most directly influence defibrillation are voltage and duration. Voltage is a critical parameter for defibrillation because its spatial derivative defines the electrical field that interacts with the heart (Fig. 1). Similarly, waveform duration is a critical parameter because the shock interacts with the heart for the duration of the waveform. Further, the heart's response to a defibrillation pulse occurs over a period that depends on the time constants of the cardiac cell membrane and possibly on other ionic, intracellular, cellular, and tissue properties. Implantable cardioverter-defibrillator (ICD) waveforms are most efficient when their phase durations are close to that of cardiac cell membrane time constants.[1-5] Thus the electrical measure of defibrillation that is most relevant physiologically is voltage (or voltage gradient) as a function of time.

Parameters that Influence ICD Design

Shock energy is the most often cited metric of shock strength and an ICD's capacity to defibrillate, but it is *not* a direct measure of shock effectiveness. For example, the maximum

Mark W. Kroll

Department of Biomedical Engineering, University of Minnesota, Minneapolis, MN, USA, mark@krolls.org

* Portions of this chapter have previously appeared in Kroll MW, Swerdlow CD. Optimizing defibrillation waveforms for ICDs. *J Interv Card Electrophysiol* 2007;18(3):247–263 and are used with permission of the publisher.

I. R. Efimov et al. (eds.), *Cardiac Bioelectric Therapy: Mechanisms and Practical Implications.*
© Springer Science+Business Media, LLC 2009

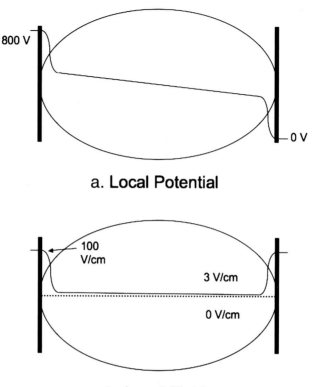

a. Local Potential

b. Local Field

Figure 1: Shock potential with respect to the right hand electrode (**a**) and the spatial derivative or electric field (**b**). The *thick vertical bars* symbolize electrodes and the oval the heart. Note that most of the voltage drop and hence the highest fields occurs close to the electrodes

shock strength of an ICD is typically in the range of 30 to 40 J. If energy were a good descriptor of defibrillation efficacy, one could defibrillate with a 9 V battery by connecting it to the heart for 20 s through large defibrillation electrodes to deliver 40 J

$$\text{Energy} = \frac{\text{Voltage}^2 \times \text{Time}}{\text{Resistance}} = \frac{9\,\text{V} \times 9\,\text{V} \times 20\,\text{s}}{40\,\Omega} = 40.5\,\text{J}.$$

Although a 9 V battery may reliably induce fibrillation,[6] it will never defibrillate.

However, the maximum energy stored in an ICD's output capacitor is a major determinant of the size of the battery and capacitor and thus of the overall size of the ICD's pulse generator. Since minimizing ICD size is an important clinical goal, designing ICDs that defibrillate with minimum stored energy is an important engineering goal.

The physics of capacitive-discharge waveforms link the energy stored in the ICD's capacitor to the voltage and duration of the delivered defibrillation waveform. For a given capacitance, stored energy is proportional to the square of voltage. (See the section on capacitive-discharge waveforms below.) Further, the time dependence of a capacitive-discharge exponential waveform is given by the system time constant τ_s, (pronounced "tau," which is the product of capacitance and pathway resistance). *Thus, in present ICDs, the value of the shock output capacitance is a key intermediary in establishing the relationship between stored energy – the key determinant of ICD size – and waveform voltage as a function of time, which is the key determinant of defibrillation efficacy.*

Principles of Capacitive Discharge Waveforms

A capacitor charged to a voltage V gives the following discharge voltage as a function of time:

$$V(t) = e^{-t/\tau_s},$$

where t is the time since the start of the discharge and τ_s is the shock system time constant, the time for voltage to decrease to $1-e^{-1}$ (about 37% of the initial value). Since

$$\tau_s = RC \text{ (where } R \text{ is the pathway resistance and } C \text{ is the ICD capacitance),}$$

voltage as a function of time is given by:

$$V(t) = e^{-t/RC}.$$

Thus a large capacitance and large load resistance result in a long discharge time. A small capacitance and small load resistance result in a short discharge time (Fig. 2a, b).

Larger electrodes have lower resistances,[7] in relationship to their macroscopic dimensions,[8] as do systems in which the housing of the ICD generator ("can") serves as a defibrillation electrode.[9] Lower voltages[10] and large heart size[11] both tend to increase the resistance. The resistance tends to increase with time[12,13] and with inspiration (assuming an extracardiac electrode is involved)[14] and also varies with a submuscular or subcutaneous location of the can electrode.[13]

Truncation

The voltage of capacitive-discharge waveforms approach zero asymptotically, and the earliest capacitive-discharge defibrillation waveforms were not truncated.[15,16] Schuder and Stoeckle[17] first reported that transthoracic defibrillation was much more effective with truncated waveforms. Subsequently, the effect of truncation on defibrillation efficacy of ICD waveforms has been studied extensively.[18–20] By definition, truncation of phase I is required to produce a single capacitor biphasic waveform.

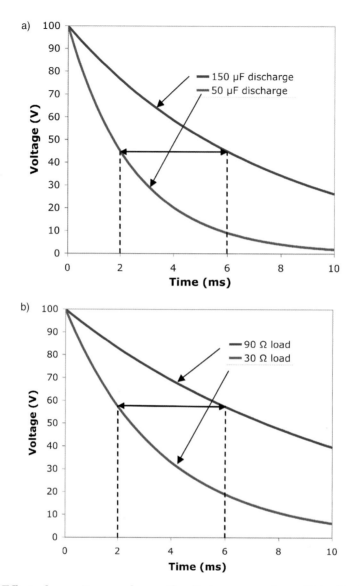

Figure 2: (a) Effect of capacitance value on the discharge waveform. Note (*horizontal double arrow*) that the time to decay to a given voltage is tripled for the 150 versus the 50 μF waveform. Capacitor is initially charged to 100 V and the pathway resistance is 50 Ω. (b) Effect of load resistance value on discharge waveform. Capacitor (110 μF) is initially charged to 100 V. Note (*horizontal double arrow*) that the time to decay to a given voltage is tripled for the 90 versus the 30 Ω load. In both cases, the capacitor is initially charged to 100 V

Stored Versus Delivered Energy

The energy stored in a capacitor is given by:

$$E_{std} = \frac{1}{2}CV^2.$$

This equation links stored energy, the key determinant of ICD size, to initial waveform voltage. Delivered energy, another term used to characterize ICDs, has no direct influence on either defibrillation or ICD design. Delivered energy is most simply calculated by subtracting the final (residual) energy stored in the capacitor at the end of the capacitive-discharge waveform from the initial stored energy:

$$E_{del} = \frac{1}{2}CV_i^2 - \frac{1}{2}CV_f^2,$$

where V_f is the "final" or trailing edge voltage. For accuracy, both V_i and V_f should be measured at the ICD's output, rather than directly from the capacitor, removing the effects of internal resistance in the ICD. Delivered energy can also be calculated by integrating the power output from the ICD:

$$E_{del} = \int_0^{End} \frac{V^2}{R}dt.$$

The two expressions for delivered energy are equivalent if capacitance is constant. In practice, the measured capacitance value tends to increase by roughly 10% or more from the leading edge value during the pulse.[21] For example, a $110\,\mu F$ capacitor may have $105\,\mu F$ of capacitance at the beginning of the shock and $115\,\mu F$ at the end. This is due to charge stored in the tunnels etched in the aluminum foil used in most ICD capacitors. Recruiting this "hidden" charge for delivery to the output circuit takes a few milliseconds during discharge of the capacitor. (There is another, less important, effect called dielectric absorption, which contributes to this increasing capacitance effect.) As this charge is recruited, the ratio of charge to voltage increases, resulting in an increased value of measured capacitance and a proportional increase in the system time constant.

The discharge curve thus departs from a single exponential curve, analogous to a double-compartment drug elimination model in physiology. Since the "C" is the effective average value this variation has little net effect except to make the τ_s less at the leading edge and greater at the trailing edge of a shock. This effect is partially offset by a possible decrease in resistance during the shock.[22]

The clinical and marketing debate over the used of stored versus delivered energy is clouded by another complication. The theoretical (ideal) stored energy discussed above is actually quite close to the delivered energy, with differences less than 10%. However, real world "delivered" energy is significantly lower due to the resistive losses in the semiconductor switching circuitry, connections, and inside the capacitor itself. The advantages and disadvantages of each measure of defibrillation efficacy are given in Table 1.

Table 1: Clinical implications of using stored versus delivered energy ratings

	Delivered energy	Stored energy
Measurement accuracy	Accurate	Estimated
Relates to safety margin	Not directly. Shortening the phase durations will often reduce the voltage defibrillation threshold. However, the delivered energy (at this defibrillation threshold voltage) is also reduced significantly giving a false impression of the safety margin as the maximum delivered energy is also reduced	Yes. The maximum stored energy is not affected by changing phase durations
Encourages good clinical practice	No. Delivered energy ratings have encouraged some manufacturers to deliver excessive phase durations, which are suboptimal, in order to increase delivered energy claims	Yes. Does not encourage the suboptimal lengthening of phase durations

Optimizing Waveforms with the RC Network Model

A simple approach, developed in the 1930s models the heart as a passive resistor–capacitor (RC) network (Fig. 3).[23,24] It has subsequently been applied to modeling defibrillation waveforms.[5,26–29] The model's parameters produce an estimate of the passive cell membrane time constant τ_m. The latter may be conceptualized as an average value in regions where defibrillation may fail because the shock field is weakest, ignoring time and voltage-dependent effects.

The RC model has are two principal assumptions: (1) The goal of a monophasic shock is to maximize the voltage change in the cardiac cell membrane at the end of the shock for a given stored energy. The same assumption applies to the first phase of a biphasic shock. (2) The goal of the second phase is to discharge the membrane potential back to the

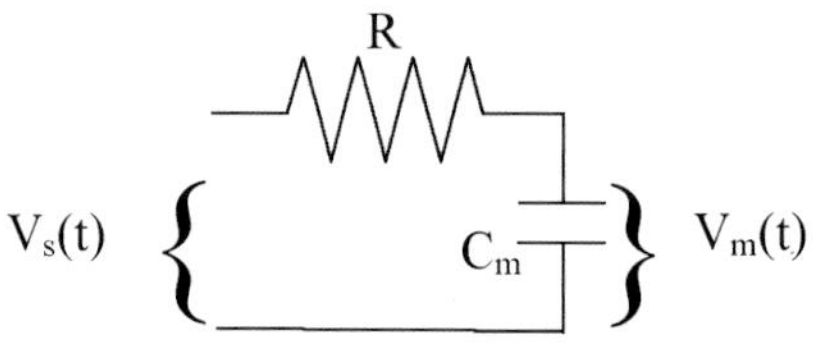

Figure 3: Resistor–capacitor membrane model for cardiac tissue. The shock voltage is $V_s(t)$ and the membrane response is given as $V_m(t)$. C_m represents the membrane capacitance and R represents the Thevenin (composite single resistance) equivalent combination of the intercellular and transmembrane resistance. The product of R and C_m gives the membrane time constant τ_m. (Used with permission of Elsevier)[25]

zero potential, removing the charge deposited by the first phase.[29] This performs several functions, with the most important probably being the discharge of the virtual electrodes. This is sometimes referred to charge burping.[30]

The empirical RC model does not distinguish among theories of defibrillation. In each of the major theories of biphasic waveform defibrillation – progressive depolarization,[31] upper limit of vulnerability,[32] and virtual electrode induced reexcitation[33,34] – the role of the first phase is to charge the cell membranes. Similarly, whatever the function of the second phase – to remove residual charge from marginally stimulated cells,[35–37] to heal cell membranes temporarily damaged (electroporated)[38] by the extreme current near the electrodes,[38–40] or to discharge the virtual electrodes[41–43] – it must return the cell membrane voltage to zero. It is not yet known if the RC model is consistent with break excitation effects.[41]

The RC model is a first-order approximation. The passive charging of the cell membrane is nonlinear, and the time constants vary depending on the local field and on the polarity of the affecting electrode.[44] It does not consider the critical roles played by tissue heterogeneity and active ionic currents in cardiac electrical activity. Nevertheless, all major predictions of this model have been verified in animal[2,4,5,30,45] and human studies[1,3,46] with impressive concordance. To date, no other model has been clinically applied successfully. *For this reason, we focus on the predictions of this model; and we use the terms optimal and optimized in relation to the predictions of RC model.*

Minimizing Shock Energy Without Electronic Constraints

Waveform optimization is most commonly considered as a problem in minimizing ICD size, and thus a problem in minimizing stored energy for capacitive-discharge waveforms. However, it is instructive to consider minimizing delivered energy in physiological terms only, with no constraints on electronics technology.

The Predicted Optimal Monophasic Shock

Consider the membrane response to the square waveform in Fig. 4a. Although the initial applied voltage is the maximum value for the waveform, the cell's membrane time constant (τ_m) limits the rate at which the cell membrane can respond.[44] Thus some of the energy associated with the high initial voltage is wasted. In contrast, the ascending waveform shown in Fig. 4b initially applies only sufficient voltage to permit the cell to respond optimally. Mathematical analysis shows that the theoretically optimal waveform begins at a nonzero percentage of the peak voltage and then rises in an exponential upward curve as shown in Fig. 4b.[27]

Unfortunately, such an ascending waveform is difficult to generate in a way that is both volumetrically and energy efficient with electronic components used in present ICDs. Thus, while an ascending waveform will minimize delivered energy,[2,26,47] stored energy might not be minimized. For the ascending waveform, an infinitely long duration does not increase its defibrillation threshold (DFT).[27] (See the chapter by Kroll and Swerdlow for further discussion.)

Now consider the capacitive-discharge waveform in Fig. 4c. The initial portion of this waveform has the same energy inefficiency as the square waveform in Fig. 2a. Further, as the pulse duration of the applied waveform increases, the membrane response voltage reaches a maximum and then decreases. The model predicts that voltage (and energy) applied after the time of maximum membrane response is wasted and may be counterproductive. For capacitive-discharge waveforms, delivering more energy by increasing waveform duration can paradoxically reduce defibrillation efficacy.[17,48] Thus, truncation is critical for capacitive-discharge exponential waveforms to achieve the first model goal of maximizing cell

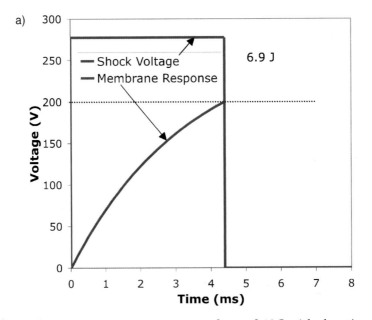

Figure 4: (a) Membrane response to square waveform of 10 J with duration of 43.75 ms, which is equal to the optimal duration of $1.25\tau_\mathrm{m}$. Impedances for Fig. 6a–c are 40 Ω, and the assumed membrane time constant is 35 ms. However, the membrane response is typically on the order of 20–100 mV, and thus the scale on the left does not apply. In all three cases the energy shown is that required to generate an equivalent membrane response of 200 arbitrary units. (b) Membrane response to ascending waveform of 10 J with duration of 7 ms. Note the decreased energy, but increased peak voltage, required compared to the square wave of Fig. 6a. (c) Membrane response to descending waveform from the optimally sized 875 μF capacitor and a 40 Ω load. Note that this clinical waveform requires more energy and voltage than both the square wave and ascending waveform. If the truncation is not at the peak (which is a common clinical problem), then the performance is further attenuated. Also, with different capacitances and resistances, this waveform is even less efficient

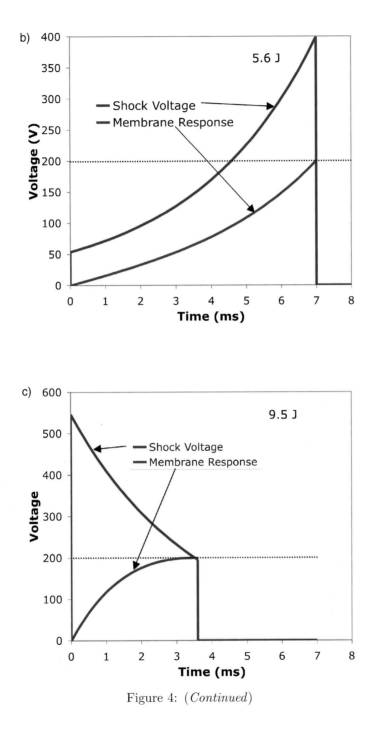

Figure 4: (*Continued*)

membrane voltage at the end of the shock. Even with predicted optimal truncation, capacitive-discharge waveforms require more voltage and energy to achieve the same membrane voltage as do square waves and ascending waveforms.

The Predicted Optimal Biphasic Shock

The charge burping hypothesis and the RC network model apply fewer constraints to phase two than to phase one. The second model assumption requires only that the second phase returns the cell membrane voltage to zero; the precise shape of phase two is unimportant. How returning the cell membrane voltage to zero facilitates defibrillation is unknown. The most likely candidates are discharge of the virtual electrodes, reducing electroporation, and discharging marginally stimulated cells in the excitable gaps.

However, unlike phase one, there is no single predicted optimal phase two for a given cell membrane and pathway resistance. Instead, the predicted optimal phase two size depends on phase one, specifically on the cell membrane voltage at the end of phase one. Phase two needs to include sufficient charge to discharge the residual membrane voltage left by phase one. The model makes no predictions regarding the benefit of optimizing the shape of phase two; to date experimental data indicate that the shape of phase two does not strongly influence defibrillation efficacy.

Optimizing Capacitive Discharge Waveforms

Optimizing Duration: Monophasic Shock and First Phase of Biphasic Shock with a Fixed Capacitance

The simplest analysis applies to a fixed capacitance. Minimizing stored energy is equivalent to minimizing leading edge (initial) voltage because the only variable is truncation of pulse duration. Figure 4c shows that predicted optimal truncation occurs at the pulse duration associated with maximal cell membrane response. This pulse duration lies between 3 and 5 ms for most present ICDs used for transvenous defibrillation.

The plot of shock strength as a function of pulse duration is known as a strength-duration curve (Fig. 5). The concept of a strength-duration curve has been applied empirically to bioelectric stimulation for over a century. The first one, Hoorweg[50] in 1892, gave the stimulation capacitor voltage required as a function of capacitance value for untruncated pulses. In 1901 Weiss[51] used truncated pulses to generate a plot of electrical charge versus duration. For her PhD thesis (1905) Marcelle Lapicque approximately duplicated Hoorweg's work. Her husband, Louis, then defined the term "chronaxie" and showed how the various formulations were essentially equivalent in 1909. The most common strength-duration curve is based on the Weiss hyperbolic equation that expresses the average current required for defibrillation (I_{avg}) in terms of pulse duration (d):

$$I_{avg} = I_r(1 + d_c/d),$$

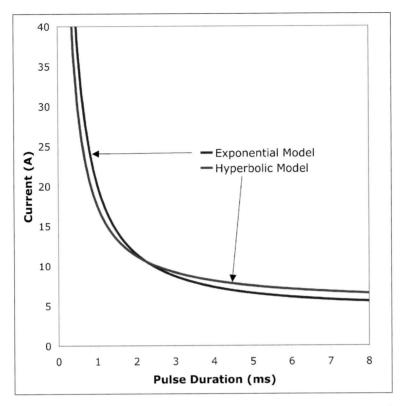

Figure 5: The plot of shock strength as a function of pulse duration is known as a strength-duration curve. The resistor–capacitor (RC) network (exponential) model predicts a strength-duration curve for capacitive-discharge waveforms as shown. The Weiss-Lapicque (hyperbolic) strength-duration curve is also shown and seen to match the exponential curve closely. The rheobase current (5 A) is that which will defibrillate for an infinitely long pulse. For capacitive-discharge shocks, the current for the hyperbolic model would refer to the average current. The hyperbolic model curve applies directly only for low tilt waveforms

where I_r is the long-duration asymptote or "rheobase" and d_c is the Lapicque "chronaxie" duration at which the required average current is twice the rheobase. For a square wave pulse, the minimum energy occurs at a pulse duration equal to the chronaxie (d_c). For a capacitive-discharge waveform, the predicted optimum duration is a weighted average of the chronaxie and the shock time constant and is given by:

$$d = 0.58d_c + 0.58RC.$$

This is a compromise between the optimal physiological duration for (square wave) defibrillation efficacy (chronaxie) and the optimal duration for the capacitor to deliver its charge (shock time constant $\tau_s = RC$).[28] Such a truncation approach has proved clinically efficacious.[3]

The chronaxie and membrane time constant for defibrillation have each been found to be in the range of 2 to 5 ms in animal[18,52–56] and in human studies.[57] The most commonly used value of membrane time constant is 3.5 ms. Theoretically:[60]

$$d_c = 0.7\tau_m.$$

The dependence of the predicted optimal duration on capacitance is illustrated by the comparison shown in Fig. 6. With a resistance of $50\,\Omega$, the capacitances of 140 and $40\,\mu F$ give shock system time constants of 7 and 2 ms, respectively. The corresponding predicted optimal durations of phase one are 5 and 2.5 ms. For any given chronaxie (or membrane time constant) and pathway resistance, there is an optimal capacitance that permits defibrillation with the lowest possible energy, provided duration is optimized for that capacitance. The

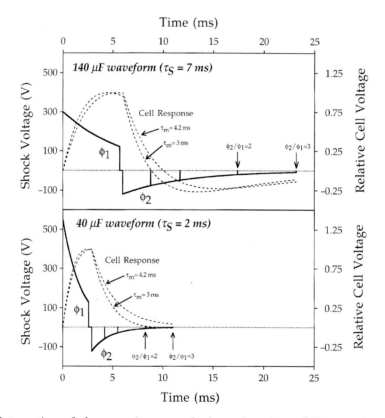

Figure 6: Interaction of the capacitance and phase durations. (The membrane response is modeled for both an assumed 3 and 4.2 ms membrane time constant.) Note that the optimal durations increase with increasing capacitance values. Note that the optimal first phase duration only changes from 5 down to 2.5 ms. (Used with permission of American Heart Association)[30]

predicted optimal pulse duration for a optimal capacitance is equal to the membrane time constant τ_{m}.[27,57]

Optimizing Capacitance

The RC model predicts that stored energy is minimized for capacitive-discharge waveforms by differentiating stored energy (or leading edge voltage) as a function of capacitance, assuming an optimal duration for capacitance. The derivative is then set equal to zero and the equation solved algebraically. This analysis shows that stored energy is minimized when the ICD's system time constant τ_{s} equals the cell membrane time constant τ_{m}. Since τ_{s} is the product of capacitance and shock pathway resistance, the model predicts that the capacitance that defibrillates with the lowest stored energy is inversely related to pathway resistance.[28] This has been verified in both animal and human experiments.[29,61–66] If we assume $\tau_{\mathrm{m}} = 3.5\,\mathrm{ms}$, the predicted optimal capacitance ranges from $117\,\mu\mathrm{F}$ for a $30\,\Omega$ pathway to $58\,\mu\mathrm{F}$ for a $60\,\Omega$ pathway.

Figure 7 shows the model's predicted effect on the stored-energy DFT of varying capacitances. The curve has a steep descending limb for lower than optimal capacitance, a relatively flat valley with a nadir at the optimal capacitance, and a gradually sloping ascending limb for higher values. These stored-energy penalty curves have important

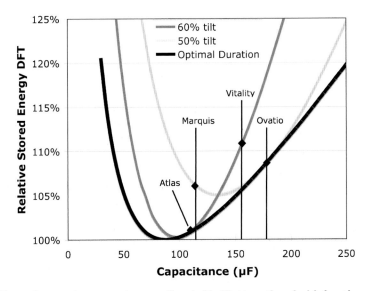

Figure 7: Effect of capacitance value on the defibrillation threshold for the most popular phase one tilts. Assumes a resistance of $50\,\Omega$ and a membrane time constant of $3.5\,\mathrm{ms}$. This is based on phase one membrane charging and assumes optimal phase two truncation, which may be generous in some cases. Included are the St. Jude Atlas® ($110\,\mu\mathrm{F}$), Medtronic Marquis® ($113\,\mu\mathrm{F}$), tantalum Boston Scientific Vitality® ($155\,\mu\mathrm{F}$), and the ELA Medical Ovatio™ ($177\,\mu\mathrm{F}$)

implications for the design of ICDs since stored energy is a critical determinant of the pulse generator size and present ICD capacitors limit maximum voltage to approximately 800 V. A modern ICD with a capacitance near 110 µF pays only a minimum energy penalty compared to the predicted optimal capacitance value of 87.5 µV.

Further, if the population mean DFT is 10.6 ± 5.2 J,[67] then the 95% percentile DFT should be 19.2 J for an assumed normal distribution. With the 110 µF capacitance value this corresponds to a voltage of about 590 V. The maximum ICD output (800 V) provides a 26% voltage and a 45% energy safety margin over this 95th percentile DFT (calculated from the maximum output down). Although the predicted optimal capacitance (87.5 µF) will reduce the stored energy DFT by 2%, the maximum output is reduced by 20%, and hence it provides a smaller *stored energy* safety margin (assuming that we are technology limited at 800 V). The model predicts that the energy penalty for 130–180 µF capacitors used in most earlier ICDs and some present ICDs[68] is in the range of 5–10%, depending on resistance. For example, a 30 Ω electrode system would be well served by a higher capacitance ICD. However, for a 70 Ω patient, higher capacitance devices are suboptimal.

Optimizing Phase Two of the Biphasic Waveform

The second model assumption is that the goal of the optimal second phase is to remove the charge deposited on myocardial cells by phase one, returning the membrane voltage to zero. The benefit of phase two can be seen in Fig. 8. The closer phase two discharges the residual membrane to zero voltage, the lower the predicted amplitude required for defibrillation in phase one. Retrospective metaanalysis[29] and prospective[30] data indicate that defibrillation efficacy is inversely related to the residual membrane voltage at the end of phase two. The phase one current required correlates with the square of the calculated residual membrane potential after phase two.

The major predictions of this theory have been supported by animal[2,4,30] and human studies.[1,46] One such prediction is that the optimal ratio of phase one to phase two is higher for larger values of τ_s (capacitance, pathway resistance, or both) and lower for lower values of τ_s.

Figure 6 illustrates the differences in predicted cell membrane responses to the electrical fields of 140 and 40 µF waveforms of equal stored energy. Phase one of the 140 µF waveform produces a weaker, but longer-lasting, field than phase one of the 40 µF waveform. The cell response to the applied 140 µF waveform is slower and continues longer. For phase two, the leading-edge voltage is a greater fraction of the phase one, leading-edge voltage, resulting in more rapid charge burping for this waveform. In addition, the phase two, negative applied voltage exceeds a minimal absolute value longer for the 140 µF waveform, resulting in a persistent negative residual membrane voltage for high ratios of phase two to phase one. The cell-response curves appear underdamped. In contrast, because the negative applied voltage decays rapidly for the 40 µF waveform, the cell response does not decrease below the relative zero value. The cell-response curves appear overdamped.

The experimentally measured effect on cell response and DFT of changing the ratio of phase one to phase two is shown in Fig. 9. For the 40 µF waveform the charge-burping hypothesis predicts that phase-duration ratios of 0.5 and 1.0 fail to return the cell membrane

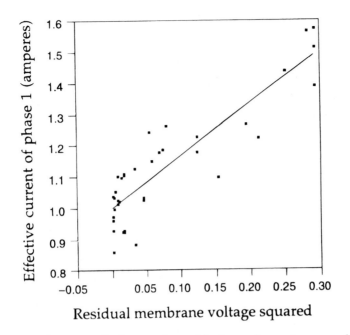

Figure 8: The closer phase two discharges the residual membrane to zero voltage, the lower the amplitude required for defibrillation in phase one. The phase one current required correlates with the square of the calculated residual membrane potential after phase two. (Used with permission of Blackwell Publishing)[29]

voltage to the preshock level and thereby leave substantial residual charge on the membrane. In contrast, there is a broad range of phase-duration ratios of $2:1$–$3:1$ that provide comparable and near-complete charge burping for either value of t_m. For $140\,\mu\mathrm{F}$ waveforms, the predictions of charge-burping theory depend strongly on the unknown value of τ_m. For τ_m of 3.0 and 4.2 ms, the predicted optimal phase-duration ratios are 0.5 and 0.75, respectively. These predictions have been confirmed experimentally.[30]

Since the goal of phase two is to reverse the membrane charging effect of phase one, there is no advantage to additional waveform phases. A methodical search of 140 different waveforms demonstrated that optimized biphasic waveforms have the lowest DFTs, and that waveforms with three or more phases had higher DFTs.

Truncation by Duration Versus Truncation by Tilt

Truncation may be defined either by waveform duration or "tilt." Tilt is defined by the expression:

$$\mathrm{Tilt} \equiv 1 - \frac{V_\mathrm{F}}{V_\mathrm{i}},$$

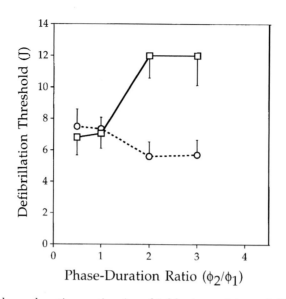

Figure 9: A fixed phase duration ratio gives highly inconsistent defibrillation thresholds (DFTs) for different capacitances. For phase two duration = 2 × phase one, the DFT varies from < 6 J to about 12 J when going from a 40 (*dashed line*) to a 140 μF capacitor (*solid line*). (Used with permission of the American Heart Association)[30]

where V_F is the final ("trailing edge") voltage and V_i is the initial ("leading edge") voltage. Consider a capacitive-discharge waveform that is truncated after one time constant (t_s) so that the final voltage is 37% of the leading edge voltage. This corresponds to a tilt of 63% (Fig. 10).

Historically, waveform truncation was first performed by tilt for engineering reasons. In Schuder's initial report by Schuder and Stoeckle,[17] transthoracic defibrillation waveforms were most effective if they were truncated after a duration equal to approximately τ_s.

Commercial ICDs use either tilt or duration for truncation, depending on the manufacturer. Medtronic, Boston Scientific, and ELA Medical devices use tilt. St. Jude Medical devices offer a choice of fixed durations and tilts. Intermedics devices (no longer sold) had a choice of fixed durations for both phases. Biotronik uses tilt for phase one and a choice of a tilt or a fixed 2 ms duration for phase two. These approaches result in different waveform durations and different changes in waveforms for varying pathway resistance.

By definition, the duration-based approach results in waveform durations predicted to be optimal by the RC network model for the assumed value of average membrane time constant (τ_m). One limitation is that, in practice, the value of τ_m is not verified. Thus the individual patient's values of τ_m, which may have a substantial effect on the predicted optimal waveform, is unknown. A second limitation is that the RC network model is a first approximation that neglects major physiological variables.

In this approach, the implanter makes an assumption about τ_m and measures the resistance of the defibrillation pathway to select the predicted optimal duration for each

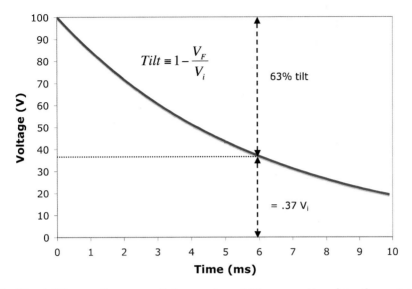

Figure 10: Fixed tilt waveforms result in a pulse width proportional to the resistance *and* capacitance. It provides an indirect method for determining pulse width. The delivered energy is proportional to the difference of the voltages (initial and final) squared

phase of a biphasic waveform. Typically, acute and chronic high-voltage lead resistances are stable within about 10%.[12,13] This sets the waveform on an individual patient basis, and the waveform is optimized to the extent that both the RC network model applies and that the value of τ_m is accurate. This approach could be automated by setting durations for each phase based on the measured resistance. Since acute ischemia may alter the membrane time constant,[71] a further refinement may be needed to adjust phase durations when ischemia is detected.

The tilt-based approach uses the same fixed predetermined values for phase one and phase two tilts in each patient, independent of pathway resistance. There is no theoretical basis to the use of tilt.

Figure 11 shows the disparate effect of changing pathway resistance on fixed-duration and fixed-tilt waveforms. Figure 11a shows that the effect of changing pathway resistance on a fixed-duration waveform is to change the trailing-edge voltage and tilt. In contrast, Fig. 11b shows that, for a tilt-based waveform, the trailing edge voltage is fixed but the durations change proportionately to the resistance.

Consider the effect of these differences on waveform optimization as predicted by the RC network model. Figure 12a shows that fixed tilt waveforms change the duration of phase one in the right direction for increasing pathway resistance, but the increase is more than theoretically required to optimize the waveform. According to the RC network model, this may leave insufficient charge on the capacitor to permit phase two to return the cell membrane voltage to 0 V. Further, Fig. 12b shows that the predicted optimal duration of

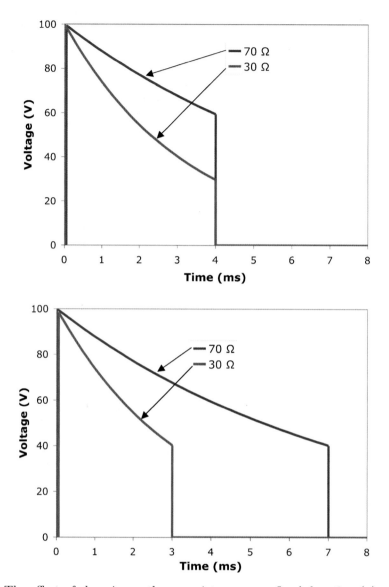

Figure 11: The effect of changing pathway resistance on a fixed-duration (**a**) waveform is to change the trailing edge voltage and tilt. For a tilt-based (**b**) waveform, the trailing edge voltage is fixed but the durations change proportionately to the resistance. The effect of these differences on waveform optimization is described in text

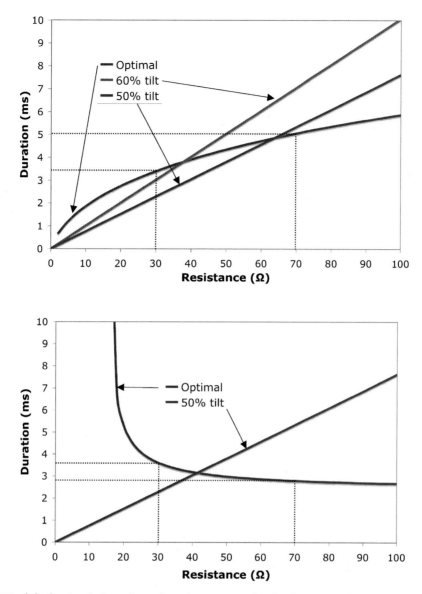

Figure 12: (a) Optimal durations for phase one of a biphasic shock assuming a 3.5 ms membrane time constant and a 110 μF capacitor. The durations given by the popular 50 and 60% tilts are also shown. Note the narrow range of optimal durations, for typical resistances of 30–70 Ω, compared to the broad swings of the tilt denominated waveforms. (b) Optimal durations for phase two as a function of resistance. These durations are compared to those produced by 50% tilt, as that is the phase two tilt used by the best-selling devices. (The Boston Scientific waveform calculates the phase two duration as two thirds of that of the first phase, giving a resulting effective tilt of 50%.) This is also based on a typical implantable cardioverter-defibrillator capacitance (110 μF) and membrane time constant of 3.5 ms. Note that the tilt-based duration adjusts to resistance changes in the opposite direction of optimal. Again, note the narrow range of the optimal durations

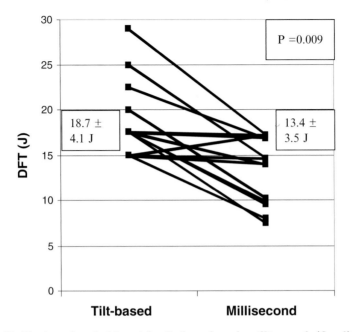

Figure 13: Defibrillation thresholds with tilt-based and millisecond (fixed) durations for each of 13 patients whose tilt-based defibrillation threshold was $\geq 15\,J$. (Used with permission of Elsevier)[1]

phase two decreases with increasing resistance, exactly opposite the response of fixed tilt waveforms.

Presently, the clinical significance of differences between tilt-based truncation and duration-based truncation is an area of controversy. Three clinical studies (two of which were funded by the manufacturer of ICDs that use duration-based truncation), reported lower DFTs using duration-based truncation than tilt-based truncation.[1,46,72] But these studies used tilt-based waveforms that are either known[3,35] or suspected[73] to be less efficient that clinically used tilt-based waveforms. One study reported that the greatest benefit for duration-based waveforms occurred in high DFT patients (Fig. 13). All three studies used capacitance values around $90\text{--}100\,\mu F$; modeling suggests that the benefit would be even greater with extremely large capacitance waveforms, which may be considered for new ICDs that utilize only subcutaneous electrodes.

Waveform Polarity

The effect of waveform polarity has been studied for transvenous defibrillation using both monophasic and biphasic waveforms. For monophasic waveforms, the right ventricular electrode should be the anode (positive), while the ICD pulse generator's housing should be the cathode.[74–76] Clinical results for biphasic waveforms are summarized in Table 2.[77] They

Table 2: Metaanalysis of studies comparing anodal versus cathodal right ventricle coils in implantable cardioverter-defibrillator therapy

Study	Can	N	Anodal DFT	Cathodal DFT	Anodal reduction (%)	Anodal better	Polarity neutral	Cathodal better
Schauerte	None	27	11.1	13.3	17	10	14	3
Shorofsky	Hot	26	11.1	12.2	9	12	6	8
Natale	None	20	16.3	21.5	24	12	6	2
Strickberger	None	15	9.9	9.5	−4	3	9	3
Keelan	Mixed	10	9.5	13.8	39	14	6	2
Olsovsky	Hot	60	7.2	8.5	15	23	26	10
Neuzner	None	32	9.38	10	6	13	11	8
Narasimhan	Mixed	22	10.5	11.05	5	7	11	2
Grouped		224	9.98	11.72	14.8	93	91	38

Taken from PACE[77]

(15% DFT reduction, $p = .00001$) show that the right ventricular electrode should be the anode for phase one of biphasic waveforms and the cathode for phase two. For biphasic waveforms, reversing polarity (right ventricle as anode) does not improve defibrillation efficacy within the measurement error of clinical DFT testing.[78]

These results are predicted by the virtual electrode hypothesis of defibrillation.[33] It predicts that postshock virtual electrodes launch new wavefronts *toward* the anode. Thus, a cathodal shock produces "expanding" wavefronts that propagate *away from* a physical right ventricular cathode, but an anodal shock produces "collapsing" wavefronts that propagate *toward* a physical right ventricular anode.[79] Thus a right ventricular cathode produces expanding and potentially proarrhythmic wavefronts, whereas a right ventricular anode produces collapsing, self-extinguishing wavefronts (Fig. 14). The effect of optimal polarity is greater for monophasic waveforms and less efficient biphasic waveforms than it is for more efficient biphasic waveforms, possibly because charge burping of efficient biphasic waveforms discharges the virtual electrodes.[74,80] An additional effect of anodal shocks may be to increase the homogeneity of membrane time constants in comparison with cathodal shocks.[81] This may, in theory, reduce the risk of refibrillation. *In today's ICDs, the right ventricular coil should be the anode for phase one of biphasic shocks.*

If the DFT is high for this electrode configuration, experts differ in opinion regarding the clinical utility of "reversing polarity." Some say that the 10–20% percent of cases in which anodal DFTs are higher than cathodal DFTs reflects the limited reproducibility of clinical DFTs rather than a true electrophysiological effect. These experts, the authors included, recommend maintaining the right ventricle as the anode for phase one and altering other components of the defibrillation system. Other experts empirically recommend reversing polarity if the anodal DFT is high, despite the lack of a conceptual framework or supporting data that exceeds the known variability of clinical DFT testing.

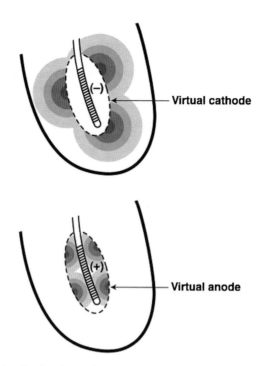

Figure 14: Cathodal shocks (*top*) produce expanding wavefronts that propagate away from the physical right ventricle (RV) coil, while anodal shocks (*bottom*) produce collapsing wavefronts that propagate toward the RV coil.(Used with permission of Blackwell Publishing)[77]

In the rare case where two epicardial patches are required, only data from older monophasic studies are available.[75,76] This suggest that the left ventricular patch should be the anode, perhaps since it directly affects more myocardium than the right ventricular patch.

Waveforms in Commercially Available ICDs

The voltages and capacitances used in commercial ICDs vary widely.[68] There are substantial disparities among their parameters, but it has been over a decade since a direct comparison of commercial waveforms has been published.[82]

Figure 15 shows the model response with $\tau_m = 3.5\,\text{ms}$ to waveforms with stored energy of 20 J delivered into a $40\,\Omega$ defibrillation pathway. The plots show waveform voltage and predicted cell membrane voltage (in arbitrary units) on the ordinate as a function of duration on the abscissa.

Figure 15a shows a St. Jude Atlas® waveform with durations programmed to result in optimal response of the model, assuming the patient's membrane time constant is estimated accurately. Phase one is truncated at the maximum membrane response. Phase

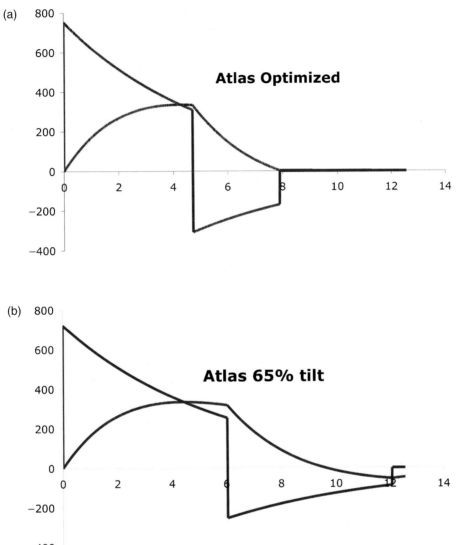

Figure 15: Various waveforms and their calculated membrane responses. The x axis is in milliseconds. This should not be relied upon for any specific patient as it is based on the mean 3.5 ms cardiac membrane τ and this is not known for a particular patient. (a) Shows a St. Jude Atlas® waveform with duration programmed to result in optimal response of the model. (b) Shows the longer St. Jude Atlas waveform with 65% tilt. (c, d) Show the Medtronic Marquis® (50% tilt) and Gem® (65% tilt) waveforms, respectively. The Boston Scientific Vitality® waveform (60/50% tilt) is shown in (e) for devices shipped with tantalum capacitors. (Used with permission of Elsevier Publishing)[83]

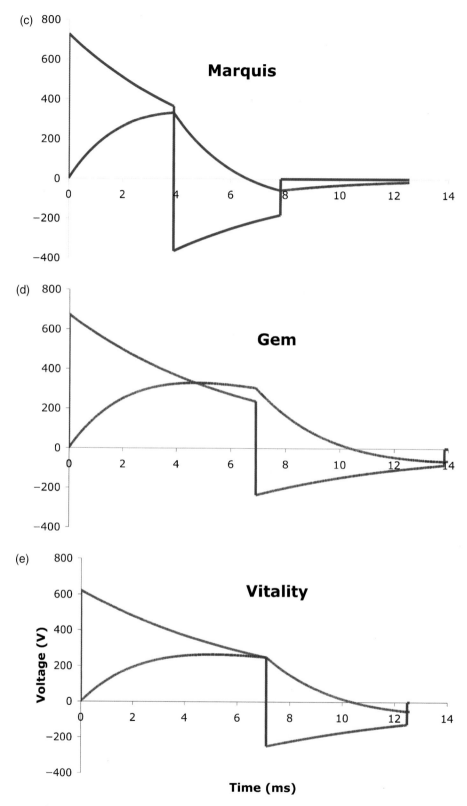

Figure 15: (*Continued*)

two is truncated when the membrane voltage returns to baseline. Figure 15b shows the longer St. Jude Atlas waveform with 65% tilt. The membrane reaches 99% of its maximum response to phase one at 4 ms, but phase one continues ineffectively for an additional 1.5 ms. The membrane voltage is below zero at the end of phase two. Recall that retrospective metaanalysis[29] and prospective[30] data indicate that defibrillation efficacy is inversely related to the residual membrane voltage at the end of phase two. In practice, the value of τ_m in an individual patient is not known and is unlikely to coincide exactly with an ICD's nominal value, as shown in Fig. 15a. However, a clinical comparison reported superior defibrillation for an estimated, "optimized" waveform (Fig. 15a) than the 65% tilt waveform that delivers a higher fraction of stored energy (Fig. 15b).[1]

Figure 15c and d show the Medtronic Marquis® (50/50% tilt) and Gem® (65/65% tilt) waveforms, respectively. In Fig. 15c, phase one is truncated just before the membrane reaches its maximum response. In contrast, Fig. 15d shows that phase one of the longer waveform continues for 2.0 ms after the membrane reaches 99% of its maximum response at 3.6 ms. A clinical comparison of 50/50% tilt and 65/65% tilt waveforms showed superior defibrillation for the 50/50% tilt waveform, which delivers a lower fraction of stored energy.

The Boston Scientific Vitality® waveform in Fig. 15e has the highest capacitance and thus the lowest leading-edge voltage for a given stored energy. It uses a 60/50% tilt waveform. Boston Scientific refers to this as a "60/40" waveform based on the percentage of time spent in each phase. Phase one continues for 1.4 ms after the membrane reaches 99% of its maximum response at 4.3 ms. The model predicts that the energy delivered after the peak is wasted. There is substantial residual voltage at the end of phase two. This waveform has not been compared clinically to any of the other waveforms; the model predicts it to be inefficient. The Vitality waveform shown is for the tantalum capacitor version. This ICD is also shipped with higher voltage aluminum capacitors predicted to result in more efficient waveforms; but details of this waveform have not been published.

The ELA Medical's Ovatio™ ICD uses a 177 μF capacitance with a 50/50% tilt waveform. Biotronik uses a 60% tilt for phase one and a choice of 50% tilt or a fixed 2 ms for phase two. Biotronik does not disclose the capacitance value for its ICDs.

Other Considerations in Optimizing Waveforms

Because ICD size reduction has been a priority, waveform optimization is often viewed as an energy minimization problem subject to constraints: higher voltage, shorter waveforms may defibrillate with lower energy, but extreme voltages may produce myocardial depression[84,85] and may exceed voltage and current limitations of semiconductor components. However, monophasic waveforms with voltages 1,540 V have been used successfully with catheters in humans.[86] And, biphasic waveforms produce less electroporation than monophasic waveforms,[38] hence the safe voltage limits have not been established for biphasic waveform transvenous defibrillation. The volumetric energy density of higher voltage capacitors allows this reduced energy to be packed in a disproportionately smaller package. If higher voltage biphasic waveform defibrillation proves safe, technology under development may permit ICDs to operate at over 1,000 V.

Presently used biphasic waveforms are substantially more effective than monophasic waveforms than the less-efficient biphasic waveforms used in the early 1990s.[82] Present ICDs and leads allow implantation without system modification more than 90% of the time. Nevertheless, ICDs prevent only approximately 60% of sudden cardiac deaths,[89] and approximately 25% of sudden deaths in ICD patients are due to failed defibrillation.[90,91] Further advances in waveform optimization may both reduce the number of difficult implants and the incidence of sudden death from failed defibrillation in ICD patients. Further, improved defibrillation efficacy may permit ICD size reduction. Finally, strong shocks delay postshock hemodynamic recovery[92] in a voltage dependent manner.[93] Postshock electromechanical dissociation is a fatal consequence of defibrillation and an important cause of sudden death in ICD patients.[90] We do not know if defibrillation waveforms can be optimized to minimize the risk of postshock electromechanical dissociation.

Waveform optimization has different priorities for external defibrillators than ICDs. For example, a sufficiently effective waveform generated by inexpensive components could facilitate distribution of automatic external defibrillators for public access defibrillation.

Shock pain correlates with peak voltage. To minimize pain, the peak voltage should be reduced[94] at the expense of delivering a long first phase. However, with first phase durations beyond 10 ms, defibrillation efficacy is reduced sufficiently that voltage requirements increase, defeating the purpose of the long waveform.[95]

With a subcutaneous or percutaneous ICD system (see the chapter by Kroll and Swerdlow) polarity is probably less relevant as there are no electrodes in direct contact with the ventricular tissue to launch new proarrhythmic wavefronts. The other waveform optimization considerations such as voltage, capacitance, and durations should all apply.

The Misunderstood Superior Vena Cava Coil

Studies of active can lead configurations[96,97] showed that the addition of the superior vena cava (SVC) coil decreases the voltage DFT, but paradoxically increases peak current more than can be explained by the reduction in DFT alone. This suggests that the vector for defibrillation is worsened with an SVC coil, but this adverse effect is more than offset by a large reduction of shock resistance.

The effect of the addition of an SVC coil on DFTs with an active can has been studied in several prospective randomized studies. Two studies by Gold et al.[98,99] showed a significant benefit with the SVC coil. Libero et al.[100] also found a significant reduction in the delivered energy DFT with the addition of an SVC coil.

Adding an SVC coil to the defibrillation pathway changes the vector, resistance, and phase durations (as they are proportional to the resistance). However, early studies all used fixed tilt waveforms, which are problematic due to the confounding effects on phase durations. As discussed previously, a limitation of fixed tilt waveforms is that they excessively increase their durations with high resistance lead systems. With a fixed duration waveform, the effect of suboptimal waveform phase durations can be neutralized by independently adjusting the durations of each phase. This isolates the phase duration effect from the effects on the resistance and electrical field (vector) in these earlier studies.

Table 3: Modeling and data driven recommendations for superior vena cava coil usage

Devices	Suggested superior vena cava usage for typical patient	Rationale
Medtronic	Begin without	The 50% tilt and capacitance values used favor a higher impedance
St. Jude Medical	With single coil impedance $\geq 60\,\Omega$ add superior vena cava coil. With $< 60\,\Omega$ single coil impedance the superior vena cava will help and hurt the defibrillation threshold in equal fractions of patients	Applies only to fixed pulse widths
Boston Scientific	Begin with	The 60% tilt and higher capacitance values used favor a lower impedance

A study designed to test the effect of an SVC coil on DFTs with fixed duration waveforms had complex findings.[101] This is not surprising since the addition of the SVC coil has competing and potentially offsetting effects on defibrillation. A benefit is the pulling of some current in a posterior direction to compete with the left pectoral can pulling current anteriorly. A negative is that current is preferably directed through the right atrium toward the SVC coil at the expense of going through the left ventricle toward the can. When the SVC coil was located in the "high" position (innominate vein–SVC junction), DFT peak voltage decreased from 430 ± 119.3 to $391.7 \pm 129.4\,\text{V}$ ($p = .01$) and stored energy was reduced from 9.9 ± 5.4 to $8.5 \pm 5.8\,\text{J}$ ($p = .03$) by programming SVC coil ON. In contrast, there was no significant benefit of the SVC coil on DFTs when the center of the coil was in the right atrial wall to SVC junction position. When the single coil shock resistance was $< 60\,\Omega$, there were no significant changes in the DFT peak voltage or stored energy with SVC coil ON. Thus, the effect of the SVC coil effect depends on waveform parameters and coil position. It should typically be used with higher resistance single-coil pathways. Suggested SVC usage is given in Table 3.

Conclusion

The electrical parameter most directly related to defibrillation is shock voltage (or voltage gradient) as a function of time. The parameter most directly related to the size of an ICD pulse generator is stored energy. The characteristics of an ICD's capacitive-discharge waveform link the electrical parameters related to physiology to those related to engineering. A simple RC network model has proved useful for designing efficient, biphasic capacitive-discharge waveforms. The right ventricular electrode should be the anode for phase one of transvenous defibrillation waveforms. Guidance can now be given for the optimal usage of the SVC coil.

References

1. Denman RA, Umesan C, Martin PT, Forbes RN, Kroll MW, Anskey EJ, Burnett HE. Benefit of millisecond waveform durations for patients with high defibrillation thresholds. *Heart Rhythm* 2006;3:536–541
2. White JB, Walcott GP, Wayland JL Jr, Smith WM, Ideker RE. Predicting the relative efficacy of shock waveforms for transthoracic defibrillation in dogs. *Ann Emerg Med* 1999;34:309–320
3. Mehdirad AA, Love CJ, Stanton MS, Strickberger SA, Duncan JL, Kroll MW. Preliminary clinical results of a biphasic waveform and an RV lead system. *Pacing Clin Electrophysiol* 1999;22:594–599
4. Schauerte P, Schondube FA, Grossmann M, Dorge H, Stein F, Dohmen B, Moumen A, Erena K, Messmer BJ, Hanrath P, Stellbrink C. Influence of phase duration of biphasic waveforms on defibrillation energy requirements with a 70-microF capacitance. *Circulation* 1998;97:2073–2078
5. Walcott GP, Walker RG, Cates AW, Krassowska W, Smith WM, Ideker RE. Choosing the optimal monophasic and biphasic waveforms for ventricular defibrillation. *J Cardiovasc Electrophysiol* 1995;6:737–750
6. Sharma AD, Fain E, O'Neill PG, Skadsen A, Damle R, Baker J, Chauhan V, Mazuz M, Ross T, Zhang Z. Shock on T versus direct current voltage for induction of ventricular fibrillation: a randomized prospective comparison. *Pacing Clin Electrophysiol* 2004;27:89–94
7. Mehdirad AA, Stohr EC, Love CJ, Nelson SD, Schaal SF. Implantable defibrillators impedance measurement using pacing pulses versus shock delivery with intact and modified high voltage lead system. *Pacing Clin Electrophysiol* 1999;22:437–441
8. Pendekanti R, Henriquez C, Tomassoni G, Miner W, Fain E, Hoffmann D, Wolf P. Surface coverage effects on defibrillation impedance for transvenous electrodes. *Ann Biomed Eng* 1997;25:739–746
9. Olsovsky MR, Shorofsky SR, Gold MR. The effect of shock configuration and delivered energy on defibrillation impedance. *Pacing Clin Electrophysiol* 1999;22:165–168
10. Weiss DN, Shorofsky SR, Peters RW, Gold MR. The effect of delivered energy on defibrillation shock impedance. *J Interv Card Electrophysiol* 1998;2:273–277
11. Kontos MC, Ellenbogen KA, Wood MA, Damiano RJ Jr, Akosah KO, Nixon JV, Stambler BS. Factors associated with elevated impedance with a nonthoracotomy defibrillation lead system. *Am J Cardiol* 1997;79:48–52
12. Schwartzman D, Hull ML, Callans DJ, Gottlieb CD, Marchlinski FE. Serial defibrillation lead impedance in patients with epicardial and nonthoracotomy lead systems. *J Cardiovasc Electrophysiol* 1996;7:697–703
13. Iskos D, Lock K, Lurie KG, Fahy GJ, Petersen-Stejskal S, Benditt DG. Submuscular versus subcutaneous pectoral implantation of cardioverter-defibrillators: effect on high

voltage pathway impedance and defibrillation efficacy. *J Interv Card Electrophysiol* 1998;2:47–52

14. Swerdlow C, Kass R, Hwang C, Gang E, Chen P, Peter C. Effect of voltage and respiration on impedance in nonthoracotomy defibrillation pathways. *Am J Cardiol* 1994;73:688–692

15. Prevost J, Batelli F. Quelques effets des decharges electriques sur le coeur des mammiferes. *J Phys Pathol Gen* 1900;2:40:52

16. Peleska B. [Transthoracic and direct defibrillation]. *Rozhl Chir* 1957;36:731–755

17. Schuder J, Stoeckle H, JAW. Transthoracic ventricular defibrillation in the dog with truncated exponential stimuli. *IEEE Trans Biomed Eng BME* 1971;18:410–415

18. Feeser S, Tang A, Kavanagh K, Rollins D, WM S, Wolf P, Ideker R. Strength-duration and probability of success curves for defibrillation with biphasic waveforms. *Circulation* 1990;82:2128–2141

19. Dixon EG, Tang AS, Wolf PD, Meador JT, Fine MJ, Calfee RV, Ideker RE. Improved defibrillation thresholds with large contoured epicardial electrodes and biphasic waveforms. *Circulation* 1987;76:1176–1184

20. Tang A, Yabe S, Wharton J, Dolker M, Smith W, Ideker R. Ventricular defibrillation using biphasic waveforms: the importance of phasic defibrillation. *J Am Coll Cardiol* 1989;13:207–214

21. Peekema, RM, Beesley, JP. Factors affecting the impedence of foil-type electrolytic capacitors. *Electrochem. Technol.* 1968;6:166

22. Malkin RA, Guan D, Wikswo JP. Experimental evidence of improved transthoracic defibrillation with electroporation-enhancing pulses. *IEEE Trans Biomed Eng* 2006;53:1901–1910

23. Blair H. On the intensity-time relations for stimulation by electric currents, I. *J Gen Physiol* 1932;15:709–729

24. Blair H. On the intensity-time relations for stimulation by electric currents, II. *J Gen Physiol* 1932;15:731–755

25. Seidl K, Denman R, JC M, Mouchawar G, Stoeppler C, Becker T, Weise U, Anskey E, Burnett H, Kroll M. Stepped defibrillation waveform is substantially more efficient than the 50/50% tilt biphasic. *Heart Rhythm* 2006;3(12):1406–1411

26. Cleland B. A conceptual basis for defibrillation waveforms. *Pacing Clin Electrophysiol* 1996;19:1186–1195

27. Fishler MG. Theoretical predictions of the optimal monophasic and biphasic defibrillation waveshapes. *IEEE Trans Biomed Eng* 2000;47:59–67

28. Kroll MW. A minimal model of the monophasic defibrillation pulse. *Pacing Clin Electrophysiol* 1993;16:769–777

29. Kroll MW. A minimal model of the single capacitor biphasic defibrillation waveform. *Pacing Clin Electrophysiol* 1994;17:1782–1792

30. Swerdlow C, Fan W, Brewer J. Charge-burping theory correctly predicts optimal ratios of phase duration for biphasic defibrillation waveforms. *Circulation* 1996;94:2278–2284

31. Dillon SM, Kwaku KF. Progressive depolarization: a unified hypothesis for defibrillation and fibrillation induction by shocks. *J Cardiovasc Electrophysiol* 1998;9:529–552

32. Chen P-S, Wolf PD, Ideker RE. The mechanism of cardiac defibrillation: a different point of view. *Circulation* 1991;84:913–919

33. Cheng Y, Mowrey KA, Van Wagoner DR, Tchou PJ, Efimov IR. Virtual electrode-induced reexcitation: a mechanism of defibrillation. *Circ Res* 1999;85:1056–1066

34. Efimov IR, Cheng Y, Yamanouchi Y, Tchou PJ. Direct evidence of the role of virtual electrode-induced phase singularity in success and failure of defibrillation. *J Cardiovasc Electrophysiol* 2000;11:861–868

35. Hodgkin A. The subthreshold potentials in a crustacean nerve fiber. *Proc R Soc Lond B* 1938;126:87–121

36. Kao CY, Hoffman BF. Graded and decremental response in heart muscle fibers. *Am J Physiol* 1958;194:187–196

37. Krassowska W, Cabo C, Knisley SB, Ideker RE. Propagation versus delayed activation during field stimulation of cardiac muscle. *Pacing Clin Electrophysiol* 1992;15:197–210

38. Tovar O, Tung L. Electroporation of cardiac cell membranes with monophasic or biphasic rectangular pulses. *Pacing Clin Electrophysiol* 1991;14:1887–1892

39. Jones JL, Jones RE. Improved defibrillator waveform safety factor with biphasic waveforms. *Am J Physiol* 1983;245:H60–H65

40. Jones JL, Jones RE. Decreased defibrillator-induced dysfunction with biphasic rectangular waveforms. *Am J Physiol* 1984;247:H792–H796

41. Anderson C, Trayanova N, Skouibine K. Termination of spiral waves with biphasic shocks: role of virtual electrode polarization. *J Cardiovasc Electrophysiol* 2000;11:1386–1396

42. Behrens S, Li C, Kirchhof P, Fabritz FL, Franz MR. Reduced arrhythmogenicity of biphasic versus monophasic T-wave shocks. Implications for defibrillation efficacy. *Circulation* 1996;94:1974–1980

43. Efimov IR, Cheng Y, Van Wagoner DR, Mazgalev T, Tchou PJ. Virtual electrode-induced phase singularity: a basic mechanism of defibrillation failure. *Circ Res* 1998;82:918–925

44. Efimov IR, Cheng YN, Biermann M, Van Wagoner DR, Mazgalev TN, Tchou PJ. Transmembrane voltage changes produced by real and virtual electrodes during monophasic defibrillation shock delivered by an implantable electrode. *J Cardiovasc Electrophysiol* 1997;8:1031–1045

45. Schauerte PN, Ziegert K, Waldmann M, Schondube FA, Birkenhauer F, Mischke K, Grossmann M, Hanrath P, Stellbrink C. Effect of biphasic shock duration on defibrillation threshold with different electrode configurations and phase 2 capacitances: prediction by upper-limit-of-vulnerability determination. *Circulation* 1999;99:1516–1522

46. Mouchawar G, Kroll M, Val-Mejias JE, Schwartzman D, McKenzie J, Fitzgerald D, Prater S, Katcher M, Fain E, Syed Z. ICD waveform optimization: a randomized, prospective, pair-sampled multicenter study. *Pacing Clin Electrophysiol* 2000;23:1992–1995

47. Shorofsky SR, Rashba E, Havel W, Belk P, Degroot P, Swerdlow C, Gold MR. Improved defibrillation efficacy with an ascending ramp waveform in humans. *Heart Rhythm* 2005;2:388–394

48. Kroll M, Lehmann M, Tchou P. Defining the defibrillation dosage. In: Kroll M, Lehmann M, eds. *Implantable Cardioverter-Defibrillator Therapy: The Engineering-Clinical Interface*. Norwell, MA: Kluwer Academic; 1996:63–88

49. Hillsley R, Walker R, Swanson D, Rollins D, Wolf P, Ideker R. Is the second phase of a biphasic waveform the defibrillating phase? *Pacing Clin Electrophysiol* 1993;16:1402–1411

50. Hoorweg J. Condensatorentladung und Auseinanderetzung mit du Bois-Reymond. *Pfugers Arch* 1892;52:87–108

51. Weiss G. Sur la possibilite' de rendre comparable entre eux les appareils survant a l'excitation electrique. *Arch Ital de Biol* 1901;35:413–446

52. Bourland JD, Tacker WA, Geddes LA. Strength duration curves for trapezoidal waveforms of various tilts for transchest defibrillation in animals. *Med Instrum* 1978;12:38–41

53. Gold J, Schuder J, Stoeckle H, Granberg T, Hamdani S, Rychlewski J. Transthoracic ventricular defibrillation in the 100 kg calf with unidirectional rectangular pulses. *Circulation* 1977;56:745

54. Wessale J, Bourland J, Tacker W, Geddes L. Bipolar catheter defibrillation in dogs using trapezoidal waveforms of various tilts. *J Electocardiol* 1980;13:359–366

55. Geddes LA, Niebauer MJ, Babbs CF, Bourland JD. Fundamental criteria underlying the efficacy and safety of defibrillating current waveforms. *Med Biol Eng Comput* 1985;23:122–130

56. Niebauer MJ, Babbs CF, Geddes LA, Bourland JD. Efficacy and safety of defibrillation with rectangular waves of 2- to 20-milliseconds duration. *Crit Care Med* 1983;11:95–98

57. Swerdlow CD, Brewer JE, Kass RM, Kroll MW. Application of models of defibrillation to human defibrillation data: implications for optimizing implantable defibrillator capacitance. *Circulation* 1997;96:2813–2822

58. Shorofsky S, Rashba E, DeGroot P, Havel W, Mugglin A, Gold M. Is the membrane time constant for defibrillation independent of the waveform? *Pacing Clin Electrophysiol* 2002;24:620 (abstract)

59. Gold MR, Shorofsky SR. Strength-duration relationship for human transvenous defibrillation. *Circulation* 1997;96:3517–3520

60. Mouchawar GA, Geddes LA, Bourland JD. Ability of the Lapicque and Blair strength-duration curves to fit experimentally obtained data from the dog heart. *IEEE Trans Biomed Eng* 1989;36:971–974

61. Hahn S, Heil J, Lin Y, Derfus D, Lang D. Improved defibrillation with small capacitance and optimized biphasic waveforms. *Circulation* 1994;90:I-175

62. Jung W, Moosdorf R, Korte T, Wolpert C, Spehl S, Bauer T, Manz M. Effect of capacitance on the defibrillation threshold in patients using a new unipolar defibrillation system. *Circulation* 1994;90(4):I-229

63. Rist K, Tchou PJ, Mowrey K, Kroll MW, Brewer JE. Smaller capacitors improve the biphasic waveform. *J Cardiovasc Electrophysiol* 1994;5:771–776

64. Leonelli FM, Kroll MW, Brewer JE. Defibrillation thresholds are lower with smaller storage capacitors. *Pacing Clin Electrophysiol* 1995;18:1661–1665

65. Swerdlow CD, Brewer JE, Kass RM, Kroll M. Estimation of optimal ICD capacitance from human strength-duration data. *J Am Coll Cardiol* 1997;96(9):2813–2822

66. Swerdlow C, Kass R, Hwang C, Chen P-S, Raissi S. Effect of capacitor size and pathway resistance on defibrillation threshold for implantable defibrillators. *Circulation* 1994;90:1840–1846

67. Sticherling C, Klingenheben T, Cameron D, Hohnloser SH. Worldwide clinical experience with a down-sized active can implantable cardioverter defibrillator in 162 consecutive patients. Worldwide 7221 ICD Investigators. *Pacing Clin Electrophysiol* 1998;21:1778–1783

68. Thammanomai A, Sweeney M, Eisenberg S. A comparison of the output characteristics of several implantable cardioverter defibrillators. *Heart Rhythm* 2006;3:1053–1059

69. Yamanouchi Y, Brewer JE, Mowrey KA, Donohoo AM, Wilkoff BL, Tchou PJ. Optimal small-capacitor biphasic waveform for external defibrillation: influence of phase-1 tilt and phase-2 voltage. *Circulation* 1998;98:2487–2493

70. Malkin RA. Large sample test of defibrillation waveform sensitivity. *J Cardiovasc Electrophysiol* 2002;13:361–370

71. Cheng Y, Mowrey KA, Nikolski V, Tchou PJ, Efimov IR. Mechanisms of shock-induced arrhythmogenesis during acute global ischemia. *Am J Physiol Heart Circ Physiol* 2002;282:H2141–H2151

72. Natarajan S, Henthorn R, Burroughs J, Esberg D, Zweibel S, Ross T, Kroll M, Gianola D, Oza A. Fixed duration "tuned" defibrillation waveforms outperform fixed 50/50% tilt defibrillation waveforms: a randomized, prospective, pair-sampled multicenter study. *Pacing Clin Electrophysiol* 2007;30:S139–S142

73. Sweeney MO, Natale A, Volosin KJ, Swerdlow CD, Baker JH, Degroot P. Prospective randomized comparison of 50%/50% versus 65%/65% tilt biphasic waveform on defibrillation in humans. *Pacing Clin Electrophysiol* 2001;24:60–65

74. Strickberger SA, Hummel JD, Horwood LE, Jentzer J, Daoud E, Niebauer M, Bakr O, Man KC, Williamson BD, Kou W, et al. Effect of shock polarity on ventricular defibrillation threshold using a transvenous lead system. *J Am Coll Cardiol* 1994;24:1069–1072

75. O'Neill PG, Boahene KA, Lawrie GM, Harvill LF, Pacifico A. The automatic implantable cardioverter-defibrillator: effect of patch polarity on defibrillation threshold. *J Am Coll Cardiol* 1991;17:707–711

76. Bardy GH, Ivey TD, Allen MD, Johnson G, Greene HL. Evaluation of electrode polarity on defibrillation efficacy. *Am J Cardiol* 1989;63:433–437

77. Kroll MW, Efimov IR, Tchou PJ. Present understanding of shock polarity for internal defibrillation: the obvious and non-obvious clinical implications. *Pacing Clin Electrophysiol* 2006;29:885–891

78. Swerdlow C, Ahern T, Chen P-S. Comparative reproducibility of defibrillation threshold and upper limit of vulnerability. *Pacing Clin Electrophysiol* 1996;19:2103–2111

79. Yamanouchi Y, Cheng Y, Tchou PJ, Efimov IR. The mechanisms of the vulnerable window: the role of virtual electrodes and shock polarity. *Can J Physiol Pharmacol* 2001;79:25–33

80. Strickberger SA, Daoud E, Goyal R, Chan KK, Bogun F, Castellani M, Harvey M, Horwood LE, Niebauer M, Man KC, Morady F. Prospective randomized comparison of anodal monophasic shocks versus biphasic cathodal shocks on defibrillation energy requirements. *Am Heart J* 1996;131:961–965

81. Mowrey KA, Cheng Y, Tchou PJ, Efimov R. Kinetics of defibrillation shock-induced response: design implications for the optimal defibrillation waveform. *Europace* 2002;4:27–39

82. Tomassoni G, Newby K, Deshpande S, Axtell K, Sra J, Akhtar M, Natale A. Defibrillation efficacy of commercially available biphasic impulses in humans. Importance of negative-phase peak voltage. *Circulation* 1997;95:1822–1826

83. Swerdlow CD. ICD waveforms: what really matters? *Heart Rhythm* 2006;3:1060–1062

84. Peleska B. Cardiac arrhythmias following condenser discharges and their dependence upon strength of current and phase of cardiac cycle. *Circ Res* 1963;13:21–32

85. Nikolski VP, Efimov IR. Electroporation of the heart. *Europace* 2005;7(Suppl 2):146–154

86. Jones DL, Klein GJ, Guiraudon GM, Sharma AD, Kallok MJ, Bourland JD, Tacker WA. Internal cardiac defibrillation in man: pronounced improvement with sequential pulse delivery to two different lead orientations. *Circulation* 1986;73:484–491

87. Russo AM, Sauer W, Gerstenfeld EP, Hsia HH, Lin D, Cooper JM, Dixit S, Verdino RJ, Nayak HM, Callans DJ, Patel V, Marchlinski FE. Defibrillation threshold testing: is it really necessary at the time of implantable cardioverter-defibrillator insertion? *Heart Rhythm* 2005;2:456–461

88. Shukla HH, Flaker GC, Jayam V, Roberts D. High defibrillation thresholds in transvenous biphasic implantable defibrillators: clinical predictors and prognostic implications. *Pacing Clin Electrophysiol* 2003;26:44–48

89. Anderson KP. Sudden cardiac death unresponsive to implantable defibrillator therapy: an urgent target for clinicians, industry and government. *J Interv Card Electrophysiol* 2005;14:71–78

90. Mitchell LB, Pineda EA, Titus JL, Bartosch PM, Benditt DG. Sudden death in patients with implantable cardioverter defibrillators: the importance of post-shock electromechanical dissociation. *J Am Coll Cardiol* 2002;39:1323–1328

91. Poole J, Johnson G, Callans D, Raitt M, Yee R, Reddy R, Wilber D, Guarnieri T, Talajic M, Marchlinski F, Lee K, Bardy G, Investigators S-H. Analysis of implantable defibrillator shock electrograms in the Sudden Cardiac Death-Heart Failure Trial. *Heart Rhythm* 2004;1:S178 (abstract)

92. Tokano T, Bach D, Chang J, Davis J, Souza JJ, Zivin A, Knight BP, Goyal R, Man KC, Morady F, Strickberger SA. Effect of ventricular shock strength on cardiac hemodynamics. *J Cardiovasc Electrophysiol* 1998;9:791–797

93. Holmes H, Bourland J, Tacker W Jr, Geddes L. Hemodynamic responses to two defibrillating trapezoidal waveforms. *Med Instrumen* 1980;14:47–50

94. Boriani G, Biffi M, Silvestri P, Martignani C, Valzania C, Diemberger I, Moulder C, Mouchawar G, Kroll M, Branzi A. Mechanisms of pain associated with internal defibrillation shocks: results of a randomized study of shock waveform. *Heart Rhythm* 2005;2:708–713

95. Boriani G, Kroll M, Biffi M, Silvestri P, Martignani C, Valzania C, Diemberger I, Moulder C, Mouchawar G, Branzi A. Plateau waveform shape allows a higher patient shock energy tolerance. *Heart Rhythm* 2006;3:S13

96. Gold M, Val-Mejias J, Leman R, Tummala R, Goyal S, Kluger J, Kroll M, Oza A. Effect of SVC coil usage and SVC electrode spacing on defibrillation thresholds. *Circulation* 2006;114:II-690

97. Gold MR, Olsovsky MR, DeGroot PJ, Cuello C, Shorofsky SR. Optimization of transvenous coil position for active can defibrillation thresholds. *J Cardiovasc Electrophysiol* 2000;11:25–29

98. Gold MR, Foster AH, Shorofsky SR. Lead system optimization for transvenous defibrillation. *Am J Cardiol* 1997;80:1163–1167

99. Gold MR, Olsovsky MR, Pelini MA, Peters RW, Shorofsky SR. Comparison of single- and dual-coil active pectoral defibrillation lead systems. *J Am Coll Cardiol* 1998;31:1391–1394

100. Libero L, Lozano IF, Bocchiardo M, Marcolongo M, Sallusti L, Madrid A, Gaita F, Trevi GP. Comparison of defibrillation thresholds using monodirectional electrical vector versus bidirectional electrical vector. *Ital Heart J* 2001;2:449–455

101. Gold M, Val-Mejias J, Leman R, Tummala R, Goyal S, Kluger J, Kroll M, Oza A. What is the optimal SVC coil usage in ICD patients? Results from a randomized, prospective multicenter study. *Heart Rhythm* 2008;5(3):394–349

Chapter 6.2

Resonance and Feedback Strategies for Low-Voltage Defibrillation

Vadim N. Biktashev

Introduction

Early experiments on defibrillation revealed that it is sometimes possible to achieve defibrillation by lower voltage pulses, if they are applied several times and are properly timed.[1] This chapter will review some ideas about detailed mechanisms and how this method may work. Most of these ideas are theoretical and tested only in numerical simulations or in a chemical model of the cardiac tissue, the Belousov–Zhabotinsky (BZ) reaction medium; only in some cases have experimentalists attempted a direct verification in cardiac preparations. The literature on the subject is vast; as the space allocated for this review is limited, the focus here will be on a few cornerstone ideas and somewhat arbitrarily selected examples.

Localized Stimulation: Induced Drift of Spiral Waves

Multiple wave sources in an excitable medium compete with one another. During such competition, the fastest source entrains increasingly more of the tissue. If the faster source is the stimulating electrode and it entrains the whole of the cardiac tissue, it would have expelled the reentrant circuits and perhaps stopped the fibrillation. However, the success of that depends on what happens to the reentry source when the high-frequency waves reach it.

This was first investigated in the chemical model of excitable tissues, the BZ reaction medium,[2] and then subsequently in more details in numerical simulations of a variant of the FitzHugh–Nagumo model.[3] Figure 1 illustrates the main concept. The first panels show the process of entrainment of the medium by the faster source, which in this particular case is the electrode located at the lower boundary of the model medium. When the entrained region reaches the spiral wave, the latter changes its nature: it is no longer a rotating source of waves, but is a dislocation in the otherwise regular field of waves

Department of Mathematics, University of Liverpool, Liverpool, UK

I. R. Efimov et al. (eds.), *Cardiac Bioelectric Therapy: Mechanisms and Practical Implications.*
© Springer Science+Business Media, LLC 2009

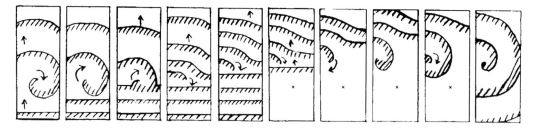

Figure 1: Enslaving (*panels 1–4*), drift (*panels 4–6*), and recovery (*panels 6–10*) of a spiral wave in the field of externally induced plane waves, in numerical experiments (schematic, similar to Ermakova et al.[3]). For comparison, the original position of the spiral rotation center is shown by a cross on panels 6–9

emitted by the fast source. Notice that it cannot disappear completely for topological reasons, as it carries a topological charge. When the approximately periodic waves are passing through a certain point in the medium, one observes oscillations of the dynamic variables at that point and can assign a phase to those oscillations. The increment of change of the phase of oscillations around a contour encircling the spiral or that is the dislocation is the same for both of them, as it cannot change as long as the oscillations persist, which they do unless the contour is crossed by the dislocation. Hence the dislocation carries this topological charge of the spiral wave. Typically it does not stay but drifts; this is sometimes called high-frequency induced drift of spirals, to distinguish it from drift caused by other mechanisms. The direction of drift depends on the parameters of the problem, in particular on the frequency of the entraining source. When the entraining source stops, the dislocation immediately turns back into a spiral wave, which locates in a new place. If the duration and direction of the induced drift are such that the dislocation reaches the place where the regular oscillations are not observed (e.g., the inexcitable border or a Wenckebach block zone), then the topological restriction is lifted and the dislocation may be eliminated, so when the high-frequency source stops, the spiral wave does not resume, and the reentry is stopped.

So the success of this method depends on the time factor: if the inexcitable border is far from the initial location of the spiral core and the induced drift speed is low, it could take a long time to expel the spiral, and if the stimulation stops earlier, it fails. Notably the amplitude of the stimulation plays a secondary role here: it should only be enough to initiate the entraining wave train; further increase of that amplitude does not enhance (at least within this particular mechanism) the chances of success. One can, however, control other parameters, such as the speed of the drift, through stimulation frequency, and its direction, through location of the stimulating electrode(s). If one uses a "grid" of synchronously working electrodes instead of a point electrode, then the distance required for the induced drift is limited by the size of the cell of this grid.[4,5]

Delocalized Stimulation: Resonant Drift of Spiral Waves

Another approach is based on an alternative idealization of the action of the electric current on cardiac tissue. Suppose, for simplicity and in the first approximation, that a reasonably spatially uniform electric field (say as produced by a transthoracic defibrillator) acts simultaneously and similarly on all cells in the tissue. Mathematically, that is equivalent to introduction into the model of a parameter that explicitly depends on time. Davydov et al.[6] considered a simplified "kinematic" description of spiral waves and predicted that if the parameters of the model are changed periodically with a period close to the rotation period of the spiral wave, then the spiral exhibits large-scale wandering, which, in the case of a precise resonance, degenerates into a drift along a straight line (Fig. 2). This theoretical prediction was supported by numerical simulations of a piecewise linear FitzHugh–Nagumo model and then immediately confirmed by experiments in BZ reaction.[7] Subsequent studies have demonstrated that this resonant drift phenomenon is not restricted to the two particular cases but can be reproduced in a wide variety of spiral wave models, including cardiac models.[9]

Following the same logic as with the high-frequency induced drift, if the excursion of the resonantly drifting vortex is large enough to bring it into an inexcitable boundary, this can lead to extermination of the spiral wave, and thus can be thought of as another low-voltage defibrillation strategy. Some difficulties in practical application of this idea are immediately obvious. As with the case of the high-frequency induced drift, one needs to know the appropriate frequency of the stimulation: the further it is from the resonance, the more compact is the trajectory of the drift. The theory proposed in Davydov et al.[6] gives the following expression for the radius of the drift trajectory R_d (up to a choice of notations):

$$R_d = \left| \frac{c_d}{\omega_s - \omega_f} \right|, \tag{1}$$

where c_d is the resonant drift speed depending on the forcing mode and magnitude, ω_f is the angular frequency of the forcing, and ω_s is the angular frequency of the spiral. So the lower the stimulation amplitude, the lower the drift speed c_d and the more precise the resonance to achieve needed R_d should be.

However, even if the resonant frequency is found, it is still not enough to eliminate the spiral. Figure 3 illustrates a simulation in a variant FitzHugh–Nagumo model in which a spiral wave drifting in a straight line reaches the vicinity of an inexcitable boundary. However, the spiral does not annihilate there, but instead turns around and drifts away from the boundary. The mechanism of such resonant repulsion has been considered in Biktashev and Holden,[10,11] where it was shown that the resonant drift can be approximately described by a system of ordinary differential equations of the form

$$\frac{d\Phi}{dt} = \omega_s(R) - \omega_f,$$
$$\frac{dR}{dt} = c_d(R)e^{i\Phi} + (C_x(R) + iC_y(R)), \tag{2}$$

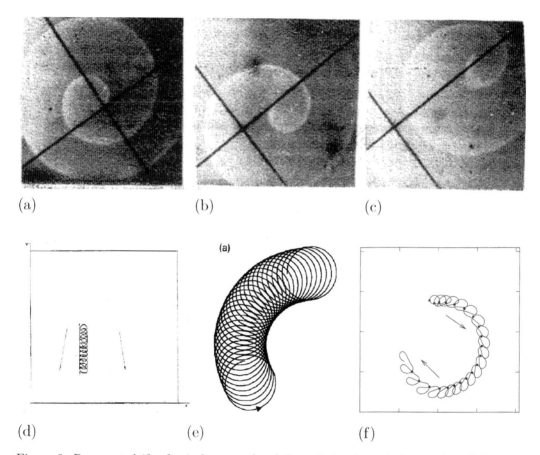

Figure 2: Resonant drift of spiral waves. (**a**–**c**) Snapshots of a spiral wave in a Belousov–Zhabotinsky (BZ) experiment at a precise resonance; *black cross* is reference. (Reprinted with permission from Agladze et al.,[7] © 1987, IEEE) (**d**) In a piecewise variant of FitzHugh–Nagumo system at a precise resonance. (Reprinted from Davydov et al.[6] with kind permission of Springer Science and Business Media) (**e**) In a kinematic model of a generic excitable medium without refractoriness, away from a precise resonance. (Reprinted with permission from Mikhailov et al.,[8] © 1994, Elsevier) (**f**) In the reaction-diffusion model with OXSOFT rabbit atrium kinetics, away from a precise resonance. (Reprinted with permission from Biktashev and Holden,[9] © 1995, Royal Society)

where $R = R(t) = X(r) + iY(t)$ is the complex coordinate of the instant center of rotation of the spiral, $\Phi = \Phi(t)$ is the phase difference between the spiral rotation and the periodic forcing, ω_s and c_d are, as before, respectively the spiral's frequency and the speed of the resonant drift, and (C_x, C_y) is the vector of the spontaneous drift of the spiral that would

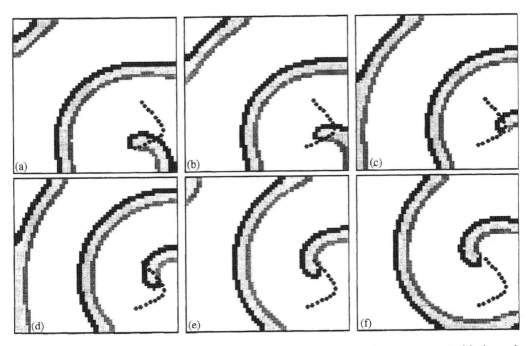

Figure 3: Mechanism of repulsion of resonantly drifting vortex from an inexcitable boundary. (Reprinted with permission from Biktashev and Holden,[10] © 1993, Elsevier) Shown are successive positions of the vortex in exactly three periods of stimulation. *Black dots* at each picture denote the positions of the vortex tip at the instant of stimulation. (**a–c**) The stimuli occur in the same rotation phase, and the trajectory is straight. (**c, d**) The natural frequency of the vortex increases near the boundary, each successive stimulus occurring at a later phase, and the direction of the drift turns. (**d–f**) The vortex goes away from the boundary, it resumes its original natural frequency, and the trajectory is again straight

happen without external perturbation, say due to spatial gradients of tissue properties or in proximity to inexcitable obstacles. If $C_x = C_y = 0$ and ω_s, $c_d = \text{const}$, then system (2) is easily solved leading to (1). In terms of system (2), the explanation of the resonant repulsion is in the dependence of its key parameters on the spatial position of the spiral, particularly $\omega_s = \omega_s(R)$. In Fig. 3, the closer the spiral is to the boundary, the higher its frequency will be. That destroys the resonance $\omega_s = \omega_f$, which by the first equation leads to an increase in Φ which means a change of the direction of the resonant drift given by $c_d e^{i\Phi}$. Such change continues until the spiral is sufficiently far from the boundary. Then $\omega_s = \omega_f$ again, and the spiral drifts along a different straight line, now away from the boundary.

Feedback-Controlled Resonant Drift

The phenomenon of resonant repulsion makes it clear that it may not be the best strategy to keep stimulation frequency constant or to change it according to a prescribed program, but this change should be determined by actual events via feedback. The feedback may be realized by monitoring activity at a point in the medium with a recording electrode. Since the frequency of real rotation of a drifting vortex is close to and changes together with the resonant frequency, the simplest control strategy is to stimulate synchronously with the monitoring of an action potential spike by recording electrode or after a fixed delay. The recorded frequency differs from the vortex frequency in the frame of reference of its core due to its motion (a Doppler effect), and, therefore, the induced motion of the vortex will not be strictly along a straight line.

The mechanism of feedback-driven resonant drift is illustrated in Fig. 4. In contrast to the case of constant frequency stimulation, the trajectory of the vortex core far from its boundaries is a curve, not a straight line, since with motion of the vortex, the phase distance from its core to the recording point changes. Close to the boundary there is no resonant repulsion. The trajectory deviates from what it would be in the absence of boundary, seemingly due to the terms C_x, C_y in the phenomenological model (2). As a result, the vortex reaches the boundary and annihilates, at a stimulation amplitude, at which constant frequency stimulation fails. Numerical simulation shows that the stimulation amplitude necessary for extinguishing the vortex by feedback-driven resonant drift can be by an order of magnitude less than that required for single-pulse defibrillation.[12]

The feedback-driven motion of the spiral can be described by an appropriate modification of the phenomenological model (2). The phase difference Φ between the spiral wave and the stimulation depends on the phase delay, required for the excitation wave emitted by the spiral rotating around a point R to reach the registration electrode location. If we denote this dependence as $\Phi = \Phi_{fb}(R)$, the third-order system (2) reduces to a second-order system:

$$\frac{dX}{dt} = C_x(X,Y) + c_d(X,Y)\cos(\Phi_{fb}(X,Y)),$$
$$\frac{dY}{dt} = C_y(X,Y) + c_d(X,Y)\sin(\Phi_{fb}(X,Y)). \tag{3}$$

An analytical expression for the function Φ_{fb} can be obtained by approximating the shape of the spiral wave by an Archimedean spiral, which allows system (3) to describe very well the behavior of the feedback-driven spirals.[11,12] Moreover, this approach can be extended to the cases when the electrode used for detection of the feedback signal is not pointlike but is spatially extended over a certain domain; variation of this domain shape and location can be a very effective tool in controlling the trajectories of the resonant drift.[13,14] System[3] is an autonomous second-order system of equations, and it is convenient to study its behavior using phase-plane analysis (Fig. 5). As it would be expected in a generic ordinary differential equation (ODE) system, there are attracting trajectories, which could be compact (i.e., attracting stationary points or limit cycles, known as resonant attractors),[13–15] or noncompact, which run away from the medium. Naturally, from the

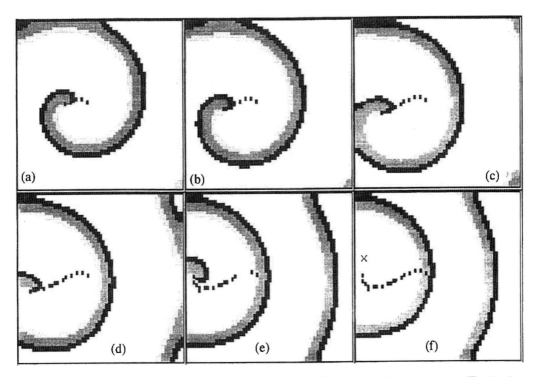

Figure 4: Mechanism of feedback-driven resonant drift, numerical experiment. Excitation patterns are shown synchronously with stimuli beginnings, which are issued synchronously with arriving wavefront to the left top corner of the preparation. Due to the feedback, each stimulus occurs at the same rotation phase, up to the phase distance from the registration point to the vortex core. Therefore, the trajectory is affected only by the usual attraction/repulsion from boundary, without resonant repulsion taking place. As a result, the vortex annihilates at the boundary. (Reprinted with permission from Biktashev and Holden,[11] © 1995, Elsevier)

practical viewpoint a resonant attractor within the tissue boundaries signifies a failure of the low-voltage defibrillation attempt, so it is preferred to avoid it.

Fibrillation, at least in some cases, is associated with multiple reentrant sources, hence the question of whether the above described feedback control strategy can cope with that. Simple simulations demonstrate that multiplicity of reentrant sources in itself is not a significant impediment to their elimination.[11] Say, for the case of point registering electrode, the feedback signal will come from the one spiral whose waves reach the electrode site, which ensures a directed drift of that spiral (Fig. 6). Cores of such "leading" spirals are circled on the figure. Other spirals may or may not annihilate during this stage. Upon reaching the boundary, the leading spiral is extinguished, and the electrode monitors the wavefront from another one, which in turn is extinguished, and so on. As a result, all the spiral waves are progressively extinguished in a time not much longer than that needed for extinguishing one.

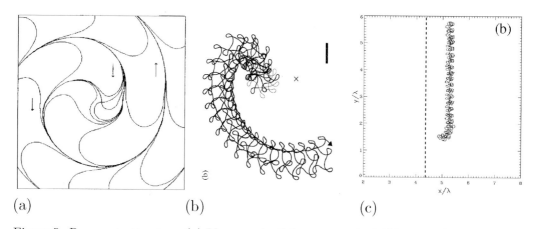

Figure 5: Resonant attractors. (a) Phase portrait for resonantly drifting spirals as predicted by the theory. (Reprinted with permission from Biktashev and Holden,[11] © 1995, Elsevier) (b) Tip trajectory computed in light-sensitive variant of the Oregonator model, with the point registering electrode (*the cross*). (Reprinted with permission from Grill et al.,[15] © 1995, American Physical Society) (c) Tip trajectory measured in an experiment with light-sensitive variant of the Belousov–Zhabotinsky (BZ) reaction with the registered electrode in the form of a straight line (*vertical dashed line*). (Reprinted with permission from Zykov et al.,[14] © 2007, World Scientific)

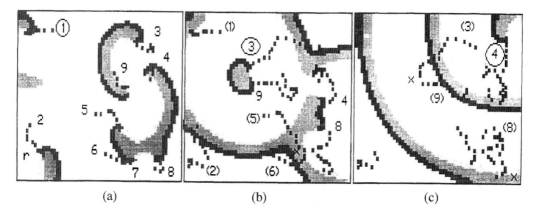

Figure 6: Evolution of multiple vortices under feedback-driven stimulation. The "leading" vortex is circled on each panel, traces of annihilated vortices are marked by digits in parentheses. (a) Vortex 1 leads, vortex 2 repulses from boundary. (b) Vortices 1, 2, 5, and 6 have annihilated vortex 3 leads. (c) Vortices 3, 8, and 9 have annihilated the only alive vortex 4 leads. Further evolution results in annihilation of vortex 4. (Reprinted with permission from Biktashev and Holden,[11] © 1995, Elsevier)

In reality, the number of spiral waves may not be fixed, and they may "multiply" via wave breakups when the resonant drift forces them out. The chances of success in that case seem to heavily depend on concrete parameters, such as the size of the medium, the rate of multiplication of spirals, and the rate of their elimination.[16]

Three-Dimensional Aspects

Another important feature of fibrillation is its three-dimensionality. Although available experimental evidence is not conclusive, there are theoretical concepts about possible specifically three-dimensional mechanisms that can contribute to fibrillation. Here the focus is on *scroll wave turbulence*, an essentially three-dimensional mechanism of multiplication of vortices, observed even in cases when a two-dimensional medium with the same properties has stable spiral waves.

Early numerical simulations of scroll waves have revealed that the scroll rings are not stationary but can contract as well as expand.[17] It was soon realized that if this behavior were extrapolated for an arbitrary shape of scroll filament, it would mean that the straight shape was unstable in favor of some more complicated behavior.[18] The earliest asymptotic theory of evolution of scroll waves with arbitrary shapes did not cover expanding rings,[19] and the first that did[20] was too complicated to clarify this question unequivocally, as the filament motion equations were linked to the evolution of scroll twist and depended on many parameters. However, it has been subsequently noted that with account of the symmetry of the problem, some of the terms in fact vanish and the dynamics of the filament shapes decouple in the main order from the dynamics of the twist. These dynamics designate a property of an excitable medium, the *filament tension*, which is positive if scroll rings collapse and negative rings expand.[21] This happens to be the most important parameter for the behavior of scrolls. Straight filaments with negative tension are indeed unstable, which could lead to self-supporting complicated behavior, where the filaments curve and extend, and then multiply when their segments annihilate on medium boundaries or with one another. It has been speculated that such complicated behavior could be relevant to fibrillation.[21,22] The first definitive observation of scroll wave turbulence as a persistent self-supporting activity mediated by negative filament tension was in the FitzHugh–Nagumo model[23] (Fig. 7a) and then in other models, including Barkley variant of the FitzHugh–Nagumo model[24] (Fig. 7b), the Oregonator model of the BZ reaction,[25] and Luo–Rudy model of ventricular tissue.[26]

An alternative mechanism with similar phenomenology was discovered by Fenton and Karma.[27,28] It is also related to curving and multiplication of scroll filaments, but it is only observed in simulations with spatially nonuniform anisotropy of the diffusion tensor, mimicking the twisted fiber structure of ventricular walls. This has been observed in the FitzHugh–Nagumo model as well as in a simplified cardiac excitation model developed by the authors for this particular purpose, since then known as the Fenton–Karma model. At the time of writing this review, its author is unaware of detailed theoretical explanation of this phenomenon, although there are theoretical developments promising that such an explanation could be obtained soon.[29]

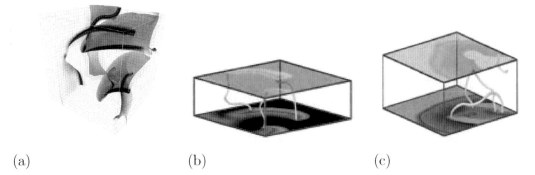

(a)   (b)   (c)

Figure 7: Three-dimensional scroll wave turbulence, (**a**, **b**) due to negative filament tension, (**c**) due to twisted anisotropy. (**a**) FitzHugh–Nagumo model: wavefronts are gray semitransparent, their edges, representing the filaments, are dark and nontransparent (same data as in Biktashev[23]). (**b**, **c**) Fenton–Karma model: shown are surface voltage distribution (top surface semitransparent), and the scroll filament between them. (Reprinted with permission from Fenton et al.,[24] © 2002, American Institute of Physics)

Although these particular mechanisms are difficult to identify in real experiments with cardiac tissue, the essentially three-dimensional nature of fibrillation, particularly ventricular fibrillation, is well known. So the question whether these or other complications caused by three-dimensionality can be overcome by low-voltage defibrillation techniques is very important. Theoretical progress here is limited but nonzero:

- Three-dimensional aspects of the high-frequency induced drift have been numerically investigated for gridlike stimulating electrodes in the already mentioned work.[4] The advantage of a gridlike stimulation extends to three dimensions, although the grid of the electrodes stays on the surface as long as the tissue is not too thick. In that case the third dimension adds little to the distance the forced vortices must travel before expulsion.

- Resonant stimulation has been studied for the negative-tension mediated scroll wave turbulence (Fig. 8) in Barkley's model.[30,31] It has been demonstrated that small oscillations of one of the parameters with a near-resonant frequency can successfully exterminate all scroll wave activity. The optimal frequency for achieving this is shifted from the solitary spiral frequency, and the decisive mechanism involved may be not resonant drift as such but inversion of the filament tension from negative to positive.

Pinning and Unpinning

The theoretical mechanisms considered above all ignored an important property of cardiac tissue, its heterogeneity. One important effect this can have on spiral and scroll waves is their "pinning" to localized inhomogeneities. This has been observed both for high-frequency

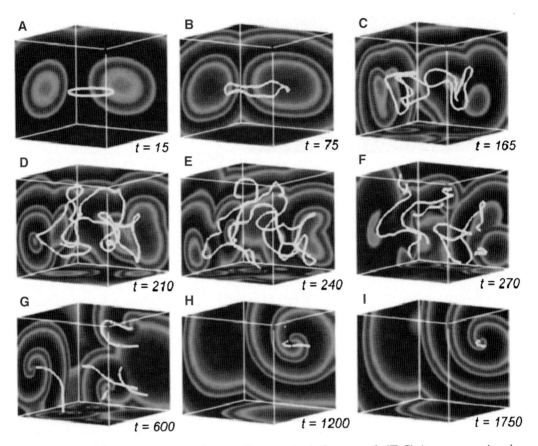

Figure 8: (**A–E**) Development of a scroll wave turbulence and (**F–I**) its suppression by delocalized periodic external forcing. Numerical simulations with Barkley model with parameters giving negative scroll filament tension, the external forcing is implemented by time-dependent modulations of the excitability, with frequency close to the frequency of free spiral waves. (Reprinted with permission from Alonso et al.,[30] © 2003, AAAS)

induced drift[2] and for "soft" drift caused by the gradient of tissue properties[32] or resonant drift with or without feedback,[33] in two as well as in three spatial dimensions (Fig. 9). The mechanism of the pinning to small and/or weak local inhomogeneities can be understood in terms of attracting, or centripetal, force by means of perturbation theory,[34] including, in three dimensions, the filament tension.[32] When the inhomogeneity is strong (e.g., an inexcitable hole), the pinning is evident for topological reasons (Fig. 9b). Obviously, if the drift was induced with the aim of expelling the vortex from the tissue, its pinning inside the tissue indicates a failure. Hence there is a question of whether it is possible to "unpin" such a pinned vortex by a low-energy intervention. If that is achieved, then it will be possible

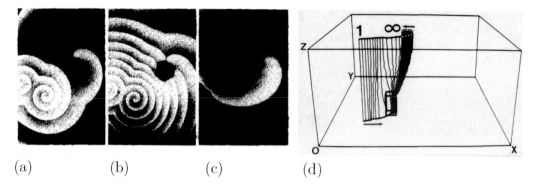

(a)   (b)   (c)   (d)

Figure 9: Pinning to an obstacle. (**a**–**c**) Pinning of high-frequency induced drift in two dimensions. Spiral wave in Belousov–Zhabotinsky (BZ) reaction rotating around an inexcitable hole (seen as a black spot in the middle frame) is entrained by a higher frequency wave train, but resumes the rotation as soon as the wave train is over. (Reprinted with permission from Krinsky et al.,[2] ©1983, Elsevier) (**d**) Pinning of gradient-induced drift in three dimensions. Scroll wave in FitzHugh–Nagumo model drifting due to spatial gradient of medium parameters is "anchored" to a localized inhomogeneity near the bottom and stops drifting. "1" is the initial position of the scroll, "∞" is the anchored stationary position in which the filament stops drifting. (Reprinted with permission from Vinson et al.,[32] ©1994, Elsevier)

to eliminate this vortex by either of the induced drifts, or it may even self-terminate via spontaneous drift.

Figure 10 gives three clues as to how unpinning could be achieved. Figure 10a illustrates that as far as small perturbations are concerned, a spiral wave is only sensitive to perturbations near its core. This is well known phenomenologically and is mathematically formalized as localization of response functions of the spiral wave.[21,35,36] Figure 10b illustrates one of the effects a bidomain structure of cardiac tissue has on the interaction of the external electric field and the spatial distribution of the transmembrane potential.[37] Despite the fact that the electrode is a point shape, the virtual electrode it produces is spread in space, has a nontrivial shape, and in some places the sign of the induced potential is opposite to the sign of the potential at the electrode. Figure 10c shows how the bidomain structure of the tissue manifests itself around an obstacle in a uniform external field.[38] The disturbance in the ohmic properties of the intracellular and extracellular domains distorts the electric field around the obstacle and creates a depolarized zone to one side of it and a hyperpolarized zone to the other side.

So if a spiral wave rotates around such an obstacle, we observe that:

- To move this spiral wave, we need to apply a stimulus in a properly chosen zone near its core which coincides with the obstacle.

- A delocalized, nearly homogeneous external electric field, by virtue of its interaction with the heterogeneity itself, produces a localized stimulus to the tissue just where it is needed, near the obstacle.

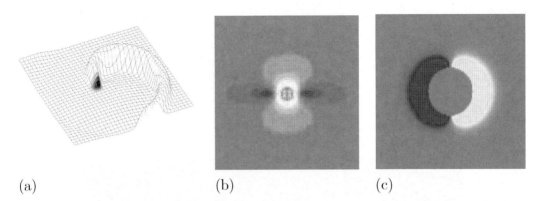

(a)   (b)   (c)

Figure 10: Localization of spiral sensitivity and of electric field action. (**a**) Response functions of a spiral wave. Elevation represents the activator variable, and the surface shade of gray represents the sum of absolute values of rotational and translational response functions (FitzHugh–Nagumo model). (Same data as in Biktasheva et al.[35]) (**b**) "Dog-bone" shape "virtual electrode" near a point electrode. Shade of gray represents instant distribution of transmembrane voltage, white is for positive and black is for negative (Bidomain Luo–Rudy model). (Reprinted with permission from Sambelashvili et al.,[37] ©2003, American Physiological Society) (**c**) "Weidmann zones" near an anatomical obstacle. Voltage distribution around a circular inexcitable hole caused by homogeneous external electric field (bidomain passive membrane model). (Reprinted with permission from Takagi et al.,[38] ©2004, American Physical Society)

That is, the stimulus is automatically delivered near to where it is needed, and one only needs to choose the timing for the Weidmann zone to superimpose with the maximum of the translational response function and to achieve a displacement of the spiral. If the displacement is large enough to get away from the zone of attraction of the inhomogeneity, this is considered unpinning.

The reasoning of referring to response functions is valid in the case when the heterogeneity is weak so a perturbation theory applies. When the heterogeneity is strong (e.g., an inexcitable hole), the reasoning is different but the result is qualitatively the same. The top row of Fig. 11 illustrates the idea qualitatively. A localized stimulus near to the core of the spiral, issued in the excitable gap, can initiate a circular wave (left panel). This circular wave breaks around the refractory zone, and one of the new wave breaks joins and annihilates with the spiral (middle panel). The other newly generated wave break curls into a spiral in another place, away from the hole (right panel). The net result is that the spiral is unpinned. To achieve that, the stimulus should be in the correct place, sufficiently close to the hole, and at the right time, in the excitable gap.

The second and third rows of Fig. 11 show numerical simulation of unpinning of a spiral by a properly timed homogeneous external electric field in a bidomain model. One can see the Weidmann zones $D+$ and $D-$ on the panel $t = 40$. The $D+$ zone serves as the localized stimulus initiating a new circular wave W (panel $t = 80$). The circular wave breaks about

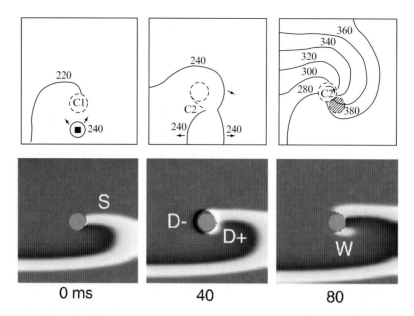

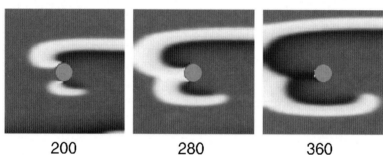

Figure 11: *Top row*: A localized stimulus issued in an appropriate phase of the spiral can shift the spiral core. If the original location was around an inexcitable hole, the new location can be away from it (i.e., the spiral gets unpinned; Piecewise-linear FitzHugh–Nagumo model). (Reprinted with permission from Krinsky et al.,[39] © 1990, Wiley–Blackwell Publishing Ltd) *Second and third rows*: Unpinning of a spiral from an inexcitable hole (bidomain FitzHugh–Nagumo model). (Reprinted with permission from Takagi et al.,[38] © 2004, American Physical Society)

the refractory tail ($t = 200$). One of the new wave breaks annihilates with the original spiral ($t = 280$). The other wave break creates a new spiral, which is unpinned from the obstacle ($t = 360$).

The possibility of unpinning a spiral wave from an obstacle using a localized stimulus close to it was recognized early.[39] It was relatively straightforward to verify it in an experiment with BZ reaction.[40] The crucial step was the idea of using a Weidmann zone as the localized stimulus.[41] It was first investigated in simulations with relatively simple models[41] and then extended to more detailed and realistic models[38,42] and verified in experiments with rabbit heart preparations.[43]

"Black-Box" Approaches

For the sake of completeness, it should be mentioned that there have been attempts to approach the problem of control of cardiac arrhythmia using generic methods of control of dynamical systems, regardless of detailed mechanisms of how the control actually works. We consider two such lines of inquiries.

Alekseev and Loskutov[44] observed that a weak parametric periodic perturbation can stabilize the chaotic behavior of a nonlinear system and turn chaos into periodic oscillations. That was done for a mathematical model of phytoplankton–zooplankton community, a system of four ordinary differential equations. This idea has been applied to a number of other model systems. In particular, its application to a two-dimensional spiral wave turbulence in a piecewise-linear FitzHugh–Nagumo model[45,46] allowed elimination of all spiral wave activity. This application involved point stimulation with a frequency small enough so waves could propagate, but larger than the frequency of the spirals. Note this is precisely the condition that is required for high-frequency induced drift of spirals. Data available do not allow us to conclude whether the detailed mechanism was indeed the high-frequency resonant drift or something different.

Ott et al.[47] have proposed that a small modification of a chaotic dynamical system can change chaos to stable periodic motion. Unlike the Alekseev and Loskutov method, their approach required that changes do not depend on time explicitly, but rather on the current state of the system (i.e., feedback). This idea was hugely popular and applied to a great variety of dynamical systems. Cardiac arrhythmias were not an exception: for example, application of this technique to ouabain-induced ventricular arrhythmia in rabbit ventricle allowed conversion of chaotic to period behavior.[48] Again, data available in their report do not allow identification of detailed mechanism; however, the proportional perturbation feedback protocol used there, although quite complicated, could have produced a nearly resonant perturbation that could cause a resonant drift.

Conclusion

A striking picture emerges from the above review. Although a wide variety of theoretical mechanisms are considered, the resulting experimental protocols required to exploit these mechanisms are not so varied. So implementation of the idea of unpinning involves a correct choice of the phase of the stimuli with respect to the spiral rotation around the hole, say to ensure that the depolarizing Weidmann zone falls within the excitable gap. A practical way to achieve that is by using some kind of feedback, and the protocol for that feedback may be close or indistinguishable from that required for resonant drift. Moreover, scanning through the phases may lead to a series of stimuli of the sort that would be needed to arrange a high-frequency resonant drift. The stimulation protocol to implement the Alekseev–Loskutov chaos control strategy seems to be indistinguishable from the one needed for high-frequency resonant drift, and the protocol for the Ott–Grebogy–Yorke strategy could produce feedback-driven resonant drift. Application of the sufficiently homogeneous external electric field, which is important for classical single-shock fibrillation, is crucial for the success of the resonant-drift approach and is also required for unpinning. Even successful experiments with low-voltage defibrillation may be interpreted in different ways; for example, the results of Pak et al.[49] are, in principle, consistent with such scenarios as high-frequency induced drift, feedback-driven resonant drift, and unpinning. So, although experimental testing of theoretical ideas as always remains a priority, there are still theoretical challenges, such as formulation of unequivocal experimental protocols and criteria that would allow us to distinguish between different mechanisms. Such a distinction hopefully will allow us to suggest possible ways to improve the efficiency of the low-voltage defibrillation.

Acknowledgments

This study has been supported in part by EPSRC grants EP/D500338/1 and EP/E016391/1 (UK) and benefited from fruitful exchanges that took place at the Cardiac Dynamics program hosted in 2007 the Kavli Institute for Theoretical Physics at the University California, Santa Barbara. The author is particularly grateful to F.H. Fenton, V.I. Krinsky, A.Y. Loskutov, A.S. Mikhailov, A.M. Pertsov, S. Sinha and V.S. Zykov for bibliographic advice.

References

1. Gurvich PL. *The Main Principles of Cardiac Defibrillation.* Moscow: Meditsina; 1975
2. Krinsky VI, Agladze KI. Interaction of rotating waves in an active chemical medium *Physica D* 1983;8:50–56
3. Ermakova EA, Krinsky VI, Panfilov AV, Pertsov AM. Interaction between spiral and flat periodic waves in an active medium. *Biofizika* 1986;31:318–323
4. Sinha S, Pande A, Pandit R. Defibrillation via the elimination of spiral turbulence in a model for ventricular fibrillation. *Phys Rev Lett* 2001;86:3678–3681
5. Pandit R, Pande A, Sinha S, Sen A. Spiral turbulence and spatiotemporal chaos: characterization and control in two excitable media. *Physica A* 2002;306:211–219
6. Davydov VA, Zykov VS, Mikhailov AS, Brazhnik PK. Drift and resonance of spiral waves in distributed media. *Sov Phys Radiophys* 1988;31:574–582
7. Agladze KI, Davydov VA, Mikhailov AS. An observation of resonance of spiral waves in distributed excitable medium. *Sov Phys JETP Lett* 1987;45:601–603
8. Mikhailov AS, Davydov VA, Zykov VS. Complex dynamics of spiral waves and motion of curves. *Physica D* 1994;70:1–39

9. Biktashev VN, Holden AV. Control of re-entrant activity by resonant drift in a two-dimensional model of isotropic homogeneous atrial tissue. *Proc Roy Soc Lond Ser B* 1995;260:211–217

10. Biktashev VN, Holden AV. Resonant drift of the autowave vortex in abounded medium. *Phys Lett A* 1993;181:216–224

11. Biktashev VN, Holden AV. Resonant drift of autowave vortices in 2D and the effects of boundaries and inhomogeneities. *Chaos Solitons Fractals* 1995;5:575–622

12. Biktashev VN, Holden AV. Design principles of a low-voltage cardiac defibrillator based on the effect of feed-back resonant drift. *J Theor Biol* 1994;169:101–112

13. Zykov VS, Engel H. Feedback-mediated control of spiral waves. *Physica D* 2004;199:243–263

14. Zykov VS, Engel H. Feedback-mediated control of spiral waves In: Schimansky-Geier L, Fiedler B, Kurths J, Schoell E, eds. *Analysis and Control of Complex Nonlinear Processes in Physics, Chemistry and Biology.* Singapore: World Scientific; 2007

15. Grill S, Zykov VS, Muller SC. Feedback-controlled dynamics of meandering spiral waves. *Phys Rev Lett* 1995;75:3368–3371

16. Sabbagh H. Stochastic properties of autowave turbulence elimination. *Chaos Solitons Fractals* 2000;11:2141–2148

17. Panfilov AV, Rudenko AN. 2 regimes of the scroll ring drift in the 3-dimensional active media. *Physica D* 1987;28:215–218

18. Brazhnik PK, Davydov VA, Zykov VS, Mikhailov AS. Vortex rings in excitable media. *Zhurnal Eksperimentalnoi I Teoreticheskoi Fiziki* 1987;93:1725–1736

19. Yakushevich LV. Vortex filament elasticity in active medium. *Studia Biophysica* 1984;100:195–200

20. Keener JP. The dynamics of 3-dimensional scroll waves in excitable media. *Physica D* 1988;31:269–276

21. Biktashev VN, Holden AV, Zhang H. Tension of organizing filaments of scroll waves. *Philos Trans R Soc Lond Ser A* 1994;347:611–630

22. Winfree AT. Electrical turbulence in three-dimensional heart muscle. *Science* 1994;266:1003–1006

23. Biktashev VN. A three-dimensional autowave turbulence. *Int J Bifurcat Chaos* 1998;8:677–684

24. Fenton FH, Cherry EM, Hastings HM, Evans SJ. Multiple mechanisms of spiral wave breakup in a model of cardiac electrical activity. *Chaos* 2002;12:852–892

25. Alonso S, Sagues F, Mikhailov AS. Negative-tension instability of scroll waves and Winfree turbulence in the Oregonator model. *J Phys Chem A* 2006;110:12063–12071

26. Alonso S, Panfilov AV. Negative filament tension in the Luo–Rudy model of cardiac tissue. *Chaos* 2007;17:015102

27. Fenton F, Karma A. Vortex dynamics in three-dimensional continuous myocardium with fiber rotation: filament instability and fibrillation. *Chaos* 1998;8:20–47

28. Fenton F, Karma A. Fiber-rotation-induced vortex turbulence in thick myocardium. *Phys Rev Lett* 1998;81:481–484

29. Verschelde H, Dierckx H, Bernus O. Covariant string dynamics of scroll wave filaments in anisotropic cardiac tissue. *Phys Rev Lett* 2007;99:168104

30. Alonso S, Sagues F, Mikhailov AS. Taming Winfree turbulence of scroll waves in excitable media. *Science* 2003;299:1722–1725

31. Alonso S, Sagues F, Mikhailov AS. Periodic forcing of scroll rings and control of Winfree turbulence in excitable media. *Chaos* 2006;16:023124

32. Vinson M, Pertsov A, Jalife J. Anchoring of vortex filaments in 3D excitable media. *Physical D* 1994;72:119–134

33. Nikolaev EV, Biktashev VN, Holden AV. On feedback resonant drift and interaction with the boundaries in circular and annular excitable media. *Chaos Solitons Fractals* 1998;9:363–376

34. Pazo D, Kramer L, Pumir A, Kanani S, Efimov I, Krinsky V. Pinning force in active media. *Phys Rev Lett* 2004;93:168303

35. Biktasheva IV, Holden AV, Biktashev VN. Localization of response functions of spiral waves in the FitzHugh–Nagumo system. *Int J Bifurcat Chaos* 2006;16(5):1547–1555

36. Biktasheva IV, Elkin Yu E, Biktashev VN. Localised sensitivity of spiral waves in the complex Ginzburg–Landau equation. *Phys Rev E* 1998;57:2656–2659

37. Sambelashvili AT, Nikolski VP, Efimov IR. Nonlinear effects in subthreshold virtual electrode polarization. *Am J Physiol Heart Circ Physiol* 2003;284:H2368–H2374

38. Takagi S, Pumir A, Efimov I, Pazó D, Nikolski V, Krinsky V. Unpinning and removal of a rotating wave in cardiac muscle. *Phys Rev Lett* 2004;93:058101

39. Krinsky VI, Biktashev VN, Pertsov AM. Autowave approaches to cessation of reentrant arrhythmias. *Ann N Y Acad Sci* 1990;591:232–246

40. Huyet G, Dupont C, Corriol T, Krinsky V. Unpinning of a vortex in a chemical excitable medium. *Int J Bifurcat Chaos* 1998;8:1315–1323

41. Pumir A, Krinsky V. Unpinning of a rotating wave in cardiac muscle by an electric field. *J Theor Biol* 1999;199:311–319

42. Takagi S, Pumir A, Pazó D, Efimov I, Nikolski V, Krinsky V. A physical approach to remove anatomical reentries: a bidomain study. *J Theor Biol* 2004;230:489–497

43. Ripplinger CM, Krinsky VI, Nikolski VP, Efimov IR. Mechanisms of unpinning and termination of ventricular tachycardia. *Am J Physiol Heart Circ Physiol* 2006;291:H184–H192

44. Alekseev VV, Loskutov AY. Control of a system with a strange attractor through periodic parametric action. *Sov Phys Dokl* 1987;32:270–271

45. Loskutov AY, Cheremin RV, Vysotskii SA. Stabilization of turbulent dynamics in excitable media by an external point action. *Dokl Phys* 2005;50:490–493

46. Loskutov AY, Vysotskii SA. New approach to the defibrillation problem: suppression of the spiral wave activity of cardiac tissue. *JETP Lett* 2006;84:524–529

47. Ott E, Grebogi C, Yorke JA. Controlling chaos. *Phys Rev Lett* 1990;64:1196–1199

48. Garfinkel A, Spano ML, Ditto WL, Weiss JN. Controlling cardiac chaos. *Science* 1992;257:1230–1235

49. Pak HN, Liu YB, Hayashi H, Okuyama Y, Chen PS, Lin SF. Synchronization of ventricular fibrillation with real-time feedback pacing: implication to low-energy defibrillation *Am J Physiol* 2003;285:H2704–H2711

Chapter 6.3

Pacing Control of Local Cardiac Dynamics

Robert F. Gilmour Jr, David J. Christini, and Alain Karma

Introduction

One approach to preventing or suppressing cardiac fibrillation is to control local cardiac electrical dynamics using externally applied electrical stimuli. This approach is predicated on the expectation that appropriate control of local dynamics will affect global dynamics and thereby prevent the initiation of reentrant excitation or terminate existing reentry. Initial efforts in this area were directed toward suppression of spatiotemporal chaos, with the objective of suppressing existing fibrillation. More recently, attempts have been made to control less complex dynamics, such as electrical alternans, with the objective of preventing fibrillation. The following sections will briefly review the strategies used to control cardiac chaos and lower dimensional dynamical behavior and discuss some potential future directions for these approaches.

Chaos Control

A number of studies[1–17] have attempted to determine whether the seemingly complex electrical activity associated with atrial and ventricular fibrillation arises from the same type of simple deterministic mechanism that gives rise to complex behavior in a variety of nonlinear dynamical systems.[18–23] In particular, investigators have asked whether key features of cardiac electrical activity may, under the appropriate experimental circumstances, undergo period doubling bifurcations that culminate in chaotic dynamics.[2,7,8,13,17] In this context,

Robert F. Gilmour Jr

Department of Biomedical Sciences, College of Veterinary Medicine, Cornell University, Ithaca, NY 14853, USA,
rfg2@cornell.edu

I. R. Efimov et al. (eds.), *Cardiac Bioelectric Therapy: Mechanisms and Practical Implications.*
© Springer Science+Business Media, LLC 2009

chaos is defined as aperiodic activity that arises in a nonlinear dynamical system as a result of a deterministic mechanism that has sensitive dependence on initial conditions.[18,23]

Several of these studies demonstrated that progressively increasing the pacing frequency induced period doubling bifurcations in isolated preparations of cardiac tissue, where a 1:1 correspondence between the pacing stimulus and the duration of the action potential was replaced by a 2:2 pattern, and subsequently by a 4:4 pattern, and so on, until at a critical frequency the periodic behavior was replaced by aperiodic (chaotic) dynamics (Fig. 1). The periodic and aperiodic dynamics were explained using a simple analytical model, in which action potential duration (APD) was a nonlinear function of the preceding rest, or diastolic, interval. For higher order period doubling and chaos to occur, it was necessary for the relationship between diastolic interval and APD, as characterized by the restitution relation, to have a region of steep slope, where APD changed rapidly with small changes in diastolic interval, and a critical point (i.e., a maxima or minima). The nature of the critical point differed according to the tissue studied and the experimental conditions.

One of the motivations for looking for a low-dimensional deterministic mechanism to explain complex dynamics is that if such a mechanism is found, then the future behavior of the system can be predicted, at least in the short term, from current behavior. In addition, altering current behavior is expected to produce predictable alterations of future behavior. Using this approach, it has been possible to control chaotic dynamics in a number of physical systems by introducing properly timed perturbations.[24–27] Control of chaos also has been demonstrated in isolated pieces of rabbit ventricular muscle by Garfinkel et al.,[5] using the chaos control strategy of Ott et al.[27]

In the latter study, cellular activation underwent period doubling bifurcations that culminated in aperiodic behavior. Poincaré maps suggested that the aperiodic behavior was chaotic, rather than random, and that the spontaneous cycle lengths during chaos fluctuated about an unstable fixed point. By determining the sequence of spontaneous cycle lengths in real time, it was possible to estimate whether the cycle lengths were approaching or diverging from the fixed point (along stable or unstable manifolds, respectively). If the cycle lengths were diverging from the fixed point, they were perturbed back into the stable manifold using an appropriately timed stimulus, whereas if the cycle lengths were converging toward the fixed point, no intervention occurred. To successfully control chaos, therefore, it was necessary to know the location of the unstable fixed point, the current spontaneous cycle length, and the most likely succeeding cycle length. This information was available because the aperiodic behavior arose from a low-dimensional deterministic system.

One limitation of the approach used by Garfinkel et al.[5] was that they could only introduce premature stimuli (postmature stimuli would have been preempted by the spontaneous activity of the preparations). Perhaps because of this limitation, or as a result of error in the fixed-point estimation,[28,29] they were not able to restore 1:1 dynamics; the best control achieved was a period 3. A similar limitation with respect to the inability to use postmature stimuli for control applied to a strategy to control low-dimensional chaos in periodically forced cardiac Purkinje fibers.[7]

To address the premature-stimulus limitation, Watanabe and Gilmour[30] subsequently developed a strategy that exploited the refractory period of cardiac tissue to permit 1:1 control of chaotic dynamics in paced ventricular muscle using both premature and

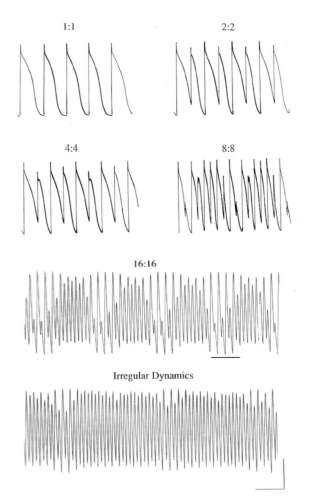

Figure 1: Action potentials recorded from an isolated canine Purkinje fiber during pacing at progressively shorter cycle lengths. Stimulus–response ratios are given above each trace and illustrate the progression from 1:1 locking through period doubling bifurcations to higher order periods, culminating in irregular (aperiodic) dynamics. Vertical calibration equals 50 mV. Horizontal calibration equals 250 ms for 1:1, 2:2, and 4:4 locking, 500 ms for 8:8 locking, and 800 ms for 16:16 locking and irregular dynamics

postmature stimuli. The control algorithm contained a learning routine, which constructed the relationship between pacing cycle length and APD as these data were acquired during simulated ventricular fibrillation. From these data, fixed points were identified. This information was then fed to an implementation routine, which delivered a brief electrical stimulus at the appropriate time (Fig. 2). The effect of the stimulus on the behavior of the system was evaluated by the learning routine, and the implementation routine was updated as needed

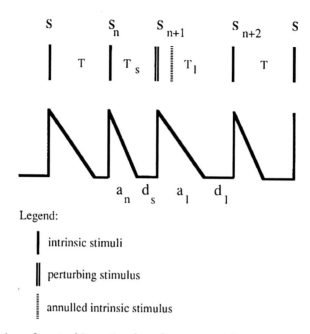

Figure 2: The timing of perturbing stimulus placement with respect to the intrinsic stimuli (S). In vivo, the intrinsic stimuli are provided by the pacemaker, and the intervals (T) between such intrinsic stimuli are nearly constant. A perturbing stimulus given at interval T_s produces an action potential a_1. Because of this action potential, the intrinsic stimulus S_{n+1} arriving at interval T as usual finds the ventricular tissue already activated and inexcitable (i.e., refractory). S_{n+1} is annulled and the $S_n S_{n+2}$ interval is partitioned into T_s and T_1

to perturb the system to the vicinity of a fixed point. The control algorithm typically established control within 1.2 s of the onset of the implementation routine (Fig. 3). Thus, it was possible to characterize the dynamics and intervene within a short enough period of time so that tissue viability would be preserved if this were an actual fibrillating ventricle.

Although the studies described above have demonstrated the feasibility of chaos control, it is uncertain whether strategies that control the local dynamics in small pieces of cardiac tissue would be capable of controlling aperiodic behavior in the whole heart, where the spatial degrees of freedom are many. Studies of ventricular fibrillation in whole hearts have suggested that the sequence of spontaneous cycle lengths during fibrillation is random, rather than deterministic.[31] Accordingly, one might question whether it is possible to identify a fixed point or to predict the sequence of cycle lengths. However, some evidence for determinism in the local dynamics during fibrillation has been reported.[6,7,31,32] In particular, Garfinkel et al.[6] have presented evidence that ventricular fibrillation results from a transition from quasiperiodicity to chaos. Nevertheless, the application of pacing-induced control of local dynamics to the termination of fibrillation in patients has yet to be demonstrated.

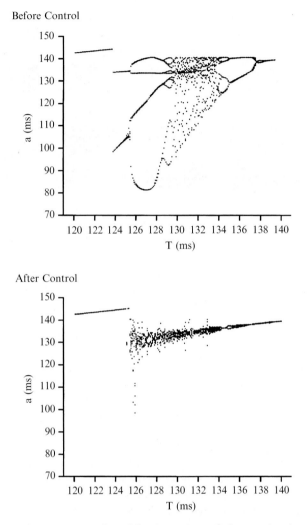

Figure 3: Bifurcation diagrams produced by iteration of the restitution function f in the unperturbed state (*upper panel*) and with control (*lower panel*). The 16th–25th iterations at $T = 120$–140 ms are shown

Alternans Control

APD Alternans

Given the substantial limitations to the control of cardiac chaos using externally applied stimuli, as discussed above, more recent efforts have focused on controlling lower dimensional electrical behavior, in particular 2:2 phase-response locking, also known as *cardiac*

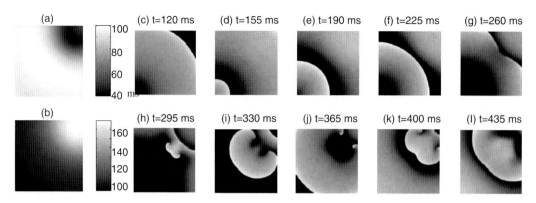

Figure 4: (**a**, **b**) show the spatial distribution of action potential durations (APDs) for two consecutive excitation waves – first is in (**a**), second in (**b**) – that originated from the *lower left corner* in a simulated 6 × 6 cm^2 cardiac monolayer. APD discordance is apparent for both waves; the inversion, from (**a**) to (**b**), of this discordance reflects alternans. (**c**–l) depict transmembrane potential (shown without units; *white* is peak amplitude, *black* is resting potential), starting 120 ms following the initiation of the wave represented by (**b**). (**c**) shows the same wave that was used for (**b**) as its wavefront (*white*) and its trailing gray refractory region move toward the *upper right corner*. Another wave, occurring at a premature time (relative to the interexcitation interval of the preceding wave sequence), appears in the *lower-left corner* of (**d**). In (**g**), this premature wavefront encroaches on the refractory tail of the preceding wave near the spatial location of the preceding wave's lengthened APD (as seen in (**b**)). This encroachment causes functional conduction block that leads to reentry into the previously excited area (**h**), and the redevelopment of a full excitation wave in the opposite direction (**i**–**j**) and sustained reentrant propagation (**l**)

alternans. Several types of alternans exist, including mechanical alternans, where the force of contraction alternates from beat to beat, and electrical alternans, where the amplitude, upstroke velocity, or duration of the action potential alternates. In addition, both mechanical and electrical alternans may be associated with alternans of intracellular calcium transients. Thus far, attempts to control alternans as an antiarrhythmic strategy have been developed primarily to suppress APD alternans.

Several studies have demonstrated that as the heart rate increases, APD first alternates concordantly (i.e., all regions of tissue exhibit the same long-short APD pattern) and then becomes spatially discordant, with areas of long-short APD alternation adjacent to areas of short-long APD alternation.[33–37] Discordant alternans produces steep gradients of repolarization that can provide the substrate for unidirectional conduction block and the initiation of reentrant excitation. This mechanism (as illustrated in Fig. 4) is the basis for the hypothesis that APD alternans is causally linked to the onset of electrical turbulence, as manifest by atrial and ventricular fibrillation.

Given that APD alternans can trigger cardiac turbulence, its elimination could be an effective means of preventing the onset of arrhythmias. In that regard, it has been shown that

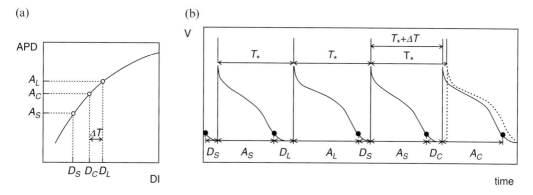

Figure 5: (**a**) Action potential duration (APD) restitution *curve* showing that APD shortens as the diastolic interval (DI) shortens. (**b**) Pacing a single cell at a short constant interval T_* causes the APD to alternate between short (AS) and long (AL); these are also shown in (**a**), with corresponding diastolic intervals DS and DL. After the third action potential, control was activated such that the next pacing interval was $T_* + \Delta T$ (as dictated by (1), with $\Delta T < 0$). As seen in (**a**), the control-shortened diastolic interval DC causes the next action potential to have APD AC, rather than the expected AL if DI had equaled DL (without control). In (**b**), the premature action potential is clearly shorter than that which would have occurred for an uncontrolled pacing interval T_* (*dotted* action potential in (**b**))

nonlinear dynamical control methods can terminate APD alternans in small preparations of frog ventricle in vitro.[38,39] In those studies, the preparations were paced initially at a constant cycle length that induced alternans. APD was monitored continuously and the difference between consecutive APDs was calculated. That difference was multiplied by a gain factor, and the resulting product was either added to or subtracted from the pacing cycle length to produce small perturbations in the pacing interval. The pacing intervals were varied until the difference in consecutive APDs was zero (i.e., alternans was eliminated). Using such an approach, APD alternans was suppressed reliably in a system that did not have spatiotemporally varying repolarization and wave propagation dynamics (the frog preparations were small enough that all cells behaved synchronously).

Nonlinear dynamical control of this type utilizes premature electrical stimulation to eliminate APD alternans by exploiting the dependence of APD on the preceding diastolic interval.[40] This property, known as *restitution*, is illustrated in Fig. 5a. To exploit restitution to eliminate APD alternans, a premature stimulus is given after a short APD, as in Fig. 5b. By shortening the diastolic interval, the stimulus shortens the next APD, relative to its value without the premature stimulus. Because that APD has been shortened, the subsequent diastolic interval will be longer than without the premature stimulus, thereby lengthening the next expected APD. Thus, through every-second-beat delivery of premature stimuli (i.e., only after the short APDs), the natural dynamics of cardiac tissue causes the long APDs to be shortened, and the short APDs to be lengthened, thereby eliminating alternans.

The precise timing of the stimulus perturbation is given by:

$$T_n = \begin{cases} T_* + \Delta T_n & \text{if } \Delta T_n < 0, \\ T_* & \text{if } \Delta T_n \geq 0, \end{cases} \tag{1}$$

where

$$\Delta T_n = (\lambda/2)(APD_n - APD_{n-1}), \tag{2}$$

T_* is the pacing period without control, λ is the feedback gain, which is a function of the nonlinearity of the system (the method of determining λ is discussed in Hall and Christini[41]), and n is the beat number.

The "if" condition in (1) dictates that the pacing period can only be shortened, which is the only way that a device can intervene in a real heart (i.e., stimulation can shorten, but not lengthen, interbeat intervals). Thus, if $\Delta Tn < 0$, a preemptive stimulus is delivered by the device (top condition of (1)); whereas if $\Delta Tn \geq 0$, a native excitation is delivered at time T_* (bottom condition of (1)). Note that in these experiments (as in Hall and Gauthier[38] and Christini et al.[42]), all native and control stimuli were delivered from the same stimulus site.

A theoretical study has suggested that the application of this method of control to larger tissues might require stimulation from multiple sites because of the complex spatiotemporal dynamics of electrophysiological repolarization.[43] This prediction has been confirmed by an analytical and modeling study of a cardiac Purkinje fiber, where control of alternans from a single pacing site was possible at sites near the pacing electrode, but ineffective at sites more than 1 cm from the stimulating electrode.[44]

The predictions from the theoretical model recently were largely confirmed in a series of studies in isolated Purkinje fibers.[42] In these studies, pacing stimuli were delivered at a period T_* to one end of an isolated canine Purkinje fiber (1.5–2.5 cm long). Transmembrane voltage signals were sampled from up to six glass microelectrodes equally spaced along the length of the fiber. Control was applied by perturbing T_* according to (1) and (2) using a real-time control system.

Quantitative results varied between fibers, but qualitative features were common to all trials. For any given fiber, the extent to which control was achieved correlated with the pacing period T_*. Specifically, for longer T_*, successful control (i.e., elimination of alternans) typically could be achieved for the entire length of the fiber (Fig. 6, $T_* = 200\,\text{ms}$). For shorter T_*, successful control extended beyond the proximal end of the fiber, but not all the way to the distal end of the fiber (Fig. 6, $T_* = 190\,\text{ms}$).

Thus, spatially uniform control of alternans was possible if alternans magnitude was small. However, as alternans magnitude increased, control became attenuated spatially. Although the prediction regarding spatial attenuation of control was correct qualitatively, it remains unclear to what quantitative extent control is limited in Purkinje fibers. This uncertainty is due to the short fiber lengths used in these experiments, which made it difficult to test the upper limits of controllable length. Furthermore, the spatial extent of such attenuation in atrial or ventricular myocardium remains to be determined.

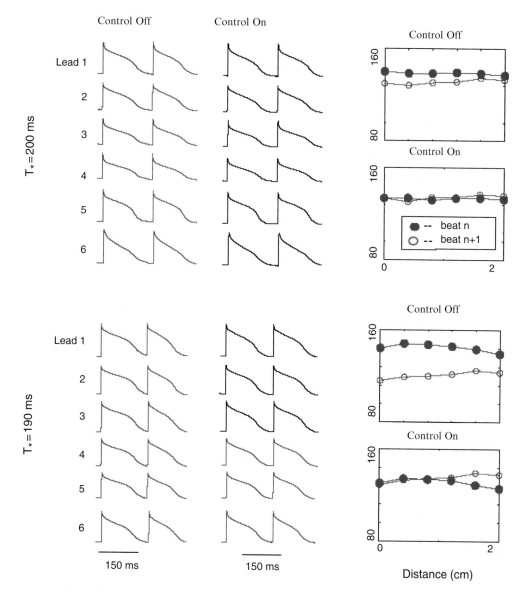

Figure 6: Data from two consecutive action potentials recorded from six microelectrodes spaced along the length of a canine Purkinje fiber. Stimulation was applied to the proximal end of the fiber near microelectrode 1. For both $T_* = 190$ ms and $T_* = 200$ ms, voltage versus time from microelectrodes 1–6 are shown in the left column (before control) and middle column (during control), and APD values computed from the six microelectrodes for the same alternate beats (as the left and middle columns) before (*top panels*) and during (*bottom panels*) control are shown in the right column. During control, stimulation was adapted according to (1)

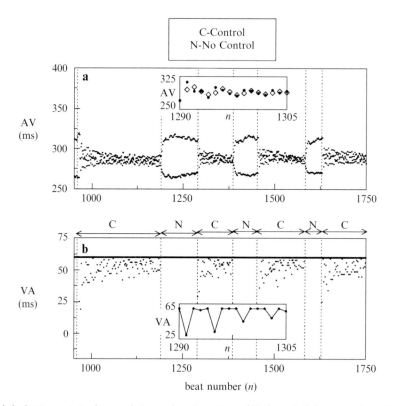

Figure 7: (a) Atrioventricular-nodal conduction time (AV) and (b) control pacing interval (VA) for a segment of a human alternans control trial. Periods of control and no control are annotated above (b). Nonlinear dynamical control perturbations applied to VA terminated the alternans in each of the control attempts shown here

Conduction Velocity Alternans

Control of other types of period-2 behavior also is possible using properly timed electrical stimuli. For example, Christini and Collins[45] have used such an approach to control atrioventricular-nodal conduction alternans, which is a period-2 alternation in atrioventricular-nodal conduction time. They used mathematical models of alternans to develop a nonlinear dynamical feedback control algorithm for electrical stimulus termination of alternans. This technique subsequently was applied to in vitro rabbit heart experiments, where it effectively controlled atrioventricular-nodal dynamics.[46] The approach was then applied successfully in the control of alternans in humans during clinical cardiac electrophysiology studies (Fig. 7).[47] A nonlinear dynamical analysis was used to adaptively compute perturbations to the timing of electrical stimuli applied to the endocardial surface of the right atrium.

References

1. Chialvo DR, Michaels DC, Jalife J. Supernormal excitability as mechanism of chaotic dynamics of activation in cardiac Purkinje fibers. *Circ Res* 1990;66:525–545
2. Chialvo DR, Gilmour RF Jr, Jalife J. Low dimensional chaos in cardiac tissue. *Nature* 1990;343:653–657
3. Chialvo DR, Jalife J. Nonlinear dynamics of rate-dependent activation in models of single cardiac cells. *Nature* 1987;330:749–752
4. Frazier DW, Wolf PD, Wharton JM, Tang ASL, Smith WM, Ideker RE. Stimulus-induced critical point. A mechanism for electrical initiation of re-entry in normal canine myocardium. *J Clin Invest* 1989;83:1039–1052
5. Garfinkel A, Spano ML, Ditto WL, Weiss JN. Controlling cardiac chaos. *Science* 1992;257:5074
6. Garfinkel A, Chen P-S, Walter DO, Karagueuzian HS, Kogan B, Evans SJ, Karpoukhin M, Hwang C, Uchida T, Gotoh M, Nwasokwa O, Sager P, Weiss JN. Quasiperiodicity and chaos in ventricular fibrillation. *J Clin Invest* 1997;99:305–314
7. Gilmour RF Jr, Watanabe M, Chialvo DR. Low dimensional dynamics in cardiac tissues. Experiments and theory. *SPIE Proc* 1993;2036:2–9
8. Gilmour RF Jr, Otani NF, Watanabe M. Memory and complex dynamics in canine cardiac Purkinje fibers. *Am J Physiol* 1997;272:H1826–H1832
9. Glass L, Guevara MR, Shrier A. Bifurcation and chaos in a periodically stimulated cardiac oscillator. *Physica D* 1983;17D:89–101
10. Guevara MR, Glass L, Shrier, A. Phase locking, period doubling bifurcations and irregular dynamics in periodically stimulated cardiac cells. *Science* 1981;214:1350–1353
11. Guevara MR, Ward G, Shrier A, Glass L. Electrical alternans and period doubling bifurcations. *IEEE Comput Cardiol* 1984;167–170
12. Lewis TJ, Guevara, MR. Chaotic dynamics in an ionic model of the propagated cardiac action potential. *J Theor Biol* 1990;146:407–432
13. Otani NF, Gilmour RF Jr. A memory model for the electrical properties of local cardiac systems. *J Theor Biol* 1997;187:409–436
14. Savino GV, Romanelli L, Gonzalez DL, Piro O, Valentinuzzi ME. Evidence for chaotic behavior in driven ventricles. *Biophys J* 1989;56:273–280
15. Sun J, Amellal F, Glass L, Billette, J. Alternans and period doubling bifurcations in atrioventricular nodal conduction. *J Theor Biol* 1995;173:79–91
16. Vinet A, Chialvo DR, Michaels DC, Jalife J. Nonlinear dynamics of rate-dependent activation in models of single cardiac cells. *Circ Res* 1990;67:1510–1524
17. Watanabe M, Otani NF, Gilmour RF Jr. Biphasic restitution of action potential duration and complex dynamics in ventricular myocardium. *Circ Res* 1995;76:915–921
18. Devaney RL. *An Introduction to Chaotic Dynamical Systems*, 2nd edn. Redwood City, CA: Addison-Wesley; 1989
19. Feigenbaum MJ. Qualitative universality for a class of nonlinear transformations. *J Stat Phys* 1978;19:25–52

20. Glass L, Mackey M. *From Clocks to Chaos. The Rhythms of Life.* Princeton, NJ: Princeton University Press; 1988
21. May RM. Simple mathematical models with very complicated dynamics. *Nature* 1976;261:459–467
22. Stone L. Period-doubling reversals and chaos in simple ecological models. *Nature* 1993;365:617–620
23. Strogatz S. *Nonlinear Dynamics and Chaos.* Reading, PA: Addison-Wesley; 1994
24. Braiman Y, Goldhirsch I. Taming chaotic dynamics with weak periodic perturbations. *Phys Rev Lett* 1991;66:2545–2548
25. Hunt ER. Stabilizing high-period orbits in a chaotic system: the diode resonator. *Phys Rev Lett* 1991;67:1953–1955
26. Singer J, Wang Y-Z, Haim HB. Controlling a chaotic system. *Phys Rev Lett* 1991;66:1123–1125
27. Ott E, Grebogi C, Yorke JA. Controlling chaos. *Phys Rev Lett* 1990;64:1196–1199
28. Christini DJ, Collins JJ. Control of chaos in excitable physiological systems: a geometric analysis. *Chaos* 1997;7:544–549
29. Christini DJ, Kaplan DT. Adaptive estimation and control method for unstable periodic dynamics in spike trains. *Phys Rev E* 2000;61:5149–5153
30. Watanabe M, Gilmour RF Jr. Strategy for control of complex low dimensional dynamics in cardiac tissue. *J Math Biol* 1996;35:73–87
31. Kaplan DT, Goldberger AL. Chaos in cardiology. *J Cardiovasc Electrophysiol* 1991;2:342–354
32. Witkowski FX, Kavanagh KM, Penkoske PA, Plonsey R, Spano ML, Ditto WL, Kaplan DT. Evidence for determinism in ventricular fibrillation. *Phys Rev Lett* 1995;75:1230–1233
33. Pastore JM, Rosenbaum DS. Role of structural barriers in the mechanism of alternans-induced reentry. *Circ Res* 2000;87:1157–1163
34. Qu Z, Garfinkel A, Chen P-S, Weiss JN. Mechanisms of discordant alternans and induction of reentry in simulated cardiac tissue. *Circulation* 2000;102:1664–1670
35. Hall K, Christini DJ, Tremblay M, Collins JC, Glass L, Billette J. Dynamic control of cardiac alternans. *Phys Rev Lett* 1997;78:4518–4521
36. Watanabe MA, Fenton FH, Evans SJ, Hastings HM, Karma A. Mechanisms for discordant alternans. *J Cardiovasc Electrophysiol* 2001;12:196–206
37. Fox JJ, Riccio ML, Hua F, Bodenschatz E, Gilmour RF Jr. Spatiotemporal transition to conduction block in canine ventricle. *Circ Res* 2002;90:289–296
38. Hall GM, Gauthier DJ. Experimental control of cardiac muscle alternans. *Phys Rev Lett* 2002;88:198102
39. Gauthier DJ, Bahar S, Hall GM. Controlling the dynamics of cardiac muscle using small electrical stimuli. In: Moss F, Gielen S, eds. *Handbook of Biological Physics: Neuro-Informatics, Neural Modeling*, vol. 4. New York: Elsevier; 2001:229–256
40. Nolasco JB, Dahlen RW. A graphic method for the study of alternation in the cardiac action potentials. *J Appl Physiol* 1968;25:191–196
41. Hall K, Christini DJ. Restricted feedback control of one-dimensional maps. *Phys Rev E* 2001;63:046204

42. Christini DJ, Karma A, Riccio ML, Culianu CA, Fox JJ, Gilmour RF Jr. Control of electrical alternans in canine cardiac Purkinje fibers. *Phys Rev Lett* 2006;96:104101–104104
43. Rappel W-J, Fenton FH, Karma A. Spatiotemporal control of wave instabilities in cardiac tissue. *Phys Rev Lett* 1999;83:456–459
44. Echebarria B, Karma A. Spatiotemporal control of cardiac alternans. *Chaos* 2002;12:923–930
45. Christini DJ, Collins JJ. Using chaos control and tracking to suppress a pathological nonchaotic rhythm in a cardiac model. *Phys Rev E* 1996;53:R49–R52
46. Hall K, Christini DJ, Tremblay M, Collins JJ, Glass L, Billette J. Dynamic control of cardiac alternans. *Phys Rev Lett* 1997;78:4518–4521
47. Christini DJ, Stein KM, Markowitz SM, Mittal S, Slotwiner DJ, Scheiner MA, Iwai S, Lerman BB. Nonlinear-dynamical arrhythmia control in humans. *Proc Nat Acad Sci USA* 2001;98:5827–5832

Chapter 6.4

Advanced Methods for Assessing the Stability and Control of Alternans

Niels F. Otani, Didier Allexandre, and Mingyi Li

Introduction

It is now widely accepted that rotating action potential waves propagating within the heart cause several types of abnormal rapid cardiac rhythm patterns. Many of these rotating waves are sustained purely through the electrical dynamics of the cardiac tissue, without the benefit of a clear anatomical obstacle around which to rotate, a phenomenon known as *functional reentry*. There have been several types of functional reentry described as possible causes of rapid cardiac rhythm, including leading circle reentry,[1] spiral wave reentry,[32] anisotropic reentry,[8] and figure-of-eight reentry.[10]

The onset of ventricular fibrillation (VF) may well be linked to factors that tend to break up these functionally reentrant waves into additional waves. One major theory suggests that a strong dependence of the action potential duration (APD) on the preceding diastolic interval (DI),[18] a phenomenon called *steep electrical restitution*, is closely correlated with the tendency for a reentrant wave to experience breakup.[38] In this theory, the steep restitution creates *alternans*, the beat-to-beat alternation of action potential parameters such as the APD or DI. When alternans is present during spiral wave rotation, the DI out in front of the rotating wave can become very short during every other rotation. As illustrated in Fig. 1, this short DI can cause a portion of the wave to block, allowing remaining segments of the wave to form additional spiral waves. The first studies of alternans on reentrant action potential waves took place in one-dimensional ring geometry.[7,14,24] This system exhibited a variation of alternans behavior called the *oscillating pulse instability*, which was found to be caused by an interaction between the dynamics associated with electrical restitution and variations in the conduction velocity, which was also assumed to depend on DI. Such was also the case when alternans was studied in finite length fibers subjected to rapid pacing.[13] In

Niels F. Otani

Department of Biomedical Sciences, College of Veterinary Medicine, Cornell University, Ithaca, NY, USA, nfo1@cornell.edu

I. R. Efimov et al. (eds.), *Cardiac Bioelectric Therapy: Mechanisms and Practical Implications.*
© Springer Science+Business Media, LLC 2009

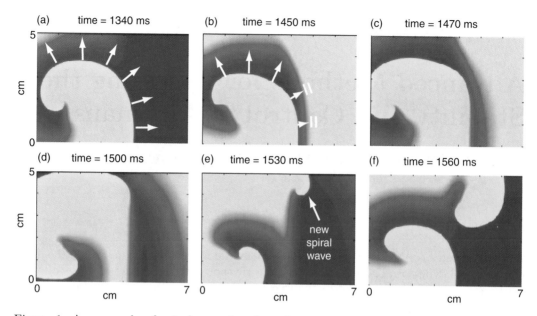

Figure 1: An example of spiral wave breakup due to steep electrical restitution (from a computer simulation). *Lighter shades* represent depolarized tissue. (**a**) A rotating spiral wave moves into a region of long diastolic interval (DI). (**b**) One rotation period later, the same spiral wave encounters a region of short DI. A portion of the wave blocks at the location indicated by the *double white lines* in (**b**), as shown in (**c**) and (**d**). In (**e**), the propagating portion of the wave forms a new spiral wave, which rotates in the opposite direction from the original wave, as shown in (**f**)

this case, in both simulation and Purkinje fiber experiments, constant rapid pacing applied to one end of the fiber resulted in alternans behavior that was either in phase throughout the system (concordant alternans) or arranged into regions that were out of phase with one another (discordant alternans). The latter were often seen to lead subsequently to block of some of the propagating action potentials. A hypothesis was subsequently put forward that the presence of discordant alternans leaves the tissue open to the block of segments of propagating wavefronts, leading to the formation of reentrant waves, subsequent block of those waves, electrical turbulence, and finally self-sustaining rapid cardiac rhythm. Substantial evidence for this theory exists; for example, it has been shown that the induction of VF can be prevented or converted into a periodic rhythm when drugs that flatten the restitution function are administered.[16,35] Pastore et al.[31] have also observed that discordant alternans degenerates into VF upon slight acceleration of the pacing frequency in guinea pig ventricular muscle.

This apparent connection between alternans and wave breakup has prompted a number of researchers to look for techniques for controlling alternans as a method for preventing VF. The vast majority of these investigations have naturally been based on these same dynamics, that is, on the dynamics of APD, DI, and conduction velocity. For example, drug-induced arrhythmias in isolated rabbit ventricular cells were stabilized by means of dynamically timed electrical stimulation based on the observed interbeat intervals.[15] Later, Hall et al.[20] showed that by adjusting the time delay of activation alternans in atrioventricular (AV) nodal conduction time could be eliminated. In this experiment, the perturbation in the time delay was chosen proportional to the difference of the conduction times for the previous two cycles. A similar control algorithm was also able to stabilize the same type of alternans in human patients.[5] In analogous fashion, if the restitution relationship between APD and DI of a small cardiac preparation is known, Watanabe and Gilmour[37] showed that alternans could be eliminated by such adjustments. Recently, a control algorithm that requires no a priori knowledge of the restitution curve was demonstrated to successfully suppress alternans.[19] All these control algorithms operated through the monitoring and then control of the various time intervals associated with the action potential.

These algorithms have exhibited a measure of success, demonstrating the importance of the concept of electrical restitution. However, they also have been plagued by the presence of stability of rhythm, or lack thereof, when restitution theory would predict the opposite, and by the inability of the underlying phenomenological model to predict when control should be successful and when it should not.[19] A number of groups have suggested that various departures from the restitution dynamics, often collectively referred to as *memory effects*, are important.[17,29,36] But even when memory is included, dynamical models have not been entirely successful in predicting behavior.[19] Another difficulty is that these methods tend not to work in tissues large enough to support discordant alternans, which is the primary target. As discovered by Echebarria and Karma,[9] methods that operate on the level of APD and DI dynamics can only control regions that have size commensurate with the size of the regions that contain in-phase alternations. This theoretical prediction is supported by the computer simulations of Rappel et al.[34] and the experiments of Christini et al.[6]

These difficulties suggest that the problem might be better examined at the level at which the fundamental dynamics occurs – that is, at the ion channel level. Treatment of the problem at this level conveys some distinct advantages. Any memory that might be present in the system is automatically included in the dynamics, and the limit on the size of the system that can be controlled is not restricted, as far as we know. Finally, operating at the ion channel level means it is possible to also take advantage of favorable features of ion channel dynamics that are not available at the APD-DI level.

Previously, study of the problem at the ion channel level was difficult due to technological limitations. The time is now right to conduct such a study. As described below, ion channel currents are now readily measured during action potentials using the current-clamped version of the perforated patch clamp technique. Several mathematical ion channel models now exist (e.g., the Luo–Rudy ion channel models,[23,28,39] the canine ventricular myocyte [CVM] model,[12] etc.) that represent a substantial improvement over their predecessors and are now able to reasonably reproduce the form and much of the dynamics of the cardiac action potential. Furthermore, with the computational power now available, it is practical to apply advanced mathematical methods to the task of unraveling the complicated interrelated dynamics of the ion channels, allowing us to extract a clear physiological, step-by-step picture of the mechanism underlying alternans and its control and other characteristics of the dynamics of action potential morphology and propagation.

What Is an Eigenmode?

An important key to this approach for studying and controlling alternans at the ion channel level lies in a mathematical construct called eigenmodes. Eigenmode theory is common in applied math, physics, and engineering, but is seldom seen in cardiac electrophysiology. In brief, the theory provides us with a method for separating the complicated behavior of certain types of systems into a set of simpler, characteristic behaviors called *eigenmodes*. Each of these eigenmodes then provides a complete description of the corresponding characteristic behavior in pure form. One ordinary example of eigenmodes comes from the theory of electromagnetic waves. Electromagnetic waves come in all frequencies, from radio waves to X-rays and beyond. Each of these frequencies is a separate eigenmode. These eigenmodes have vastly different properties from one another – radio waves, microwaves, visible light, and X-rays have different wavelengths and differ widely in the degree to which they are absorbed, scattered, reflected by, and/or propagate through various materials. These properties may all be diagnosed once the structure of the eigenmode in the given material is known. Other examples of eigenmodes include sound waves of every frequency, the vibrational modes of entities as diverse as stars, bridges, and molecules, and the quantum wave functions of electron orbitals in atoms.

In order for eigenmode theory to be applicable, the behavior of the system under study must generally be divisible into two components: a *steady state* component, and a *perturbation*, which is the term that generally refers to any disturbance to the steady state. Each of these two components must have certain properties. The steady state component, as the name suggests, must be unchanged when viewed at regularly spaced time intervals. There are two variations here: either this time interval is infinitesimal, meaning that the state may be viewed at any time, which requires that the steady state be exactly the same all the time, or the time interval is finite, in which case the state of the system is allowed to change, provided it then changes back in time for the next viewing time. The condition on the perturbation is simply that it must be small in some sense.

If the behavior of the system is divisible in this way, it can be shown mathematically (with a couple of extra technical conditions not discussed here) that there always exists a set of special perturbations, each of which grows, decays, and/or oscillates by a constant factor from one viewing time to the next, and each of which is, apart from this factor, identical from one viewing time to the next. These special perturbations are the eigenmodes, and the constant factor associated with each of these eigenmodes is called its *eigenvalue*. These eigenvalues each have two components: one that gives the frequency at which the corresponding eigenmode oscillates, and one that gives the exponential rate of growth or decay of the eigenmode in time. When the eigenvalue indicates decay, the corresponding eigenmode is called *stable*. It will thus effectively disappear over time. If the eigenmode is growing exponentially, it is called *unstable*. These are the modes that are normally of concern.

As an example, consider the case of sound waves bouncing around inside a room. The steady state for this case is simply the room with no sound in it. The perturbations are the sound waves. All sound waves of normal listening volume are small enough to satisfy the "smallness" condition for the perturbation. The eigenmodes are then simply the sound waves at each frequency. The eigenvalues are the frequencies themselves together with the rate at which each eigenmode wave exponentially decreases in amplitude. The eigenmode itself consists of the special set of changes, at every point in space, in air pressure, density, and fluid velocity relative to their steady state values, which together embody the propagating sound wave at the given frequency. Each of these quantities oscillates with this same (eigenvalue) frequency and decreases exponentially in amplitude with the same (eigenvalue) decay rate. Consequently, the proportionality of the amplitude of all these quantities with one another remains identical for all times, thus satisfying the requirement that the eigenmode remains unchanged apart from an overall scaling factor given by the eigenvalue.

There exists a nice, geometric method for visualizing the workings of the eigenmode formulation. The idea is to represent any general perturbation as a single vector living in a very high dimensional space. This vector is the sum of component vectors, each of which represents the amplitude of one of the dynamical variables, as shown schematically in Fig. 2a. (The two component vectors shown in each panel are meant to represent the usually much larger number of dynamical variables actually present.) Examples of dynamical variables are the variations in density, pressure, and fluid velocity at every point in space, as in the sound wave example, or variations in the membrane potential, gating variables, and ion concentrations and/or ion currents, for the case discussed later in this chapter. For most perturbations, this vector continuously changes length and direction as time passes, as illustrated by the successive panels in Fig. 2a. Eigenmode theory says that any general perturbation that is small enough may be written as the vector sum of so-called *eigenvectors*, as illustrated in Fig. 2b. Again, the number of eigenvectors is usually much larger than two; but only two are shown here for clarity. As depicted in Fig. 2b–d, each of these eigenvectors has the properties that (1) its direction remains unchanged and (2) its length increases or decreases by a constant factor given by the eigenvalue, from one viewing time to the next. From Fig. 2c, d, we see that this invariance in direction forces the amplitudes of the dynamical variables to maintain the same proportionality relative to one another at every viewing time and also forces each of the dynamical variables associated with the eigenmode to grow or decay with same constant factor as the eigenvector itself.

The usefulness of the eigenmode technique should be clear from Fig. 2. The behavior of the dynamical variables and vector representation of a typical perturbation can appear to be very complicated, with the dynamical variables changing sign and fluctuating in a complicated way, and the vector changing direction, and shortening and lengthening seemingly at random, as suggested by Fig. 2a. In contrast, as shown in Fig. 2b–d, when the perturbation is decomposed into eigenmodes, arbitrary perturbations are seen to be composed of a set of very simple behaviors, each of which grows or decays exponentially in amplitude and whose dynamical variables maintain constant proportionality to one another.

In particular, the eigenmode decomposition makes it clear that, in order to control arbitrary perturbations, it suffices to control the unstable eigenmodes, either by modifying the system so that all modes are rendered stable, or by adding a "control" disturbance that zeroes out the unstable mode(s). Both of these approaches are potentially relevant to the problem; thus both are currently under study. The former falls within the discipline of *control theory* and is used extensively in several areas of engineering. When applied to the

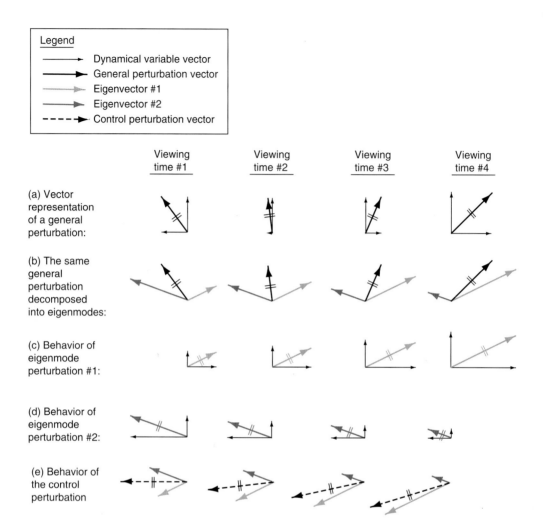

Figure 2: Graphical description of the eigenmode technique. Each panel shows the decomposition of the vector with *two small lines* cutting across its length into the other two vectors displayed. (**a**) Representation of a general perturbation as the sum of vectors (two shown) whose amplitudes are those of the constituent disturbances to individual dynamical variables, at four regularly spaced viewing times. (**b**) Representation of the same general perturbation as a vector sum of eigenvectors, at the same viewing times. (**c**, **d**) The first and second eigenvectors for the same general perturbation and their decompositions into vectors representing the dynamical variables. (**e**) The decomposition into eigenvectors of the perturbations created when control is applied at the first viewing time

cardiac electrophysiology problem, it has the potential for providing a rigorous basis on which to develop drug, electrical, and gene therapies that yield inherent modifications to the tissue that render it resistant to the development of alternans.

This chapter will concentrate on the other technique, which has been more extensively studied. Specifically, the chapter focuses on a method of electrical intervention that, when combined with an existing disturbance, zeroes out the amplitude of the unstable alternans eigenmode(s). The method by which this may be achieved is illustrated in Fig. 2e. In this case, the goal is to eliminate eigenmode perturbation 1, which as shown in Fig. 2c is the unstable mode. We are usually not free to apply control disturbances to any particular dynamical variable; for example, for the case of electrical intervention, it is possible to directly modify the membrane potential, but modification of the gating variables, ion concentrations, and so forth can only occur indirectly through the effect of the modification of the membrane potential on these quantities. Suppose, in the illustrated example, disturbances to the membrane potential are represented by horizontal vectors. As with any other vector, a horizontal vector may be decomposed into eigenvectors, as shown in the first panel of Fig. 2e. Suppose that the magnitude of the control disturbance to the membrane potential is chosen so that its eigenvector 1 component is exactly equal and opposite to the corresponding existing eigenvector component at viewing time 1 (compare eigenvector 1 in Fig. 2c, e). We observe that, not only will the two exactly cancel at viewing time 1, but they will cancel at all subsequent viewing times, since both the previously existing eigenvector 1 and that resulting from the control disturbance grow at the same rate. Thus we see that eigenmode theory may be used to determine the proper amplitude for a control disturbance that will completely eliminate an unwanted, unstable mode. Note that this disturbance does not, in general, cancel other eigenvectors. In the example shown, eigenvector 2 is not zeroed out. However, it is the nature of eigenmode 2, as determined by its eigenvalue, that this mode damps out. Thus, for this example, eigenmode 1 is zeroed out, and eigenmode 2 damps out; thus arbitrary disturbances may be controlled.

It is important to note that the eigenmode formulation is technically only valid for small perturbations. In practice, however, the technique often tells us a lot about larger amplitude disturbances as well. For example, sonic booms or blast waves created by explosions are sound waves that are too large in amplitude for the eigenmode theory to be strictly valid, yet these waves still propagate via essentially the same mechanism as their smaller amplitude counterparts. In both cases, they propagate through the imbalance between regions of higher and lower density, with variations of pressure acting as the restoring force.

Characterization and Control of Alterans in Isolated Cardiac Myocytes

Application of the Eigenmode Method

We now show how the eigenmode formulation may be applied to the task of diagnosing the mechanism responsible for alternans in action potential morphology when isolated cardiac cells are subjected to constant external electrical pacing. In this case, the steady state consists of action potentials generated by the pacing that are identical to one another (often called 1:1 or period-1 behavior). The membrane potential trace and the traces of all other dynamical quantities are identical from one action potential to the next in this state. The perturbation then consists of the departure of the membrane potential and all other dynamical quantities (i.e., the currents, concentrations, gating variables, and so forth) from their steady state counterparts.

An example of this separation of the behavior into a steady state and a perturbation is shown in Fig. 3 using data obtained from a computer simulation that employs the CVM model developed by Fox et al.[12] The figure shows the special case in which the perturbation is the alternans eigenmode. Two successive action potentials are shown, with the assumption that the behavior continues over a much longer series of action potentials. Figure 3a shows both the steady-state behavior of the membrane potential, and the membrane potential when the alternans eigenmode has been added as a perturbation to the steady state. The membrane potential perturbation $\delta V(t)$ associated the alternans eigenmode is then just the difference between the two traces in Fig. 3a. It is plotted separately in Fig. 3b. Note that the steady state action potentials are identical, as they must be, to be considered a steady state. The traces of all the other dynamical variables are also identical from one action potential to the next during steady state behavior (not shown). The other feature of note is that the alternans eigenmode membrane potential perturbation shown in Fig. 3b is identical from one action potential to the next, apart from a negative scaling factor. Thus the trace associated with the second action potential has the same shape as the trace associated with the first, except that the former is upside down and has an amplitude slightly larger than the latter. Any other dynamical quantity from the alternans eigenmode will also show the same kind of behavior. For example, Fig. 3c shows the perturbation to the potassium-delayed rectifier current δI_{Kr} associated with the alternans perturbation. Its trace for the second action potential is also a flipped over, slightly amplified version of its trace for the first action potential.

Figure 3d shows how this behavior is consistent with the vector-based graphical description of eigenmodes just presented. The eight gray vectors shown are the alternans eigenvectors corresponding to the eight times indicated. Each eigenvector was constructed by summing two vectors of (signed) length equal to the alternans eigenmode perturbations δV and δI_{Kr} at the given time. (As before, the eigenvectors shown are two-dimensional representations of the actual eigenvectors, which exist in a much higher dimensional space. The actual eigenvector is the vector sum of all the vectors representing perturbations to all the dynamical variables.) Each of the last four eigenvectors shown were constructed exactly one pacing period after the times for the first four eigenvectors. If the viewing times are also chosen to be separated by exactly one pacing period, the eigenvectors behave as expected. For example, if the viewing times are chosen to coincide with the times of the first and fifth eigenvector insets, shown in Figure 3d, we see that the eigenvector in this fifth inset points in exactly the same (actually in exactly the opposite) direction as the eigenvector in the first inset. This is therefore the first eigenvector multiplied by a negative constant (which is given by the eigenvalue), as advertised. Similar statements could also have been made about the eigenvectors shown in the second and sixth insets, or the third and seventh insets, and so on, if the viewing times had been chosen to coincide with the times of those

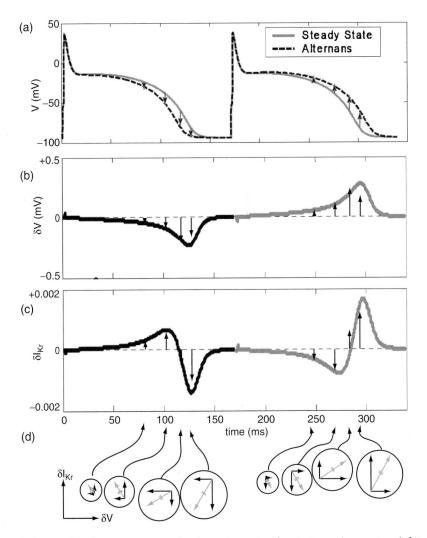

Figure 3: Relationship between perturbations to a steady state action potential trace and vectors for the alternans eigenmode for an isolated cell using the canine ventricular myocyte (CVM) model. (a) Membrane potential versus time for the steady state case (*solid line*) and the steady state to which has been added a pure alternans eigenmode perturbation (*dashed line*). The perturbation has been exaggerated for purposes of visibility. (b) Perturbation to the membrane potential versus time for the alternans eigenmode. This perturbation is the difference between the traces in (a). Thus, the darker portion of the trace is the perturbation to the first action potential shown in (a); the lighter portion is the perturbation to the second action potential. The *arrows* indicate the perturbation from the steady state at eight different times and would be proportional to the *arrows* appearing in (a) if the trace in the latter had not been exaggerated. (c) Perturbation to the I_{Kr} current in the alternans eigenmode. (d) Vector representation of the alternans eigenmode at eight times during the two action potentials. The *arrows pointing horizontally* represent perturbations of the membrane potential (δV); *arrows that point vertically* represent perturbations to I_{Kr}. These *arrows* are equal in length to their counterparts in (b) and (c). The *gray arrows* represent the alternans eigenmode as a function of time and, in each case are the vector sum of the other two *arrows* (modified from Li and Otani, Fig. 2)[26]

pairs of insets. The steady state values of the membrane potential (cf. Fig. 3a) and all other dynamical variables (not shown) also turn out to be identical from one viewing time to the next, since all steady state action potentials are identical.

We note that the eigenvector can in general change direction in between viewing times. This motion is, in fact, very useful – it provides detailed information about the dynamics of the eigenmode. For example, a detailed study of how perturbations in the dynamical variables that comprise the alternans eigenmode ebb and flow yields the full mechanism by which alternans maintains itself. This study may be conducted through an examination of the plots of the perturbations to all the dynamical variables, two examples of which are shown in Fig. 3b, c.

The Ion Channel Mechanism Underlying Alternans

So far, our group has conducted this type of study on two ion channel models: the Beeler–Reuter model[4] and the CVM model[12] used to create Fig. 3. Here we present a brief description of the alternans mechanism found in the CVM model,[30] which is the more modern, detailed, and realistic model of the two. A detailed description of the alternans mechanism found in the Beeler–Reuter model appears elsewhere.[25]

The primary mechanism involved in producing alternans in the CVM model resides within the calcium cycling subsystem of the cell, depicted schematically by the portion of the flow diagram below the dashed line in Fig. 4. Briefly, at the beginning of every other action potential, the level of calcium-dependent inactivation is lower than average (i.e., lower than its steady state value). This causes the influx of calcium through the L-type calcium channel to be higher than average, triggering a larger than average calcium-induced calcium release from the sarcoplasmic reticulum. The enhanced calcium influx and release together result in a higher-than-average concentration of calcium in the intracellular space, which increases calcium-dependent inactivation to a higher-than-average value by the beginning of the next action potential. The entire mechanism can then repeat itself with opposite polarity during the next action potential. Thus, the dynamics of calcium cycling has the ability to create the alternation of all the dynamical quantities that is consistent with alternans behavior. This observation is consistent with the views of other researchers.[12,33]

The eigenmode analysis, however, has more to say about the alternans mechanism. Careful study shows that the alternation would decay exponentially with time were this the only operative mechanism. The decay is due to a negative feedback mechanism within the calcium cycling dynamics. Specifically, the elevated level of calcium-dependent inactivation present toward the end of the first action potential acts to reduce the L-type calcium current, which in turn reduces the degree of inactivation that is presented to the next action potential. The analysis then shows that this damping mechanism is counteracted by additional dynamics associated with the membrane potential, as shown in the portion of Fig. 4 above the dashed line. In this additional mechanism, the enhanced L-type calcium current elevates the plateau membrane potential above its steady state value. This higher-than-average membrane potential results in a lower-than-average inward rectifier potassium current (I_{K1}) due to a negatively sloped I–V curve. A lower-than-average rapid delayed rectifier current (I_{Kr}) is generated as well. The reduction of these two repolarizing currents tends to reinforce the elevation of the membrane potential above its steady state value. This

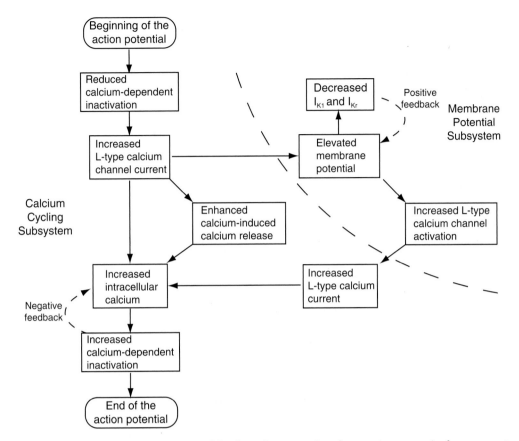

Figure 4: The mechanism responsible for alternans in the canine ventricular myocyte (CVM) model as diagnosed by eigenmode theory (modified from Otani et al., Fig. 1, with permission from Elsevier)[30]

is therefore an *amplification* mechanism, whereby a small disturbance in the membrane potential early in the plateau phase is amplified through most of the remainder of the action potential. The higher membrane potential increases the activation of the L-type calcium channel (the *d* gate), which increases calcium influx and props up the calcium concentration, counteracting the effects produced by the previously mentioned negative feedback in the calcium cycling dynamics. Thus, alternans in the CVM model originates in the calcium cycling subsystem, but is sustained with help from the membrane ion channel dynamics.

The eigenmode formulation defines not only the behavior of the membrane potential as a function of time for each mode, but that of all the other dynamical variables as well. Thus, these other variables should behave as predicted by the eigenmode method in experiments. One example of this agreement can be demonstrated by comparing the results of recent experiments of Hua and Gilmour[22] to the theory. In these experiments, the action potential clamp method was used to determine the behavior of I_{Kr} during APD alternans. Specifically,

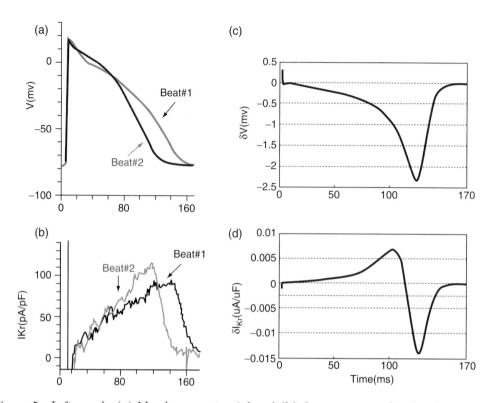

Figure 5: *Left panels*: (**a**) Membrane potential and (**b**) I_{Kr} current on for the eleventh and twelfth beats (labeled beats 1 and 2) obtained experimentally using the action potential clamp method. *Right panels*: perturbations in the (**c**) membrane potential and (**d**) I_{Kr}, versus time obtained computationally for the alternans eigenmode in the canine ventricular myocyte (CVM) ion channel model. The theory predicts that the traces in (**c**) and (**d**) should be proportional to the difference between beat 2 and beat 1 in (**a**) and (**b**), respectively (modified with permission from Hua and Gilmour, Fig. 2)[22]

the membrane potential was recorded from regularly paced (cycle length equals 170 ms) isolated cells exhibiting alternans behavior. These recordings were then used as command potentials in the presence and absence of the I_{Kr} blocker E-4031 (5 µM). The subtraction current, presumed to be the I_{Kr} current, for two consecutive action potentials is shown in Fig. 5b, along with the command membrane potentials for those beats (Fig. 5a). The current is seen to be smaller for the longer duration action potential (beat 1) through the early portion of the action potential ($t = 20$–120 ms), but is larger after that ($t = 120$–170 ms). This result is consistent with the perturbation I_{Kr} current associated with the alternans eigenmode obtained for the CVM model, shown in Fig. 5d. As expected, the perturbation current is approximately proportional to the difference between the traces shown in Fig. 5b, being positive for $t = 20$–120 ms, and negative thereafter ($t = 120$–170 ms). The observed behavior is also consistent with the alternans mechanism just described. For example, in the beat 1 trace in Fig. 5b, the I_{Kr} current during the plateau is seen to be smaller than during beat 1. In an unclamped cell, this would tend to elevate the membrane potential in the later stages of the plateau and during repolarization, consistent with the higher beat 1 membrane potential appearing in Fig. 5a, and consistent with the positive feedback loop of the alternans mechanism appearing in the upper right corner of Fig. 4.

Development and Testing of a Control Algorithm

We next turn our attention to the problem of how to control the alternans dynamics just described through the application of small amplitude electrical stimuli. Technical details of these ideas appear in the Appendix and in Li and Otani,[26] here a conceptual description is provided. The approach is to employ the eigenvector-canceling technique depicted in Fig. 2e as described above. For this specific case, the goal is to cancel the alternans eigenmode shown in Fig. 3 using an externally applied electrical stimulus. We are free to apply the stimulus at any time during the action potential. Whenever the stimulus is applied, the goal is always to cancel the alternans eigenvector present at the given time. For example, if the stimulus were applied at any of the eight times illustrated in Fig. 3d, the goal would be to cancel the eigenvector shown in the inset corresponding to the chosen time. In patch-clamp experiments, the application of a brief current pulse through the pipette effectively discontinuously changes the membrane potential by an amount approximately equal to $-I_0 \Delta t / C_m$, where I_0 and Δt are the amplitude and duration of the current pulse, and C_m is the capacitance of the cell membrane. Thus, application of a current stimulus is approximately equivalent to introducing a membrane potential perturbation.

Since the alternans eigenvector changes direction and magnitude throughout the action potential (as illustrated in Fig. 3d), as do all the other eigenvectors, it is obvious that the current needed to cancel the alternans eigenvector at different times during the action potential will also change. When this current is plotted as a function of time through the action potential, a surprising result is obtained. We might have expected that, since the APD is determined largely by when repolarization occurs, the APD might be most easily adjusted by applying the stimulus during the repolarization phase (phase 3). However, Fig. 6 shows that the best time to deliver the stimulus (that is, the time when the current required is the smallest) is actually early in the plateau phase. Additional analysis reveals that the positive feedback mechanism shown in the upper right-hand corner of Fig. 4 is responsible for this paradoxical result. The positive feedback loop amplifies the effect of any stimulus applied early in the plateau phase, which thereby reduces the current required to make changes in repolarization later in the action potential. The amplification is, in fact, quite dramatic for the CVM model: as is evident from Fig. 6b, the stimulus charge requirement is hundreds of times smaller than the charge required late in phase 3.

These predictions were tested by applying the calculated stimuli to the CVM model. When a small amplitude alternans mode was initiated in the system with pacing interval 170 ms, a single stimulus applied in the early plateau (at 17 ms after the pacing stimulus) with amplitude given by the theory completely eliminated alternans, as expected. We were also interested to see whether these stimuli would be effective for the large amplitude alternans. Accordingly, in another simulation, alternans was allowed to grow until its

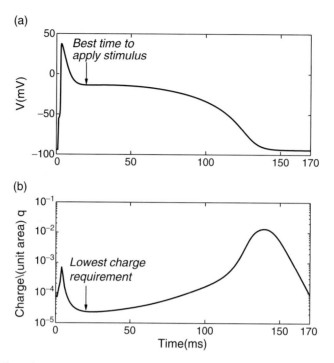

Figure 6: (b) The charge per unit membrane surface area $q = I_0 \Delta t/(\text{Surface area})$ (μA ms cm^{-2}) required to eliminate alternans of a given amplitude versus stimulus application time during the action potential in the canine ventricular myocyte (CVM) model. (a) shows the membrane potential, V, as a function of time, for reference (modified from Li and Otani, Fig. 4)[26]

amplitude stabilized. A stimulus was then applied on every other action potential, 16 ms after the pacing stimulus, with the amplitude predicted by the theory. We found that the perturbation associated with alternans was nearly eliminated by the first stimulus. Since any remaining perturbations were then small, they were effectively controlled by the application of the next two to three control stimuli.

These tests suggested a control stimulus algorithm that could be effective in experiments, even if knowledge of the ion channel dynamics for a given cell was incomplete. The membrane potential was first recorded during the repolarization phase (specifically, 135 ms after the pacing stimulus for the case shown) of two successive action potentials, as illustrated by Fig. 7. The difference between these membrane potentials, $V_1 - V_2$, was considered to be a measure of the amplitude of the alternans mode. A stimulus proportional to $V_1 - V_2$ was then applied to the early plateau phase of the following membrane potential. In simulations, the control stimulus was applied as a fixed current of 10 μA μF^{-1} with a duration of $0.12(V_1 - V_2)$ ms (with the membrane potential given in mV). This protocol was very effective against alternans in the CVM model, effectively eliminating them almost immediately. (Note the evenness of the last two action potentials in Fig. 7 compared to the first two.) The mechanism

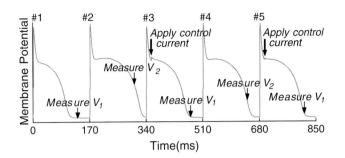

Figure 7: The control stimulus protocol. The membrane potential trace shown is the actual one obtained from the control scheme. Note the reduction in alternans amplitude between the first and last pairs of action potentials. The initially small effect of the stimulus on the action potential is visible on action potentials 3 and 5 (reproduced from Li and Otani, Fig. 3)[26]

by which alternans was eliminated was found to be similar to that observed in the tests described above, and similar to that predicted by the theory.

Note that the control stimulus produces almost no immediate change to the membrane potential itself in these studies – the disturbance to the membrane potential is barely visible on the third and fifth action potentials shown in Fig. 7. The effect is far from insignificant, however. Many of the dynamic variables (e.g., d and X_{Kr}) are markedly changed when the stimulus is applied. This in turn results in substantial changes in the perturbation dynamics compared to the controlled case, eventually resulting in a strong modification to the membrane potential much later in time, in the repolarization phase.

To determine whether current pulses applied during the early plateau phase of the action potential have the ability to suppress electrical alternans, as predicted by the eigenmode analysis described above, a small number of experiments were conducted ($n = 4$) in small preparations of canine endocardial muscle and Purkinje fibers.[27] Small preparations (2–3 mm long $\times$ 1–2 mm wide $\times$ 1 mm thick) were used to allow approximately simultaneous delivery of current to the entire preparation. Both pacing and control stimuli were delivered using a bipolar electrode having an interelectrode spacing of 3 mm. The constant pacing interval was chosen short enough to generate APD alternans in the absence of control stimuli. Figure 8 shows a case in which hyperpolarizing 100 μA constant-current pulses of 1.0 ms duration were delivered 15 ms after the upstroke of every other action potential during alternans activity. Delivery of the current pulse during action potentials with shorter-than-normal APDs tended to increase the alternans magnitude, as was the case between times 1 and 2 in Fig. 8, whereas delivery of the current pulse during action potentials with long APDs markedly reduced the alternans magnitude (between times 2 and 3 in the figure). When the control stimulus was turned off, alternans reappeared, but the magnitude of the alternans was smaller than before delivery of the control stimulus (following time 3). The behavior was found to be repeatable after a period of equilibration.

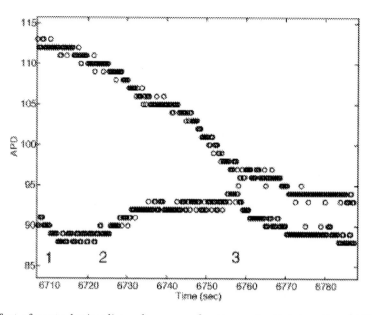

Figure 8: Effect of control stimuli on alternans of action potential duration (APD) in canine ventricular muscle. *Left panel*: APD plotted as a function of time during pacing at a cycle length (CL) of 150 ms. In the absence of a control stimulus, APD alternans occurred at this CL (beginning of record). At 1, a hyperpolarizing control stimulus was delivered to the short duration action potential of the short-long pairs. At 2, the control stimulus was switched to the long duration action potential. The control stimulus was turned off at 3 (reproduced from Li et al., Fig. 5, copyright IEEE, 2003)[27]

Characterization and Control of Spiral Wave Instabilities

Nature of Spiral Wave Instabilities

The eigenmode method can also be applied to the case of rotating action potential waves (spiral waves) in two spatial dimensions by employing the version of eigenmode theory that assumes the viewing time interval is infinitesimal (as described above). Technical details have been published previously[2] and also appear in abbreviated form in the Appendix. To find the steady state and eigenmodes, the theoretical approach, as described by Barkley,[3] for a spiral wave system was applied. The three-variable Fenton–Karma model[11] was used as the underlying ion channel model. It was modified so that it exhibited both unstable alternans eigenmodes and also eigenmodes that characterize the tendency of the spiral wave to meander. The model was then used to study the control of these unstable modes.

The steady state for this case was simply a rigidly rotating spiral wave (i.e., a wave that rotates with constant angular velocity without changing form). If viewed in the frame

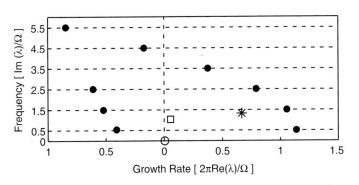

Figure 9: Eigenvalues for the two-dimensional, modified three-variable Fenton–Karma model. The *solid dots*, the *asterisk*, the *open square*, and the *open circle* denote the alternans eigenvalues, the meandering mode eigenvalue, the eigenvalue associated with the translational symmetry, and the eigenvalue associated with rotational symmetry, respectively (modified from Allexandre and Otani, Fig. 2, copyright American Physical Society)[2]

of reference rotating with the wave, such a wave appears to be completely stationary and unchanging at all times, thus satisfying the requirement for a steady state previously discussed when the viewing time interval is infinitesimal.

The role of perturbations in this case was then to modify this rigid waveform. Inclusion of perturbations thus allowed the wave to widen and/or narrow, and speed up and/or slow down, as it rotated. Furthermore, these alterations did not necessarily apply to the wave as a whole; it was possible for some portions of the wave to widen while others narrowed, for example. Addition of perturbations also made it possible for the spiral wave tip to simultaneously move toward or away from the center of rotation, creating a meandering pattern commonly seen in spiral wave computer simulations. The profile of the wave could also be changed by the presence of perturbations.

When the eigenmode theory was applied, it was found that the total number of eigenmodes was tremendous – equal to the total number of points in the system times the number of variables. In fact, the former is technically infinite; but remains finite although large in the computer calculation due to the spatial discretization scheme used in the analysis. Fortunately, only a small number of these modes are unstable. The eigenvalues of these unstable modes (along with a few of the most prominent stable modes) are shown in Fig. 9. Of all the alternans eigenmodes (represented by the solid dots), four were found to be unstable, those lying to the right of the dashed vertical line. There was also one unstable meandering eigenmode (represented by the asterisk). All the alternans modes had one property in common: at every point in the tissue through which the spiral wave rotated, the APD of the wave alternated between being slightly longer and slightly shorter than the steady state APD, each time the wave came around, consistent with the definition of alternans. The alternans modes differed from one another through their spatial structure – that is, the size, shape, and locations of the regions that differed in phase relative to one another were different for each of the different modes.

Elimination of Alternans in a Rotating Spiral Wave

As with the single cell case, eigenmode theory also provided us with information about when and where control stimuli might best be applied. Most of the eigenmodes were found to be most sensitive to modification when the stimulus was situated close to the center of rotation, in the recovery phase of the spiral wave. The stimulus location and timing were chosen accordingly. To simplify the study, the initial perturbation to the steadily rotating wave was chosen in a special way – it was calculated so that a single stimulus would eliminate all the unstable alternans modes. The development of a plan to kill all the alternans modes when an arbitrary perturbation is present is somewhat more complicated, and is a topic currently under investigation. The results for the case of the specially chosen initial conditions are shown in Fig. 10. The upper panels show that the alternans modes are indeed unstable, leading to increasingly large perturbations as shown in Fig. 10c, d. In contrast, when a single stimulus is applied at the location outlined by the small circle in Fig. 10e with the timing and amplitude provided by the theory to a simulation that is otherwise identical, the result is the near-complete suppression of alternans for four rotational periods of the spiral wave, as shown in the four lower panels of Fig. 10.

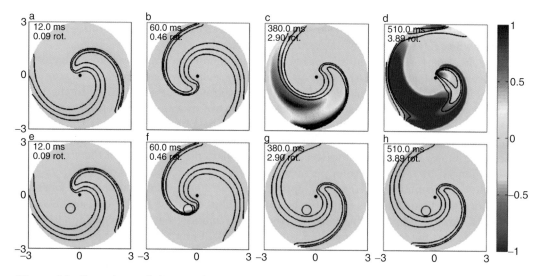

Figure 10: Snapshots of the membrane potential perturbation at several selected times, for the case where no control stimulus is applied (*top panels*) and for the case in which a control stimulus is applied at time $t = 10$ ms (*bottom panels*). The two cases were initialized with specially chosen, identical perturbations. Viewed in color, the color shading gives amplitude of the perturbation. Viewed in *black and white*, the *darker shades* correspond to the larger perturbations. Level contours of the total membrane potential (steady state plus linearized perturbation) are shown as *black lines*. A small *black circle* was drawn in each of the lower subplots to highlight the region in which the stimulus was applied (from Allexandre and Otani, Fig. 8, copyright American Physical Society)[2]

Perhaps the most surprising aspect of these studies is that a single stimulus at a single location can affect the dynamics over such a large region. This assertion stands despite the fact that the initial conditions are specially chosen – the simulation still represents a clear example of how a point stimulus can influence an area of linear dimension much larger than the space constant, which is the usual decay length associated with perturbations in the membrane potential in excitable tissue. The preliminary explanation for this phenomenon is that the effect of the stimulus must use the dynamics of the spiral wave itself to spread its influence, effectively "surfing" on the wave to propagate across the system. Further study of this effect is ongoing.

Summary and Implications for Treatment of Cardiac Arrhythmias

This chapter has demonstrated that eigenmode methods can be used to diagnose the ion channel basis for alternans and other disturbances to action potential behavior, once a mathematical model representative of the functioning of the ion channels is provided. When applied to isolated cells, the method provides a complete picture of which quantities play the important roles in generating and sustaining behavior such as electrical alternans, and when during the course of the action potential they are involved. Among the quantities available for analysis are the membrane potential, the ion channel gates and currents, and the ion concentrations in both buffered and free forms, in both the intracellular space and compartments of the sarcoplasmic reticulum. We have shown that, for the two ion channel models studied, a complete, step-by-step description of the mechanism responsible for alternans may be extracted from the analysis. For the CVM ion channel model, the mechanism is primarily tied to calcium handling, but requires help from the dynamics of other channels in the cell membrane in order to be sustainable. Since many cardiac drugs work at the ion channel level, this type of understanding should allow for improved pharmacological therapies that are based on the actual mechanism involved in alternans, that, for example, can target one of the key steps involved in creating and/or sustaining alternans.

The eigenmode method also allows us to determine how best to control phenomena such as alternans through electrical means. For example, for the CVM model, the best time to apply control stimuli is early in the plateau phase of the action potential, a surprising result. This case thus demonstrates the usefulness of the eigenmode method in providing guidance regarding the amplitude, sign, and timing of the control stimulus that, at times, can run counter to intuition. The method has the potential for guiding research toward new strategies for control algorithms. For example, the analysis of the CVM model has shown the possibility that the cardiac cells' own internal dynamics can contain an amplification mechanism, which might allow creation of new algorithms that require less energy.

Not only can the eigenmode method be applied to individual cells, but it can also be applied to cardiac tissue of finite size on which propagate various action potential waveforms of relevance to many tachyarrhythmias. This chapter has demonstrated the application of these methods to rotating spiral waves, which are thought to be present in some form in both ventricular tachycardia and VF. The method revealed that, when the underlying ion channel model was a modification of the Fenton–Karma three-variable model, spiral waves exhibit several unstable modes, including four alternans modes, each with its own spatial structure of the alternans phase, and a spiral wave meandering mode. The analysis also showed that most of these modes were most easily modified through stimuli applied close to the center of spiral wave rotation, during the recovery phase. When a single stimulus of amplitude and timing calculated from the theory was applied in this region, it was found that, at least for a special case, alternans were almost completely eliminated over the entire spiral wave. These results lead to two conclusions: (1) Spiral waves are more easily controlled using stimuli close to their centers of rotation, and most interestingly, (2) it appears possible to control alternans over a very large region (e.g., over a region much larger than the space constant) using properly placed and timed stimuli. The latter may be due to dynamics at the ion channel level, which again demonstrates the usefulness of operating at this level. Of course, both of these conclusions require additional testing, in both experiments and computer simulations employing more realistic ion channel models and more general initial conditions. Nevertheless, these two results can be viewed with some optimism, as the first is likely to be generic to spiral waves in general, while the second may be cautiously hypothesized to be is caused by the ability of perturbations to propagate across the face of action potential wavefronts, the essential dynamics of which is handled well in the current model.

Appendix: Mathematical Details

This appendix provides a summary of the mathematics on which the descriptions in this chapter are based. For more information, please see Li and Otani[25,26] for a description of the theory in isolated cells, and Allexandre and Otani[2] for additional details on the methods used for the two-dimensional spiral wave.

Theory of alternans control in isolated cells. The mathematics of the eigenmode method used for the single cell case was fairly straightforward. Consider an isolated cell to which identical electrical stimuli are applied with regular time interval T. This system may be assumed to be described by differential equations of the form,

$$d\mathbf{u}(t)/dt = \mathbf{f}(\mathbf{u}(t)) + \mathbf{i}(t), \tag{1}$$

where $\mathbf{u}(t)$ is a vector of the dynamical variables at time t, $\mathbf{i}(t)$ accounts for the applied stimuli, and $\mathbf{f}(\mathbf{u})$ is a vector-valued function. Define $\mathcal{M}(t)$ to be an operator that returns a vector $\mathbf{u}(t + T)$ of dynamical variables as a function of these same dynamical variables $\mathbf{u}(t)$ a time T earlier. Thus,

$$\mathbf{u}(t + T) = \mathcal{M}(t)(\mathbf{u}(t)). \tag{2}$$

The steady state solution $\mathbf{u}_0(t)$ to this mapping, defined as the function satisfying $\mathbf{u}_0(t) = \mathcal{M}(t)(\mathbf{u}_0(t))$ for all t, may be obtained in two steps. First, we solve for $\mathbf{u}_0(t_0)$ at some particular time t_0 by applying the Broyden method, a root solver similar to the secant method, to the function, $\mathbf{F}(\mathbf{u}_0(t_0), t_0)) \equiv \mathbf{u}_0(t_0) - \mathcal{M}(t_0)(\mathbf{u}_0(t_0))$. The entire steady state solution, $\mathbf{u}_0(t)$ can then be obtained by integrating the differential equation (1) forward starting from initial conditions $\mathbf{u}_0(t_0)$.

We next construct the linear mapping that relates small perturbations $\delta\mathbf{u}(t + T)$ of the steady state at time $t + T$ to perturbations $\delta\mathbf{u}(t)$ at a time T earlier. Specifically, the elements of the matrix $\mathbf{M}$ in the formula,

$$\delta\mathbf{u}(t + T) = \mathbf{M}(t) \cdot \delta\mathbf{u}(t) \qquad (3)$$

are obtained by perturbing each of the components of $\mathbf{u}(t)$ very slightly away from the steady state $\mathbf{u}_0(t)$, one at a time, and observing what perturbations to $\mathbf{u}_0(t)$ result a time T later. We then calculate the eigenvalues λ_i and eigenvectors $\mathbf{v}_i(t_0)$, $i = 1, \ldots, N$ of the N-dimensional matrix $\mathbf{M}(t_0)$ at some particular time, t_0. The eigenmodes $\mathbf{v}_i(t)$, $i = 1, \ldots, N$ are then constructed using $\mathbf{u}(t_0) = \mathbf{u}_0(t_0) + \varepsilon\mathbf{v}_i(t_0)$ as the initial conditions in (1), where ε is chosen very small, and then solving for $\mathbf{v}_i(t) = (\mathbf{u}(t) - \mathbf{u}_0(t))/\epsilon$.

To find the amplitude of the control stimulus required to cancel the alternans eigenmode at any particular time t, we begin by noting that, generally, any vector may be written as a linear combination of eigenmodes, so that, in particular, the perturbation vector may be written as,

$$\delta\mathbf{u}(t) = c_1\mathbf{v}_1(t) + c_2\mathbf{v}(t) + \cdots, \qquad (4)$$

where $\mathbf{v}_1(t)$ is defined to be the alternans eigenmode, $\mathbf{v}_2(t)$, $\mathbf{v}_3(t)$, ... are the remaining eigenmodes, and c_1, c_2, ... are constants. Similarly, the effect of an applied control stimulus on all the dynamical variables may be expressed as another vector perturbation function $\delta\mathbf{s}(t)$, which can also be expressed as a sum of eigenvectors:

$$\delta\mathbf{s}(t) = s_1\mathbf{v}_1(t) + s_2\mathbf{v}_2(t) + \cdots. \qquad (5)$$

The alternans eigenmode may then be eliminated by simply choosing the control stimulus so that $s_1 = -c_1$. Applying the control stimulus would then add $\delta\mathbf{s}(t)$ to $\delta\mathbf{u}(t)$, zeroing out the coefficient of the alternans mode, $\mathbf{v}_1(t)$, completely killing it, as suggested by the sum of vectors in Fig. 2c, e. A very short duration control stimulus applied at time t may be approximated as discontinuous jump $\Delta V = I_0\Delta t/C$ in the membrane potential, where I_0/C is the applied current per unit capacitance (positive inward), and Δt is the stimulus duration. Defining the first component in these vectors to be the one containing the membrane potential, the control stimulus perturbation at time t is then:

$$\delta\mathbf{s}(t) = [I_0\Delta t/C, 0, 0, \ldots]^T. \qquad (6)$$

Dotting the *left* alternans eigenmode, $\mathbf{w}_1(t)$, into both (4) and (5), using the fact that $\mathbf{w}_i(t) \cdot \mathbf{v}_j(t) = 0$ except when $i = j$, and setting $s_1 = -c_1$, yields

$$I_0\Delta t = -C\frac{\mathbf{w}_1(t) \cdot \delta\mathbf{u}(t)}{w_{11}(t)} \qquad (7)$$

as the charge delivered by the stimulus that will exactly annihilate the alternans mode if delivered at time t, where $w_{11}(t)$ is the first component of $\mathbf{w}_1(t)$.

Characterization and control of unstable eigenmodes of rotating spiral waves. To apply eigenmode methods to the problem of spiral wave instability and control, we begin by transforming the governing partial differential equations to the rotating frame:

$$\partial \mathbf{u}/\partial t = \Omega \partial \mathbf{u}/\partial \theta + \mathbf{D} \cdot \nabla^2 u + \mathbf{f}(\mathbf{u}) \equiv \mathcal{G}(\mathbf{u}), \tag{8}$$

where $\mathbf{u}(x, y, t)$ is now a vector containing the dynamical variables as functions of both time and space, $\theta = \tan^{-1}(y/x)$ is the azimuthal direction, Ω is the angular frequency of the rotating frame, which is set equal to the steady state spiral wave rotation frequency, $\mathbf{D}$ is a matrix containing the gap junction conductances, and $\mathbf{f}(\mathbf{u})$ now contains the Fenton–Karma model ion channel dynamics. A typical spiral wave will appear to be approximately stationary in this frame of reference; thus, it is reasonable to expect that a steady state solution exists. We can iteratively solve for this solution, $\mathbf{u}_0(x, y)$, by setting the right-hand side of (8) equal to zero and using the Newton–Raphson method. There exists rotational symmetry in the problem, implying that any solution rotated around the origin by any angle is also a solution. We take advantage of this symmetry by choosing the value of one variable at one point, effectively selecting one of these redundant solutions, and in its place, treat Ω as an unknown. This enables us to find a steady state solution and the angular frequency at the same time. If (8) is then linearized about this steady state, the following equation is obtained:

$$\partial \delta \mathbf{u}/\partial t = (\partial \mathcal{G}(\mathbf{u}_0)/\partial \mathbf{u}) \cdot \delta \mathbf{u}, \tag{9}$$

where $\partial \mathcal{G}(\mathbf{u}_0)/\partial \mathbf{u}$ is the Jacobian of the function $\mathcal{G}$, defined in (8) and evaluated at the steady state $\mathbf{u}_0$. The desired eigenmodes are then just the eigenvectors of this Jacobian. When discretized, this Jacobian is in general a very large sparse matrix. Fortunately, it suffices to calculate the fastest growing 100 or so eigenvectors and eigenvalues. This is accomplished through the use of the method described by Henry and Hakim.[21] This method approximates the subspace spanned by the M fastest growing eigenmodes by repeatedly integrating the perturbation equations from specially chosen initial conditions. A coordinate system is then defined for the subspace, and the eigenvector problem is then solved in this space. This calculation is fast, since the relevant matrix is only $M \times M$.

The calculation yielded four unstable alternans modes ($\text{Re}(\lambda) > 0$), as shown in Fig. 9, together with their complex conjugates (not shown). In the rotating frame, these modes had eigenfrequencies that were approximate half-integer multiples of the wave rotation angular frequency ($\pm 0.5\Omega$, $\pm 1.5\Omega$, $\pm 2.5\,\Omega$, etc.). This was to be expected: the frequencies must be approximately half-integer to re-create an alternans pattern – that is, a pattern that repeats once every two times the wave rotates. When the eigenmodes were plotted, they were found to be consistent with alternans dynamics, in that the morphology of the action potential width alternated between narrow and wide (not shown).

The best location in which to apply the control stimulus was obtained by calculating the left eigenmodes of the Jacobian, which were obtained in a manner analogous to the right eigenmodes. This location varied from one eigenmode to the next, but for most of the unstable eigenmodes, the optimal location was in the recovery region of the spiral wave, close to the center of rotation. The stimulus location was therefore chosen in this region. The canceling of the four unstable alternans eigenmodes, plus one unstable meandering mode, together with their complex conjugates, requires, in general, five separate stimuli. The optimal timing for all these stimuli is a somewhat complex calculation, which is reserved for future study. To simplify the current investigation, we elected instead to choose amplitudes for the eigenmodes that would allow simultaneous annihilation of all the unstable eigenmodes using a single stimulus. This was, admittedly a specialized case, which, nevertheless illustrated that it is possible for a single stimulus to affect alternans behavior over the very large region (relative to the space constant) typically covered by a rotating spiral wave.

References

1. Allessie MA, Bonke FIM, Schopman FJG. Circus movement in rabbit atrial muscle as a mechanism of tachycardia, III. The "leading circle" concept: a new model of circus movement in cardiac tissue without the involvement of an anatomical obstacle. *Circ Res.* 1977;41:9–18

2. Allexandre D, Otani NF. Preventing alternans-induced spiral wave breakup in cardiac tissue: An ion-channel-based approach. *Phys Rev E* 2004;70:061903

3. Barkley D. Linear stability analysis of rotating spiral waves in excitable media. *Phys Rev Lett* 1992;68(13):2090–2093

4. Beeler GW, Reuter H. Reconstruction of the action potential of ventricular myocardial fibres. *J Physiol* 1977;268(1):177–210

5. Christini DJ, Stein KM, Markowitz SM, Mittal S, Slotwiner DJ, Scheiner MA, Iwai S, Lerman BB. Nonlinear-dynamical arrhythmia control in humans. *Proc Natl Acad Sci USA* 2001;98(10):5827–5832

6. Christini DJ, Riccio ML, Culianu CA, Fox JJ, Karma A, Gilmour RF Jr. Control of electrical alternans in canine cardiac Purkinje fibers. *Phys Ref Lett* 2006;96:104101

7. Courtemanche M, Glass L, Keener JP. Instabilities of a propagating pulse in a ring of excitable media. *Phys Rev Lett* 1993;70(14):2182–2185

8. Dillon SM, Allessie MA, Ursell PC, Wit AL. Influences of anisotropic tissue structure on reentrant circuits in the epicardial border zone of subacute canine infarcts. *Circ Res* 1988;63:182–206

9. Echebarria B, Karma A. Spatiotemporal control of cardiac alternans. *Chaos* 2002;12(3):923–930

10. El-Sherif N. Reentrant mechanisms in ventricular arrhythmias. In: Zipes DP, Jalife J, eds. *Cardiac Electrophysiology: From Cell to Bedside*, 2nd edn. Philadelphia: W.B. Saunders; 1995:567–582

11. Fenton F, Karma A. Vortex dynamics in three-dimensional continuous myocardium with fiber rotation: filament instability and fibrillation. *Chaos* 1998;8(1):20–47

12. Fox JJ, McHarg JL, Gilmour RF Jr. Ionic mechanism of electrical alternans. *Am J Physiol Heart Circ Physiol* 2002;282(2):H516–H530

13. Fox JJ, Riccio ML, Hua F, Bodenschatz E, Gilmour RF Jr. Spatiotemporal transition to conduction block in canine ventricle. *Circ Res* 2002;90(3):289–296

14. Frame LH, Simson MB. Oscillations of conduction, action potential duration, and refractoriness: a mechanism for spontaneous termination of reentrant tachycardias. *Circulation* 1988;78:1277–1287

15. Garfinkel A, Spano ML, Ditto WL, Weiss JN. Controlling cardiac chaos. *Science* 1992;257:1230–1235

16. Garfinkel A, Kim YH, Voroshilovsky O, Qu ZL, Kil JR, Lee MH, Karagueuzian HS, Weiss JN, Chen PS. Preventing ventricular fibrillation by flattening cardiac restitution. *Proc Natl Acad Sci USA* 2000;97(11):6061–6066

17. Gilmour RF Jr, Otani NF, Watanabe M. Memory and complex dynamics in cardiac Purkinje fibers. *Am J Physiol* 1997;272:H1826–H1832

18. Guevara MR, Ward G, Shrier A, Glass L. Electrical alternans and period-doubling bifurcations. *IEEE Comput Cardiol* 1984;167–170

19. Hall GM, Gauthier DJ. Experimental control of cardiac muscle alternans. *Phys Rev Lett* 2002;88(19):198102

20. Hall K, Christini DJ, Tremblay M, Collins JJ, Glass L, Billette J. Dynamic control of cardiac alternans. *Phys Rev Lett* 1997;78(23):4518–4521

21. Henry H, Hakim V. Scroll waves in isotropic excitable media: linear instabilities, bifurcations, and restabilized states. *Phys Rev E* 2002;65(4):046235

22. Hua F, Gilmour RF Jr. Contribution of I_{Kr} to rate-dependent action potential dynamics in canine endocardium. *Circ Res* 2004;94:810–819

23. Hund T, Rudy Y. Rate dependence and regulation of action potential and calcium transient in a canine cardiac ventricular cell model. *Circulation* 2004;110(20):3168–3174

24. Karma A, Levine H, Zou X. Theory of pulse instabilities in electrophysiological models of excitable tissues. *Physica D* 1994;73:113–127

25. Li M, Otani NF. Ion channel basis for alternans and memory in cardiac myocytes. *Ann Biomed Eng* 2003;31(10):1213–1230

26. Li M, Otani NF. Controlling alternans in cardiac cells. *Ann Biomed Eng* 2004;32(6):784–792

27. Li M, Gilmour RF, Riccio ML, Otani NF. Controlling alternans in cardiac cells. *Comput Cardiol* 2003;30:9–12

28. Luo C-H, Rudy Y. A dynamic model of the cardiac ventricular action potential I. Simulations of ionic currents and concentration changes. *Circ Res* 1994;74:1071–1096

29. Otani NF, Gilmour RF Jr. Memory models for the electrical properties of local cardiac systems. *J Theor Biol* 1997;187(3):409–436

30. Otani NF, Li M, Gilmour RF Jr. What can nonlinear dynamics teach us about the development of ventricular tachycardia/ventricular fibrillation? *Heart Rhythm* 2005;2:1261–1263

31. Pastore JM, Girouard SD, Laurita KR, Akar FG, Rosenbaum DS. Mechanism linking t-wave alternans to the genesis of cardiac fibrillation. *Circulation* 1999;99(10):1385–1394

32. Pertsov AM, Davidenko JM, Salomonsz R, Baxter WT, Jalife J. Spiral waves of excitation underlie reentrant activity in isolated cardiac muscle. *Circ Res* 1993;72(3):631–650

33. Pruvot EJ, Katra RP, Rosenbaum DS, Laurita KR. Role of calcium cycling versus restitution in the mechanism of repolarization alternans. *Circ Res* 2004;94(8):1083–1090

34. Rappel W-J, Fenton F, Karma A. Spatiotemporal control of wave instabilities in cardiac tissue. *Phys Rev Lett* 1999;83(2):456–459

35. Riccio ML, Koller ML, Gilmour RF Jr. Electrical restitution and spatiotemporal organization during ventricular fibrillation. *Circ Res* 1999;84(8):955–963

36. Tolkacheva EG, Romeo MM, Guerraty M, Gauthier DJ. Condition for alternans and its control in a two-dimensional mapping model of paced cardiac dynamics. *Phys Rev E* 2004;69:031904
37. Watanabe M, Gilmour RF Jr. Strategy for control of complex low-dimensional dynamics in cardiac tissue. *J Math Biol* 1996;35(1):73–87
38. Weiss JN, Garfinkel A, Karagueuzian HS, Qu ZL, Chen PS. Chaos and the transition to ventricular fibrillation – a new approach to antiarrhythmic drug evaluation. *Circulation* 1999;99(21):2819–2826
39. Zeng J, Laurita KR, Rosenbaum DS, Rudy Y. Two components of the delayed rectifier K^+ current in ventricular myocytes of the guinea pig type, theoretical formulation and their role in repolarization. *Circ Res* 1995;77:140–152

Chapter 6.5

The Future of the Implantable Defibrillator

Mark W. Kroll and Charles D. Swerdlow

As successful as the implantable cardioverter-defibrillator (ICD) has been, the therapy is far from perfect. The device implantations are nontrivial and implant testing still has some morbidity and a relatively rare mortality associated with it. Partly due to the high effectiveness of ICDs, the largest morbidity associated with this therapy is psychiatric due to the pain of shocks especially – but not exclusively – due to inappropriate shocks. In spite of the dramatic positive impact on sudden death, patients with ICDs can still die from sudden death because of high defibrillation threshold fibrillation or nonshockable rhythms such as pulseless electrical activity. This chapter will discuss possibilities for addressing these therapy limitations.

Sensing and Detection

Reduction of Ventricular Oversensing

Oversensing is defined as sensing of unintended nonphysiological signals or physiological signals that do not accurately reflect local depolarization.[1] Nonphysiological signals usually arise from extracardiac electromagnetic interference. Electrical artifacts are a common cause of oversensing from leads with insulation failure or intermittent fracture resulting in "make-break" potentials. Physiological signals may be intracardiac (P, R, or T waves) or extracardiac (myopotentials). Oversensing often results in characteristic patterns of near-field (pace-sense) and far-field (shock) electrograms (EGMs).[2,3] In ICD patients, most oversensing results in detection of sufficiently rapid signals that inappropriate detection of ventricular fibrillation (VF) occurs. Oversensing accounts for approximately one third of inappropriate shocks in studies of chronic ICD systems.[4]

Charles D. Swerdlow

Division of Cardiology, Department of Medicine, Cedars-Sinai Medical Center, Los Angeles, CA, swerdlow@ucla.edu

I. R. Efimov et al. (eds.), *Cardiac Bioelectric Therapy: Mechanisms and Practical Implications.*
© Springer Science+Business Media, LLC 2009

Two strategies may permit reduction of inappropriate shocks caused by oversensing. The first relates to comparison of the sensing EGM and far-field EGMs. R waves sensed on the near-field EGM that are not present on the far-field EGM likely represent oversensing (e.g., T waves, diaphragmatic myopotentials, pace-sense lead failure).

The second requires use of digital signal processing technology to discriminate true R waves from oversensed events. For example, digital signal processing has been used successfully to discriminate far-field R waves from P waves.[5] Similar algorithms could be developed to discriminate R waves from T waves and 60 Hz electromagnetic interference, based on signal frequency content.[1]

Digital signal processing methods may also identify signals related to insulation or conductor failure in electrodes. These are the most serious causes of oversensing because a shock into a faulty electrode may achieve sufficient voltage at the heart to induce VF (if applied in the vulnerable period), but not sufficient voltage to defibrillate. An algorithm that predicts subclinical lead failures has been validated.[6–8] ICD manufacturers should design pulse generators that detect lead failures reliably and protect patients against their adverse consequences.

Active SVT-VT Discrimination

Presently, ICD algorithms that discriminate ventricular tachycardia/ventricular fibrillation (VT/VF) from supraventricular tachycardia (SVT) passively analyze information derived from a sequence of sensed atrial and ventricular EGMs, including rate, regularity, atrioventricular (AV) association and patterns, and ventricular EGM morphology. Active pacing maneuvers provide unique advantages for SVT–VT discrimination and are commonly applied in the electrophysiology lab. They were not incorporated into early detection algorithms because of concerns regarding proarrhythmia and the complexity of interpreting responses. It is now recognized that conservative burst ventricular pacing at ∼90% of the tachycardia cycle length has a low (1–2%) risk of proarrhythmia.

In addition to terminating most monomorphic VTs, burst ventricular pacing terminates more than 50% of inappropriately detected pathological SVTs with a 1:1 AV relationship.[9] During other SVTs, concealed retrograde conduction of ventricular antitachycardia pacing may slow the ventricular response by causing AV conduction delay or block. Active discrimination represents a paradigm shift in design of detection algorithms from "diagnose before intervening" to "treat first; analyze only those tachycardias that persist after treatment." In dual chamber algorithms, the principal value of active discrimination applies to tachycardias with 1:1 AV association. Atrial, ventricular, or combined atrial and ventricular pacing may be applied. The latter may be most useful.[10,11]

Hemodynamic Sensors for ICDs

Presently, ICDs do not differentiate directly between hemodynamically stable and unstable tachycardias. Historically, detection durations and therapy sequences have been programmed aggressively to minimize potential for syncope, but this results in delivery of unnecessary shocks. Implantable hemodynamic sensors integrated with the detection and therapy decision process may reduce unnecessary shocks for hemodynamically stable VT and SVT. They may also be useful to prevent inappropriate shocks in response to oversensing or to ensure appropriate shocks in rare cases of undersensing of VF. A reliable measure of hemodynamic stability would obviate the need for duration-based "safety-net" features that override SVT–VT discriminators. Presently, these programmable features deliver therapy if an arrhythmia satisfies the ventricular rate criterion for a sufficiently long duration even if discriminators indicate SVT.

Mixed venous oxygen saturation, right atrial pressure, right ventricular pressure, subcutaneous photoplethysmography, endocardial accelerometers, and impedance measurements have been proposed as methods for discrimination of hemodynamically stable versus unstable tachycardias (Fig. 1).[12–21] Subcutaneous photoplethysmography technology has been described and tested in acute and chronic animal models. These studies have found a good correlation between mean arterial pressure and photoplethysmography pulse amplitude and demonstrated the feasibility of discriminating perfusing (stable) from nonperfusing (unstable) tachycardias.[22,23] Implantable systems for ambulatory hemodynamic monitoring using right ventricular pressure and mixed venous oxygen sensors has been described.[24]

A recent prospective clinical study with right ventricle (RV) pressure monitoring using the Medtronic Chronicle B[TM] have reported the utility of the sensor for heart failure monitoring.[25] This device has the capability of recording RV pressure waveforms during tachycardias detected using rate combined with interval analysis. Episodes of recorded spontaneous VF demonstrate substantial changes in RV pressure waveforms (Fig. 2). Many factors influence the hemodynamic stability of a tachyarrhythmia. Developing reliable metrics that discriminate stable versus unstable tachyarrhythmias for integration into ICD algorithms remains a major challenge.

Implant Testing

For 25 years the accepted method for ICD implantation has included induction of VF to ensure that the ICD will sense, detect, and defibrillate VF. Occasionally, it causes complications, and rarely it causes death. In the early era of less efficient ICDs, the value of defibrillation testing seemed self-evident. Today, better understanding of defibrillation, improved technology, and use of ICDs for primary prevention of VT or VF have led some to question the need for either defibrillation testing or any assessment of defibrillation efficacy at ICD implantation.[26,27]

The goal of implant testing is to determine the optimal balance between implant safety and long-term benefits of ICD therapy. Experts consider testing less critical for left pectoral ICDs than they did 10 years ago. Sensing of VF is reliable if the R wave $\geq$5–7 mV.[28–32] ICD generator failures are rare. Defibrillation is judged adequate by commonly used safety margin implant criteria in ~95% of patients. Low programmed first shock strength (intended to minimize risk of syncope) is less important because the incidence of spontaneous VT/VF

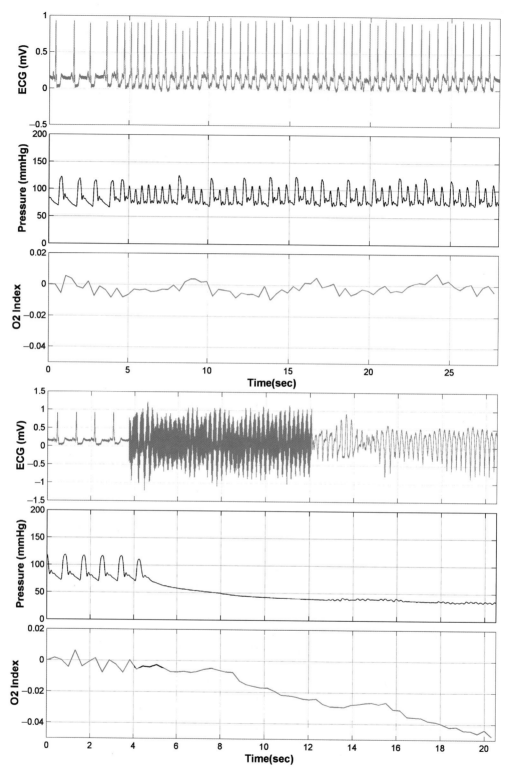

Figure 1: (*Continued*)

is lower, antitachycardia pacing terminates most episodes of rapid VT, and charge times are faster in most ICDs.

Conventional testing probably rejects less than 3–5% of prophylactic ICD patients correctly (true negative).[33] Rigorous testing increases the fraction of true negative test results, but also increases implant complexity and risk. But most implanters, patients, and families have near zero tolerance for sudden cardiac death caused by preventable, failed defibrillation. Experts disagree about optimal implant testing because data are insufficient to define the optimal trade-off between accuracy and risk. Implant testing is in a state of evolution. The major trend is away from rigorous defibrillation threshold (DFT) testing and toward limited safety margin testing or no testing. A minor trend is toward substitution of vulnerability testing based on the upper limit of vulnerability (ULV) for defibrillation testing. Implantation of ICDs without testing of defibrillation efficacy has been proposed but is not an accepted standard.

Vulnerability Testing

The ULV Hypothesis of Defibrillation

The ULV is the weakest shock strength at or above which VF is not induced when the shock is delivered during the vulnerable period. The ULV hypothesis of defibrillation[34–38] postulates both that local vulnerable periods exist during VF and that the ULV in VF is (approximately) equal to the ULV in normal rhythm. It proposes that successful defibrillation must fulfill two sequential requirements: First the shock must interrupt all VF wavefronts. Then it must not reinitiate VF. The ULV hypothesis also requires that the ULV during VF exceeds the shock strength required to stop all VF wavefronts.

According to the ULV hypothesis, a shock always defibrillates if it terminates all VF wavefronts and prevents reinitiation of VF. The latter requirement implicitly includes both spatial and temporal components: The shock must not reinitiate VF even if the spatial region of weakest field strength (lowest voltage gradient) is temporally coincident with the local vulnerable period. The minimum required shock strength is the ULV during VF. The response to a shock that stops all wavefronts but is weaker than the ULV varies depending

---

Figure 1: Investigational photoplethysmography sensor. Recordings are made from an investigational sensor during electrophysiology laboratory testing. The sensor is mounted on the housing of an ICD emulator and placed in the pocket during implant testing. Each panel shows surface ECG (upper tracing), arterial pressure (middle tracing), and photoplethysmographic oxygen (O_2) index of tissue perfusion (lower tracing). The first panel shows the onset of atrial pacing at cycle length 400 ms. The arterial pressure remains stable, and the O_2 index retains its phasic component with a mean value near the baseline normalized value of zero. The second panel shows the onset of VF induced by 50 Hz current. With the onset of 50 Hz stimulation, the arterial pressure drops abruptly and the O_2 index loses its phasic component. About two seconds later, the O_2 index begins a steep monotonic decline

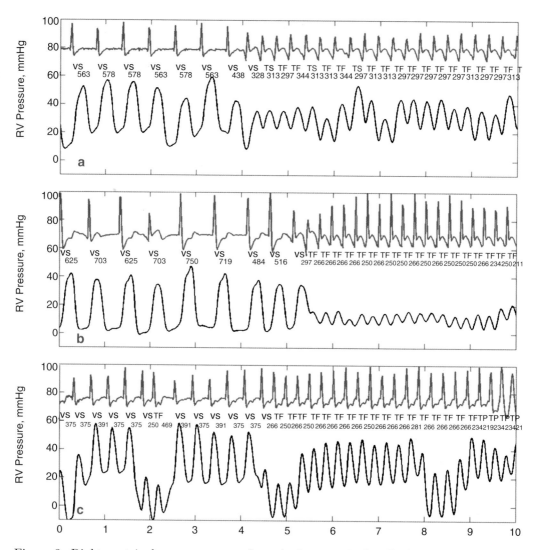

Figure 2: Right ventricular pressure waveform during ventricular fibrillation. Stored EGM and pressure tracing from investigational ICD with hemodynamic sensor (Medtronic "Chronicle ICD"). In each panel, the upper tracing shows the shock electrogram recorded between the right ventricular (RV) coil and left pectoral ICD housing. The marker channel below it shows the interval classification and interval duration in milliseconds. The lower tracing shows RV pressure recorded from the implanted hemodynamic sensor in millimeters of mercury. Horizontal axis shows time in seconds. Intervals are labeled VS (sinus zone), TS (VT zone), TF (Fast VT zone). (a) Onset of VT at cycle length 300 ms. The patient was asymptomatic prior to antitachycardia pacing. RV systolic pressure falls by less than half. (b) Onset of VT at cycle length 250 ms. The patient presented with syncope. RV systolic pressure drops abruptly and remains below a third of the baseline value. (c) Rapidly conducted atrial fibrillation at cycle length 260 ms. Inappropriate antitachycardia pacing (TP markers) occurs for the last four beats. There is only a slight reduction in RV systolic pressure at shorter cycle lengths. The patient had no alteration of consciousness. Tracings provided by Dr. Michael Sweeney

on the unpredictable fibrillatory pattern of preshock activation and repolarization in the region of weakest field strength. If the shock occurs in the local vulnerable period, it reinitiates VF and is unsuccessful. Otherwise it terminates VF and is successful. Thus the ULV hypothesis predicts that defibrillation will be probabilistic on a macroscopic level. The ULV hypothesis of defibrillation does not depend on a specific cellular or tissue mechanism for defibrillation, but rather on a class of possible mechanisms that result in shock-initiated refibrillation.

The ULV and Vulnerability Safety Margin

The ULV–DFT correlation has been validated in multiple animal[34,39,40] and human studies.[41–46] It remains strong and invariant, within experimental error, over a wide range of conditions.[47] Clinically, vulnerability testing can be applied to either a patient-specific strategy (which requires initiation of one VF episode) or to a safety margin strategy. The latter strategy has attracted interest because it permits assessment of defibrillation efficacy without inducing VF in 75–90% of ICD recipients[31,48,49] It has been validated in a large, prospective multicenter study.[32]

Clinical vulnerability safety margin testing has been reviewed for details.[47] Briefly, T-wave shocks are delivered at several coupling intervals to ensure that the most vulnerable part of the cardiac cycle is scanned.[50] If VF is not induced, the shock strength exceeds the ULV, which approximates the shock strength associated with a 90% probability of defibrillation (E_{90}).[51] Because the ULV is more reproducible than the DFT, determination of the ULV (which requires one induction of VF) provides greater statistical power for clinical research with fewer episodes of VF.[52,53]

Limitations of vulnerability testing. Vulnerability testing reduces those risks of implant testing related to VF or circulatory arrest, cerebral hypoperfusion,[54–57] and post-VF fatal electromechanical dissociation. There is a higher probability of significant hypotension after a single fibrillation-defibrillation episode than after three T-wave shocks that do not induce VF (8% vs. 2%, $p=.006$).[58] However, the vulnerability method does not reduce risks caused by shocks alone. Both defibrillation and vulnerability testing can cardiovert atrial fibrillation, resulting in thromboembolism. The principal limitations of vulnerability testing are that (1) it requires general anesthesia or deep sedation for 3–4 min, (2) VF is induced in 5–25% of patients, depending on the safety margin required,[59] and (3) it does not assess sensing of VF. However, sensing of VF is reliable if the baseline R wave exceeds 5–7 mV.[28–32]

State of the Art

Evidence-Based Implant Testing

VF should be induced to assess sensing in ~5% of ICD recipients. Defibrillation or vulnerability testing is indicated in 20–40% of recipients who can be identified as having a higher than usual probability of an inadequate defibrillation safety margin based on patient-specific factors. At least one high output shock should usually be delivered at the time of generator replacement to identify lead failure modes that cannot be identified with

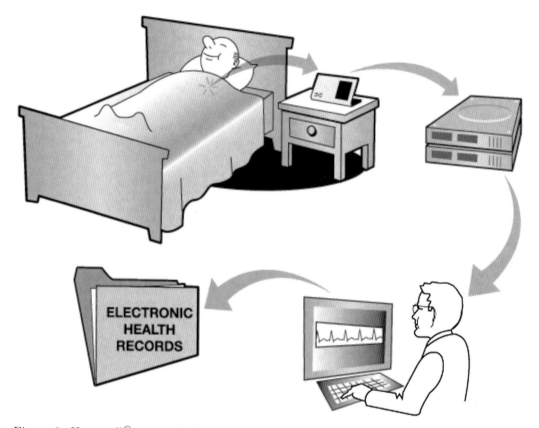

Figure 3: Housecall® remote follow-up system. The newest remote follow-up system communicates with an RF link to the patient's ICD. Gathered data are then automatically transmitted over a phone line to a database for analysis by trained professionals and stored in the clinic's electronic health records

low-output pulses.[60] On the other hand, implant testing is too risky in ~5% of ICD recipients and may not be worth the risks in 10–30% more. In 25–50% of ICD recipients, implant testing cannot presently be identified as either critical or contraindicated.[33] Prospective data are needed to address this important clinical issue. Introduction of ICDs with subcutaneous electrodes will further increase the need for objective data, as these ICDs lack an efficient method for inducing VF.

Legal, regulatory, and training considerations. Assessing defibrillation efficacy at implantation of ICDs is now the legal standard of practice. Labeling on all U.S. manufactured ICDs recommends assessment of defibrillation efficacy at implant and programming the first VF shock with a 10 J safety margin. The Heart Rhythm Society also recommends implant defibrillation testing.[61]

Training requirements for ICD implantation attract great interest because they may substantively affect whether, in the future, ICDs are implanted primarily by electrophysiologists with extensive training in defibrillation testing or primarily by cardiologists with limited or no training in defibrillation testing. Thus training requirements may have a substantial influence on the number and qualifications of implanters. To the extent that more implanters results in more implants, training requirements may impact sales of ICDs. And to the extent that methods of implant testing (or no testing) influence training requirements, there is an implicit link between implant testing, who implants ICDs, and the economics of the medical device industry.[62]

After the Implant

A wireless remote patient monitoring system significantly lowers the follow-up burden on the patient and physician. The system enables a physician to quickly evaluate and communicate with an ICD patient, even if the two are thousands of miles apart. Programmable alerts allow the physician to be notified quickly over the telephone or internet in the event of a issue that requires medical attention. The transtelephonic ICD follow-up provided by the Merlin.net[TM] internet-based remote monitoring system (Fig. 3) appears to be more comprehensive, less intrusive, and more desirable than routine follow-up visits. Patients consider this follow-up more than acceptable and indicated high degrees of satisfaction with the convenience, ease of use, and reliability of transtelephonic monitoring. All ICD manufacturers now offer some type of remote follow-up system. Impedances, R-wave amplitudes, and battery levels can be easily monitored. Obviously, DFTs are not checked, but those are almost never checked in clinic visits anyway.

Novel Waveform Strategies

The conventional clinical wisdom is that the introduction of the biphasic waveform in 1990 was the ultimate triumph of defibrillation waveform research. However, recent work has demonstrated the potential of novel waveforms to significantly reduce the DFT even further, reduce shock pain, and even to possibly treat pulseless electrical activity.

Defibrillation Threshold Reduction

The single-capacitor, biphasic direct discharge waveform has been optimized sufficiently that further reductions in DFT will likely require major changes in defibrillation waveforms. The predicted optimal monophasic waveform for delivered energy is an ascending waveform beginning at a nonzero fraction of the peak voltage. An ascending ramp beginning at zero volts is not optimal as it wastes some energy at the lowest voltages without substantially charging the cell membranes. Nevertheless, such a waveform has been demonstrated to improve defibrillation in comparison with an efficient, clinically used waveform.[63] This type of waveform can be achieved by adding a high-frequency chopping circuit with a smoothing inductor to the shock output circuit. It is not yet known if the inefficiency incurred by

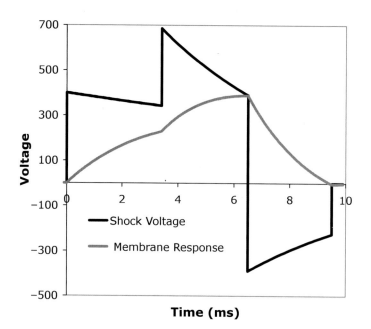

Figure 4: Stepped waveform and predicted membrane response. The stepped waveform (black tracing) has two positive phases that more efficiently charge the cardiac myocyte membranes. The predicted membrane response is shown in the gray tracing. The first step is formed by partially discharging two capacitors in parallel followed by the second step with the capacitors in series. The negative phase is conventional

the circuitry required to generate this waveform justifies the improvement in defibrillation efficacy.

However, the predicted optimal ascending waveform for delivered energy can be approximated by a three-part "stepped" waveform using only capacitors in parallel and series: The first portion is positive with two capacitors in parallel, the second is positive with the capacitors in series, and the last portion is negative, also with the capacitors in series. Such a waveform is shown in a recent study that reported a 40% reduction in DFT for a stepped waveform in comparison with an efficient, clinically used waveform when used with lower impedance lead systems (Fig. 4).[64]

Another possibility for lowering the DFT is the use of a left-sided auxiliary pulse.[65,66] The possibility of combining auxiliary pulses and the stepped waveform have yet been investigated. However, the probability of the DFT being cut by 50% from present levels is high. This could allow very small devices of 15 J output to compete with the present "lower" energy 30 J devices. Perhaps more exciting is the possibility of an ICD with the present 35 J "high energy" output having the equivalent of a 70 J performance. This could essentially eliminate the high DFT problem patients and make it far easier to rationalize implants with no threshold testing.

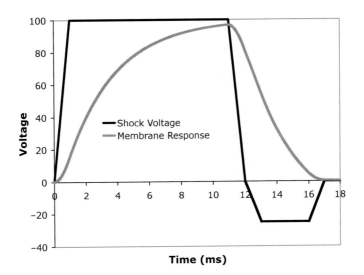

Figure 5: Plateau waveform for pain reduction. The plateau waveform (black tracing) reduces pain by significantly lowering the peak voltage. The efficient membrane response (gray tracing) also correctly predicts low defibrillation thresholds

Cardioversion Pain Reduction

It appears that the pain of a defibrillation shock could be significantly reduced. This would be beneficial for making atrial cardioversion more acceptable, thus reducing the false shocks delivered to the ventricle. But, besides that, the actual ventricular-delivered shock could be made much more tolerable. Shock pain appears to be primarily (but not exclusively) due to the peak voltage of the shock.[67] This inspired the testing of a "plateau" or flat-topped waveform, which has been shown to increase the energy tolerance by a factor of nearly 4:1, at least in low-energy shocks.[68] The plateau waveforms are predicted to have low DFTs based on their modeled membrane response, as seen in Fig. 5. These energy efficiency predictions have been confirmed for cardioversion whether performed externally[69–71] or internally.[72–74]

The prepulse inhibition approach appears to offer a significant opportunity for pain reduction.[75,76] For a gross oversimplification one can state that the human pain detection system has a refractory period of approximately 100 ms. Thus, a small, noticeable but tolerable, shock delivered 100 ms before the main shock will significantly reduce pain. This is obviously a very tempting approach to combine with the plateau waveforms for overall pain reduction. Such a combination has not yet been clinically evaluated. Were such a combination to work synergistically, one could predict a pain threshold shift of approximately an order of magnitude. Thus a patient who would tolerate a 2 J (conventional waveform) shock for cardioversion might be willing to tolerate a 20 J shock. More modestly, a patient might have the toleration limit moved from 1 up to 10 J.

Medium Voltage Therapy

The use of voltages between those for pacing therapy and defibrillation therapy is relatively unexplored. These "medium" voltages are in the range of 20–200 V and are delivered between large electrodes such as the RV coil and the can. Such voltages, along with fairly complex long waveforms, have been demonstrated to give cardiac output even in the presence of VF.[77,78] Although the relative contribution of the contractions of the skeletal muscles and of the cardiac myocytes has not been well delineated, it does appear that this could allow patients to survive temporarily without defibrillation. This presents an opportunity for a prophylactic "super pacemaker" as well as methods for maintaining cardiac output in the presence of a "nonshockable" rhythm such as asystole.

The use of medium voltage therapy has also demonstrated, in an animal model, the ability to convert pulseless electrical activity into sinus rhythm.[79] Thus medium voltage therapy presents a tantalizing, if minimally demonstrated, approach to rhythms presently considered untreatable.

Novel Packaging Strategies

Reducing device-related morbidity and simplifying the implant procedure as well as patient follow-up have been and remain the major goals of ICD therapy. Two novel designs are currently being investigated that may aid in achieving these goals. The first utilizes a subcutaneous approach without transvenous electrodes. The second device is implanted percutaneously and the entire system resides in the vasculature. Ironically, both have at least a portion of the generator located in the abdomen. The irony of these novel approaches is that one eschews the veins while the other is purely venous, including the generator.

Subcutaneous ICDs

Much of the morbidity associated with the present ICD systems is related to the presence of transvenous defibrillation and sensing leads. An ICD that uses sensing and shock electrodes only in the subcutaneous (or submuscular) tissue would eliminate specific problems associated with transvenous leads. Further, such an ICD might be implanted without fluoroscopy in any surgical suite, thus simplifying the implant procedure. Early studies indicate that defibrillation can be achieved in pediatric patients[80–83] and the majority of adults[84,85] using subcutaneous electrodes with shock strengths that are in the range of present technology. To date, this has been achieved by using high-capacitance waveforms with maximum voltages near 800 V, although higher voltage/lower capacitance waveforms would likely be more efficient for high-resistance defibrillation pathways. Subcutaneous ICDs must rely on subcutaneous EGMs for sensing and detection of VF. In one version, correlation waveform analysis, using two different channels of subcutaneous EGMs, is used to detect fast VT/VF and avoid inappropriate detection of myopotential noise and electromagnetic interference.[86] There are no published data on sensing and detection performance of algorithms in subcutaneous ICDs under investigation, but there is a substantial literature on subcutaneous EGMs based on implantable loop recorders.[87,88]

It is too early to know what fraction of patients will be defibrillated reliably by subcutaneous ICDs or how well long-term sensing and detection will perform using subcutaneous electrodes. Such ICDs also have important inherent limitations: They cannot perform bradycardia pacing or antitachycardia pacing. In contrast to transvenous ICD, which treat more than 70% of ventricular tachyarrhythmias with painless pacing, all therapies for subcutaneous ICDs are shocks. The reliability with which VF can be induced to test defibrillation efficacy is unknown. If induction of VF requires a temporary transvenous electrode, fluoroscopy will be required for the implant.

Percutaneous, Fully Transvenous ICD

One new company has engineered an ICD that leverages familiar percutaneous interventional techniques for a time-efficient implant of this catheter-like device. The ICD is a series of thin titanium cylinders, each containing either batteries, capacitors, or circuitry, all connected by flexible couplers allowing low-impact maneuvering of anatomical angles. Positioned within the vena cava and anchored distally, the ICD also utilizes a fully integrated RV ICD lead. Early testing indicates efficient defibrillation and reliable sensing through both conventional and novel vectors. Advantages of this device in addition to the implant simplicity include that it is invisible to the patient, leaves no scar, has safety pacing and ATP capabilities, simplified follow-up capabilities tuned to the needs of the primary prevention patient, and, due to the modular design, can be readily iterated to a broader cardiac rhythm management platform.

Conclusion

Implantable defibrillator technology has achieved major successes in the therapy of patients with ventricular arrhythmias. However, major challenges with psychiatric morbidity, implant complications, and residual mortality remain to be conquered. With newer technologies on the horizon, we are confident that many of these challenges will be met.

References

1. Swerdlow C, Gillberg J, Olson W. Sensing and detection. In: Ellenbogen K, Kay G, Lau C, Willkoff B, eds. *Clinical Cardiac Pacing, Defibrillation, and Resynchronization Therapy.* Philadelphia: Saunders; 2007:75–160
2. Gunderson B, Patel A, Bounds C. Automatic identification of implantable cardioverter-defibrillator lead problems using intracardiac electrograms. *Comput Cardiol* 2002;29:121–124

3. Swerdlow C, Shivkumar K. Implantable cardioverter defibrillators: clinical aspects. In: Zipes DP, Jalife J, eds. *Cardiac Electrophysiology: From Cell to Bedside*. Philadelphia: W.B. Saunders; 2004:980–993

4. Poole J, Johnson G, Callans D, Raitt M, Yee R, Reddy R, Wilber D, Guarnieri T, Talajic M, Marchlinski F, Lee K, Bardy G, SCD-HeFT Investigators. Analysis of implantable defibrillator shock electrograms in the Sudden Cardiac Death-Heart Failure Trial. *Heart Rhythm* 2004;1:S178 (abstract)

5. Theres H, Sun W, Combs W, Panken E, Mead H, Baumann G, Stangl K. P wave and far-field R wave detection in pacemaker patient atrial electrograms. *Pacing Clin Electrophysiol* 2000;23:434–440

6. Gunderson BD, Gillberg JM, Wood MA, Vijayaraman P, Shepard RK, Ellenbogen KA. Development and testing of an algorithm to detect implantable cardioverter-defibrillator lead failure. *Heart Rhythm* 2006;3:155–162

7. Gunderson BD, Patel AS, Bounds CA, Ellenbogen KA. Automatic identification of clinical lead dysfunctions. *Pacing Clin Electrophysiol* 2005;28(Suppl 1):S63–S67

8. Gunderson BD, Patel AS, Bounds CA, Shepard RK, Wood MA, Ellenbogen KA. An algorithm to predict implantable cardioverter-defibrillator lead failure. *J Am Coll Cardiol* 2004;44:1898–1902

9. Wathen MS, Volosin KJ, Sweeney MO, Khalighi K, Canby RC, Machado C, Adkisson WO, Rubenstein DS, Otterness MF, Stark AJ, Gillberg JM, DeGroot PJ. Ventricular antitachycardia pacing by implantable cardioverter defibrillators reduces shocks for inappropriately detected supraventricular tachycardia. *Heart Rhythm* 2004;1 (abstract)

10. Ridley DP, Gula LJ, Krahn AD, Skanes AC, Yee R, Brown ML, Olson WH, Gillberg JM, Klein GJ. Atrial response to ventricular antitachycardia pacing discriminates mechanism of 1:1 atrioventricular tachycardia. *J Cardiovasc Electrophysiol* 2005;16:601–605

11. Saba S, Baker L, Ganz L, Barrington W, Jain S, Ngwu O, Christensen J, Brown M. Simultaneous atrial and ventricular anti-tachycardia pacing as a novel method of rhythm discrimination. *J Cardiovasc Electrophysiol* 2006;17:695–701

12. Bordachar P, Garrigue S, Reuter S, Hocini M, Kobeissi A, Gaggini G, Jais P, Haissaguerre M, Clementy J. Hemodynamic assessment of right, left, and biventricular pacing by peak endocardial acceleration and echocardiography in patients with end-stage heart failure. *Pacing Clin Electrophysiol* 2000;23:1726–1730

13. Hegbom F, Hoff PI, Oie B, Folling M, Zeijlemaker V, Lindemans F, Ohm OJ. RV function in stable and unstable VT: is there a need for hemodynamic monitoring in future defibrillators? *Pacing Clin Electrophysiol* 2001;24:172–182

14. Kaye G, Astridge P, Perrins J. Tachycardia recognition and diagnosis from changes in right atrial pressure waveform – a feasibility study. *Pacing Clin Electrophysiol* 1991;14:1384–1392

15. Khoury D, McAlister H, Wilkoff B, Simmons T, Rudy Y, McCowan R, Morant V, Castle L, Maloney J. Continuous right ventricular volume assessment by catheter measurement of impedance for antitachycardia system control. *Pacing Clin Electrophysiol* 1989;12:1918–1926

16. Sharma AD, Bennett TD, Erickson M, Klein GJ, Yee R, Guiraudon G. Right ventricular pressure during ventricular arrhythmias in humans: potential implications for implantable antitachycardia devices. *J Am Coll Cardiol* 1990;15:648–655

17. Wood M, Ellenbogen KA, Lu B, Valenta H. A prospective study of right ventricular pulse pressure and dP/dt to discriminant-induced ventricular tachycardia from supraventricular and sinus tachycardia in man. *Pacing Clin Electrophysiol* 1990;13:1148–1157

18. Ellenbogen KA, Lu B, Kapadia K, Wood M, Valenta H. Usefulness of right ventricular pulse pressure as a potential sensor for hemodynamically unstable ventricular tachycardia. *Am J Cardiol* 1990;65:1105–1111

19. Ellenbogen KA, Wood MA, Kapadia K, Lu B, Valenta H. Short-term reproducibility over time of right ventricular pulse pressure as a potential hemodynamic sensor for ventricular tachyarrhythmias. *Pacing Clin Electrophysiol* 1992;15:971–974

20. Plicchi G, Marcelli E, Marini S. An endocardial acceleration sensor for sustained ventricular tachycardia detection. *Europace Suppl* 2002;3:96 (abstract)

21. Whitman T, Sheldon T, McFadden S. Endocardial acceleration measurements in tachycardia induced heart failure in canines. *Pacing Clin Electrophysiol* 2002;24:569 (abstract)

22. Nabutovsky Y, Bjorling A, Ghaffari-Farazi T, Noren K, Bornzin G. A novel algorithm for VF detection from subcutaneously implanted leads. *Heart Rhythm.* 2005 (abstract);2:S124–S125

23. Turcott R, Pavek T. Detection of hemodynamically unstable arrhythmias using subcutaneous photoplethysmography. *Heart Rhythm* 2005;2:S83 (abstract)

24. Bennett T, Kjellstrom B, Taepke R, Ryden L. Development of implantable devices for continuous ambulatory monitoring of central hemodynamic values in heart failure patients. *Pacing Clin Electrophysiol* 2005;28:573–584

25. Cleland JG, Coletta AP, Freemantle N, Velavan P, Tin L, Clark AL. Clinical trials update from the American College of Cardiology meeting: CARE-HF and the Remission of Heart Failure, Women's Health Study, TNT, COMPASS-HF, VERITAS, CANPAP, PEECH and PREMIER. *Eur J Heart Fail* 2005;7:931–936

26. Strickberger SA, Klein GJ. Is defibrillation testing required for defibrillator implantation? *J Am Coll Cardiol* 2004;44:88–91

27. Neuzner J. Is DFT testing still mandatory? *Herz* 2005;30:601

28. Ellenbogen KA, Wood MA, Stambler BS, Welch WJ, Damiano RJ. Measurement of ventricular electrogram amplitude during intraoperative induction of ventricular tachyarrhythmias. *Am J Cardiol* 1992;70:1017–1022

29. Glikson M, Luria D, Friedman PA, Trusty JM, Benderly M, Hammill SC, Stanton MS. Are routine arrhythmia inductions necessary in patients with pectoral implantable cardioverter defibrillators? *J Cardiovasc Electrophysiol* 2000;11:127–135

30. Panotopoulos P, Krum D, Axtell K, Dhala A, Sra J, Akhtar M, Deshpande S. Ventricular fibrillation sensing and detection by implantable defibrillators: is one better than the others? A prospective, comparative study. *J Cardiovasc Electrophysiol* 2001;12:445–452

31. Swerdlow CD. Implantation of cardioverter defibrillators without induction of ventricular fibrillation. *Circulation* 2001;103:2159–2164

32. Day JD, Doshi RN, Belott P, Birgersdotter-Green U, Behboodikhah M, Ott P, Glatter KA, Tobias S, Frumin H, Lee BK, Merillat J, Wiener I, Wang S, Grogin H, Chun S, Patrawalla R, Crandall B, Osborn JS, Weiss JP, Lappe DL, Neuman S. Inductionless or limited shock testing is possible in most patients with implantable cardioverter-defibrillators/cardiac resynchronization therapy defibrillators: results of the multicenter ASSURE Study (Arrhythmia Single Shock Defibrillation Threshold Testing Versus Upper Limit of Vulnerability: Risk Reduction Evaluation With Implantable Cardioverter-Defibrillator Implantations). *Circulation* 2007;115:2382–2389

33. Swerdlow CD, Russo AM, Degroot PJ. The dilemma of ICD implant testing. *Pacing Clin Electrophysiol* 2007;30:675–700

34. Chen P-S, Shibata N, Dixon E, Martin R, Ideker R. Comparison of the defibrillation threshold and the upper limit of ventricular vulnerability. *Circulation* 1986;73:1022–1028

35. Chen P-S, Shibata N, Dixon EG, Wolf PD, Danleley ND, Sweeney MB, Smith WM, Ideker RE. Activation during ventricular defibrillation in open-chest dogs. *J Clin Invest* 1986;77:810–823

36. Chen P-S, Shibata N, Wolf P, Dixon EG, Danieley ND, Sweeney MB, Smith WM, Ideker RE. Epicardial activation during successful and unsuccessful ventricular defibrillation in open chest dogs. *Cardiovasc Rev Rep* 1986;7:625–648

37. Chen P-S, Wolf PD, Ideker RE. The mechanism of cardiac defibrillation: a different point of view. *Circulation* 1991;84:913–919

38. Chen P-S, Wolf PD, Melnick SD, Danieley ND, Smith WM, Ideker RE. Comparison of activation during ventricular fibrillation and following unsuccessful defibrillation shocks in open chest dogs. *Circ Res* 1990;66:1544–1560

39. Fabritz CL, Kirchhof PF, Behrens S, Zabel M, Franz MR. Myocardial vulnerability to T wave shocks: relation to shock strength, shock coupling interval, and dispersion of ventricular repolarization. *J Cardiovasc Electrophysiol* 1996;7:231–242

40. Malkin R, Idriss S, Walker R, Ideker R. Effect of rapid pacing and T-wave scanning on the relation between the defibrillation and upper-limit-of-vulnerability dose-response curves. *Circulation* 1995;92:1291–1299

41. Bessho R, Tanaka S. Measurement of the upper limit of vulnerability during defibrillator implantation can substitute defibrillation threshold measurement. *Int J Artif Organs* 1998;21:151–160

42. Birgersdotter-Green U, Undesser K, Fujimura O, Feld GK, Kass RM, Mandel WJ, Peter CT, Chen PS. Correlation of acute and chronic defibrillation threshold with upper limit of vulnerability determined in normal sinus rhythm. *J Interv Card Electrophysiol* 1999;3:155–161

43. Chen PS, Feld GK, Kriett JM, Mower MM, Tarazi RY, Fleck RP, Swerdlow CD, Gang ES, Kass RM. Relation between upper limit of vulnerability and defibrillation threshold in humans. *Circulation* 1993;88:186–192

44. Hui RC, Rosenthal L, Ramza B, Nsah E, Lawrence J, Tomaselli G, Berger R, Calkins H. Relationship between the upper limit of vulnerability determined in normal sinus rhythm

and the defibrillation threshold in patients with implantable cardioverter defibrillators. *Pacing Clin Electrophysiol* 1998;21:687–693

45. Hwang C, Swerdlow CD, Kass RM, Gang ES, Mandel WJ, Peter CT, Chen PS. Upper limit of vulnerability reliably predicts the defibrillation threshold in humans. *Circulation* 1994;90:2308–2314

46. Kirilmaz A, Dokumaci B, Uzun M, Kilicaslan F, Dinckal MH, Yucel O, Karaca M. Detection of the defibrillation threshold using the upper limit of vulnerability following defibrillator implantation. *Pacing Clin Electrophysiol* 2005;28:498–505

47. Swerdlow C, Shehata M, Chen P. Using the upper limit of vulnerability to assess defibrillation efficacy at implantation of ICDs. *Pacing Clin Electrophysiol* 2007;30:258–270

48. Day J, Doshi R, Belott P, Birgersdotter-Green U, Behboodikhah M, Ott P, Glatter K, Lee B, Frumin H, Crandall B, Osborn J, Weiss J, Lappe J, Valderrabano M, Urratio C, McGuire M, Hahn S. Most patients may safely undergo inductionless or limited shock testing at ICD implantation. *Heart Rhythm* 2005;2:S232 (abstract)

49. Swerdlow C, Shivkumar K, Zhang J. Determination of the upper limit of vulnerability using implantable cardioverter-defibrillator electrograms. *Circulation* 2003;107:3028–3033

50. Swerdlow C, Martin D, Kass R, Davie S, Mandel W, Gang E, Chen P. The zone of vulnerability to T-wave shocks in humans. *J Cardiovasc Electrophysiol* 1997;8:145–154

51. Swerdlow C, Ahern T, Kass R, Davie S, Mandel W, Chen P-S. Upper limit of vulnerability is a good estimator of shock strength associated with 90% probability of successful defibrillation in humans with transvenous implantable cardioverter defibrillators. *J Am Coll Cardiol* 1996;27:1112–1117

52. Swerdlow C, Ahern T, Chen P-S. Comparative reproducibility of defibrillation threshold and upper limit of vulnerability. *Pacing Clin Electrophysiol* 1996;19:2103–2111

53. Swerdlow CD, Kass RM, O'Connor ME, Chen PS. Effect of shock waveform on relationship between upper limit of vulnerability and defibrillation threshold. *J Cardiovasc Electrophysiol* 1998;9:339–349

54. Singer I, Edmonds H Jr. Changes in cerebral perfusion during third-generation implantable cardioverter defibrillator testing. *Am Heart J* 1994;127:1052–1057

55. Singer I, Lang D. Defibrillation threshold: clinical utility and therapeutic implications. *Pacing Clin Electrophysiol* 1992;15:932–949

56. de Vries JW, Bakker PF, Visser GH, Diephuis JC, van Huffelen AC. Changes in cerebral oxygen uptake and cerebral electrical activity during defibrillation threshold testing. *Anesth Analg* 1998;87:16–20

57. Vriens EM, Bakker PF, Vries JW, Wieneke GH, Van Huffelen AC. The impact of repeated short episodes of circulatory arrest on cerebral function. Reassuring electroencephalographic (EEG) findings during defibrillation threshold testing at defibrillator implantation. *Electroencephalogr Clin Neurophysiol* 1996;98:236–242

58. Day JD, Doshi RN, Belott P, Birgersdotter-Green U, Behboodikhah M, Ott P, Glatter KA, Tobias S, Frumin H, Lee BK, Merillat J, Wiener I, Wang S, Grogin H, Chun S, Patrawalla R, Crandall B, Osborn JS, Weiss JP, Lappe DL, Neuman S. Inductionless

or limited shock testing is possible in most patients with implantable cardioverter-defibrillators/cardiac resynchronization therapy defibrillators: results of the multicenter ASSURE Study (Arrhythmia Single Shock Defibrillation Threshold Testing Versus Upper Limit of Vulnerability: Risk Reduction Evaluation With Implantable Cardioverter-Defibrillator Implantations). *Circulation.* 2007;115(18):2382–2389.

59. Swerdlow CD, Shehata M, Chen PS. Using the upper limit of vulnerability to assess defibrillation efficacy at implantation of ICDs. *Pacing Clin Electrophysiol* 2007;30:258–270

60. Ellenbogen KA, Wood MA, Shepard RK, Clemo HF, Vaughn T, Holloman K, Dow M, Leffler J, Abeyratne A, Verness D. Detection and management of an implantable cardioverter defibrillator lead failure: incidence and clinical implications. *J Am Coll Cardiol* 2003;41:73–80

61. Curtis AB, Ellenbogen KA, Hammill SC, Hayes DL, Reynolds DW, Wilber DJ, Cain ME. Clinical competency statement: training pathways for implantation of cardioverter defibrillators and cardiac resynchronization devices. *Heart Rhythm* 2004;1:371–375

62. Swerdlow CD. Reappraisal of implant testing of implantable cardioverter defibrillators. *J Am Coll Cardiol* 2004;44:92–94

63. Shorofsky SR, Rashba E, Havel W, Belk P, Degroot P, Swerdlow C, Gold MR. Improved defibrillation efficacy with an ascending ramp waveform in humans. *Heart Rhythm* 2005;2:388–394

64. Seidl K, Denman R, Moulder J, Mouchawar G, Stoeppler C, Becker T, Weise U, Anskey J, Burnett H, Kroll W. Stepped defibrillation waveform is substantially more efficient than the 50/50% tilt biphasic. *Heart Rhythm* 2006;3:1406–1411

65. Kenknight BH, Walker RG, Ideker RE. Marked reduction of ventricular defibrillation threshold by application of an auxiliary shock to a catheter electrode in the left posterior coronary vein of dogs. *J Cardiovasc Electrophysiol* 2000;11:900–906

66. Walker RG, Kenknight BH, Ideker RE. Critically timed auxiliary shock to weak field area lowers defibrillation threshold. *J Cardiovasc Electrophysiol* 2001;12:556–562

67. Boriani G, Biffi M, Silvestri P, Martignani C, Valzania C, Diemberger I, Moulder C, Mouchawar G, Kroll M, Branzi A. Mechanisms of pain associated with internal defibrillation shocks: results of a randomized study of shock waveform. *Heart Rhythm* 2005;2:708–713

68. Boriani G, Kroll M, Biffi M, Silvestri P, Martignani C, Valzania C, Diemberger I, Moulder C, Mouchawar G, Branzi A. Plateau waveform shape allows a higher patient shock energy tolerance. *Heart Rhythm* 2006;3:S13

69. Niebauer MJ, Chung MK, Brewer JE, Tchou PJ. Reduced cardioversion thresholds for atrial fibrillation and flutter using the rectilinear biphasic waveform. *J Interv Card Electrophysiol* 2005;13:145–150

70. Niebauer MJ, Brewer JE, Chung MK, Tchou PJ. Comparison of the rectilinear biphasic waveform with the monophasic damped sine waveform for external cardioversion of atrial fibrillation and flutter. *Am J Cardiol* 2004;93:1495–1499

71. Mittal S, Ayati S, Stein KM, Schwartzman D, Cavlovich D, Tchou PJ, Markowitz SM, Slotwiner DJ, Scheiner MA, Lerman BB. Transthoracic cardioversion of atrial

fibrillation: comparison of rectilinear biphasic versus damped sine wave monophasic shocks. *Circulation* 2000;101:1282–1287

72. Manoharan G, Evans N, Allen D, Anderson J, Adgey J. Comparing the efficacy and safety of a novel monophasic waveform delivered by the passive implantable atrial defibrillator with biphasic waveforms in cardioversion of atrial fibrillation. *Circulation* 2004;109:1686–1692

73. Manoharan G, Evans N, Kidwai B, Allen D, Anderson J, Adgey J. Novel passive implantable atrial defibrillator using transcutaneous radiofrequency energy transmission successfully cardioverts atrial fibrillation. *Circulation* 2003;108:1382–1388

74. Walsh SJ, Manoharan G, Escalona OJ, Santos J, Evans N, Anderson JM, Stevenson M, Allen JD, Adgey AA. Novel rectangular biphasic and monophasic waveforms delivered by a radiofrequency-powered defibrillator compared with conventional capacitor-based waveforms in transvenous cardioversion of atrial fibrillation. *Europace* 2006;8:873–880

75. Swerdlow NR, Stephany NL, Talledo J, Light G, Braff DL, Baeyens D, Auerbach PP. Prepulse inhibition of perceived stimulus intensity: paradigm assessment. *Biol Psychol* 2005;69:133–147

76. Swerdlow NR, Blumenthal TD, Sutherland AN, Weber E, Talledo JA. Effects of prepulse intensity, duration, and bandwidth on perceived intensity of startling acoustic stimuli. *Biol Psychol* 2007;74:389–395

77. Gilman B, Kroll M. Electrically induced chest constrictions during ventricular fibrillation produce blood flow. *J Am Coll Cardiol* 2007;49(9), Supp 1:230A

78. Gilman B, Kroll M, Wang P, Kroll K. Electrically induced chest constrictions during ventricular fibrillation produce blood flow via thoracic-only pump mechanism. *Heart Rhythm* 2007;4(5) Supp;S134

79. Rosborough JP, Deno DC. Electrical therapy for post defibrillatory pulseless electrical activity. *Resuscitation* 2004;63:65–72

80. Berul CI, Triedman JK, Forbess J, Bevilacqua LM, Alexander ME, Dahlby D, Gilkerson JO, Walsh EP. Minimally invasive cardioverter defibrillator implantation for children: an animal model and pediatric case report. *Pacing Clin Electrophysiol* 2001;24:1789–1794

81. Luedemann M, Hund K, Stertmann W, Michel-Behnke I, Gonzales M, Akintuerk H, Schranz D. Implantable cardioverter defibrillator in a child using a single subcutaneous array lead and an abdominal active can. *Pacing Clin Electrophysiol* 2004;27:117–119

82. Madan N, Gaynor JW, Tanel R, Cohen M, Nicholson S, Vetter V, Rhodes L. Single-finger subcutaneous defibrillation lead and "active can": a novel minimally invasive defibrillation configuration for implantable cardioverter-defibrillator implantation in a young child. *J Thorac Cardiovasc Surg* 2003;126:1657–1659

83. Snyder CS, Lucas V, Young T, Darling R, Dalal G, Davis JE. Minimally invasive implantation of a cardioverter-defibrillator in a small patient. *J Thorac Cardiovasc Surg* 2007;133:1375–1376

84. Andrew AG, Warren MS, Margaret AH, Derek TC, Francis DM, Ian GC, Iain CM, David JW, Riccardo C, Gust HB. A prospective, randomized comparison in humans of defibrillation efficacy of a standard transvenous ICD system with a totally subcutaneous ICD system (The S-ICD® system). *Heart Rhythm* 2005;2:1036

85. Burke MC, Coman JA, Cates AW, Lindstrom CC, Sandler DA, Kim SS, Knight BP. Defibrillation energy requirements using a left anterior chest cutaneous to subcutaneous shocking vector: implications for a total subcutaneous implantable defibrillator. *Heart Rhythm* 2005;2:1332–1338
86. Bardy G. Subcutaneous implantable defibrillator. In: Malik M, ed. *Dynamic Electrocardiography*. 2004 Blackwell-Futura
87. Krahn AD, Klein GJ, Yee R, Norris C. Maturation of the sensed electrogram amplitude over time in a new subcutaneous implantable loop recorder. *Pacing Clin Electrophysiol* 1997;20:1686–1690
88. Chrysostomakis SI, Klapsinos NC, Simantirakis EN, Marketou ME, Kambouraki DC, Vardas PE. Sensing issues related to the clinical use of implantable loop recorders. *Europace* 2003;5:143–148

Chapter 6.6

Lessons Learned from Implantable Cardioverter-Defibrillators Recordings

Jeff Gillberg, Troy Jackson, and Paul Ziegler

Introduction

The diagnostic capability of the implantable cardioverter-defibrillator (ICD) has undergone substantial changes since the first devices were designed in the 1980s. The earliest ICDs provided only counters to confirm the number of shocks delivered and had no diagnostics that could be used to confirm the ventricular rate or rhythm of treated episodes.[1] The availability of simple diagnostic information, such as ventricular rate and patterns of ventricular intervals, in the few seconds surrounding delivered therapy was a major step forward in providing information necessary to understand the nature of the rhythms being treated. However, the addition of stored cardiac electrogram (EGM) signals to complement and confirm ventricular rate and interval pattern information has been the crucial advance that has allowed clinicians, scientists, and engineers to confirm appropriate ICD function and to improve their understanding of the cardiac rhythms treated by ICDs in the ambulatory setting.

The memory capacity of ICDs has increased dramatically since the initial introduction of stored electrograms. The first ICDs with stored EGM had minimal capacity for storing a total of <1min of ventricular electrogram data, with $\leq$ 5s for each treated episode. Today's modern ICDs have capacity for recording $\geq$ 20 min of EGMs spanning several treated episodes, each with 2–5 min of electrogram recording.[2] Other clinically important diagnostics in modern ICDs include programmed detection and therapy parameters, time/date for detected episodes to help correlate ICD therapy with clinical symptoms, long-term trends of arrhythmia episodes, therapy success counters, EGMs for nonsustained tachycardias, episodes that the ICD classified as supraventricular tachycardia (SVT) and withheld therapy, and logs of up to several hundred episodes to capture episodes when the stored EGM memory capacity of the device is exceeded. In addition to the information stored

Jeff Gillberg
CRDM Research, Medtronic, Inc., Minneapolis, MN, USA, jeff.gillberg@medtronic.com

I. R. Efimov et al. (eds.), *Cardiac Bioelectric Therapy: Mechanisms and Practical Implications.*
© Springer Science+Business Media, LLC 2009

directly related to cardiac tachyarrhythmias and ICD therapies, ICDs may store important diagnostics such as patient's activity, heart rate variability, atrial and ventricular EGM amplitude, and information on device self-checks such as pacing thresholds, lead impedance, and battery voltage.

The rich information available in ICD recordings has provided clinicians, scientists, and engineers with a wealth of knowledge that continues to result in improvements to ICD therapy. This chapter presents some of the lessons learned from ICD recordings regarding cardiac tachyarrhythmias and ICD therapies over the past decade. In the first section, we present some additional background information to familiarize the reader with ICD recordings, and in particular, the cardiac electrogram. In the remaining sections, we discuss lessons learned using ICD recordings from appropriately treated ventricular tachyarrhythmia episodes, inappropriately treated ICD episodes (including supraventricular tachyarrhythmias), and appropriately treated atrial tachyarrhythmia episodes.

ICD Electrograms

EGMs are recordings of the potential difference between two implanted electrodes over time. This is analogous to the surface electrocardiogram (ECG), but because EGMs are recorded from implanted electrodes, their appearance can be quite different depending on the location of the implanted electrodes and their proximity to cardiac tissue. An implanted ICD system will have multiple electrodes located in several positions in the heart, with EGMs measured between various pairs of electrodes or between individual electrodes and the ICD housing or "can." *Near-field* EGMs are measured between closely spaced bipolar pairs of electrodes on leads in the heart. Typical amplitudes of near-field EGMs are approximately ten times the amplitude of surface ECG signals (5–20 mV for ventricular near-field EGMs and 1–3 mV for atrial near-field EGMs). Near-field EGMs tend to have higher frequency content and accentuate the local wavefronts of depolarization and repolarization that pass the electrode at the tip of the lead, and thus are relatively immune to non-local cardiac or extracardiac signals. Exceptions to this may occur due to several factors, including wider bipolar electrode spacing, unfavorable electrode locations, and large non-local potentials that may increase the relative amplitude of non-local activity seen on the near-field EGM (e.g., ventricular depolarizations on the atrial near-field EGM and diaphragmatic myopotentials on ventricular near-field EGM).[3,4] Because of their relative immunity to non-cardiac potentials, ICD circuits process near-field EGMs to perform *sensing* (i.e., to determine the timing of cardiac depolarizations) in order to provide the most accurate rate estimates for automatic therapy decisions.[5] *Far-field* EGMs in an ICD system are measured from the defibrillation electrodes and are recorded for diagnostic purposes or for automatic morphology analysis during the tachyarrhythmia detection process.[6,7] The amplitude of far-field ventricular EGMs is typically 2–15 mV when one of the electrodes is the right ventricular coil. When both electrodes are relatively distant from the ventricular chamber (e.g., superior vena cava (SVC) coil to can), signal amplitudes are dramatically reduced and more similar to the amplitudes of surface ECGs (i.e., 0.5–2 mV). Far-field EGMs tend to have lower frequency content than near-field signals and are more similar in appearance to the surface ECG since they provide a more global view of cardiac depolarization/repolarization. Far-field EGMs are also more susceptible to recording extracardiac potentials (e.g., myopotentials are frequently apparent on far-field EGMs in signals with the ICD housing as one of the electrodes).[8] Figure 1 presents an X-ray of a typical single chamber ICD with example near-field and far-field EGM recordings during spontaneous tachycardia.

Interpretation of ICD Recordings

The interpretation of ICD recordings is ideally done in conjunction with patient-specific clinical data (e.g., age, cardiovascular history, arrhythmia history), along with knowledge of patient activities and symptoms at the time of the ICD recorded event. Although there are still circumstances where patient-specific clinical information is helpful, the addition of EGM signals to ICD recordings provides valuable information to allow for highly accurate interpretations of proper device function as well as arrhythmia diagnosis. In one of the earliest reports on the use of ICD recordings to diagnose arrhythmias leading to ICD shock, Hook and Marchlinski[9] analyzed ventricular rate, regularity, and EGM morphology compared to baseline to determine the cause of ambulatory shocks in three patients. A study of 241 ICD patients demonstrated that unnecessary ICD shocks could be diagnosed more often with ICDs having stored EGM capability than by Holter or telemetry monitoring in patients having devices without stored EGMs.[10] Using the criteria described by Hook, Callans et al.[11] demonstrated that qualitative analysis of near-field and far-field EGM recordings can discriminate between ventricular tachycardia (VT) and SVT for 91–94% of VT episodes. The errors in rhythm diagnosis using EGMs can be attributed to several factors, including changes in cardiac conduction (e.g., bundle branch block),[12] idiopathic changes in EGM morphology during normally conducted SVT,[13] lack of EGM morphology change during VT, and EGM morphology changes after ICD shock.[14] Despite these potential limitations, the analysis of ICD recordings is used to adjust medical therapy or ICD programming to achieve significant reductions of inappropriate ICD therapy.[15] The atrial EGM information in dual chamber and cardiac resynchronization ICDs has further improved the diagnostic accuracy of ICD recordings by providing a direct measurement of atrial activation for rhythm interpretation.[16,17]

Figure 2 depicts the decision process for analyzing a typical ICD recording from a detected tachycardia episode. Since patient-specific clinical data are often not complete, experts rely heavily on the ICD recording to determine the rhythm diagnosis. All tachycardia detection algorithms utilize the measured rate (or cardiac intervals) as a foundation; therefore, the first step is to verify appropriate sensing by the device to ensure the rhythm detected was truly a tachycardia and not caused by oversensing of physiologic or non-physiologic signals, causing the measured heart rate to be higher than the actual heart rate. The EGMs are inspected and correlated with the sensing markers and/or the measured rate. As shown in Fig. 2, appropriate sensing can be confirmed by ensuring the device marker is associated with only true cardiac depolarizations (Fig. 2a) and that no extra sensing markers are associated with non-depolarization EGM waveforms (as in Fig. 2b which shows oversensing due to a compromise in the right ventricle (RV) tip or RV ring conductor in the ICD lead). Once the presence of a tachycardia is confirmed, the EGMs,

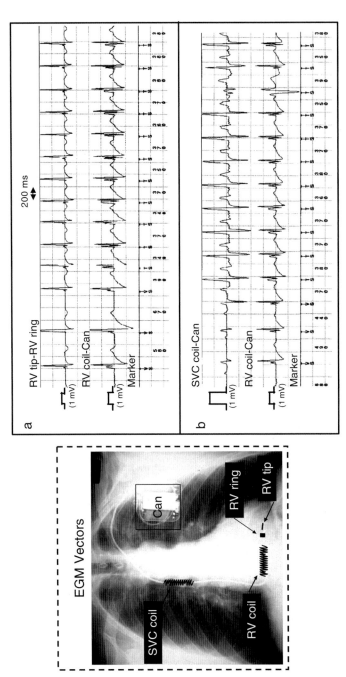

Figure 1: X-ray of an implanted implantable cardioverter-defibrillator (ICD) system with the ICD housing ("can") in the upper chest and the tip of the intracardiac lead implanted in the apex of the right ventricle. The tip, ring, and coil electrodes are integrated into a single ICD lead. (a) shows near-field (right ventricle [RV] tip-RV ring) and far-field (RV coil-can) electrogram (EGM) signals during two beats of normal rhythm (*left*) and spontaneous tachycardia. (b) shows two beats of normal rhythm (*left*) followed by the same tachycardia from the same patient as (a). Due to its closer proximity to atrial tissue, the far-field EGM measured from the superior vena cava (SVC) coil to the can electrode (SVC coil-can) revealed the presence of P waves (atrial depolarizations) and helped to determine that the spontaneous rhythm was an atrial tachycardia. The marker tracing at the bottom of tracings (a) and (b) indicates the timing of ventricular depolarizations as sensed by the ICD, with the numbers indicating the number of milliseconds between depolarizations (VS = ventricular sense, TS = tachycardia sense)

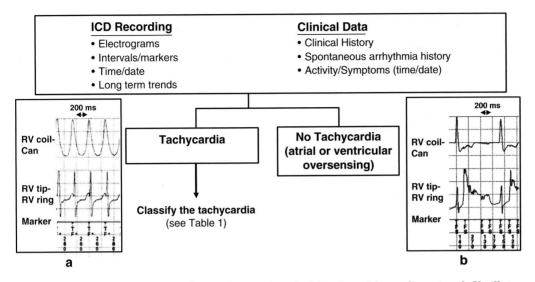

Figure 2: The decision process for analyzing a typical implantable cardioverter-defibrillator (ICD) recording from a detected tachycardia episode. (a) shows appropriate sensing is confirmed by correlating the depolarizations in the EGM with the sensing markers. (b) shows an event recording during oversensing (extra sensing markers not associated with true ventricular depolarizations) due to a compromise in the right ventricle (RV) tip or RV ring conductor in the ICD lead

device markers, and measured intervals are analyzed to "classify" the tachycardia according to established criteria. Since no single criteria alone is definitive, experts will weigh the evidence from several different criteria including EGM morphology, rate, regularity, and atrioventricular association to make a final determination of tachycardia classification.[15,18,19] Table 1 presents a summary of the published criteria for EGM analysis for the purpose of adjudicating ICD detected tachycardia episodes.

Lessons Learned from ICD Treatment of Ventricular Tachyarrhythmias

Incidence of Ventricular Tachyarrhythmias

The application of ICD therapy for reducing sudden cardiac death has also allowed the characterization of tachyarrhythmias in a large number of subjects. Examining ICD recordings from treated arrhythmias illustrates the therapeutic role played by the device. Because the characteristics of patients receiving ICDs have undergone dramatic shifts over time, the incidence of various tachyarrhythmias cannot be captured by any one study. The initial patients who received ICDs were survivors of sudden cardiac death who were unresponsive to drug treatment. ICDs were a therapy of last resort. The current patient population comprises

Table 1: Criteria for adjudicating implantable cardioverter-defibrillator detected tachycardia episodes

	Ventricular EGM only					Atrial and ventricular EGM		
	Ventricular cycle length ≤ 260 mS	Ventricular EGM morphology Same as baseline	Sudden ventricular rate increase	Irregular ventricular intervals	Beat–beat ventricular EGM morphology variability	Ventricular rate < atrial rate (no undersensing)	Chamber of tachycardia onset = atrium	Atrial rate ≥ ventricular rate with atrioventricular association
Evidence for SVT	-[a]	++	+	++	+[b]	---	++	++
Evidence for VT/VF	++	-[c]	+	+	++	+++	-	+[d]

EGM, electrogram; SVT, supraventricular tachycardia; VT/VF, ventricular tachyarrhythmias and ventricular fibrillation; AF, atrial fibrillation

Evidence supporting a particular classification is categorized as very strong, strong, or weak by the symbols "+++," "++," and "+", respectively. Evidence *refuting* a particular classification is categorized as very strong, strong, or weak by the symbols "−−," "−," and "−" respectively

[a] Rapidly conducted atrial fibrillation may have ventricular cycle length ≤ 260 mS

[b] Beat–beat morphology variability can result from conduction aberrancy during AF

[c] ~ 5% of VTs will have EGMs similar to baseline

[d] VT with 1:1 retrograde conduction has atrioventricular association

a combination of indications for ICD therapy, and a large number have no history of cardiac arrest or ventricular tachyarrhythmia. Examining the tachyarrhythmia incidence in studies that led to major changes in ICD indications provides a sense of what ICDs encounter in the most common clinical applications.

The Antiarrhythmics Versus Implantable Defibrillators (AVID) trial established ICDs as superior to antiarrhythmic drugs for improving survival in patients with documented serious arrhythmias.[20] This result changed ICDs from a therapy of last resort to a first-line therapy against sudden cardiac death. The patients in the AVID trial are currently described as "secondary prevention" patients. These are patients for whom the ICD is prescribed for ventricular fibrillation (VF) or for ventricular tachycardia (VT) and syncope or for VT in the setting of depressed cardiac function and symptoms. There were 216 patients with prior VF and 276 patients with VT-related reasons for therapy who were studied for an average of 31 months.[21]

These two groups (VF or VT history) in the study exhibited different distributions of VT and VF, but VT rhythms were encountered in a significant portion of the VF group. Eighty-nine subjects (20%) had at least one episode of VF treated, and 230 subjects (54%) had at least one treated VT episode. Thus, monomorphic VT (MVT) was the most commonly treated rhythm both in the number of patients treated for it and in the total number of episodes observed during the study. Arrhythmia history predicted differences in arrhythmia incidence. Patients were more likely to be treated for the tachyarrhythmia that caused them to receive their ICD. Subjects from the non-VF group were more than twice as likely to have subsequent VT (74% vs. 30%), while the group with prior VF was more likely to have VF (28% vs. 18%). Surprisingly the proportion of patients in both groups that were treated for both VT and VF was not significantly different ($\sim$ 18%).

After AVID, ICD usage was further expanded to a new class of patients determined for the purpose of "primary prevention". These patients are treated with ICD therapy because of clinical characteristics that place them at high risk of sustained tachyarrhythmias and sudden death. The role of the ICD is to stop the *first* occurrence of a serious tachyarrhythmia. This is in contrast to secondary prevention patients for whom a significant tachyarrhythmia has already been observed. The primary prevention patient profile evolved through a series of studies that applied ICD therapy for increasingly expanded clinical conditions. A key condition of all primary prevention indications is reduced ventricular function. This is determined by measuring the left-ventricular ejection fraction (LVEF). LVEF is the volume of blood ejected from the left ventricle by a contraction divided by the volume just prior to contraction expressed as a percentage. The LVEF that defined reduced function in primary prevention studies ranged from 30 to 40%. Reduced function in conjunction with other clinical aspects has been used to identify patients who could benefit from prophylactic ICD therapy.

Two key primary prevention trials are the Multicenter Automatic Defibrillator Implantation Trial (MADIT) and the Multicenter Unsustained Tachycardia Trial (MUSTT). There are subtle differences in the details between the patient populations, but both studies found ICD therapy significantly improved survival in their populations. These patients all had coronary artery disease, reduced ventricular function, asymptomatic, unsustained ventricular tachycardia, and had VT or VF induced during an electrophysiology study. After the success of ICD therapy in MADIT and MUSTT, an additional trial, the Multicenter Automatic Defibrillator Implantation Trial II (MADIT-II) established a further expansion of the primary prevention indication. The patients in MADIT-II received ICDs on the basis of having a prior myocardial infarction and an LVEF $\leq 30\%$, removing the requirement to demonstrate that VT or VF can be induced during an electrophysiology study. MADIT-II ICD diagnostic data demonstrated that as patient populations had expanded, VT had remained the most commonly treated tachyarrhythmia.[22] In the MADIT-II ICD cohort, 169 patients of 719 received an appropriate ICD therapy. The first appropriate therapy in the population was dominated by VT, with 82% of patients having the first appropriate therapy for VT. The remaining 18% had a first therapy for VF.

The PainFREE Rx II study, roughly 4 years after AVID, enrolled both primary and secondary prevention patients and provided an example of arrhythmia incidence in a combined population.[23] There were 334 secondary prevention patients and 248 primary prevention patients enrolled in the study. There was no significant difference in the distribution of VT, Fast VT (FVT, VT with cycle length $< 320\,\mathrm{ms}$), and VF between the primary and secondary prevention groups based on episode classification from 191 patients with true ventricular arrhythmias. In the primary prevention population, 14% of the detected ventricular arrhythmias were VF, while 10% of the secondary prevention arrhythmias were VF. The FVT rhythms accounted for 35% of the ventricular arrhythmias in both populations while the remainder was VT.

The most recent expansion in primary prevention patients resulted from the Sudden Cardiac Death in Heart Failure Trial (SCD-HeFT). There were 829 subjects in the ICD therapy arm and the only criteria for ICD therapy were New York Heart Association (NYHA) class II or III; chronic, stable congestive heart failure; and an LVEF $\leq 35\%$.[24] There were 177 patients who received shock therapy for VT and/or VF: 109 patients had therapy for VT, and 68 patients received VF therapy.[25] In this expansive new primary prevention patient population VT is still a dominant rhythm, but the gap between VT and VF rates in terms of number of patients is less than in prior studies. It remains to be seen in reports of the episode incidence if the gap also narrows between the rates of VT and VF episodes.

Consistently across the general ICD patient populations, the device is more likely to treat VT than VF. This has held up across all of the expansions of the main indications for ICD therapy. The most recent expansion of ICD indication, the SCD-HeFT population, showed a greater percentage of patients with VF than prior studies. Despite this shift, VT still represents a majority of episodes. There are other less common indications for ICD therapy, such as long QT syndrome, that do have different arrhythmia distributions. But in a general ICD population, VT remains the most common tachyarrhythmia.

Therapy Efficacy and Failure Modes

ICDs are the practical embodiment of many aspects of electrotherapy. They combine low-energy pacing stimulation and high-energy countershock therapy in the treatment of VF and VT. The ICD has provided successful therapy for the reduction of sudden cardiac death in a number of different patient populations.[20,24,26] It was not obvious that implanted devices capable of automatically delivering electrical therapy would be an effective mode of treatment. ICD diagnostic information has been used to establish the role of ICDs in clinical medicine and has guided improvements in the practical application of electrotherapy. It has illustrated how electrotherapies fail in ambulatory use and highlighted where those failure modes agree or differ with laboratory evaluations. In some cases ICD diagnostics have revealed aspects of therapy that cannot be observed in the laboratory.

Therapy Efficacy: Defibrillation

The defibrillation shocks delivered by ICDs were optimized through acute experiments, while diagnostics had an insignificant role. The most important improvement in ICD therapy was the development of the biphasic defibrillation shock waveform. Biphasic waveforms reduced the energy requirements for successful defibrillation, allowing pectoral implant of the ICD and the use of transvenous shocking electrodes. This was a vast improvement over abdominally implanted ICDs with epicardial patch electrodes. ICD diagnostics confirmed the system's defibrillation efficacy during ambulatory use.

The first pectoral-endocardial ICD system delivered successful defibrillation therapy in the ambulatory setting for 99% of the detected spontaneous fibrillation episodes.[27] The high rate of successful defibrillation has been maintained across the different patient populations, including the typical ICD patient population, comprising both primary and secondary prevention patients.[28] Although the overall efficacy of defibrillation by ICDs is high, reviewing ICD recordings shows that the ability to provide multiple shocks in an episode of VF is of vital importance for overall defibrillation efficacy. For example, in the PainFREE Rx II trial the first defibrillation shock was set to 10 J more than the defibrillation threshold measured at implant. This shock energy succeeded in 87% of the first shocks for VF.[29] The subsequent shocks were at the full output capability of the device; an example of a multiple-shock episode is shown in Fig. 3. None of the episodes where the first shock failed required more than three additional shocks to convert. The overall shock efficacy was 100%. The most recent shock performance reporting is from the Low Energy Safety Study (LESS).[28] The full-output capability of the device resulted in a first shock defibrillation success rate of 97%. This was compared to programming the first shock of the device to a rigorous defibrillation threshold measurement (DFT++). DFT++ also resulted in 97% first shock success. In LESS, the overall efficacy of defibrillation, including multiple attempts, was 100%.

In addition to verifying programming strategies and corroborating acute study results, ICD diagnostics motivated important improvements for automatic shock delivery algorithms. Initial ICD designs were committed to shock delivery once VF was identified because of concerns that EGM amplitude during VF might become too small for accurate device detection. However, diagnostic data showed high rates of spontaneous termination of detected episodes during the capacitor-charging phase of therapy delivery.[30] EGM amplitude was also robust enough for accurate device rhythm classification during extended durations of VF. This combination of factors has lead to extending the amount of time required for tachycardia detection before classifying a rhythm and changing shock delivery algorithms to reconfirm the presence of the tachyarrhythmia after charging.

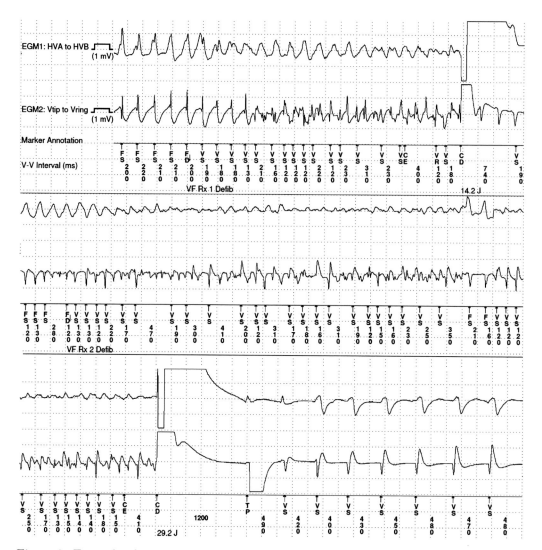

Figure 3: Example of multiple shocks to convert spontaneous ventricular fibrillation (VF). The three sections proceed from *top* to *bottom*. The *upper* electrogram (EGM) trace is measured from the shocking coil to the implantable cardioverter-defibrillator (ICD) can; the *lower* trace is the near-field sensing EGM. The intervals measured by the device from the Vtip-Vring EGM are given in milliseconds. "CD" markers indicate shock delivery with delivered energy measured by the device below the marker. The successful second shock was at the 30 J full-output capability of the device

When it comes to the survival of patients with ICDs, its high efficacy makes it difficult for any single study to reflect aspects of ICD therapy needing improvement. An analysis by Mitchell et al.[31] used patient data from a number of trials over a 5-year period to determine why some ICD patients still suffer sudden cardiac death. There were 90 deaths categorized as "sudden cardiac," of which the cause could be assigned for 68. The majority (81%) of these sudden deaths began with VT or VF. The reasons for therapy failure were a mix of technical failures or clinical conditions. Technical failures were VT or VF falling into the therapeutic programming of the device but with no device response or persistence of VT/VF after a therapy delivery that was not recognized by the device. The clinical scenarios included exhaustion of the maximum number of shocks without terminating VT/VF or incessant VT/VF that was appropriately detected and effectively treated by the ICD but immediately returned to arrhythmia (Fig. 4 is an example). A unique clinical failure is post-shock electromechanical dissociation (EMD), in which the device restores a normal electrical rhythm but not sufficient mechanical function. The dominant mode of sudden cardiac death was post-shock EMD (20 cases), followed by the inability to terminate the arrhythmia (17 cases), and incessantly recurring VT/VF (9 cases). It may be just as important for future device therapies to avoid or correct post-shock EMD as it is for improved shock efficacy when looking to increase the ability of devices to reduce sudden cardiac death.[32]

Therapy Efficacy: Cardioversion

The use of cardioversion therapy, where the shock is synchronized to the depolarization of the ventricles, to terminate ventricular tachycardia provides efficacy similar to defibrillation therapy.[33] There are notable differences in the factors affecting efficacy. During fibrillation or polymorphic VT (PVT) the preshock state of the heart is more complex than in tachycardia. This deemphasizes the role that synchronization of shock delivery plays in defibrillation efficacy and increases the amount of energy required for effective therapy. However, for monomorphic VT, the state of the heart is simpler, and timing effects influence both the necessary energy to terminate the rhythm and the incidence of unfavorable shock failures such as acceleration or disruption of the VT to VF (shown in Fig. 4).[34,35] Shocks delivered late in relation to the onset of the surface ECG R wave have a better efficacy and lower acceleration rate than those delivered early.[36] This pronounced role for timing may explain the inability to terminate VT with full-output cardioversion observed in some cases. Cardioversion shock delivery by ICDs is synchronized to an intracardiac bipolar EGM. This will have a variable relationship to ECG-based shock timing and will not be the optimal time for all VTs.

Shock therapy in the ambulatory setting, where patient circumstances are uncontrollable, can have other unexpected results. Energy-dependent effects have also included a situation where higher energy shocks (24 J) would consistently convert a fast VT to a slower VT, but treating the fast rhythm with a 3 J shock reproducibly converted to sinus rhythm.[37] Additionally, high-energy shocks will sometimes result in either a brief self-terminating tachycardia or a new sustained ventricular tachycardia.[38-40]

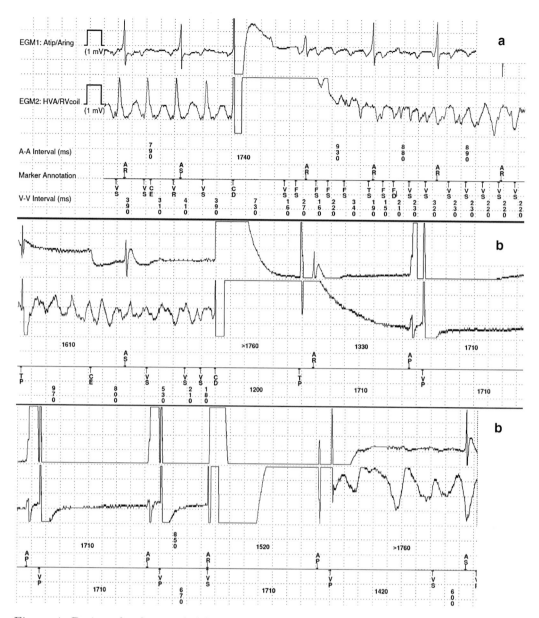

Figure 4: Patient death recorded by implantable cardioverter-defibrillator (ICD) diagnostics. The top signal is the atrial near-field electrogram (EGM). Atrial intervals for intrinsic events ("AS" or "AR") and paces "AP" are above the marker line. The second signal is the shock coil to ICD can EGM. Ventricular intervals are measured from the rate-sensing bipolar EGM (not shown) and are below the marker line. Markers ending in "P" are pace events, while the remainder are intrinsic events except for "CE" for end of charging, and "CD" for charge delivered (i.e., a shock). A number of individual episodes were recorded by the device, which demonstrates continued reinitiation of the tachyarrhythmia. In this series, a cardioversion therapy accelerates ventricular tachycardia (VT) to ventricular fibrillation (VF) (**a**). The VF was successfully terminated, but arrhythmias continued to reinitiate after successful therapies. In (**b**) a spontaneous VF is converted but resumes after a few pacing cycles. The recording ends, as the EGM amplitude is too small to be detected by the device.

Therapy Efficacy: Antitachycardia Pacing

In addition to terminating rhythms by high-voltage shocks, ICDs are also capable of terminating tachyarrhythmias by pacing-strength stimulation. Antitachycardia pacing (ATP) works through the extinguishing of reentrant activity by overdrive pacing. By pacing faster than the tachycardia rate, the activations driven from the pacing site capture increasing areas of the ventricles. If the reentrant circuit is entered by paced activations and is driven to an unsustainable rate, the resulting conduction block terminates the tachycardia.[41] However, ATP is ineffective for polymorphic tachycardias and fibrillation.[42] ATP therapy can be applied using many different algorithmic methods that set the timing of each pacing pulse.[43,44] ICD diagnostics have played a vital role in understanding the different aspects of ATP therapy and in broadening its application.

Specialized pacemakers, not ICDs, were the first devices to apply automatic ATP.[45] However, like shock therapies, ATP has a number of possible failure modes. It can fail to terminate the tachyarrhythmia or only slow the tachycardia rate. ATP can also accelerate the rhythm to a faster tachycardia or fibrillation (see Fig. 5 for an example). Acceleration failures resulting in lethal rhythms indicated that shock backup was needed for automatic ATP devices. Thus, ATP for ventricular tachyarrhythmias is now exclusively delivered by ICDs.

The efficacy of ATP for monomorphic ventricular tachycardia (MVT), the predominant rhythm treated by ICDs, is the same as low-energy cardioversion.[46] In recent large studies, ATP efficacy for MVT was approximately 90%.[35,47] The rate of ATP failures that result in acceleration of the rhythm is related to ATP aggressiveness, the amount by which the tachycardia is overdriven.[44] In studies using predominantly burst pacing (single-cycle length stimulation trains) at 88% of the tachycardia cycle length, acceleration ranged from 2 to 3% of treated episodes.

The initial ICD trials proved ATP was a reliable therapy option and established that ATP success in the laboratory setting carried over to the ambulatory setting.[48] Many of the major events that drove increased ATP utilization would not have been possible without ICD diagnostic data. The first major expansion in ATP use was triggered by findings that ATP efficacy was not completely predicted by induced tachycardia efficacy. A patient could benefit from ATP without having demonstrated successful ATP in the laboratory. This also meant that tailoring ATP parameters based on laboratory testing was not required, and empirically programmed parameters were sufficient.[49] Another limitation of laboratory studies of ATP was demonstrated by the discovery that ATP efficacy for spontaneous MVT exceeds the efficacy for induced MVT in the laboratory.[50,51] A partial explanation for these findings came from examination of ICD electrograms of both induced and spontaneous episodes. It was found that the MVT induced in the laboratory for a patient was often different from the tachycardia EGM morphology of the ambulatory episodes (see examples in Fig. 6).[52]

The large proportion of rapid MVT ($> 200\,\text{bpm}$) observed in ICD diagnostics, coupled with the efficacy of empirically programmed ATP, motivated an investigation of the application of ATP for rapid MVT.[42] Prior programming strategies reflected concerns that syncope

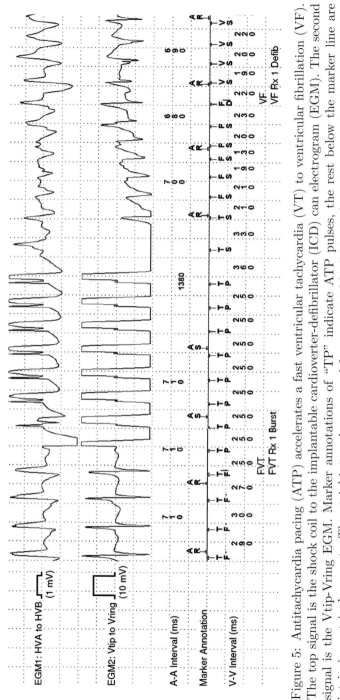

Figure 5: Antitachycardia pacing (ATP) accelerates a fast ventricular tachycardia (VT) to ventricular fibrillation (VF). The top signal is the shock coil to the implantable cardioverter-defibrillator (ICD) can electrogram (EGM). The second signal is the Vtip-Vring EGM. Marker annotations of "TP" indicate ATP pulses, the rest below the marker line are intrinsic ventricular events. The atrial intervals measured from an atrial lead bipole (waveform not shown) are all due to intrinsic events and are shown above the marker line. The pacing train prior to acceleration ("TP" markers) consists of eight pulses at 88% of the average VT cycle length

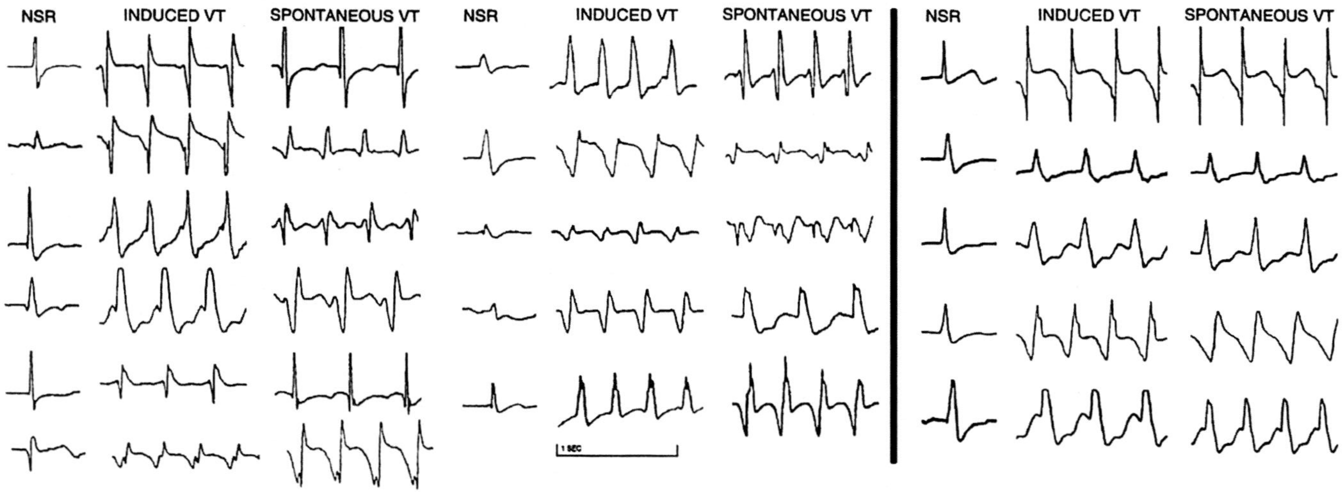

Figure 6: Far-field electrogram (EGM) examples of normal sinus rhythm (NSR), induced ventricular tachycardia (VT), and spontaneous VT. Each group of three EGMs represents one patient. EGM scale is consistent for signals from the same patient. The *heavy line* separates patients into those with an EGM different between induced and spontaneous VTs (on the *left*) from those for which it was the same (on the *right*) (Adapted from Figs. 1–2 Monahan et al. 1999)[52]

and related morbidity would increase if ATP was attempted for rapid tachyarrhythmias, either due to greater acceleration or a cycle-length dependent efficacy. Therefore, cardioversion was considered the appropriate first therapy for rapid tachyarrhythmias.[33] To develop a new strategy, previous ICD studies of ATP were analyzed, and a conservative ATP algorithm was developed that attempted to balance efficacy with acceleration risk. The algorithm used 88% of the tachycardia cycle length as the pacing cycle and delivered an eight-pulse train. The efficacy of this ATP algorithm for rapid VT was about 75% (an example episode is shown in Fig. 7) and carried no additional risk of syncope or acceleration compared to using cardioversion for the initial therapy.[35,42] As ICD indications have expanded, this ATP algorithm has continued to demonstrate 75% efficacy for rapid MVT.[47]

The ability of ATP to successfully terminate so many of the rhythms encountered by ICDs is encouraging for painless treatment of patients. However, given the high incidence of MVT over the course of a patient's life with ICD therapy, even an average efficacy of 90% will not eliminate painful shock therapy for MVT. This should motivate the continued evolution of ATP. Other ICD advancements have targeted increasing the overall utilization of ATP. Devices that attempt ATP during the charging phase of high-voltage therapies have been introduced.[53] Beyond the technical considerations, additional evolution of ATP will require addressing factors discovered through ICD diagnostics, such as the reduced efficacy of ATP linked to elevated heart rates prior to tachycardia.[54] From a utilization and impact perspective, the painless termination of ventricular tachycardia must be considered the most successful electrical therapy developed for these arrhythmias.

Investigating the Causes of Tachyarrhythmia

The data from continuous rhythm monitoring provided by ICDs added a new tool for investigating how spontaneous arrhythmias occur. Prior to ICDs, data on spontaneous arrhythmias came from wearable ECG systems. Holter monitors, worn for a day or two, provided continuous recordings, but capturing a tachyarrhythmia was rare. ICDs have substantially increased the longitudinal observation of arrhythmia incidence. Additionally, the population of ICD patients has significantly increased over time, providing a large pool of subjects. Many diagnostic evaluations were first performed on Holter data, and then the same techniques were applied to ICD data. As ICD memory capacity increased, novel analyses have been developed.

A simple piece of information about a tachyarrhythmia is when it occurs. Analyses of sudden cardiac death patterns illustrated a circadian variation, with more deaths reported in the morning and during the rest of the day.[55] These findings were considered strong, but limited by the bias from having observers reliably relate the time of death. A number of ICD studies have demonstrated similar circadian variation in the genesis of tachyarrhythmias in different patient populations.[56–63] Each analysis documented a circadian variation in the occurrence of ventricular tachyarrhythmias where arrhythmia incidence was significantly higher during the day than at night. Many reports point to the hours between 6:00 A.M. and 12:00 P.M. as the region of peak arrhythmia density.[56,58–60,62,64,65] The nonuniform distribution of arrhythmias favoring the waking hours confirmed a strong relationship

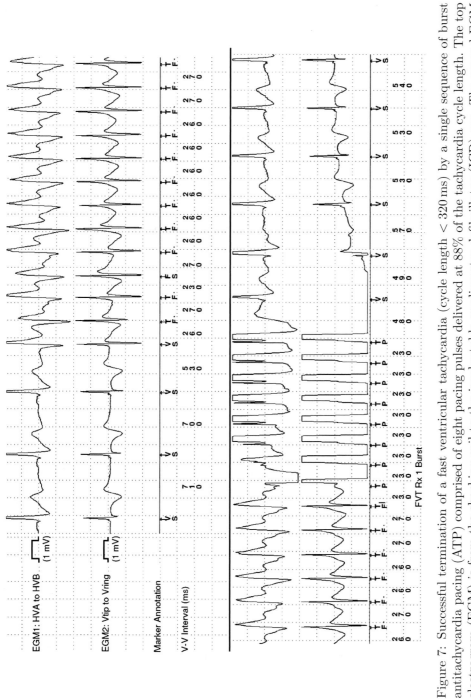

Figure 7: Successful termination of a fast ventricular tachycardia (cycle length < 320 ms) by a single sequence of burst antitachycardia pacing (ATP) comprised of eight pacing pulses delivered at 88% of the tachycardia cycle length. The top electrogram (EGM) is from the shocking coil to the implantable cardioverter-defibrillator (ICD) can. The second EGM is the near-field EGM (Vtip-Vring). Marker annotations of "TP" indicate ATP pulses, the rest of the annotations are intrinsic ventricular events

between sympathetic autonomic activity and the initiation of tachyarrhythmia, potentially leading to sudden cardiac death.

The link between sympathetic autonomic tone and tachyarrhythmia has also been suggested as an important contributor to the annual variation in the occurrence rate of tachycardia recorded by ICDs.[66] Winter had the highest mortality rate. Treatment with ICD therapy significantly lowers mortality during the highest-risk season of the year. An analysis using temperature effects showed that thermal extremes also increase the detected arrhythmia rate.[57] Taken together, these studies again demonstrate the link between periods of high sympathetic excitation and an increased rate of arrhythmia. These investigations have provided strong evidence for the theory that the bulk of sudden cardiac deaths are caused by tachyarrhythmias.

The transition from normal rhythm to tachyarrhythmia is often captured by ICDs, providing a view into what happens in the 10–20s prior to the arrhythmia. The stored EGM and cardiac interval information allows the identification of premature ventricular complexes (PVCs) and other rhythm abnormalities. Additionally, the type of tachyarrhythmia (such as MVT or PVT or VF) can often be identified, including cases where the rhythm transitions between types. The bulk of the analyses on patterns of initiation have been performed using data from single-chamber ICDs. Without information on the atrial activity it can be challenging to determine whether a premature complex is a PVC or a conducted premature atrial complex. Another challenging aspect to the analysis of initiation is identifying if the complex at the initiation of a tachycardia has the same or different morphology as the rest of the tachycardia. Despite these limitations the large number of subjects with ICD diagnostics allows statistical analyses to characterize how tachyarrhythmias start.

PVCs, pauses, and short-long-short (SLS) sequences were associated with the onset of arrhythmias by a number of analyses of the initiation of tachyarrhythmias.[58,67–70] The most common initiation pattern is a late-coupled PVC (i.e., a PVC with a cycle length greater than half of the preceding normal cycle). Late-coupled PVCs have been reported for up to 85% of episode initiations.[70] The SLS sequence was thought to be associated with PVT, but ICD studies showed it was prevalent in the initiation of both MVT and PVT. SLS initiation ranged from as little as 2% to as much as 25% of the recorded episodes.[67,70] Methodologies and classifications are not uniform between studies, making comparisons difficult. Studies that use an additional category of "sudden onset" give different results. *Sudden onset* is defined as the first beat of a tachyarrhythmia having the same EGM morphology and cycle length for the initial late-coupled beat as the rest of the tachycardia. Examples of all of these patterns are shown in Fig. 8. Sudden onset is the initiation in about one quarter of the episodes in these studies. SLS remains similar in proportion, but the extrasystolic initiations, while still dominant, are reduced.[58,69] The relative proportions are found to vary little across different disease states, although PVT has been associated with more early coupled PVCs and SLS sequences than MVT. Within each patient, a common finding across studies is that the initiation sequence is very consistent. Roughly 80% of patients have an exclusive mode of tachyarrhythmia onset.

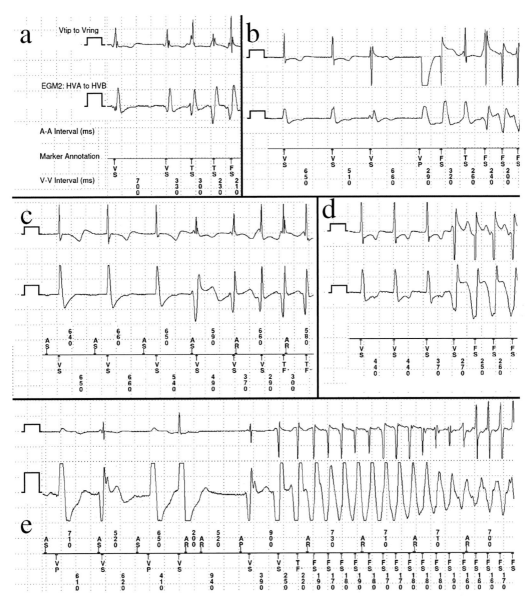

Figure 8: Examples of ventricular tachyarrhythmia onset patterns. Each frame is identified by letter, and the layout is the same for all frames: near-field sensing electrogram (EGM) is the top trace, shock coil to can is the second trace, and each square pulse is 2-mV high and 200-ms wide. The annotations ending with "P" are pacing, all other events are intrinsic. (a) Short-coupled premature ventricular complex (PVC) at 330 ms (0.47 prematurity) initiates ventricular tachycardia (VT) at 230 ms. The complex immediately before the PVC is identical to sinus rhythm and is at the sinus cycle length of 700 ms. (b) A pause started by a PVC is terminated by a rate-smoothing pace followed by ventricular fibrillation (VF). (c) Late-coupled PVC at 540 ms (0.81 prematurity) initiates VT. (d) Sudden onset of VT, unlike the late-coupled initiation, the first complex is very similar to the VT and the first to second VT complex interval of 270 ms is nearly identical to the 260 ms VT cycle length. (e) Short-long-short initiation of PVT by a short coupled PVC at 410 ms followed by 940 ms pause and a short interval of 390 ms.

Devices themselves introduced new types of arrhythmia onset into analyses. The bradycardia pacing support functionality of ICDs interacts with the intrinsic rhythm at the onset of some tachycardias, as shown in Fig. 8b. Sometimes the pacing delivered by the device is inappropriate due to failure to sense intrinsic activity. Inappropriate pacing has the ability to initiate both VF and VT,[69] but pacing that is appropriate to provide heart rate support has also been associated with the initiation of tachycardia.[69,71] Regardless of the mode used, pacing can produce (or at least allow) the same SLS sequence seen prior to tachycardia.[72] In addition to activation patterns created by pacing, a subject could be vulnerable to pace stimulation itself. Although pacing as a cause of arrhythmia can only be inferred from the retrospective view provided by ICD diagnostics, there has been at least one controlled study that found that in a cohort of 150 consecutive patients, 13 (8.6%) had arrhythmias where the onset was only pacing related. Using a crossover trial design where subjects were randomized between 60 bpm and pacing deactivated, it was shown that arrhythmias in these patients only occurred during the active pacing periods.[73]

Despite extensive review of patterns of onset, the findings of ICDs have been strong confirmation of prior knowledge from Holter studies, not new observations. The dominance of PVC-initiated arrhythmias demonstrates the potential for these events to cause arrhythmias. However, the same coupling intervals and morphologies are observed in nonarrhythmic recordings as well. The initiation of tachycardia is multifactorial, and short-term triggers are only a part. Additional work that moves beyond the immediate rhythm aspects is needed.

As ICD memory increased, the ability to store thousands of cardiac intervals prior to the detection of a tachyarrhythmia added to the available data. This opened up the evaluation of the autonomic system with heart-rate variability (HRV) analysis. A number of different HRV measures have been applied to ICD interval recordings. The results of standard linear system measures of HRV, both frequency and time domain, have been mixed. Some studies report significant changes in the HRV signals suggestive of sympathetic dominance prior to tachycardia,[74–76] while others have reported no changes in the HRV signal.[77–80] Evidence for increased sympathetic modulation, while inconsistent in HRV analysis, is supported by the consistent appearance of increased heart rates prior to many tachyarrhythmias.[81,82]

The introduction of nonlinear methods for analyzing HRV, such as symbolic dynamics, detrended fluctuation analysis, and fractal self-similarity measures,[74,80] are less thoroughly reported, but have shown significant initial results. Some of the new techniques are capable of using shorter time series than the traditional HRV measures and focus on different aspects of heart rhythm modulation. This may make them better suited to tracking arrhythmia risk in more detail. None of these methods have yet to undergo prospective evaluation in an ICD-based study and therefore their performance as predictors of tachycardia remains unknown.

As ICD EGM storage continues to increase, analysis of the EGM, rather than cardiac intervals, is expected to provide more information regarding the genesis of arrhythmias. ICD EGMs have already demonstrated QT interval changes prior to tachycardias.[83] Additionally, ICD EGMs have been shown to provide sufficient information for T-wave alternans analysis.[84,85] The ability to combine EGM-derived information with heart rate dynamics may increase the ability to identify the periods where arrhythmia risk is highest. In the future sufficient information may provide for the guidance of preventative therapies.

Lessons Learned from Inappropriately Treated ICD Episodes

The fundamental clinical goal for an ICD is to prevent sudden cardiac death. This requires ICD sensing and detection algorithms to achieve high sensitivity for VT/VF detection, often at the expense of rhythm misclassification and therapy being delivered for non-VT/VF events. Investigators have reported that 10–40% of patients in clinical studies experience inappropriate ICD therapy, depending on patient population, study duration, and ICD detection programming.[23,34,86–89] The clinical consequences of inappropriate ICD therapy vary, but in the worst cases can result in proarrhythmia,[90,91] reduced patient quality of life, and significant psychological consequences. Reduced quality of life is especially associated with frequent appropriate or inappropriate ICD shocks.[92–94] Analyses of inappropriately treated ICD episodes have revealed that the most common reasons include rapidly conducted SVT, such as atrial fibrillation and sinus tachycardia, detection of nonsustained VT, and ventricular oversensing.[89,95,96] Clinicians have a variety of options for reducing the likelihood of inappropriate ICD therapy, including reprogramming the detection and therapy parameters available in the ICD, prescribing adjunctive medical therapy (e.g., beta-blockers to control rate during SVT), and invasive procedures to modify ICD system hardware (as a last resort).[19] The sections that follow present more detail on each of the three major causes of inappropriately treated episodes observed from ICD recordings.

Inappropriate Detection Due to Oversensing

ICD sensing circuits are designed to be highly sensitive so that low amplitude EGM waveforms during fibrillation can be sensed adequately.[5] As a result, oversensing of cardiac and noncardiac signals in ICDs occurs and is one of the major sources of inappropriate ICD therapy. Oversensing on the ventricular sensing channel of an ICD (ventricular oversensing) causes inappropriate VT/VF detection due to overestimation of the true cardiac rate. Oversensing on the atrial sensing channel (atrial oversensing) may lead to failures of dual chamber SVT discriminators to properly withhold VT/VF detection during SVT. Ventricular oversensing is generally a much more serious clinical concern than atrial oversensing, as it is more likely to result in inappropriate ICD therapy. Analyses of long-term studies of chronically implanted ICDs have reported that 7–11% of all ICD-detected VF episodes were due to ventricular oversensing of the intrinsic rhythm.[95,97] The most commonly reported sources of ventricular oversensing include T-waves, sensing lead fractures, diaphragmatic myopotentials, and electromagnetic interference, with P-wave oversensing and double-counting of R-waves reported less frequently.[4,19,95,97–105] Figure 9a shows an example of an ICD recording with T-wave oversensing resulting in inappropriate detection and ATP therapy. In this case, the T-wave oversensing resulted in inappropriate ICD therapy that was proarrhythmic, inducing polymorphic VT that was promptly terminated by the device. Figure 9b–d present ICD recordings from ventricular oversensing episodes caused by lead

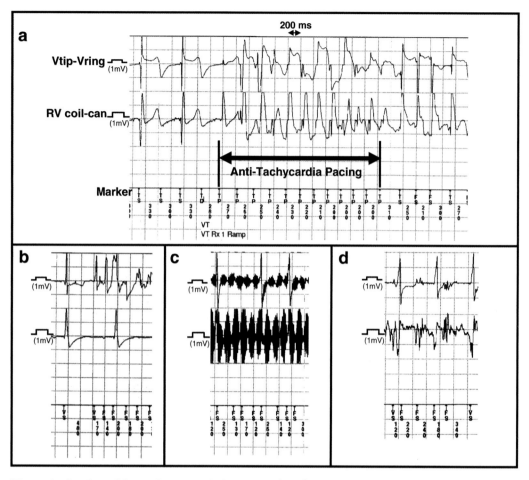

Figure 9: Implantable cardioverter-defibrillator (ICD) recordings from ventricular oversensing episodes. Tracings are Vtip-Vring (*top*), right ventricle (RV) coil-can (*middle*), and device markers for all panels. Numbers are measured intervals in milliseconds. (**a**) T-wave oversensing with inappropriate therapy and proarrhythmia (see text). (**b**) Ventricular oversensing due to lead fracture. (**c**)Ventricular oversensing due to electromagnetic interference. (**d**) Ventricular oversensing due to myopotential noise

fracture (Fig. 9b), electromagnetic interference (Fig. 9c), and myopotential oversensing (Fig. 9d). Device reprogramming can sometimes correct ventricular oversensing due to T-waves, P-waves, diaphragmatic myopotentials, or R-wave double-counting. However, in all cases of sensing lead fracture and in some cases of oversensing caused by small R-waves, an invasive procedure to replace/reposition the sensing lead is required.[19]

Inappropriate Detection and Therapy Due to Nonsustained VT/VF

ICDs detect tachyarrhythmias based on rate and duration. Detection durations are programmable in number of beats or in duration, depending on ICD manufacturer, with typical nominal values ranging from 12 beats up to 3 s. If a detected tachycardia spontaneously terminates during ICD reconfirmation (typically during or just after the device charges its capacitors for high-voltage therapy), the ICD may or may not recognize that the tachycardia has terminated. In some cases, PVCs, oversensing, and/or high intrinsic rates may "fool" the ICD into believing that the tachycardia is still present, resulting in an inappropriate shock. In a preliminary analysis of the shocks in the SCD-HeFT, Poole reported that nearly 3% of all shocks delivered were for nonsustained VT.[51] Wathen et al.[35] reported that 34% of all VTs faster than 320 ms terminated spontaneously after being detected using a programmed detection duration of 18 beats, and Gunderson et al.[30] has suggested that longer detection durations may provide reduction in inappropriate detection and therapy for self-terminating VT. ICD manufacturers have made some improvements to reconfirmation algorithms over the years, including analysis of intervals during capacitor charging, to make algorithms less prone to confirm the presence of tachyarrhythmia based on one or two fast intervals. Figure 10 presents examples of two spontaneously terminating VT episodes, one that received a shock due to premature ventricular contractions during the VT reconfirmation period and one where an improved reconfirmation algorithm aborted therapy successfully.

Inappropriate Detection Due to Supraventricular Tachycardia

Special algorithms for discrimination of VT/VF and SVT with rapid ventricular rate are incorporated into ICDs with the aim of reducing inappropriate detection and therapy.[5,19,106] Clinically optimized combinations of ventricular rate, regularity, and onset information initially formed the basis for single chamber ICD detection with the best SVT discrimination capability[107,108] and are now combined with EGM morphology analysis methods to further improve discrimination.[7,109–111] Dual-chamber and cardiac resynchronization therapy devices also incorporate information from the atrial EGM to improve the specificity and sensitivity of VT detection. Explicit or implicit calculation of atrial rate relative to ventricular rate, measures of atrioventricular association, and atrioventricular patterns derived from the atrial timing measured relative to the ventricular timing can provide additional detection specificity. Sensitivity for VT detection is improved by applying the ventricular regularity or EGM morphology discriminators only when the atrial rate is confirmed to be equal to or higher than the ventricular rate, eliminating false-negative detection of obvious VT (when the ventricular rate is faster than the atrial rate).[112,113]

The high level of sophistication in discrimination algorithms is driven by the need for ICDs to detect and treat life-threatening VT or VF under all circumstances, including the challenging scenario of double tachycardia (simultaneous atrial and ventricular tachyarrhythmia), VT with 1:1 retrograde conduction, and sinus tachycardia that arises during VT. Figure 11 presents examples of two challenging spontaneous tachyarrhythmias that are appropriately detected despite SVT discriminators being enabled. The fact that SVT

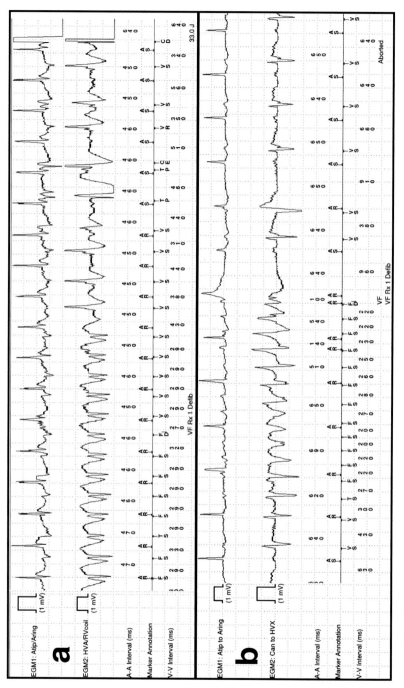

Figure 10: Self terminating ventricular tachycardia (VT) episodes. (a) Shows a shock delivered inappropriately due to two premature ventricular complex (PVC) events during the implantable cardioverter-defibrillators (ICD) reconfirmation period (following the "charge end" (CE) annotation), two ventricular cycles within the treatable range of the device (350 then 340 ms) trigger a shock. This occurs because of the lack of an algorithm to abort shocks during capacitor charging (the period from FD to CE annotations). (b) Shows appropriate operation of an algorithm to recognize spontaneous termination during charging and abort the shock when at least four of the last five ventricular intervals are considered nonarrhythmic. Note that the abort is annotated prior to the appearance of a CE annotation

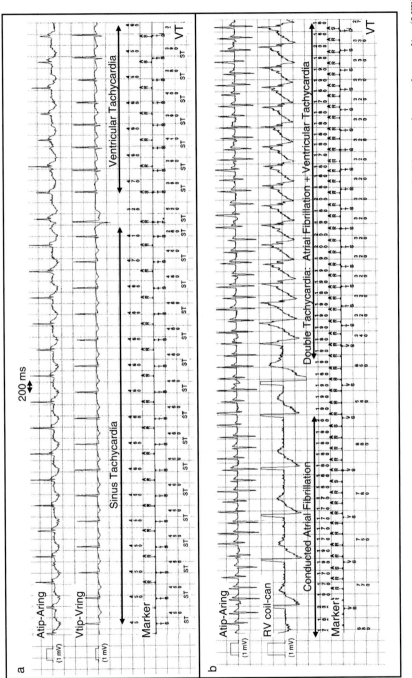

Figure 11: Challenging spontaneous tachyarrhythmias that are appropriately detected. Ventricular tachycardia (VT) detection occurs on the right-hand side of each tracing at the label "VT." (a) Shows an episode of ongoing sinus tachycardia for which implantable cardioverter-defibrillator (ICD) therapy is being withheld. As indicated by the labeling, VT started spontaneously as evidenced by the slight rate change, atrioventricular dissociation, and subtle change in electrogram (EGM) morphology (initial deflection is more negative during VT). (b) is an example of spontaneous VT during ongoing atrial fibrillation. Note the dramatic EGM morphology change and regularization of ventricular rate with atrioventricular dissociation during VT

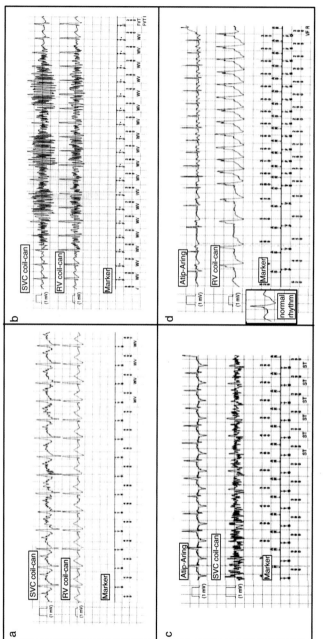

Figure 12: Examples of supraventricular tachycardia (SVT) discriminator success and failure. (**a**) Sinus tachycardia (120 bpm) for which therapy is appropriately withheld by an electrogram (EGM) morphology template-matching algorithm. The implantable cardioverter-defibrillator (ICD) withheld therapy because the EGM morphology on the right ventricle (RV) coil-can EGM was sufficiently close to the EGM morphology during slow rate sinus rhythm. (**b**) Example of sinus tachycardia (160 bpm) with transient myopotential noise on both far-field EGM signals. The ICD initially withheld therapy (prior to the myopotential noise), but then inappropriately detected VT because the myopotential noise caused the RV coil-can EGM morphology to no longer match the noise-less intrinsic EGM morphology template. (**c**) Example of sinus tachycardia (155 bpm) with myopotential noise on the superior vena cava (SVC) coil-can EGM with ICD therapy appropriately withheld. In this example, sinus tachycardia is identified by the atrioventricular timing relationships established from the near-field atrial and ventricular electrodes, and the noisy far-field EGM does not cause inappropriate detection. (**d**) Example of sudden onset atrial tachycardia at 200 bpm with conduction aberrancy. Despite the 1:1 relationship, SVT could not be appropriately discriminated from sinus tachycardia due to the sudden onset. EGM morphology matching would not improve discrimination performance without matching to a template of the aberrant beats during tachycardia. Normal rhythm EGM morphology from the RV coil-can is inset

discrimination algorithms in ICDs maintain high sensitivity for VT/VF detection even in these challenging scenarios leads to less-than-perfect performance in withholding unnecessary therapy for true SVT episodes. Studies have demonstrated that these algorithms can reduce the number of inappropriately detected VT/VF episodes by 50–90% compared to rate-detection alone, with negligible loss in sensitivity for VT and no loss in sensitivity for VF.[107,109–111,114–118] Analysis of ICD recordings has revealed that failures of SVT discriminators for reducing inappropriate therapies can be caused by nonoptimal parameter settings, implicit or explicit rate override criteria that do not allow discriminators to be applied for very rapid SVT (typically faster than 180 bpm), and failures that are inherent in a particular algorithm design.[114,115,117,119] Figure 12 presents examples of successful and unsuccessful operation of SVT discriminators.

Inappropriate ICD Therapies and Changing Patient Population

The high proportion of primary prevention patients now receiving ICDs seems to be causing a relative increase in the prevalence of SVT versus VT in ICD patients, thus lowering the positive predictive value of VT/VF detection compared to earlier studies with secondary prevention patients. This has resulted in renewed concern for inappropriate therapy (especially shocks) in ICD patients, since the shift in patient population has resulted in a relative increase of inappropriate shocks compared to appropriate shocks. Despite improvements in the specificity of SVT discrimination algorithms, recent prospective studies with spontaneous tachycardias in ICD patients have reported positive predictive values for VT/VF detection of only 60–70% for modern, optimized ICD detection algorithms.[114,119] Studies such as the Primary Prevention Parameters Evaluation (PREPARE) trial are being conducted in an attempt to reduce ICD morbidity caused by shocks through selecting optimal ICD detection and therapy parameters that reduce overtreatment of self-terminating tachycardias, improving discrimination of SVTs from VT/VF and maximizing the use of antitachycardia pacing therapy to terminate tachyarrhythmias.[120]

Lessons Learned from Appropriately Treated AT/AF Episodes

Over the past decade, much has been learned about the treatment of atrial tachycardias and atrial fibrillation (AT/AF) from data collected by implantable devices. This section presents some of the lessons learned regarding the use of stored EGMs to assess the performance of devices designed to treat AT/AF and the efficacy of device-based therapies for the management of patients with AT/AF.

Atrial Tachyarrhythmia Detection and Termination Accuracy

The foundation for all device-based treatments of AT/AF and its associated diagnostic information is the ability to accurately and reliably detect the arrhythmia. Algorithms for detecting AT/AF must be designed for high specificity to avoid overtreatment of nonsustained atrial tachyarrhythmias. The desired time course for automatic therapy for atrial tachyarrhythmias may vary from several minutes to several hours, depending on patient symptoms and acceptance of the therapies. This is in contrast to automatic detection and therapy for ventricular tachyarrhythmias, which must be performed with high sensitivity and within several seconds to avoid loss of patient consciousness and arrhythmic death.

High specificity for AT/AF detection has been achieved by use of more sophisticated detection algorithms, which incorporate atrial rate estimations with pattern-based algorithms to recognize atrial tachyarrhythmias with higher atrial rate than ventricular rate (e.g., >1:1 A:V pattern) and reject far-field R-wave oversensing on the atrial sensing channel. These algorithms also include methods for discrimination of AT (organized atrial tachycardia) from AF (atrial fibrillation, or disorganized atrial tachycardia). AT/AF discrimination algorithms are important for guiding therapies, since AT rhythms are more likely to respond to atrial antitachycardia pacing.

Early research efforts were directed at quantifying the detection accuracy so physicians could be confident that devices were treating true arrhythmias and that the diagnostic data provided by the device were valid. The performance of this rate and pattern-based AT/AF detection algorithm was prospectively evaluated in 58 patients using a custom telemetry Holter device to simultaneously record ECG and device markers for 24 hours. The results of this analysis validated the continuous detection of AT/AF with a sensitivity of 100% and a specificity of 99.9% (116 hours of AT/AF, 1,290 hours of non-AT/AF).[121] Further evaluation of AT/AF detection performance has been performed in prospective evaluations of implanted devices, providing AT/AF therapy by analyzing the portion of EGM data that is automatically stored for a limited number of episodes at the time of detection. The positive predictive value of AT/AF detection has been reported to range from 95 to 99%, depending on the population studied.[122,123] Figure 13a presents an example of continuous AT/AF detection with successful atrial antitachyarrhythmia pacing therapy, and Fig. 13b presents an example of atrial undersensing that resulted in delayed AT/AF detection.

Equally important to detecting the initiation of an atrial arrhythmia is the ability to accurately and reliably detect its termination. This allows implantable devices to accurately calculate the duration of specific episodes and to tabulate the cumulative percentage of time spent in AT/AF (AT/AF burden). These metrics have important clinical implications since a physician may classify a patient's arrhythmia status as being paroxysmal, persistent, or permanent based in part on the episode duration and AT/AF burden reported by the device. Incorrect classification of the patient's arrhythmia status could lead to prescribing inappropriate therapies. Providing EGM information at the termination of an episode allows physicians to verify that the device correctly identified the end of the arrhythmia. Undersensing of the atrial signal is one of the primary causes of inappropriate episode termination (Fig. 13b). The rate of appropriate detection of sinus rhythm at the termination of an AT/AF episode has been shown to be 92% in an ICD population.[124]

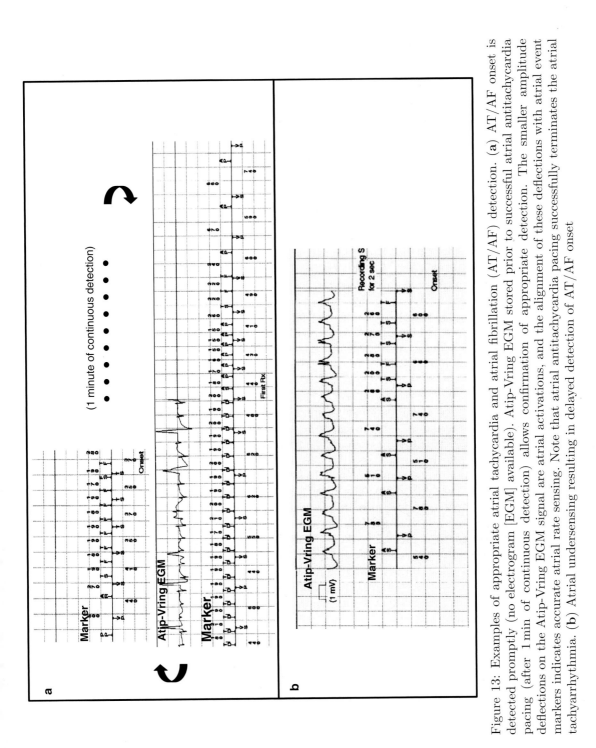

Figure 13: Examples of appropriate atrial tachycardia and atrial fibrillation (AT/AF) detection. (a) AT/AF onset is detected promptly (no electrogram [EGM] available). Atip-Vring EGM stored prior to successful atrial antitachycardia pacing (after 1 min of continuous detection) allows confirmation of appropriate detection. The smaller amplitude deflections on the Atip-Vring EGM signal are atrial activations, and the alignment of these deflections with atrial event markers indicates accurate atrial rate sensing. Note that atrial antitachycardia pacing successfully terminates the atrial tachyarrhythmia. (b) Atrial undersensing resulting in delayed detection of AT/AF onset

Efficacy of Device-Based Therapies for AT/AF

Many modern implantable devices offer features that are designed to terminate ongoing atrial arrhythmias. Some pacemakers and ICDs are capable of delivering low-voltage pacing stimuli intended to interrupt the reentrant activation pattern of certain atrial arrhythmias. This pacing strategy is known as antitachycardia pacing (ATP). In addition, ICDs are capable of delivering high-voltage defibrillation shocks to terminate AT/AF episodes. Clinical research has taught us several lessons on how to improve the efficacy and acceptance of these device-based therapies.

AT/AF Therapy Efficacy: Impact of Early Recurrence of Atrial Fibrillation

One of the challenges in device-based management of AT/AF is the issue of early recurrences of atrial fibrillation (ERAF). ERAF occurs when an AT/AF episode terminates (either spontaneously or in response to a therapy) and is shortly followed by another episode of AT/AF. The time interval over which a recurrence may be classified as ERAF is somewhat arbitrary. The incidence of ERAF following an atrial shock has been reported to be 17% within 1 m, 30% within 1 h, and 43% within 1 day.[125] Very sudden ERAF can confuse the device into thinking that a therapy was unsuccessful when in fact it was effective in terminating the arrhythmia (albeit briefly). The EGM tracing in Fig. 14a shows an AT/AF episode that is treated with an ICD shock. The arrhythmia converts to sinus rhythm for two beats and then quickly reverts to AT/AF. The device reported this as an unsuccessful shock since the device-based definition for successful termination (five beats of sinus rhythm) was not satisfied. Without an EGM tracing at the time of therapy delivery, the physician may have incorrectly concluded that the shock energy was not sufficient to defibrillate the heart. In actuality, the shock was successful in terminating the arrhythmia, but its effect was short-lived due to almost instantaneous ERAF. The EGM tracing in Fig. 14b is from the same patient and same episode. After waiting a longer period of time, a shock with identical energy output is able to successfully terminate the episode without ERAF, and the device declares that the episode was successfully terminated after five beats of sinus rhythm. This example illustrates the findings of earlier studies that reported that the incidence of ERAF could be decreased by delaying a shock for 24 h instead of shocking the arrhythmia within a few hours of its initiation and that the most potent predictor of ERAF was an episode duration less than 3 h.[125,126] Another implication of ERAF is that the true efficacy of an episode's first shock may actually be higher than the ~85% that has been reported based on device classification alone.[127]

Atrial ATP Therapy Efficacy

The percentage of episodes that terminate after ATP is applied (ATP efficacy) has been reported to range from 40 to 58% in AT/AF populations to as high as 67% in atrial flutter populations.[126–128] However, ATP efficacy by itself may not provide an accurate indication of the success of the therapy for several reasons. First, ATP efficacy does not account

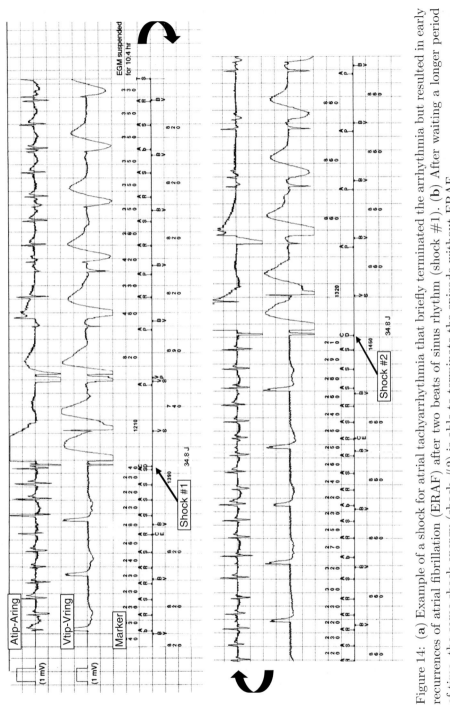
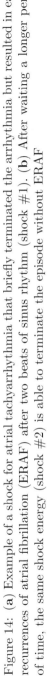

Figure 14: (a) Example of a shock for atrial tachyarrhythmia that briefly terminated the arrhythmia but resulted in early recurrences of atrial fibrillation (ERAF) after two beats of sinus rhythm (shock #1). (b) After waiting a longer period of time, the same shock energy (shock #2) is able to terminate the episode without ERAF

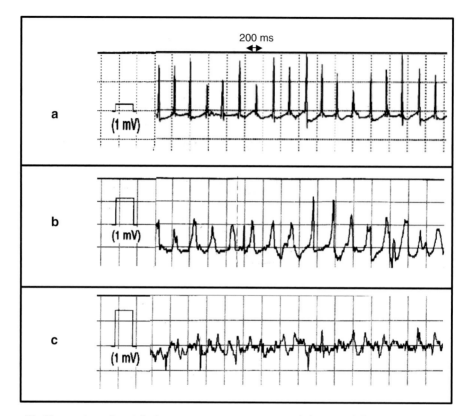

Figure 15: Examples of atrial electrogram tracings with (a) high, (b) intermediate, and (c) low degrees of organization

for the potentially large percentage of episodes in which treatment is not attempted. It is important to recognize that ATP is generally delivered to slower, more regular rhythms. Therefore, a patient with predominantly fast, irregular rhythms may not receive many attempts with ATP therapy. Even if those few ATP attempts were highly successful, it is unlikely that it would have a clinically relevant impact on the overall arrhythmia burden. A second reason that ATP efficacy may be a poor endpoint is that treating arrhythmias early can give the illusion that efficacy is higher due to the increased likelihood of spontaneous terminations that would be inadvertently attributed to the device therapy. To differentiate between a true and spontaneous termination, the EGM tracing must be examined and the ATP therapy should cleanly terminate the arrhythmia within 1 s of its completion.

Despite the limitations of device-classified ATP efficacy as an endpoint, clinical research has shown that individual patients who had high ATP efficacy (defined as ≥60%) were found to have significant reductions in AT/AF burden when ATP was activated.[129] In contrast, patients with low ATP efficacy had no change in AT/AF burden during the ATP active phase of the trial. EGM data from implantable devices have also provided important clues as to the types of rhythms in which ATP is effective. One study classified atrial tachyarrhythmias into groups of high, intermediate, or low degrees of organization. Figure 15 presents EGM examples of rhythms with these different classifications. ATP was shown to be effective in terminating 62% of highly organized rhythms, 34% of rhythms with intermediate organization, and 0% of rhythms with low organization.[130] Device manufacturers have utilized this research to improve the delivery scheme for ATP therapies. Initially, atrial ATP therapy sequencing mimicked the sequencing used for ventricular ATP. This resulted in atrial ATP delivery schemes preferentially delivering therapies toward the beginning of AT/AF episodes. Consequently, all scheduled therapies were frequently exhausted within a few minutes of episode detection, leaving none available to treat the episode later if the rhythm should become more organized. This observation led to the development of new approaches for scheduling atrial ATP therapies. Medtronic's Reactive ATP® algorithm specifically looks for rhythms with high organization and delivers the therapy regardless of when it occurs within the episode. Reactive ATP makes use of two lessons learned from AT/AF diagnostic data. First, it provides an opportunity to treat rhythms later in the chronology of the episode when the likelihood of ERAF is reduced. Second, it provides an opportunity to treat the rhythm when the degree of organization is high, which has been shown to result in greater efficacy.

Atrial Defibrillation Shock Efficacy

One of the most effective treatments for AT/AF is atrial defibrillation. This therapy has been shown to terminate 76–87% of AT/AF episodes[122,123] and has also resulted in a significant reduction in AT/AF burden. One study showed that atrial therapies (including shocks) significantly reduced AT/AF burden from 58.5 h per month to 7.8 h per month.[131] Another study demonstrated that the median duration of successfully treated episodes was 8.9 min compared to 144 min for episodes where the therapy failed.[123]

The main limitation of atrial defibrillation is poor patient acceptance of the therapy since it is usually painful and the arrhythmia is not immediately life threatening. However, since the long-term detrimental effects of AT/AF on stroke risk, mortality, and hospitalization are well documented,[132] physicians and device manufacturers have spent considerable effort in trying to improve the acceptance of this highly effective therapy.

One lesson learned from clinical research is that lower energy shocks are as painful as higher energy shocks.[133] This same study also indicated that a second shock is perceived as more painful than the first shock regardless of the energy. Consequently, in order to minimize shock discomfort, the number of shocks required to terminate AT/AF should be minimized. Programming the device to deliver atrial shocks with full energy output beginning with the first shock rather than successively increasing the energy output can facilitate this.

Other approaches to minimize the discomfort associated with atrial defibrillation shocks are to sedate the patient prior to delivering the shock or program the device to deliver the shock automatically at night while the patient is sleeping. One study showed that nitrous oxide significantly reduced preshock anxiety by 48%, shock-related intensity by 45%, pain by 60%, and discomfort by 78% compared to control shocks.[134] In contrast, night shocks resulted in no change in these parameters. A separate study demonstrated that atrial cardioversion with oral sedation significantly reduced shock recall by 77%, therapy dissatisfaction by 57–71%, shock discomfort by 61–73%, shock pain by 79–83%, and shock intensity by 73–77% compared to automatic night cardioversion without sedation.[135] These studies indicate that sedation significantly improves atrial shock acceptability, and that shocks without sedation are significantly less acceptable, even when performed while sleeping. Additional studies are required to determine if widespread use of these techniques to minimize shock discomfort will significantly improve clinical outcomes in AT/AF patients.

Conclusion

In this chapter we have seen that the rich information available in ICD recordings has enabled clinicians, scientists, and engineers to gain a wealth of knowledge. The importance of various aspects of ICD recordings, including sensed cardiac intervals, markers, and electrogram signals, has been illustrated through examples and findings presented from widespread clinical investigations. Important discoveries about arrhythmias in ambulatory patients, the performance of tachyarrhythmia detection algorithms, and the efficacy of device-delivered therapies have provided the impetus for evolutionary improvements to the ICD and to improvements in the medical management of ICD patients.

Despite the vast knowledge gained over the past decade, there is more to discover about arrhythmias and their treatment. As technology evolves, ICD data capacity will grow and devices will likely incorporate information from various sensors (implanted and external) to further elucidate the nature of cardiac arrhythmias and allow the development of improved strategies for their management. Discoveries regarding the genesis of cardiac arrhythmias in ambulatory patients may some day lead to the development of algorithms to monitor an individual patient's arrhythmic risk over time and to automatically invoke preventative therapies as needed.

References

1. Marchlinski FE, Callans DJ, Gottlieb CD, et al. Benefits and lessons learned from stored electrogram information in implantable defibrillators. *J Cardiovasc Electrophysiol* 1995;6(10 Pt 1):832–851
2. Israel CW, Barold SS. Pacemaker systems as implantable cardiac rhythm monitors. *Am J Cardiol* 2001;88(4):442–445

3. Weretka S, Becker R, Hilbel T, et al. Far-field R wave oversensing in a dual chamber arrhythmia management device: predisposing factors and practical implications. *Pacing Clin Electrophysiol* 2001;24(8 Pt 1):1240–1246

4. Sweeney MO, Ellison KE, Shea JB, et al. Provoked and spontaneous high-frequency, low-amplitude, respirophasic noise transients in patients with implantable cardioverter defibrillators. *J Cardiovasc Electrophysiol* 2001;12(4):402–410

5. Ellenbogen KA, Kay G, Lau C-P, et al. *Cardiac Pacing, Defibrillation and Resynchronization Therapy*, 3rd ed. Philadelphia: Saunders/Elsevier, 2007

6. Gold MR, Shorofsky SR, Thompson JA, et al. Advanced rhythm discrimination for implantable cardioverter defibrillators using electrogram vector timing and correlation. *J Cardiovasc Electrophysiol* 2002;13(11):1092–1097

7. Swerdlow CD, Brown ML, Lurie K, et al. Discrimination of ventricular tachycardia from supraventricular tachycardia by a downloaded wavelet-transform morphology algorithm: a paradigm for development of implantable cardioverter defibrillator detection algorithms. *J Cardiovasc Electrophysiol* 2002;13(5):432–441

8. Luthje L, Vollmann D, Rosenfeld M, et al. Electrogram configuration and detection of supraventricular tachycardias by a morphology discrimination algorithm in single chamber ICDs. *Pacing Clin Electrophysiol* 2005;28(6):555–560

9. Hook BG, Marchlinski FE. Value of ventricular electrogram recordings in the diagnosis of arrhythmias precipitating electrical device shock therapy. *J Am Coll Cardiol* 1991;17(4):985–990

10. Grimm W, Flores BF, Marchlinski FE. Electrocardiographically documented unnecessary, spontaneous shocks in 241 patients with implantable cardioverter defibrillators. *Pacing Clin Electrophysiol* 1992;15(11 Pt 1):1667–1673

11. Callans DJ, Hook BG, Marchlinski FE. Use of bipolar recordings from patch-patch and rate sensing leads to distinguish ventricular tachycardia from supraventricular rhythms in patients with implantable cardioverter defibrillators. *Pacing Clin Electrophysiol* 1991;14(11 Pt 2):1917–1922

12. Sarter BH, Hook BG, Callans DJ, et al. Effect of bundle branch block on local electrogram morphologic features: implications for arrhythmia diagnosis by stored electrogram analysis. *Am Heart J* 1996;131(5):947–952

13. Hallett N, Monahan K, Casavant D, et al. Inadequacy of qualitative implantable cardioverter defibrillator electrogram analysis to distinguish supraventricular from ventricular tachycardia due to electrogram changes during normally conducted complexes. *Pacing Clin Electrophysiol* 1997;20(6):1723–1726

14. Nayak HM, Tsao L, Santoni-Rugiu F, et al. A pitfall in using far-field bipolar electrograms in arrhythmia discrimination in a patient with an implantable cardioverter defibrillator. *Pacing Clin Electrophysiol* 1997;20(11):2864–2866

15. Hook BG, Callans DJ, Kleiman RB, et al. Implantable cardioverter-defibrillator therapy in the absence of significant symptoms. Rhythm diagnosis and management aided by stored electrogram analysis. *Circulation* 1993;87(6):1897–1906

16. Fan K, Lee K, Lau CP. Dual chamber implantable cardioverter defibrillator benefits and limitations. *J Interv Card Electrophysiol* 1999;3(3):239–245

17. Greenberg RM, Degeratu FT. Use of atrial and ventricular electrograms from a dual chamber implantable cardioverter defibrillator to elucidate a complex dysrhythmia. *Pacing Clin Electrophysiol* 1998;21(10):2002–2004

18. Marchlinski FE, Gottlieb CD, Sarter B, et al. ICD data storage: value in arrhythmia management. *Pacing Clin Electrophysiol* 1993;16(3 Pt 2):527–534

19. Swerdlow CD, Friedman PA. Advanced ICD troubleshooting: Part I. *Pacing Clin Electrophysiol* 2005;28(12):1322–1346

20. AVID Investigators. A Comparison of Antiarrhythmic-drug therapy with implantable defibrillators in patients resuscitated from near-fatal ventricular arrhythmias. *N Engl J Med* 1997;337(22):1576–1584

21. Raitt MH, Klein RC, Wyse DG, et al. Comparison of arrhythmia recurrence in patients presenting with ventricular fibrillation versus ventricular tachycardia in the Antiarrhythmics Versus Implantable Defibrillators (AVID) trial. *Am J Cardiol* 2003;91(7): 812–816

22. Singh JP, Hall WJ, McNitt S, et al. Factors influencing appropriate firing of the implanted defibrillator for ventricular tachycardia/fibrillation: findings from the Multicenter Automatic Defibrillator Implantation Trial II (MADIT-II). *J Am Coll Cardiol* 2005;46(9):1712–1720

23. Sweeney MO, Wathen MS, Volosin K, et al. Appropriate and inappropriate ventricular therapies, quality of life, and mortality among primary and secondary prevention implantable cardioverter defibrillator patients: results from the Pacing Fast VT REduces Shock ThErapies (PainFREE Rx II) trial. *Circulation* 2005;111(22):2898–2905

24. Bardy GH, Lee KL, Mark DB, et al. Amiodarone or an implantable cardioverter-defibrillator for congestive heart failure. *N Engl J Med* 2005;352(3):225–237

25. Poole JE, Johnson GW, Callans DJ, et al. Rhythm precursors in those treated for ventricular tachycardia or ventricular fibrillation in SCD-HeFT. *Heart Rhythm* 2005;2(5 Suppl 1):S39–S40

26. Moss AJ, Zareba W, Hall WJ, et al. Prophylactic implantation of a defibrillator in patients with myocardial infarction and reduced ejection fraction. *N Engl J Med* 2002;346(12):877–883

27. Bardy GH, Yee R, Jung W. Multicenter experience with a pectoral unipolar implantable cardioverter-defibrillator. Active Can Investigators. *J Am Coll Cardiol* 1996;28(2):400–410

28. Gold MR, Higgins S, Klein R, et al. Efficacy and temporal stability of reduced safety margins for ventricular defibrillation: primary results from the Low Energy Safety Study (LESS). *Circulation* 2002;105(17):2043–2048

29. Sweeney MO, DeGroot PJ, Stark AJ, et al. Relationship between defibrillation threshold, programmed energy, and first shock efficacy for fast ventricular tachycardia and ventricular fibrillation in PainFREE Rx II. *Circulation* 2004;110(17 Suppl):1–835

30. Gunderson BD, Abeyratne AI, Olson WH, et al. Effect of programmed number of intervals to detect ventricular fibrillation on implantable cardioverter-defibrillator aborted and unnecessary shocks. *Pacing Clin Electrophysiol* 2007;30(2):157–165

31. Mitchell LB, Pineda EA, Titus JL, et al. Sudden death in patients with implantable cardioverter defibrillators: the importance of post-shock electromechanical dissociation. *J Am Coll Cardiol* 2002;39(8):1323–1328

32. Anderson KP. Sudden cardiac death unresponsive to implantable defibrillator therapy: an urgent target for clinicians, industry and government. *J Interv Card Electrophysiol* 2005;14(2):71–78

33. Neglia JJ, Krol RB, Giorgberidze I, et al. Evaluation of a programming algorithm for the third tachycardia zone in a fourth-generation implantable cardioverter-defibrillator. *J Interv Card Electrophysiol* 1997;1(1):49–56

34. McVeigh K, Mower MM, Nisam S, et al. Clinical efficacy of low energy cardioversion in automatic implantable cardioverter defibrillator patients. *Pacing Clin Electrophysiol* 1991;14(11 Pt 2):1846–1849

35. Wathen MS, DeGroot PJ, Sweeney MO, et al. Prospective randomized multicenter trial of empirical antitachycardia pacing versus shocks for spontaneous rapid ventricular tachycardia in patients with implantable cardioverter-defibrillators: Pacing Fast Ventricular Tachycardia Reduces Shock Therapies (PainFREE Rx II) trial results. *Circulation* 2004;110(17):2591–2596

36. Li HG, Yee R, Mehra R, et al. Effect of shock timing on efficacy and safety of internal cardioversion for ventricular tachycardia. *J Am Coll Cardiol* 1994;24(3):703–708

37. Chinushi M, Aizawa Y, Higuchi K. Ventricular tachycardia initiated by high energy cardioversion in a patient with an implantable cardioverter defibrillator. *Heart* 1997;77(4):373–374

38. Cates AW, Wolf PD, Hillsley RE, et al. The probability of defibrillation success and the incidence of postshock arrhythmia as a function of shock strength. *Pacing Clin Electrophysiol* 1994;17(7):1208–1217

39. Duru F, Candinas R. Potential proarrhythmic effects of implantable cardioverter-defibrillators. *Clin Cardiol* 1999;22(2):139–146

40. Zivin A, Souza J, Pelosi F, et al. Relationship between shock energy and postdefibrillation ventricular arrhythmias in patients with implantable defibrillators. *J Cardiovasc Electrophysiol* 1999;10(3):370–377

41. Josephson ME. *Clinical Cardiac Electrophysiology: Techniques and Interpretations*, 3rd ed. Philadelphia: Lippincott Williams & Wilkins, 2002

42. Wathen MS, Sweeney MO, DeGroot PJ, et al. Shock reduction using antitachycardia pacing for spontaneous rapid ventricular tachycardia in patients with coronary artery disease. *Circulation* 2001;104(7):796–801

43. Fisher JD, Zhang Z, Kim SG, et al. Comparison of burst pacing, autodecremental (ramp) pacing, and universal pacing for termination of ventricular tachycardia. *Arch Mal Coeur Vaiss* 1996;89(Spec No 1):135–139

44. Peinado R, Almendral J, Rius T, et al. Randomized, prospective comparison of four burst pacing algorithms for spontaneous ventricular tachycardia. *Am J Cardiol* 1998;82(11):1422–1425, A1428–1429

45. Fisher JD, Johnston DR, Furman S, et al. Long-term efficacy of antitachycardia pacing for supraventricular and ventricular tachycardias. *Am J Cardiol* 1987;60(16):1311–1316

46. Bardy GH, Poole JE, Kudenchuk PJ, et al. A prospective randomized repeat-crossover comparison of antitachycardia pacing with low-energy cardioversion. *Circulation* 1993;87(6):1889–1896

47. Wilkoff BL, Ousdigian KT, Sterns LD, et al. A comparison of empiric to physician-tailored programming of implantable cardioverter-defibrillators: results from the prospective randomized multicenter EMPIRIC trial. *J Am Coll Cardiol* 2006;48(2):330–339

48. Porterfield JG, Porterfield LM, Smith BA, et al. Conversion rates of induced versus spontaneous ventricular tachycardia by a third generation cardioverter defibrillator. The VENTAK PRx Phase I Investigators. *Pacing Clin Electrophysiol* 1993;16(1 Pt 2):170–173

49. Schaumann A, von zur Mu hF, Herse B, et al. Empirical versus tested antitachycardia pacing in implantable cardioverter defibrillators: a prospective study including 200 patients. *Circulation* 1998;97(1):66–74

50. Gillis AM, Leitch JW, Sheldon RS, et al. A prospective randomized comparison of autodecremental pacing to burst pacing in device therapy for chronic ventricular tachycardia secondary to coronary artery disease. *Am J Cardiol* 1993;72(15): 1146–1151

51. Poole JE, Johnson GW, Callans DJ, et al. Analysis of implantable defibrillator shock electrograms in the sudden cardiac death-heart failure trial. *Heart Rhythm* 2004;1(1 Suppl 1):S178–S179

52. Monahan KM, Hadjis T, Hallett N, et al. Relation of induced to spontaneous ventricular tachycardia from analysis of stored far-field implantable defibrillator electrograms. *Am J Cardiol* 1999;83(3):349–353

53. Schoels W, Steinhaus D, Johnson WB, et al. Optimizing implantable cardioverter-defibrillator treatment of rapid ventricular tachycardia: Antitachycardia pacing therapy during charging. *Heart Rhythm* 2007;4(7):879–885

54. Kouakam C, Lauwerier Bened, Klug D, et al. Effect of elevated heart rate preceding the onset of ventricular tachycardia on antitachycardia pacing effectiveness in patients with implantable cardioverter defibrillators. *Am J Cardiol* 2003;92(1):26–32

55. Muller JE, Ludmer PL, Willich SN, et al. Circadian variation in the frequency of sudden cardiac death. *Circulation* 1987;75(1):131–138

56. Englund A, Behrens S, Wegscheider K, et al. Circadian variation of malignant ventricular arrhythmias in patients with ischemic and nonischemic heart disease after cardioverter defibrillator implantation. European 7219 Jewel Investigators. *J Am Coll Cardiol* 1999;34(5):1560–1568

57. Fries RP, Heisel AG, Jung JK, et al. Circannual variation of malignant ventricular tachyarrhythmias in patients with implantable cardioverter-defibrillators and either coronary artery disease or idiopathic dilated cardiomyopathy. *Am J Cardiol* 1997;79(9):1194–1197

58. Grimm W, Walter M, Menz V, et al. Circadian variation and onset mechanisms of ventricular tachyarrhythmias in patients with coronary disease versus idiopathic dilated cardiomyopathy. *Pacing Clin Electrophysiol* 2000;23(11 Pt 2): 1939–1943

59. Lampert R, Rosenfeld L, Batsford W, et al. Circadian variation of sustained ventricular tachycardia in patients with coronary artery disease and implantable cardioverter-defibrillators. *Circulation* 1994;90(1):241–247

60. Mallavarapu C, Pancholy S, Schwartzman D, et al. Circadian variation of ventricular arrhythmia recurrences after cardioverter-defibrillator implantation in patients with healed myocardial infarcts. *Am J Cardiol* 1995;75(16):1140–1144

61. Taneda K, Aizawa Y, the Japanese ICDSG. Absence of a morning peak in ventricular tachycardia and fibrillation events in nonischemic heart disease: analysis of therapies by implantable cardioverter defibrillators. *Pacing Clin Electrophysiol* 2001;24(11):1602–1606

62. Tofler GH, Gebara OC, Mittleman MA, et al. Morning peak in ventricular tachyarrhythmias detected by time of implantable cardioverter/defibrillator therapy. The CPI Investigators. *Circulation* 1995;92(5):1203–1208

63. Wood MA, Simpson PM, London WB, et al. Circadian pattern of ventricular tachyarrhythmias in patients with implantable cardioverter-defibrillators. *J Am Coll Cardiol* 1995;25(4):901–907

64. Behrens S, Galecka M, Bru gT, et al. Circadian variation of sustained ventricular tachyarrhythmias terminated by appropriate shocks in patients with an implantable cardioverter defibrillator. *Am Heart J* 1995;130(1):79–84

65. Lee AKY, Mardini M, Ross DL, et al. Factors affecting diurnal variability of ventricular tachyarrhythmias detected by multiprogrammable implantable cardioverter-defibrillators. *Heart Lung Circ* 2004;13(3):256–260

66. Page RL, Zipes DP, Powell JL, et al. Seasonal variation of mortality in the Antiarrhythmics Versus Implantable Defibrillators (AVID) study registry. *Heart Rhythm* 2004;1(4):435–440

67. Meyerfeldt U, Schirdewan A, Wiedemann M, et al. The mode of onset of ventricular tachycardia: a patient-specific phenomenon. *Eur Heart J* 1997;18(12): 1956–1965

68. Roelke M, Garan H, McGovern BA, et al. Analysis of the initiation of spontaneous monomorphic ventricular tachycardia by stored intracardiac electrograms. *J Am Coll Cardiol* 1994;23(1):117–122

69. Saeed M, Link MS, Mahapatra S, et al. Analysis of intracardiac electrograms showing monomorphic ventricular tachycardia in patients with implantable cardioverter-defibrillators. *Am J Cardiol* 2000;85(5):580–587

70. Taylor E, Berger R, Hummel JD, et al. Analysis of the pattern of initiation of sustained ventricular arrhythmias in patients with implantable defibrillators. *J Cardiovasc Electrophysiol* 2000;11(7):719–726

71. Roelke M, O'Nunain S, Osswald S, et al. Ventricular pacing induced ventricular tachycardia in patients with implantable cardioverter defibrillators. *Pacing Clin Electrophysiol* 1995;18(3 Pt 1):486–491

72. Sweeney MO, Ruetz LL, Belk P, et al. Bradycardia Pacing-induced short-long-short sequences at the onset of ventricular tachyarrhythmias: a possible mechanism of proarrhythmia? *J Am Coll Cardiol* 2007;50(7):614–622

73. Himmrich E, Przibille O, Zellerhoff C, et al. Proarrhythmic effect of pacemaker stimulation in patients with implanted cardioverter-defibrillators. *Circulation* 2003;108(2):192–197

74. Lombardi F, Porta A, Marzegalli M, et al. Heart rate variability patterns before ventricular tachycardia onset in patients with an implantable cardioverter defibrillator. Participating Investigators of ICD-HRV Italian Study Group. *Am J Cardiol* 2000;86(9):959–963

75. Mani V, Wu X, Wood MA, et al. Variation of spectral power immediately prior to spontaneous onset of ventricular tachycardia/ventricular fibrillation in implantable cardioverter defibrillator patients. *J Cardiovasc Electrophysiol* 1999;10(12):1586–1596

76. Sierra G, Molin F, Savard P, et al. Characterization of ventricular tachycardias based on time and frequency domain analyses of cycle length variability in patients with implantable cardioverter defibrillator. *Can J Cardiol* 1999;15(11):1223–1228

77. Baumert M, Baier V, Haueisen J, et al. Forecasting of life threatening arrhythmias using the compression entropy of heart rate. *Methods Inf Med* 2004;43(2):202–206

78. Baumert M, Wessel N, Schirdewan A, et al. Scaling characteristics of heart rate time series before the onset of ventricular tachycardia. *Ann Biomed Eng* 2007;35(2):201–207

79. Burri H, Chevalier P, Arzi M, et al. Wavelet transform for analysis of heart rate variability preceding ventricular arrhythmias in patients with ischemic heart disease. *Int J Cardiol* 2006;109(1):101–107

80. Wessel N, Ziehmann C, Kurths J, et al. Short-term forecasting of life-threatening cardiac arrhythmias based on symbolic dynamics and finite-time growth rates. *Phys Rev E* 2000;61(1):733–739

81. Meyerfeldt U, Wessel N, Schutt H, et al. Heart rate variability before the onset of ventricular tachycardia: differences between slow and fast arrhythmias. *Int J Cardiol* 2002;84(2–3):141–151

82. Nemec J, Hammill SC, Shen WK. Increase in heart rate precedes episodes of ventricular tachycardia and ventricular fibrillation in patients with implantable cardioverter defibrillators: analysis of spontaneous ventricular tachycardia database. *Pacing Clin Electrophysiol* 1999;22(12):1729–1738

83. Diem BorH, Stellbrink C, Michel M, et al. Temporary disturbances of the QT interval precede the onset of ventricular tachyarrhythmias in patients with structural heart diseases. *Pacing Clin Electrophysiol* 2002;25(10):1413–1418

84. Armoundas AA, Albert CM, Cohen RJ, et al. Utility of implantable cardioverter defibrillator electrograms to estimate repolarization alternans preceding a tachyarrhythmic event. *J Cardiovasc Electrophysiol* 2004;15(5):594–597

85. Paz O, Zhou X, Gillberg J, et al. Detection of T-wave alternans using an implantable cardioverter-defibrillator. *Heart Rhythm* 2006;3(7):791–797

86. Dorian P, Newman D, Thibault B, et al. A randomized clinical trial of a standardized protocol for the prevention of inappropriate therapy using a dual chamber implantable cardioverter defibrillator. *Circulation* 1999;1:I–786 (abstract)

87. Bansch D, Steffgen F, Gronefeld G, et al. The 1 + 1 trial: a prospective trial of a dual- versus a single-chamber implantable defibrillator in patients with slow ventricular tachycardias. *Circulation* 2004;110(9):1022–1029

88. Alter P, Waldhans S, Plachta E, et al. Complications of implantable cardioverter defibrillator therapy in 440 consecutive patients. *Pacing Clin Electrophysiol* 2005;28(9):926–932

89. Daubert J, Zareba W, Cannom D, et al. Inappropriate Implantable Cardioverter-Defibrillator Shocks in MADIT-II: Frequency, Mechanisms, Predictors and Survival Impact. *J Am Coll Cardiol* 2008;51: 1357–1365

90. Healy E, Goyal S, Browning C, et al. Inappropriate ICD therapy due to proarrhythmic ICD shocks and hyperpolarization. *Pacing Clin Electrophysiol* 2004;27(3): 415–416

91. Vollmann D, Luthje L, Vonhof S, et al. Inappropriate therapy and fatal proarrhythmia by an implantable cardioverter-defibrillator. *Heart Rhythm* 2005;2(3): 307–309

92. Schron EB, Exner DV, Yao Q, et al. Quality of life in the antiarrhythmics versus implantable defibrillators trial: impact of therapy and influence of adverse symptoms and defibrillator shocks. *Circulation* 2002;105(5):589–594

93. Sears SE Jr, Conti JB. Understanding implantable cardioverter defibrillator shocks and storms: medical and psychosocial considerations for research and clinical care. *Clin Cardiol* 2003;26(3):107–111

94. Sears SF, Lewis TS, Kuhl EA, et al. Predictors of quality of life in patients with implantable cardioverter defibrillators. *Psychosomatics* 2005;46(5): 451–457

95. Poole J, Johnson G, Callans D, et al. Analysis of implantable cardioverter-defibrillator shock electrograms in the Sudden Cardiac Death Heart Failure trial. *Heart Rhythm* 2004; (Suppl):S178

96. Klein RC, Raitt MH, Wilkoff BL, et al. Analysis of implantable cardioverter defibrillator therapy in the Antiarrhythmics Versus Implantable Defibrillators (AVID) Trial. *J Cardiovasc Electrophysiol* 2003;14(9):940–948

97. Gunderson BD, Gillberg J, Swerdlow C. Importance of oversensing in inappropriate detection of ventricular fibrillation by chronically implanted ICDs. Heart Rhythm 2004; 1:S244

98. Achtelik M, Bocchiardo M, Trappe HJ, et al. Performance of a new steroid-eluting coronary sinus lead designed for left ventricular pacing. *Pacing Clin Electrophysiol* 2000;23(11 Pt 2):1741–1743

99. Babuty D, Fauchier L, Cosnay P. Inappropriate shocks delivered by implantable cardiac defibrillators during oversensing of activity of diaphagmatic muscle. *Heart* 1999; 81(1):94–96

100. Doshi RN, Goodman J, Naik AM, et al. Initial experience with an active-fixation defibrillation electrode and the presence of nonphysiological sensing. *Pacing Clin Electrophysiol* 2001;24(12):1713–1720

101. Garg A, Wadhwa M, Brown K, et al. Inappropriate implantable cardioverter defibrillator discharge from sensing of external alternating current leak. *J Interv Card Electrophysiol* 2002;7(2):181–184

102. Gurevitz O, Fogel RI, Herner ME, et al. Patients with an ICD can safely resume work in industrial facilities following simple screening for electromagnetic interference. *Pacing Clin Electrophysiol* 2003;26(8):1675–1678

103. Manolis AG, Katsivas AG, Vassilopoulos CV, et al. Implantable cardioverter defibrillator-an unusual case of inappropriate discharge during showering. *J Interv Card Electrophysiol* 2000;4(1):265–268

104. Peters RW, Cooklin M, Brockman R, et al. Inappropriate shocks from implanted cardioverter defibrillators caused by sensing of diaphragmatic myopotentials. *J Interv Card Electrophysiol* 1998;2(4):367–370

105. Weretka S, Michaelsen J, Becker R, et al. Ventricular oversensing: a study of 101 patients implanted with dual chamber defibrillators and two different lead systems. *Pacing Clin Electrophysiol* 2003;26(1 Pt 1):65–70

106. Swerdlow CD, Friedman PA. Advanced ICD troubleshooting: Part II. *Pacing Clin Electrophysiol* 2006;29(1):70–96

107. Brugada J, Mont L, Figueiredo M, et al. Enhanced detection criteria in implantable defibrillators. *J Cardiovasc Electrophysiol* 1998;9(3):261–268

108. Swerdlow CD, Chen PS, Kass RM, et al. Discrimination of ventricular tachycardia from sinus tachycardia and atrial fibrillation in a tiered-therapy cardioverter-defibrillator. *J Am Coll Cardiol* 1994;23(6):1342–1355

109. Gold MR, Kim J, Bocek J, et al. Rhythm dscrimination using a new electrogram (EGM) vector timing and correlation (VTC)algorithm. *Pacing and Clin Electrophsyiol* 2001;24:577

110. Gronefeld GC, Schulte B, Hohnloser SH, et al. Morphology discrimination: a beat-to-beat algorithm for the discrimination of ventricular from supraventricular tachycardia by implantable cardioverter defibrillators. *Pacing Clin Electrophysiol* 2001;24(10):1519–1524

111. Glikson M, Swerdlow CD, Gurevitz OT, et al. Optimal combination of discriminators for differentiating ventricular from supraventricular tachycardia by dual-chamber defibrillators. *J Cardiovasc Electrophysiol* 2005;16(7):732–739

112. Aliot E, Nitzsche R, Ripart A. Arrhythmia detection by dual-chamber implantable cardioverter defibrillators. A review of current algorithms. *Europace* 2004;6(4):273–286

113. Swerdlow CD. Supraventricular tachycardia-ventricular tachycardia discrimination algorithms in implantable cardioverter defibrillators: state-of-the-art review. *J Cardiovasc Electrophysiol* 2001;12(5):606–612

114. Klein GJ, Gillberg JM, Tang A, et al. Improving SVT discrimination in single-chamber ICDs: a new electrogram morphology-based algorithm. *J Cardiovasc Electrophysiol* 2006;17(12):1310–1319

115. Wilkoff BL, Kuhlkamp V, Volosin K, et al. Critical analysis of dual-chamber implantable cardioverter-defibrillator arrhythmia detection: results and technical considerations. *Circulation* 2001;103(3):381–386

116. Boriani G, Biffi M, Dall'Acqua A, et al. Rhythm discrimination by rate branch and QRS morphology in dual chamber implantable cardioverter defibrillators. *Pacing Clin Electrophysiol* 2003;26(1 Pt 2):466–470

117. Lee MA, Corbisiero R, Nabert DR, et al. Clinical results of an advanced SVT detection enhancement algorithm. *Pacing Clin Electrophysiol* 2005;28(10):1032–1040

118. Bailin SJ, Niebauer M, Tomassoni G, et al. Clinical investigation of a new dual-chamber implantable cardioverter defibrillator with improved rhythm discrimination capabilities. *J Cardiovasc Electrophysiol* 2003;14(2):144–149

119. Friedman PA, McClelland RL, Bamlet WR, et al. Dual-chamber versus single-chamber detection enhancements for implantable defibrillator rhythm diagnosis: the detect supraventricular tachycardia study. *Circulation* 2006;113(25):2871–2879

120. Wilkoff BL, Stern R, Williamson B, et al. Design of the primary prevention parameters evaluation (PREPARE) trial of implantable cardioverter defibrillators to reduce patient morbidity [NCT00279279]. *Trials* 2006;7:18

121. Swerdlow CD, Schsls W, Dijkman B, et al. Detection of atrial fibrillation and flutter by a dual-chamber implantable cardioverter-defibrillator. For the Worldwide Jewel AF Investigators. *Circulation* 2000;101(8):878–885

122. Schoels W, Swerdlow CD, Jung W, et al. Worldwide clinical experience with a new dual-chamber implantable cardioverter defibrillator system. *J Cardiovasc Electrophysiol* 2001;12(5):521–528

123. Gold MR, Sulke N, Schwartzman DS, et al. Clinical experience with a dual-chamber implantable cardioverter defibrillator to treat atrial tachyarrhythmias. *J Cardiovasc Electrophysiol* 2001;12(11):1247–1253

124. Purerfellner H, Gillis AM, Holbrook R, et al. Accuracy of atrial tachyarrhythmia detection in implantable devices with arrhythmia therapies. *Pacing Clin Electrophysiol* 2004;27(7):983–992

125. Schwartzman D, Musley SK, Swerdlow C, et al. Early recurrence of atrial fibrillation after ambulatory shock conversion. *J Am Coll Cardiol* 2002;40(1):93–99

126. Schwartzman D, Musley S, Koehler J, et al. Impact of atrial fibrillation duration on postcardioversion recurrence. *Heart Rhythm* 2005;2(12):1324–1329

127. Swerdlow CD, Schwartzman D, Hoyt R, et al. Determinants of first-shock success for atrial implantable cardioverter defibrillators. *J Cardiovasc Electrophysiol* 2002;13(4):347–354

128. Schuchert A, Boriani G, Wollmann C, et al. Implantable dual-chamber defibrillator for the selective treatment of spontaneous atrial and ventricular arrhythmias: arrhythmia incidence and device performance. *J Interv Card Electrophysiol* 2005;12(2):149–156

129. Gillis AM, Koehler J, Morck M, et al. High atrial antitachycardia pacing therapy efficacy is associated with a reduction in atrial tachyarrhythmia burden in a subset of patients with sinus node dysfunction and paroxysmal atrial fibrillation. *Heart Rhythm* 2005;2(8):791–796

130. Israel CW, Ehrlich JR, Gronefeld G, et al. Prevalence, characteristics and clinical implications of regular atrial tachyarrhythmias in patients with atrial fibrillation: insights from a study using a new implantable device. *J Am Coll Cardiol* 2001;38(2):355–363

131. Euler DE, Friedman PA. Atrial arrhythmia burden as an endpoint in clinical trials: is it the best surrogate? Lessons from a multicenter defibrillator trial. *Card Electrophysiol Rev* 2003;7(4):355–358

132. Wolf PA, Mitchell JB, Baker CS, et al. Impact of atrial fibrillation on mortality, stroke, and medical costs. *Arch Intern Med* 1998;158(3):229–234

133. Steinhaus DM, Cardinal DS, Mongeon L, et al. Internal defibrillation: pain perception of low energy shocks. *Pacing Clin Electrophysiol* 2002;25(7):1090–1093
134. Ujhelyi M, Hoyt RH, Burns K, et al. Nitrous oxide sedation reduces discomfort caused by atrial defibrillation shocks. *Pacing Clin Electrophysiol* 2004;27(4):485–491
135. Boodhoo L, Mitchell A, Ujhelyi M, et al. Improving the acceptability of the atrial defibrillator: patient-activated cardioversion versus automatic night cardioversion with and without sedation (ADSAS 2). *Pacing Clin Electrophysiol* 2004;27(7):910–917

Index